CDC

HEALTH INFORMATION FOR INTERNATIONAL TRAVEL

THE YELLOW BOOK

2016

DISCARD

CDC

HEALTH INFORMATION FOR INTERNATIONAL TRAVEL

THE YELLOW BOOK

2016

Editor in Chief
Gary W. Brunette, MD, MS

Chief Medical Editor
Phyllis E. Kozarsky, MD

Medical Editors
Nicole J. Cohen, MD, MS
Mark D. Gershman, MD
Alan J. Magill, MD
Stephen M. Ostroff, MD
Edward T. Ryan, MD
David R. Shlim, MD
Michelle Weinberg, MD, MPH
Mary Elizabeth Wilson, MD

Managing Editor
Megan Crawley O'Sullivan, MPH

Technical Editor
Ronnie Henry

US DEPARTMENT OF HEALTH AND HUMAN SERVICES
Public Health Service
Centers for Disease Control and Prevention
National Center for Emerging and Zoonotic Infectious Diseases
Division of Global Migration and Quarantine
Atlanta, Georgia

OXFORD
UNIVERSITY PRESS

Oxford University Press is a department of the University of
Oxford. It furthers the University's objective of excellence in research,
scholarship, and education by publishing worldwide.

Oxford   New York

Auckland   Cape Town   Dar es Salaam   Hong Kong   Karachi
Kuala Lumpur   Madrid   Melbourne   Mexico City   Nairobi
New Delhi   Shanghai   Taipei   Toronto

With offices in

Argentina   Austria   Brazil   Chile   Czech Republic   France   Greece
Guatemala   Hungary   Italy   Japan   Poland   Portugal   Singapore
South Korea   Switzerland   Thailand   Turkey   Ukraine   Vietnam

Oxford is a registered trademark of Oxford University Press in the UK
and certain other countries.

Published in the United States of America by
Oxford University Press
198 Madison Avenue, New York, NY 10016

ISBN 978–0–19–937915–6

1 2 3 4 5 6 7 8 9
Printed in the United States of America
on acid-free paper

Oxford University Press is proud to pay a portion of its sales for this book to the CDC Foundation. Chartered
by Congress, the CDC Foundation began operations in 1995 as an independent, nonprofit organization fos-
tering support for CDC through public-private partnerships. Further information about the CDC Foundation
can be found at www.cdcfoundation.org. The CDC Foundation did not prepare any portion of this book and
is not responsible for its contents.

Suggested Citation
Centers for Disease Control and Prevention. CDC Health Information for International Travel 2016. New York: Oxford University Press; 2016.

Readers are invited to send comments and suggestions regarding this publication to Gary W. Brunette, Editor in Chief, Centers for Disease Control and Prevention, Division of Global Migration and Quarantine (E-03), Travelers' Health Branch, 1600 Clifton Road NE, Atlanta, GA 30333, USA.

Disclaimers
Both generic and trade names (without trademark symbols) are used in this text. In all cases, the decision to use one or the other was made based on recognition factors and was done for the convenience of the intended audience. Therefore, the use of trade names and commercial sources in this publication is for identification only and does not imply endorsement by the US Department of Health and Human Services, the Public Health Service, or CDC.

References to non-CDC Internet sites are provided as a service to readers and do not constitute or imply endorsement of these organizations or their programs by the US Department of Health and Human Services, the Public Health Service, or CDC. CDC is not responsible for the content of these sites. URL addresses were current as of the date of publication.

Notice
This material is not intended to be, and should not be considered, a substitute for medical or other professional advice. Treatment for the conditions described in this material is highly dependent on the individual circumstances. While this material is designed to offer accurate information with respect to the subject matter covered and to be current as of the time it was written, research and knowledge about medical and health issues are constantly evolving, and dose schedules for medications and vaccines are being revised continually, with new side effects recognized and accounted for regularly. Readers must, therefore, always check the product information and clinical procedures with the most up-to-date published product information and data sheets provided by the manufacturers and the most recent codes of conduct and safety regulation. Oxford University Press and the authors make no representations or warranties to readers, express or implied, as to the accuracy or completeness of this material, including without limitation that they make no representations or warranties as to the accuracy or efficacy of the drug dosages mentioned in the material. The authors and the publishers do not accept, and expressly disclaim, any responsibility for any liability, loss, or risk that may be claimed or incurred as a consequence of the use and/or application of any of the contents of this material.

The Publisher is responsible for author selection and the Publisher and the Author(s) make all editorial decisions, including decisions regarding content. The Publisher and the Author(s) are not responsible for any product information added to this publication by companies purchasing copies of it for distribution to clinicians.

For additional copies, please contact Oxford University Press. Order online at www.oup.com/us.

Contents

1 INTRODUCTION 2

2 THE PRE-TRAVEL CONSULTATION 28

3 INFECTIOUS DISEASES RELATED TO TRAVEL 150

7

INTERNATIONAL TRAVEL WITH INFANTS & CHILDREN ... 538

8

ADVISING TRAVELERS WITH SPECIFIC NEEDS 560

APPENDICES 634

INDEX 645

PHOTO CREDITS 659

List of Boxes, Figures, Maps, & Tables, by Topic

DISEASES, CONDITIONS, & VACCINES

General Travel Health Risks

General Vaccine Information

Acute Mountain Sickness and Altitude Illness

Deep Vein Thrombosis and Pulmonary Embolism

Dengue

Dermatologic Conditions

Diarrheal Illnesses

Escherichia coli

LIST OF BOXES, FIGURES, MAPS, & TABLES, BY TOPIC | xiii

RESOURCES

General Resources

Insect Avoidance

Pre-Travel Consultation

Water Treatment

SPECIAL POPULATIONS

Cruise Ship Passengers

LIST OF MAPS

Disease Maps

Destination and Reference Maps

Editorial Staff

Editor in Chief: Gary W. Brunette
Chief Medical Editor: Phyllis E. Kozarsky
Medical Editors: Nicole J. Cohen, Mark D. Gershman, Alan J. Magill, Stephen M. Ostroff, Edward T. Ryan, David R. Shlim, Michelle Weinberg, and Mary Elizabeth Wilson
Managing Editor: Megan Crawley O'Sullivan
Technical Editor: Ronnie Henry
Design and Production Editor: Kelly Holton
Editorial Assistant: Julie Ephgrave
Cartographer: R. Ryan Lash
Assistant Cartographer: C. Virginia Lee

CDC Contributors

Alexander, James P.
Anderson, Alicia
Ansari, Armin
Arguin, Paul M.
Armstrong, Gregory L.
Averhoff, Francisco
Bair-Brake, Heather
Ballesteros, Michael F.
Barbre, Kira A.
Beavers, Suzanne
Benenson, Gabrielle A.
Benoit, Tina J.
Bialek, Stephanie R.
Blaney, David D.
Bowen, Anna
Bresee, Joseph
Brogdon, William G.
Brooks, John T.
Brown, Clive M.
Brunette, Gary W.
Buff, Ann M.
Burke, Heather
Cantey, Paul T.
Chen, Tai-Ho
Chiller, Tom M.
Cohen, Nicole J.
Czarkowski, Alan G.
Dhara, V. Ramana
Dubray, Christine
Duong, Krista Kornylo
Dykewicz, Clare A.

Ederer, David J.
Epperson, Scott
Erskine, Stefanie K.
Fiebelkorn, Amy Parker
Fischer, Marc
Flannery, Brendan
Fox, LeAnne M.
Gaines, Joanna
Galloway, Renee L.
Galland, G. Gale
Gargano, Julia Warner
Garrison, Laurel E.
Gastañaduy, Paul A.
Gee, Jay E.
Geissler, Aimee L.
Gerber, Susan I.
Gershman, Mark D.
Goodson, James L.
Gould, L. Hannah
Grant, Althea M.
Green, Michael D.
Griffin, Patricia M.
Grosse, Scott D.
Guerra, Marta A.
Hall, Aron J.
Han, Pauline V.
Hanlon, Cathleen A.
Henry, Ronnie
Herwaldt, Barbara L.
Hills, Susan L.
Hlavsa, Michele C.

Holtzman, Deborah
Illig, Petra A.
Iwamoto, Martha
Jentes, Emily S.
Jones, Jeffrey L.
Kharod, Grishma A.
Kidd, Sarah E.
Kile, James C.
Knust, Barbara
Kozarsky, Phyllis E.
Kroger, Andrew T.
Kutty, Preeta K.
Lebo, Emmaculate J.
Lee, Amanda W.
Liang, Jennifer L.
Lippold, Susan A.
LoBue, Philip
Lopman, Ben
Lyss, Sheryl
MacNeil, Jessica R.
Mahon, Barbara E.
Malilay, Josephine
Maloney, Susan A.
Marano, Nina
Margolis, Harold S.
Marienau, Karen J.
Marin, Mona
Marston, Chung K.
Martin, Diana L.
McQuiston, Jennifer
Mead, Paul S.

Meites, Elissa
Meyer, Sarah A.
Mintz, Eric
Mitruka, Kiren
Mody, Rajal
Montgomery, Susan
Montiel, Sonia H.
Morgan, Oliver W
Moro, Pedro L.
Morof, Diane F.
Mullan, Robert J.
Murphy, Trudy V.
Nasci, Roger S.
Nelson, Christina A.
Nelson, Noele P.
Newton, Anna E.
Nguyen, Duc B.,
Olson, Christine K.
O'Reilly, Ciara E.
Powers, Ann M.
Rabe, Ingrid B.

Reef, Susan E.
Reyes, Nimia L.
Reynolds, Mary G.
Rollin, Pierre E.
Routh, Janell A.
Roy, Sharon L.
Schmid, D. Scott
Shadomy, Sean V.
Sharp, Tyler M.,
Shealy, Katherine R.
Skoff, Tami H.
Sleet, David A.
Sobel, Jeremy
Sotir, Mark J.
Spruit-McGoff, Kathryn E.
Staples, J. Erin
Steele, Stefanie F.
Stoddard, Robyn A.
Stoney, Rhett J.
Strikas, Raymond A.
Tan, Kathrine R.

Teo, Chong-Gee
Tiller, Rebekah
Tiwari, Tejpratap S. P.
Tomashek, Kay M.
Traxler, Rita M.
Villarino, Margarita E.
Wallace, Gregory S.
Warren, Dora
Wassilak, Steven G. F.
Waterman, Stephen H.
Watson, John C.
Watson, John T.
Weinberg, Michelle
Weinberg, Nicholas
Wilson, Todd W.
Wirtz, Robert A.
Wolkin, Amy F.
Woodhall, Dana M.
Workowski, Kimberly
Xiao, Lihua
Yoder, Jonathan S.

External Contributors

Adler, Tina Westat — National Center for Complementary and Integrative Health Clearinghouse, Rockville, MD

Ansdell, Vernon E. — University of Hawaii, Honolulu, HI

Backer, Howard D. — California Emergency Medical Services Authority, Sacramento, CA

Barbeau, Deborah Nicolls — Tulane University, New Orleans, LA

Barnett, Elizabeth D. — Boston University School of Medicine and Boston Medical Center, Boston, MA

Benenson, Michael W. — Armed Forces Research Institute of the Medical Sciences, Bangkok, Thailand (retired)

Borwein, Sarah T. — TravelSafe Medical Centre, Hong Kong, China

Bowron, Christopher S. — University of Minnesota, Minneapolis, MN

Carroll, I. Dale — The Pregnant Traveler, Spring Lake, MI

Chen, Lin H. — Mount Auburn Hospital-Travel Medicine Center, Cambridge, MA, and Harvard Medical School, Boston, MA

Connor, Bradley A. — Weill Medical College of Cornell University, New York, NY

DeRomaña, Inés — University of California System, Education Abroad Program, Santa Barbara, CA

DuPont, Herbert L. — University of Texas Health Science Center, School of Public Health, Houston, TX

Ejike-King, Lacreisha — Office of Minority Health, US Department of Health and Human Services, Rockville, MD

Fairley, Jessica K. — Emory University School of Medicine, Atlanta, GA

Freedman, David O. — Shoreland, Inc., Milwaukee, WI

Gracia, J. Nadine — Office of Minority Health, US Department of Health and Human Services, Rockville, MD

Gushulak, Brian D. — Migration Health Consultants, Cheltenham, Canada

Hackett, Peter H. — Institute for Altitude Medicine, Telluride, CO, and Altitude Research Center, University of Colorado Denver School of Medicine, Denver, CO

Hamer, Davidson H.	Center for Global Health and Development Boston University; Department of Global Health, Boston University School of Public Health and Section of Infectious Diseases, Boston Medical Center, Boston, MA
Hochberg, Natasha S.	Section of Infectious Diseases, Boston University School of Medicine, Boston, MA
Kain, Kevin C.	University of Toronto, Toronto, Canada
Keystone, Jay S.	University of Toronto, Toronto, Canada
Killen, Jack	National Center for Complementary and Integrative Health, National Institutes of Health, Bethesda, MD (consultant)
Kotton, Camille Nelson	Massachusetts General Hospital and Harvard University, Boston, MA
LaRocque, Regina C.	Massachusetts General Hospital and Harvard Medical School, Boston, MA
Law, Catherine	National Center for Complementary and Integrative Health, National Institutes of Health, Bethesda, MD
Libman, Michael.	McGill University, Centre for Tropical Disease, Montreal, Canada
Ludwig, Grant	US Department of State
Maalim, Salahudin M.	University of Minnesota, Minneapolis, MN
Magill, Alan J.	Walter Reed Army Institute of Research, Experimental Therapeutics, Silver Spring, MD
Neumann, Karl	Weill Medical College of Cornell University and New York Presbyterian Hospital/Cornell Medical Center, New York, NY
Nilles, Eric J.	Division of Health Securities and Emergencies, World Health Organization, Suva, Fiji
Nord, Daniel A.	Divers Alert Network, Durham, NC
Offit, Paul	The Children's Hospital of Philadelphia, Philadelphia, PA
Ostroff, Stephen M.	Food and Drug Administration, Silver Spring, MD
Pedone, Bettina N.	Arthur Ashe Student Health & Wellness Center, University of California, Los Angeles, CA
Reisenauer, Amy K.	Hawaii Permanente Medical Group, Wailuku, HI
Rhodes, Gary	Center for Global Education, University of California, Los Angeles, CA
Rosselot, Gail A.	Travel Well of Westchester, Inc., Briarcliff Manor, NY
Ryan, Edward T.	Massachusetts General Hospital and Harvard University, Boston, MA
Shlim, David R.	Jackson Hole Travel and Tropical Medicine, Jackson Hole, WY
Staat, Mary Allen	International Adoption Center, Cincinnati Children's Hospital Medical Center, Cincinnati, OH
Stauffer, William M.	University of Minnesota, Minneapolis, MN, and CDC, Atlanta, GA
Thigpen, Michael C.	National Institutes of Health, Rockville, MD
Valk, Thomas H.	VEI Inc., Marshall, VA
Wangu, Zoon	Division of Pediatric Infectious Diseases, UMass Memorial Children's Medical Center, Worcester, MA
Wilson, Mary Elizabeth	Harvard School of Public Health, Boston, MA
Wu, Henry M.	Emory University, Department of Medicine, Atlanta, GA
Youngster, Ilan	Children's Hospital Boston and Harvard University, Boston, MA

All contributors have signed a statement indicating that they have no conflicts of interest with the subject matter or materials discussed in the document(s) that they have written or reviewed for this book and that the information that they have written or reviewed for this book is objective and free from bias.

Acknowledgments

The *CDC Health Information for International Travel 2016* editorial team gratefully acknowledges all the authors and reviewers for their commitment to this new edition. We extend sincere thanks to the following people for their contributions to the production of this book:

- Elise Beltrami, Clive Brown, and Scott Santibanez for their extensive review of the text.
- Amanda W. Lee, Laurie Dieterich, and Crystal Polite for their assistance in preparing the text for publication.
- Stephanie Brantman for freely lending her graphic design expertise to help refine the cartographic styles used throughout the book.
- Michael Johansson for his assistance in procuring and evaluating the data utilized to produce all dengue disease maps.

Preface

To stay on the cutting edge of travel health information, this latest edition of *CDC Health Information for International Travel* has been extensively revised. The book serves as a guide to the practice of travel medicine, as well as the authoritative source of US government recommendations for immunizations and prophylaxis for foreign travel. As international travel continues to become more common in the lives of US residents, having at least a basic understanding of the medical problems that travelers face has become a necessary aspect of practicing medicine. The goal of this book is to be a comprehensive resource for clinicians to find the answers to their travel health–related questions.

CENTERS FOR DISEASE CONTROL AND PREVENTION
Thomas R. Frieden, MD, MPH, Director

NATIONAL CENTER FOR EMERGING AND ZOONOTIC INFECTIOUS DISEASES
Beth P. Bell, MD, MPH, Director

DIVISION OF GLOBAL MIGRATION AND QUARANTINE
Martin S. Cetron, MD, Director
Gary W. Brunette, MD, MS, Chief, Travelers' Health Branch
Phyllis E. Kozarsky, MD, Expert Consultant, Travelers' Health Branch
Megan Crawley O'Sullivan, MPH, Health Communications Specialist, Travelers' Health Branch

Introduction

INTRODUCTION TO TRAVEL HEALTH & THE YELLOW BOOK

Amanda W. Lee, Phyllis E. Kozarsky

TRAVEL HEALTH

The number of people traveling internationally has continued to grow substantially in the past decade. According to the World Tourism Organization, there were >1 billion worldwide international tourist arrivals in 2013, an increase of 5% from 2012 and >57% from 2003. In 2013, US residents made >61.5 million trips with at least 1 night outside the United States. The importance of protecting the health of individual travelers, as well as safeguarding the health of the communities to which they return, cannot be overstated. International travel takes on many forms, including tourism, business, study abroad, research, visiting friends and relatives, ecotourism, adventure, medical tourism, mission work, and responding to international disasters. Travelers are as unique as their itineraries, covering all age ranges and having a variety of preexisting health concerns and conditions. The infectious disease risks that travelers face are dynamic—some travel destinations have become safer, while in other areas, new diseases have emerged and other diseases have reemerged.

The risk of becoming ill or injured during international travel depends on many factors, such as the region of the world visited, a traveler's age and health status, the length of the trip, and the diversity of planned activities. CDC provides international travel health information to address the range of health risks a traveler may face, with the aim of assisting travelers and clinicians to better understand the measures necessary to prevent illness and injury during international travel. This publication and the CDC Travelers' Health website (www.cdc.gov/travel) are the 2 primary avenues of communicating CDC's travel health recommendations.

HISTORY AND ROLES OF THE YELLOW BOOK

CDC Health Information for International Travel ("The Yellow Book") has been a trusted resource since 1967. Originally, it was a small pamphlet published to satisfy the International Sanitary Regulations' requirements and the International Health Regulations (IHR), adopted by the World Health Organization (WHO) in 1951 and 1969, respectively; the IHR were completely revised in 2005. The purpose of the IHR is to ensure maximum security against the international spread of diseases, with minimum interference with world travel and commerce. A copy of the current IHR and supporting information can be found on the WHO website (www.who.int/csr/ihr/en).

In addition to reporting public health events of international concern, the United States must also inform the public about health requirements for entering other countries, such as the necessity of being vaccinated against yellow fever. The Yellow Book and the CDC Travelers' Health website aim to communicate these requirements under the IHR (2005). Although this publication includes the most current available information at the time of printing, requirements can change. The CDC Travelers' Health website (www.cdc.gov/travel) may be checked for regularly updated information to ensure that requirements for international travel are known and met.

The Yellow Book is written primarily for clinicians, including physicians, nurses, and pharmacists. Others, such as people in the travel industry, multinational corporations, missionary and volunteer organizations, and individual travelers, can also find a wealth of information here.

This text is authored by subject-matter experts from within CDC and outside the agency. The guidelines presented in this book are evidence-based and supported by best practices. Internal text citations have not been included; however, a bibliography is included at the end of each section for those who would like to obtain more detailed information. The CDC Travelers' Health program and the CDC Foundation are pleased to partner with Oxford University Press, Inc., to publish the 2016 edition. In addition to the printed copy, a searchable, online version of the Yellow Book can be found on the CDC Travelers' Health website (www.cdc.gov/yellowbook).

CONTACT INFORMATION FOR CDC

Questions, comments, and suggestions for CDC Travelers' Health, including comments about this publication, may be made through the CDC-INFO contact center, toll-free at 800-CDC-INFO (800-232-4636) 8 AM to 8 PM Eastern Time (Monday–Friday, closed on holidays) or by visiting www.cdc.gov/info to submit your question through an online e-mail form.

Pre-Travel or Post-Travel Clinical Questions

Since CDC is not a medical facility, clinicians needing assistance with preparing patients for international travel should consider referral to a travel clinic or a clinic listed on the International Society of Travel Medicine (ISTM) website (www.istm.org).

Clinicians with post-travel health questions regarding their patients may consider referral to a clinic listed on the ISTM website, the American Society of Tropical Medicine and Hygiene website (www.astmh.org), or a medical university with specialists in infectious diseases.

Because of the complexity of some travel-related diseases, Box 1-1 lists contact information for providers needing clinical assistance.

BOX 1-1. CDC CONTACT INFORMATION FOR CLINICIANS

CDC-INFO National Contact Center
All topics for clinicians and general public *(English and Spanish)*
- 8 AM to 8 PM Eastern, M–F: toll-free at 800-CDC-INFO (800-232-4636)
- E-mail form: www.cdc.gov/info

CDC Emergency Operations Center
Emergency or urgent patient care assistance *(Note: This line is not intended for use by the general public.)*
- Available 24/7: 770-488-7100

(continued)

BOX 1-1. CDC CONTACT INFORMATION FOR CLINICIANS (continued)

CDC Drug Service
Distribution of special biologic agents and drugs
- Formulary: www.cdc.gov/laboratory/drugservice/formulary.html
- 8 AM to 4:30 PM Eastern, M–F: 404-639-3670
- After hours/weekends/holidays: 770-488-7100
- E-mail: drugservice@cdc.gov

Chikungunya, Japanese Encephalitis, Tickborne Encephalitis, and Yellow Fever
Assistance with diagnostic testing for these diseases and for questions about antibody response to yellow fever vaccination
- Division of Vectorborne Diseases, 8 AM to 4:30 PM Mountain, M–F: 970-221-6400
- Viral Special Pathogens Branch can also assist for tickborne encephalitis, 8:30 AM to 5:30 PM Eastern, M–F: 404-639-1115
- After hours/weekends/holidays: 770-488-7100
- State or local health departments may be able to assist: www.cdc.gov/mmwr/international/relres.html

Dengue
Dengue diagnostic testing assistance
- 8 AM to 5 PM Atlantic (office in Puerto Rico), M–F: 787-706-2399
- After hours/weekends/holidays: 770-488-7100
- Clinical/laboratory guidance: www.cdc.gov/Dengue/clinicalLab/index.html

Malaria Hotline
Assistance with diagnosis or management of suspected cases of malaria
- 9 AM to 5 PM Eastern, M–F: 770-488-7788 or toll-free at 855-856-4713
- Emergency consultation after hours/weekends/holidays: 770-488-7100, ask for a Malaria Branch clinician

Parasitic Diseases (other than malaria)
Hotline
Assistance with evaluation and treatment of patients suspected to have a parasitic disease
- 8 AM to 4 PM Eastern, M–F: 404-718-4745
- Emergency consultation after hours/weekends/holidays: 770-488-7100, ask for an on-call clinician in Parasitic Diseases
- E-mail: parasites@cdc.gov

DPDx
Online parasitic diseases diagnostic assistance service for laboratorians, pathologists, and other health professionals
- www.cdc.gov/dpdx/contact.html

Rickettsial Diseases
Diagnostic and treatment assistance
- 8 AM to 4:30 PM Eastern, M–F: 404-639-1075

Viral Hemorrhagic Fevers
Diagnosis
Consultation for diagnosis and reporting suspected cases in or requiring evacuation to the United States
- 8:30 AM to 5:30 PM Eastern, M–F: 404-639-1115
- Emergency consultation after hours/weekends/holidays: 770-488-7100

(continued)

Treatment

Requests for ribavirin through the Food and Drug Administration (FDA) from Valeant Pharmaceuticals

- Providers should request through FDA at 301-736-3400
- Simultaneously notify Valeant at 800-548-5100, ext. 5 (domestic) or 949-461-6971 (international)

BIBLIOGRAPHY

1. United Nations World Tourism Organization. UNWTO World Tourism Barometer, Vol. 12 (January). Madrid: United Nations World Tourism Organization; 2014 [cited 2014 Aug 7]. Available from: http://dtxtq4w60xqpw.cloudfront.net/sites/all/files/pdf/unwto_barom14_01_jan_excerpt.pdf.

2. US Department of Commerce, Office of Travel and Tourism Industries. 2013 Monthly US Outbound Air Travel to International Regions. Washington, DC: US Department of Commerce; 2014 [cited 2014 Aug 8]. Available from: http://travel.trade.gov/view/m-2013-0-001/index.html.

3. World Health Organization. International Health Regulations (2005). 2nd ed. Geneva: World Health Organization; 2008 [cited 2014 Aug 8]. Available from: http://www.who.int/ihr/9789241596664/en/index.html.

PLANNING FOR HEALTHY TRAVEL: CDC TRAVELERS' HEALTH WEBSITE AND MOBILE APPLICATIONS

Kathryn E. Spruit-McGoff, Ronnie Henry

TRAVELERS' HEALTH WEBSITE

Updated in 2013, the CDC Travelers' Health website contains 2 separate portals with different content for travelers and clinicians (Figure 1-1). Travelers and clinicians also have the ability to select the type of traveler (such as "traveling with children" or "immunocompromised traveler"), which allows them to receive customized health recommendations for those specific populations. Revised travel notice levels are based on the level of the health threat and precautions that travelers can take to protect themselves. Other updates include information centers with resources for clinicians, travelers, and the travel industry, and a directory of travel-related illnesses.

Destination Pages

The most popular feature of the Travelers' Health website are the "destination pages" (Figure 1-2). Each destination page has a clinician and traveler view that can be easily toggled back and forth. Destination pages provide health recommendations for a particular destination and include the following information:

- Vaccine and medicine recommendations
- Stay healthy and safe/patient counseling information:
  > Eat and drink safely (preventing foodborne and waterborne illnesses)
  > Prevent bug bites (preventing vectorborne infections)

1

FIGURE 1-1. CDC TRAVELERS' HEALTH WEBSITE HOMEPAGE

> Stay safe outdoors (avoiding injury and illness during outdoor activities)
> Keep away from animals (avoiding injuries from animals and zoonotic infections)
> Reduce your exposure to germs (general hygiene measures for avoiding respiratory and other infections)
> Avoid sharing body fluids (preventing bloodborne infections)
> Know how to get medical care while traveling (finding care overseas)
> Select safe transportation (international road safety)
> Maintain personal security (avoiding becoming a victim of violence or crime)
• Healthy travel packing list
• Travel health notices
• Post-travel health information

Information Centers

The **clinician information center** (wwwnc.cdc.gov/travel/page/clinician-information-center) includes useful resources such as clinical updates on travel medicine–related topics, travel medicine–related journal articles, continuing education courses on travel medicine, and in-clinic quick links, which include immunization and special population content (Figure 1-3).

The **traveler information center** (wwwnc.cdc.gov/travel/page/common-travel-health-topics) consists of a series of printable fact sheets that cover >40 travel health topics written in plain language for the international traveler. Topics include travel health insurance, jet lag, motion sickness, cruise ship travel, and travel to high altitudes. The traveler information center functions as a traveler-focused version of the Yellow Book.

The **travel industry information center** (wwwnc.cdc.gov/travel/page/travel-industry-information-center) contains specific guidelines for the air travel and cruise ship industries. It includes information on reporting illnesses and deaths among travelers, managing ill crew members, and other guidance.

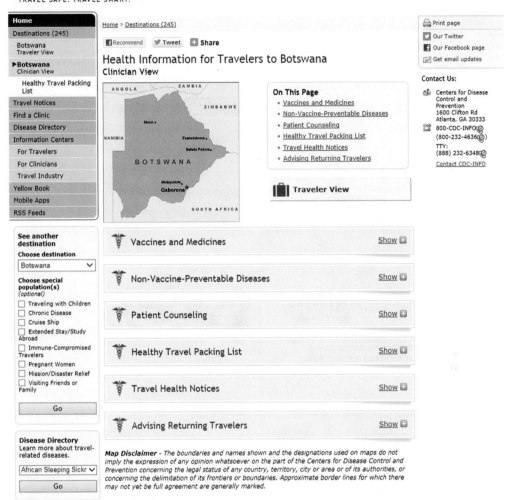

FIGURE 1-2. CDC TRAVELERS' HEALTH WEBSITE SAMPLE DESTINATION PAGE

Disease Directory

The disease directory (wwwnc.cdc.gov/travel/diseases) is an ever-expanding list of diseases that may be related to travel. It is intended to be a resource on rare as well as common infections, the risk to travelers, and what travelers can do to prevent them.

Travel Notices

CDC posts travel health notices about disease outbreaks and international events (such as natural disasters or mass gatherings) that may affect the health of travelers (Figure 1-4). The notices include information about what the situation or health risk is, who is affected, how travelers can protect their health, and links for more information. Travel health notices can be found at wwwnc.cdc.gov/travel/notices.

CDC posts notices only about confirmed events from official sources. Serious consideration is given to the impact, both

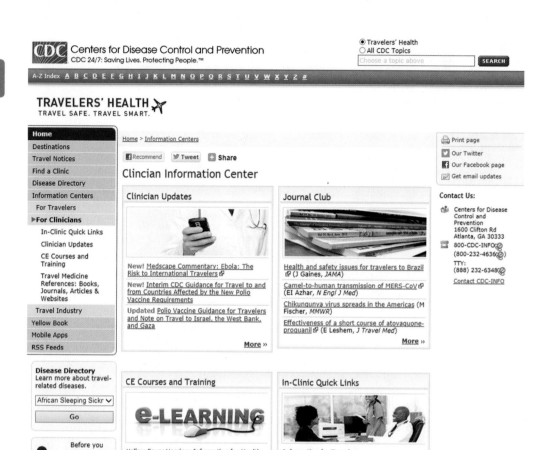

FIGURE 1-3. CDC TRAVELERS' HEALTH WEBSITE CLINICIAN INFORMATION CENTER

positive and negative, before posting a notice. To determine whether to post a notice, CDC uses a standard decision tool that is based on the 2005 International Health Regulations and consensus from agency experts. CDC also uses disease-specific criteria to help determine when a notice should be posted.

CDC issues different types of notices for international travelers. As of April 5, 2013, these definitions have been refined to make the announcements more easily understood by travelers, health care providers, and the general public. See Table 1-1 for the revised definitions. Notices are assigned different levels based on their health recommendations. All notices describe levels of risk for the traveler along with recommended preventive measures to take at each level of risk.

MOBILE APPLICATIONS

CDC has developed 2 mobile applications for travelers, *Can I Eat This?* and *TravWell*, in

FIGURE 1-4. CDC TRAVELERS' HEALTH WEBSITE SAMPLE TRAVEL NOTICE

addition to the mobile version of the Yellow Book. All are available for iOS and Android devices and can be accessed from wwwnc. cdc.gov/travel/page/apps-about.

Can I Eat This?

CDC's *Can I Eat This?* application is intended to help international travelers avoid travelers' diarrhea by guiding their food and drink choices. Travelers can select the country they are in and answer a few simple questions about what they are eating or drinking, and the application will tell them whether it is likely to be safe. In addition to helping guide their on-the-spot decisions, *Can I Eat This?* also teaches travelers about

Table 1-1. CDC Travel Notice Definitions

NOTICE LEVEL	TRAVELER ACTION	OUTBREAK/EVENT EXAMPLE (HYPOTHETICAL)
Level 1: Watch	Reminder to follow **usual** precautions for this destination.	**Dengue in Panama—Outbreak Watch:** Because dengue is endemic to Panama, this notice signifies a slightly higher rate of dengue cases than expected. Travelers are to follow "usual" insect precautions. **Olympics in London—Event Watch:** There may be possible health conditions in London that could affect travelers during the Olympics, such as measles. Travelers are to follow usual health precautions, making sure they are up-to-date on their measles vaccine, follow traffic safety laws, and use sunscreen.
Level 2: Alert	Follow **enhanced** precautions for this destination.	**Yellow Fever in Brazil—Outbreak Alert:** Because an outbreak of yellow fever is occurring in Brazil outside the reported yellow fever risk areas, this is a change in "usual" precautions. Travelers should follow "enhanced precautions" for that risk area by receiving the yellow fever vaccine. **Flooding in El Salvador—Event Alert:** There are possible conditions that could affect the health of the traveler and parts of the destination's infrastructure could be compromised. Travelers are to follow special precautions for flooding.
Level 3: Warning	Avoid all nonessential travel to this destination.	**SARS in Asia—Outbreak Warning:** Because SARS spreads quickly and has a high case-fatality ratio, a warning notice signifies a high chance a traveler could be infected. Travelers should avoid this destination if possible. **Earthquake in Haiti—Event Warning:** The destination's infrastructure (including sanitation and transportation) cannot support travelers at this time.

general principles regarding safe food and water. All recommendations are stored locally on the user's device, so no international data connection is needed to use the application when traveling.

TravWell

CDC's *TravWell* is a companion to the Travelers' Health destination pages. It allows users to build an itinerary and receive destination-specific vaccine and medicine recommendations. For each itinerary, it also generates a customizable, destination-specific to-do list and packing list. *TravWell* also prompts users to set reminders for healthy behaviors, such as taking malaria prophylaxis or getting booster doses of vaccines. It also provides users with a place to store electronic copies of health-related travel documents, such as prescriptions or vaccination records.

TRAVEL EPIDEMIOLOGY

Mark J. Sotir, Regina C. LaRocque

Travelers are an epidemiologically important population because of their mobility, the potential for exposure to diseases and other adverse health outcomes outside their home country, and the possibility that they will either import nonendemic diseases into their country of origin or export nonendemic diseases to the country they visit. International tourist arrivals exceeded 1 billion in 2012 and are projected to increase to almost 2 billion by 2030, so the public health impact of travel will only increase. Increasing travel to destinations in Asia (arrivals up 7% from 2011 to 2012) and Africa (arrivals up 6% from 2011 to 2012) will place more travelers at risk for a variety of travel-related conditions, including malaria, dengue, measles, and other tropical or vaccine-preventable infections.

To provide optimal pre-travel advice, preventive measures, and education to travelers, health care providers must be familiar with basic epidemiologic concepts and the epidemiology and geographic distribution of relevant diseases and conditions. Risk can be assessed by examining both past and current disease trends. However, there are limitations to the data available for making such an assessment. Knowledge of the precise risk for a particular disease in a specific location, especially pertinent for a traveler, remains elusive for many destinations despite decades of interest and improvements in global surveillance efforts.

Information regarding the actual risk for travelers (often expressed as number of events per 100,000 travelers) is limited for a number of reasons. It is difficult to obtain an accurate numerator (number of cases of disease among travelers) and denominator (number of travelers overall or travelers to a specific destination who are susceptible to infection and illness). Many travelers to a specific location who become infected have already returned to their home country by the time they develop signs and symptoms, so will not be included in the surveillance data of the country of exposure even if reporting is optimal. Similarly, diseases with short incubation periods or brief durations may have resolved by the time a traveler returns home and thus may not be counted in surveillance data of the traveler's country of origin. If the illness is mild, the traveler may never seek health care, or diagnostic tests may not be performed to accurately diagnose the cause. Travelers often visit multiple locations, and it may be difficult to determine where the exposure occurred. A denominator for all travelers to a specific location that could be used to calculate incidence is also generally problematic. Even when available, denominator data are typically estimates provided only at the country or region level and not at the local destination level.

Frequently quoted studies on the incidence of infection in travelers are based on extrapolations of limited data, collected in limited samples of travelers. In addition, these studies were often conducted >20 years ago and might be of limited relevance to current travelers. These studies also use a variety of methodologic designs, each with its own set of strengths and weaknesses, making the findings difficult to compare or combine. They have also, for the most part, only examined a few key diseases or conditions and have combined all travelers regardless of destination. Many have been single-clinic or single-destination studies that lead to conclusions that are not applicable to groups of travelers with different local, national, or cultural backgrounds.

A number of factors are relevant to epidemiologic data on travel-related diseases and adverse health events. First, the characteristics of the disease itself must be considered, including mode of transmission, incubation period, signs and symptoms, duration of illness, and diagnostic testing. Second, the presence, frequency, seasonality, and geographic distribution of the disease need to be assessed; these might change over time because of outbreaks, emergence or reemergence in new areas or populations, successful public health interventions, or other factors. Third, travelers represent a unique subset of people, and their exposures, behaviors, and disease susceptibility might differ dramatically from those of the local population at a tourist destination. Along with demographic characteristics, additional travel-specific factors that should be considered include trip length, destinations (both current and previous), specific travel itineraries, and purpose of travel. Fourth, travelers themselves are a heterogeneous group, and different subgroups of travelers might have different risks because of activities, behaviors, and other factors during travel. For example, travelers visiting friends and relatives (VFR travelers) have consistently demonstrated higher proportions of serious febrile illness, particularly malaria, when compared with other types of travelers. Finally, preparation before travel, especially use of preventive measures such as vaccines, also factors into the epidemiology of travel illnesses.

During the past 2 decades, the most relevant data on travel-related disease occurrence have come from surveillance of travelers themselves. Data on disease incidence in local populations may identify the most important diseases to monitor in a country, but their relevance to travelers who have different risk behaviors, eating habits, accommodations, knowledge of preventive measures, and activities is usually limited. Surveillance data that either focus on travelers or collect data on illnesses that affect travelers, and incorporate some of the travel-specific variables described above in their data collection methods, are more useful in describing travel-related disease patterns and risks.

One example of a surveillance data source is the GeoSentinel Surveillance Network, an ongoing collaborative effort between the International Society of Travel Medicine (ISTM) and CDC. GeoSentinel is a global provider-based network of travel and tropical medicine clinics that has been systematically collecting data on travel-related illnesses since 1997. As of 2014, GeoSentinel had 57 participating clinics on 6 continents, with a database of >200,000 records on patients with a confirmed or probable travel-related diagnosis. Details of the data collection instrument, diagnostic categories, and patient classification methods used in GeoSentinel have

recently been published in a CDC *Morbidity and Mortality Weekly Report* (MMWR) surveillance summary. Further information on GeoSentinel can be found at: www.istm.org/geosentinel.

Recent data from the GeoSentinel network indicate that Asia (32.6%) and sub-Saharan Africa (26.7%) were the most common regions where travel-related illnesses were acquired (Figure 1-5). The most frequently identified illness categories were gastrointestinal (34.0%), febrile (23.3%), and dermatologic (19.5%) problems. Malaria, dengue, enteric fever, spotted-fever group rickettsioses, chikungunya, and nonspecific viral syndromes were the most frequent contributors to the acute systemic febrile illness category. *Falciparum* malaria was most commonly acquired in West Africa, while enteric fever was most often contracted on the Indian subcontinent; leptospirosis, scrub typhus, and murine typhus were principally acquired in Southeast Asia. More than two-thirds of dengue infections were acquired in Asia, mostly Thailand, Indonesia, and India; seasonality of dengue varied according to destination. Common skin and soft tissue infections, mosquito bites (often infected), and allergic dermatitis were the most common skin conditions affecting travelers. Among the more exotic diagnoses, hookworm-related cutaneous larva migrans, leishmaniasis, myiasis, and tungiasis were the most important. The relative frequency of many diseases varied by travel destination and reason for travel, and VFR travelers had a disproportionately high prevalence of serious febrile illness (malaria) and low rates of seeking advice before travel (18.3%). Only 40.5% of all ill GeoSentinel travelers reported pre-travel medical visits.

Although GeoSentinel and similar traveler surveillance networks, such as TropNet in Europe, offer advantages over disease-specific studies or data collated at single centers, these networks have limitations. The data are based on a convenience sample of ill returned travelers visiting specialist clinics. This group may not reflect the experience of healthy travelers, those with mild or self-limited illness who visit other providers, or those who do not seek health care when ill. In addition, there are differences in patient populations and travel destinations among the GeoSentinel participating

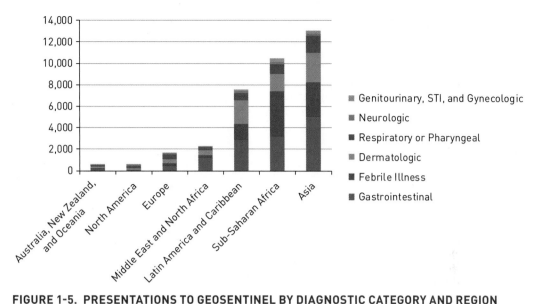

FIGURE 1-5. PRESENTATIONS TO GEOSENTINEL BY DIAGNOSTIC CATEGORY AND REGION (2007–2011)[1]

[1] Data from Leder K, Torresi J, Libman MD, Cramer JP, Castelli F, Schlagenhauf P, et al. GeoSentinel surveillance of illness in returned travelers, 2007–2011. Ann Intern Med. 2013 Mar 19;158(6):456–68.

sites. Because of a lack of a true denominator in GeoSentinel data, they cannot be used to determine absolute or relative risks. However, they show the relative frequency and range of illnesses seen in wide samples of ill travelers.

Another valuable source of epidemiologic data is Global TravEpiNet (GTEN), a US-based provider network formed in 2009 that systematically collects information on travelers presenting to a consortium of 26 clinics, including specialized travel clinics, primary care and public health sites, and pharmacy-based practices. GTEN providers evaluate the health characteristics and pre-travel health care of travelers and document these in a central electronic database; >51,000 records have been collected as of January 1, 2014. GTEN does not capture information on travelers who seek pre-travel care overseas, and participating sites may not be representative of clinical practice in all parts of the United States. More information on Global TravEpiNet, its web tools, and its membership can be found at www.healthful.travel.

Data from 13,235 travelers seen from 2009 through 2011 in GTEN clinics indicated that India, South Africa, and China were the most common destinations for US travelers seeking pre-travel health care, and more than one-third of trips occurred in June, July, and August. Travelers seen in sampled GTEN clinics ranged in age from 1 month to 94 years, with a median of 35 years. The median duration of travel was 14 days, although 22% of travelers pursued trips of >28 days, and 3% of travelers pursued trips of >6 months. A total of 75% were traveling to malaria-endemic countries, and 38% were visiting yellow fever–endemic countries. Immunocompromising conditions, such as HIV infection and AIDS, organ transplant, or receipt of immunocompromising medications, were present in 3% of GTEN travelers.

Travel medicine is still a nascent field. Correspondingly, travel epidemiology and its accompanying methods are also still evolving. Although efforts to collect and distribute data on illnesses in travelers have been successful, challenges and limitations remain. National population-based surveys, or even the addition of questions related to travel, including illness and adverse outcomes experienced during or after travel, might yield promising new data to further define rates and risk in travelers. In 2010, the ISTM research committee published a report summarizing travel medicine research priorities; applied epidemiology, including the work of networks such as GeoSentinel and GTEN, can contribute to providing data to address some of these priorities, including:

- What is the benefit of pre-travel counseling (for example, what counseling leads to safer sexual behaviors and fewer road travel accidents, animal bites, drownings, and other noninfectious threats to health)?
- How effective is the pre-travel encounter in ensuring that the traveler is up-to-date with locally relevant immunizations (which may or may not be considered travel immunizations)?

- What are the risks during medical tourism (such as bloodborne pathogens, nosocomial infections, and procedure complications)?
- Do long-term travelers behave differently than short-term travelers?
- Do travelers who develop traveler's diarrhea take their standby antibiotics?
- Is the repeated or long-term use of permethrin and other insecticides safe in the ways that travelers use them (on clothing, for example)?
- What is the role of travelers in the spread of emerging infections such as chikungunya?

BIBLIOGRAPHY

1. Adachi K, Coleman MS, Khan N, Jentes ES, Arguin P, Rao SR, et al. Economics of malaria prevention in US travelers to West Africa. Clin Infect Dis. 2014 Jan;58(1):11–21.
2. Behrens RH, Carroll B. The challenges of disease risk ascertainment using accessible data sources for numbers of travelers. J Travel Med. 2013 Sep–Oct;20(5):296–302.
3. CDC. Malaria surveillance—United States, 2011. MMWR Surveill Summ. 2013 Nov 1;62(5):1–17.
4. Harvey K, Esposito DH, Han P, Kozarsky P, Freedman DO, Plier DA, et al. Surveillance for travel-related disease—GeoSentinel Surveillance System, United States, 1997–2011. MMWR Surveill Summ. 2013 Jul 19;62:1–23.
5. LaRocque RC, Rao SR, Lee J, Ansdell V, Yates JA, Schwartz BS, et al. Global TravEpiNet: a national consortium of clinics providing care to international travelers—analysis of demographic characteristics, travel destinations, and pretravel healthcare of high-risk US international travelers, 2009–2011. Clin Infect Dis. 2012 Feb 15;54(4):455–62.
6. Leder K, Torresi J, Libman MD, Cramer JP, Castelli F, Schlagenhauf P, et al. GeoSentinel surveillance of illness in returned travelers, 2007–2011. Ann Intern Med. 2013 Mar 19;158(6):456–68.
7. Leder K, Wilson ME, Freedman DO, Torresi J. A comparative analysis of methodological approaches used for estimating risk in travel medicine. J Travel Med. 2008 Jul–Aug;15(4):263–72.
8. Sotir M, Freedman D. Basic epidemiology of infectious diseases, including surveillance and reporting. In: Zuckerman J, Leggat P, Brunette G, editors. Essential Travel Medicine. Chichester, UK: John Wiley & Sons; Forthcoming 2015.
9. Talbot EA, Chen LH, Sanford C, McCarthy A, Leder K, Research Committee of International Society of Travel Medicine. Travel medicine research priorities: establishing an evidence base. J Travel Med. 2010 Nov–Dec;17(6):410–5.
10. United Nations World Tourism Organization. UNWTO Tourism Highlights, 2013 ed. [Internet]. Madrid: World Tourism Organization; 2013 [cited 2014 Aug 8]. Available from: http://www.e-unwto.org/content/hq4538/?p=537baabf5c5d4cb0a1a08132a5066cff&pi=15.

Perspectives

THE ROLE OF THE TRAVELER IN TRANSLOCATION OF DISEASE
Stephen M. Ostroff

Since people began moving from one place to another, they have offered free passage to microorganisms on themselves, in their belongings, or on their conveyances. The consequences of such microbial hitchhiking have, at times, altered the course of history. Among the more notable examples are the great plagues that swept into Europe from Asia during the Middle Ages, the introduction of smallpox to the Americas by European explorers, and the reverse movement of syphilis into Europe in those same returning explorers.

Although the movement of pathogens by travelers is not a new phenomenon, today's increasing pace and scale of global human movement have enhanced the opportunities and speed for disease spread. HIV infection, which generally takes years for symptoms to develop, spread to every corner of the world less than a decade after it was recognized in the early 1980s. In the 21st century, no place on earth is more than a day from any other location. Even diseases with short incubation periods have unprecedented opportunities for rapid spread through human movement. What follows are vivid examples of this phenomenon from the last several years that demonstrate how crucial travel has become to the spread of emerging diseases. They also remind us that all travelers, regardless of the purpose, duration, or distance of the journey, should take steps to prevent bringing more than luggage to and from their destinations.

MIDDLE EAST RESPIRATORY SYNDROME (MERS)
MERS was first identified in September 2012 by Dutch researchers who analyzed specimens from a Saudi Arabian patient who had died of severe pneumonia. The same month, a second case of this disease was diagnosed in a Qatari citizen with pneumonia. Thus after only 2 cases, it became clear that MERS could spread through international travelers. This phenomenon has since been seen repeatedly. Even though all known cases of MERS have been linked to exposure in countries on or near the Arabian Peninsula, through mid-2014 MERS has been diagnosed among travelers in other parts of the Middle East, Europe, North Africa, Asia, and North America (Map 1-1). Some of these travel-associated cases have resulted in limited person-to-person transmission.

MAP 1-1. DISTRIBUTION OF CONFIRMED CASES OF MIDDLE EAST RESPIRATORY SYNDROME BY REPORTING COUNTRY[1]

[1] Adapted from Figure 2 in: European Centre for Disease Prevention and Control. Epidemiological update: Middle East respiratory syndrome coronavirus (MERS-CoV). 25 Nov 2013 [cited 2014 Sep 26]. Available from: http://www.ecdc.europa.eu/en/press/news/_layouts/forms/News_DispForm.aspx?List=8db7286c-fe2d-476c-9133-18ff4cb1b568&ID=913.

MERS is caused by a newly recognized coronavirus; the earliest confirmed human cases occurred in a cluster of respiratory illnesses at a hospital in Zarga, Jordan, in April 2012. MERS represents the second coronavirus to cause a major global health concern in the last 10 years. In 2003, the severe acute respiratory syndrome (SARS) coronavirus produced a transcontinental outbreak that resulted in 8,098 illnesses with a case-fatality ratio of 9.5% before ending later that year. In one of the most astonishing examples of how travel can promote disease spread, the global dissemination of SARS occurred through just 10 guests of a Hong Kong hotel whose stay overlapped with that of a Chinese physician who was ill during his stay and quickly died of the disease. After their exposure but before illness onset, the 10 hotel guests boarded planes bound for different countries, igniting major chains of transmission at destinations as far away as Toronto, Canada.

SARS and MERS both may cause an acute respiratory illness characterized by severe pneumonia (although milder infections have been described), both have been transmitted in hospital settings (including to health care workers), and both have overlapping age distributions in adults with few infections found in children. However, MERS has proven to be more lethal. Among the first 837 laboratory-confirmed cases of MERS, a total of 291 (34.8%) have died from the illness.

Efforts are underway to understand the source and mode of transmission of MERS to humans. Serologic investigations have found the MERS coronavirus and similar coronaviruses are widely distributed in camels. Some people who later developed MERS had exposure to camels that had detectable MERS virus, which suggests that camels may play a role in spreading the virus or may even be an animal reservoir. Understanding risk factors for exposure is critical to developing preventive and therapeutic strategies, especially given that the Middle East is a hub for global travel, including tourism, a substantial foreign workforce, and the pilgrimage to Mecca and other religious events that bring millions of visitors to Saudi Arabia annually. Travel to areas affected by MERS offers major opportunities for ongoing international spread of this disease.

INFLUENZA

The last few years have been notable for a steady stream of newly recognized influenza A viruses causing human disease. This trend has implications for all international travelers. The most high-profile example is the 2009 variant of influenza A (H1N1) that produced the first flu pandemic of the 21st century. This virus initially appeared in early 2009 in central Mexico, where it caused a sizeable outbreak of respiratory disease. But it was not recognized as a new flu variant until it crossed over the US border in April 2009 and the first cases appeared in southern California. The virus proved to be easily transmissible, especially among children, affording rapid spread. After recognition, travelers with pandemic H1N1 who had visited Mexican tourist destinations were quickly detected elsewhere in the world, and an analysis of air traffic patterns found a strong correlation between the volume of air travel from Mexico and the likelihood that H1N1 was identified in a destination during the early stages of the pandemic. Through travelers, the virus quickly spread globally, and within only 2 months the outbreak was designated a pandemic by the World Health Organization. Although the pandemic has come and gone, the virus remains in circulation as the seasonal influenza A (H1N1) subtype and was the predominant influenza strain in the United States in 2013–2014.

Avian influenza A (H5N1) has also been a major global concern, although its epidemiologic features have been considerably different than the pandemic virus and less affected by travel. This virus first produced a limited-scale outbreak in Hong Kong in 1997, and then no human illness from H5N1 was seen for several years. The virus resurfaced in Vietnam and Thailand in 2003 and has been in continuous circulation in poultry and wild birds ever since. Since 2003, human disease has been relatively infrequent, with only 650 confirmed cases reported through the end of 2013. However, people in whom there is a recognized case of H5N1 infection almost always have severe pneumonia, and the disease has an overall case-fatality ratio of 59%. This figure is even more remarkable in light of the fact that most cases have been in children and young adults (median age 18 years). Most deaths from seasonal influenza occur in the elderly.

The virus has been found in birds in >60 countries encompassing parts of Asia, Europe, the Middle East, and Africa, and international movement in conveyances and animals has been documented and may explain some of its geographic spread. The 3 countries with the most human illnesses (Indonesia, Vietnam, and Egypt) account for 76% of all cases and are all major tourist destinations, although to date no tourism-associated illnesses have been identified in international visitors to these countries. This is because close contact with infected poultry is generally considered necessary for exposure; sustained human-to-human transmission has not been observed. In January 2014, the first H5N1 illness was documented in North America in a Canadian citizen who had traveled to Beijing for a 3-week visit and became ill with pneumonia and encephalitis on the way home. The patient, who died, had no known history of poultry exposure while in Beijing and the source of infection is unknown. This case demonstrates that H5N1 can be a risk for travelers, reinforcing the recommendation to avoid contact with live poultry in areas affected by this virus.

The third major influenza virus to recently emerge is avian influenza A (H7N9). This virus was first detected as a cause of human illness in March 2013 in eastern China, with cases seen in Shanghai and adjacent provinces. The number of identified cases rose sharply over the spring of 2013, then diminished until a second wave of infections occurred during the winter and spring of 2014. Through early April 2014 a total of 418 confirmed cases had been identified, with a 30% case-fatality ratio. People reported to have H7N9 infection have been considerably older (mean age of 55 years) than those reported to have H5N1.

Most avian influenza viruses that have been linked to human disease have also produced large-scale die-offs in poultry (they are highly pathogenic viruses). Therefore, poultry outbreaks allow the identification of locations where humans are at risk of exposure and infection. In contrast, H7N9 does not exhibit this characteristic, making it very difficult to know where and when it is circulating. To date, almost all cases have occurred in people in eastern and southern China, with illness often linked to exposure to live poultry in wet markets. Cases have been identified in Hong Kong and Taiwan among travelers to and from affected areas of mainland China. In addition, a Chinese traveler was diagnosed with the disease while on a visit to Malaysia.

CHIKUNGUNYA VIRUS

Exotic mosquito-transmitted infections, particularly malaria and dengue fever, have long been major travel health concerns. Compounding the challenges of vectorborne diseases to travelers, a number of mosquito-transmitted viruses have recently expanded their geographic range through movement in infected mosquitoes, infected reservoir hosts such as birds, or infected people. The most notable contemporary example is the translocation of West Nile virus into the Western Hemisphere in 1999. Since an apparent single introduction into New York City, the virus has relentlessly spread throughout most of the Western Hemisphere and now produces disease annually throughout the mainland United States.

Chikungunya is a less well-known virus that, like West Nile virus before it, has recently become established in the Western Hemisphere. First identified in Tanzania in the 1950s, chikungunya causes fever accompanied by severe muscle and joint pain. Until the 21st century, chikungunya virus was largely confined to east Africa and Asia, where it produced small, localized outbreaks of disease. Beginning in 2005, it began to spread across the islands of the Indian Ocean to the Indian subcontinent, producing massive outbreaks involving hundreds of thousands of people in locations such as Réunion, Mauritius, and southern India. The transmission cycle of this virus includes only mosquitoes and humans, and infected travelers likely contribute to the movement of this virus. This was confirmed when the virus was introduced to Italy in 2007 through an infected traveler from India, resulting in 205 locally acquired cases in several adjacent towns near Ravenna on the Adriatic Coast. Local transmission of chikungunya also occurred in southeast France in 2010 but did not persist in either of the European locations. Chikungunya also spread eastward into other parts of Asia and even the western Pacific Islands, where locally acquired human disease has occurred.

Over the last few decades, cases of chikungunya have been occasionally diagnosed in the Western Hemisphere among travelers to or from affected areas (especially south Asia). But until late 2013, there was no evidence of local acquisition in the Western Hemisphere until disease suddenly appeared on the French side of the island of Saint Martin in the Caribbean, a major tourist destination, in people with no travel history. From what appears to be a single introduction, chikungunya has hopscotched across the islands of the Caribbean and even to the mainland of South and Central America, producing local outbreaks of disease. As of August 2014, locally acquired human illness has been detected in the Caribbean as far north as the Bahamas, and travel-associated cases have been detected elsewhere, including >600 in the United States (mainly Florida). Less than a year after its introduction, almost 600,000 confirmed and suspected cases of chikungunya have been reported from the Caribbean, with the largest number of cases in the Dominican Republic, Haiti, and on the French islands of Guadeloupe and Martinique. As of August 2014, 6 locally acquired cases of chikungunya have been reported in the United States, all in south Florida. These findings illustrate the potential for chikungunya to become established in some areas of the North American mainland.

CHOLERA IN THE CARIBBEAN

In October 2010, cholera unexpectedly appeared in Haiti for the first time in recorded history. The cholera outbreak struck 10 months after the devastating January 2010 Haiti earthquake, which killed an estimated 316,000 people. The *Vibrio cholerae* strain (toxigenic serogroup O1, serotype Ogawa, biotype El Tor) responsible for the outbreak did not genetically resemble the Latin American outbreak strain that appeared in the early 1990s or strains occasionally found along the coast of the Gulf of Mexico. Instead, it closely resembled strains that had been recently circulating in south Asia and Africa. Among the hypotheses to explain how the organism arrived in Haiti included the potential inadvertent introduction of cholera by Nepalese troops serving as part of the United Nations peacekeeping force housed upstream of the area where the first cases were recognized. Given Haiti's widespread poverty, poor sanitation, and population displacement in the aftermath of the earthquake, cholera spread rapidly. In just weeks, thousands of cases were occurring throughout the country, and the outbreak has persisted with gradually decreasing intensity despite efforts to improve sanitary measures. As of August 2014, >700,000 cases of cholera, including almost 400,000 hospitalizations and 8,579 (1.2%) deaths, had been reported from Haiti, which has a population of only about 10 million people. Cholera has also spread to other countries in the region, in particular the Dominican Republic, which shares the island of Hispaniola with Haiti and saw its first cases in November 2010. Since then, more than 31,000 cases have been reported by the Dominican Republic. In 2012, cholera was recognized in Cuba, where >700 cases have been seen, and in the fall of 2013 it was reported in Mexico along the coastal Gulf of Mexico, where 187 cases were identified.

Cholera has been detected in other countries in travelers to or from Haiti, including in the United States, but these other locations generally have good sanitation infrastructure and the risk of local spread is considered low.

CHILDHOOD VACCINE-PREVENTABLE DISEASES

Vaccination programs are considered among the most cost effective of public health interventions and have substantially reduced the global prevalence of childhood infectious diseases. In the United States, year-round indigenous measles and rubella transmission were declared eliminated in 2000 and 2004, respectively, and the incidence of diseases such as mumps and rubella is dramatically decreased compared with their incidence in the pre-vaccine era. The region of the Americas is certifying regional elimination of measles and rubella. Poliomyelitis is the second vaccine-preventable disease (after smallpox) targeted to be intentionally eradicated; in early 2014 India was certified as polio-free by the World Health Organization. However, most vaccine-preventable diseases are highly transmissible and can easily spread in unvaccinated travelers who become infected. The importance of travelers in the spread of vaccine-preventable diseases is evidenced by importations and associated outbreaks of measles in the United States every year and importations of wild poliovirus into Equatorial Guinea and Brazil.

Measles

Outside the Western Hemisphere, measles continues to circulate because of low vaccination coverage. In the United States, measles cases and outbreaks continue to be reported, despite measles being declared eliminated. Unvaccinated US residents traveling abroad, international visitors, and overseas adoptees have become infected while abroad and have brought the virus to the United States. These importations have ignited domestic outbreaks at the local level because of suboptimal levels of population immunity in some US communities, particularly in areas where parents elect not to vaccinate their children for religious, philosophical, or personal reasons. From 2001 through 2008, the reported median number of measles cases identified in the United States (56 cases per year) was low, but the number of cases has since risen sharply. In 2011, a total of 220 cases of measles were reported. Among these cases, 90% were linked to importation (the source for the remaining 10% could not be established). During 2014, the United States has had the highest number of reported measles cases since 1994; by August 22, 592 measles cases had been reported. In 2014, 99% of cases were associated with importation (the remainder had unknown source) from at least 18 countries. Among 49 instances of direct importation (the source case for an outbreak), 45 (92%) involved US residents returning from abroad (49% from the Philippines), while the other 5 (8%) were foreign visitors to the United States. The largest outbreak (378 cases) started when members of an Amish community were infected while visiting the Philippines (where a large outbreak of measles was occurring at the time), returned to Ohio, and introduced measles into Amish communities with low vaccination coverage.

In February 2014, an outbreak of measles occurred in Europe on a cruise ship sailing the western Mediterranean. A total of 27 cases (22 confirmed and 5 probable cases) of measles were identified, mostly among the crew. However, 4 passengers, including 2 infants, also contracted the disease. The virus strain responsible for the cruise ship outbreak is similar to measles viruses circulating in the Philippines.

Polio

In 1988, the World Health Assembly targeted poliomyelitis for eradication. Through the use of large-scale vaccination campaigns, by 2012 this goal appeared to be in sight, as only 223 cases of wild-type polio were reported from 5 countries, and the disease was endemic in only 3 countries (Afghanistan, Nigeria, and Pakistan). However, in 2013, the number of cases rose by 86% (to 414 cases), mostly in Pakistan. Polio was also identified in 5 countries in the Middle East and Africa, where it had not recently circulated. These countries include Syria and Somalia, locations marked by civil and humanitarian crises. The appearance of polio in these locations most likely represents importation through travel from an endemic country. In the early part of 2014, the number of identified cases had more than doubled (from 34 to 82) compared with the same period of 2013, and disease was identified in 2 additional countries (Iraq and Equatorial Guinea). As a result, on May 5, 2014, the World Health Organization declared polio to represent a public health emergency of international concern under the International Health Regulations and recommended that countries known to be exporting polio (Pakistan, Syria, and Cameroon) ensure departing residents and long-term visitors receive a dose of polio vaccine before travel and encouraged countries where the virus was present but there was no evidence of exportation to implement similar policies.

These examples highlight the diversity of opportunities for microbial movement afforded by travel, and the pivotal role travel has played in many of today's major emerging disease threats. No amount of vigilance is likely to eliminate such opportunities, especially since microbes can be silent travelers. However, all travelers should be knowledgeable about the risks at their destinations and take precautions to prevent the spread of disease.

BIBLIOGRAPHY

1. Bermingham A, Chand MA, Brown CS, Aarons E, Tong C, Langrish C, et al. Severe respiratory illness caused by a novel coronavirus, in a patient transferred to the United Kingdom from the Middle East, September 2012. Euro Surveill. 2012;17 (40):20290.

2. Cassadou S, Boucau S, Petit-Sinturel M, Huc P, Leparc-Goffart I, Ledrans M. Emergence of chikungunya fever on the French side of Saint Martin island, October to December 2013. Euro Surveill. 2014 Apr 3;19(13).

3. CDC. Measles—United States, 2011. MMWR Morb Mortal Wkly Rep. 2012 Apr 20;61:253–7.

4. CDC. Measles—United States, January 1–May 23, 2014. MMWR Morb Mortal Wkly Rep. 2014 Jun 6;63(22):496–9.

5. Charrel R, Leparc-Goffart I, Gallian P, de Lamballerie X. Globalization of Chikungunya: 10 years to invade the world. Clin Microbiol Infect. 2014 Jul;20(7):662–3.

6. Chen LH, Wilson ME. The role of the traveler in emerging infections and magnitude of travel. Med Clin North Am. 2008 Nov;92(6):1409–32, xi.

7. Cheng VC, To KK, Tse H, Hung IF, Yuen KY. Two years after pandemic influenza A/2009/H1N1: what have we learned? Clin Microbiol Rev. 2012 Apr;25(2):223–63.

8. European Centre for Disease Prevention and Control. Updated rapid risk assessment: severe respiratory disease associated with Middle East respiratory syndrome coronavirus (MERS-CoV). 9th update ed. Stockholm: European Centre for Disease Control; 2014 [cited

2014 Jun 12]. Available from: http://www.ecdc.europa.eu/en/publications/Publications/Middle-East-respiratory-syndrome-coronavirus-risk-assessment-25-April-2014.pdf.

9. Khan K, Arino J, Hu W, Raposo P, Sears J, Calderon F, et al. Spread of a novel influenza A (H1N1) virus via global airline transportation. N Engl J Med. 2009 Jul 9;361(2):212–4.

10. Liu J, Xiao H, Wu Y, Liu D, Qi X, Shi Y, et al. H7N9: a low pathogenic avian influenza A virus infecting humans. Curr Opin Virol. 2014 Apr;5:91–7.

11. Moturi EK, Porter KA, Wassilak SG, Tangermann RH, Diop OM, Burns CC, et al. Progress toward polio eradication—worldwide, 2013–2014. MMWR Morb Mortal Wkly Rep. 2014 May 30;63(21):468–72.

12. Nasci R. Movement of chikungunya virus into the Western Hemisphere. Emerg Infect Dis. 2014 Aug;20(8):1394–5.

13. Raj VS, Osterhaus AD, Fouchier RA, Haagmans BL. MERS: emergence of a novel human coronavirus. Curr Opin Virol. 2014 Apr;5:58–62.

14. Stoddard ST, Morrison AC, Vazquez-Prokopec GM, Paz Soldan V, Kochel TJ, Kitron U, et al. The role of human movement in the transmission of vector-borne pathogens. PLoS Negl Trop Dis. 2009 Jul 21;3(7):e481.

15. World Health Organization. Cumulative number of confirmed human cases of avian influenza A(H5N1) reported to WHO. Geneva: World Health Organization; 2012 [cited 2014 Jun 9]. Available from: http://www.who.int/influenza/human_animal_interface/H5N1_cumulative_table_archives/en/index.htm.

16. World Health Organization. Map and epidemiological curve of confirmed human cases of avian influenza A(H7N9). World Health Organization; 2014 [cited 2014 Jun 11]. Available from: http://who.int/influenza/human_animal_interface/influenza_h7n9/Data_Reports/en/.

17. Zaki AM, van Boheemen S, Bestebroer TM, Osterhaus AD, Fouchier RA. Isolation of a novel coronavirus from a man with pneumonia in Saudi Arabia. N Engl J Med. 2012 Nov 8;367(19):1814–20.

Perspectives

WHY GUIDELINES DIFFER

Alan J. Magill, David R. Shlim

INTRODUCTION

Numerous international, national, and professional organizations publish guidelines and recommendations that assist travel health providers in giving the best possible advice to prospective travelers. The CDC Yellow Book is one example of published recommendations. However, it is quickly apparent

Perspectives sections are written as editorial discussions aiming to add depth and clinical perspective to the official recommendations contained in the book. The views and opinions expressed in this section are those of the authors and do not necessarily represent the official position of CDC.

to both clinicians and patients that guidelines and recommendations differ, sometimes dramatically. Conflicting messages from authoritative sources may confuse patients and clinicians and undermine the credibility of the source. It can be unsettling for patients to receive travel medicine advice, vaccines, and an antimalarial drug prescription from a provider, only to find that the recommendations conflict with what they have obtained from other sources or even heard from other advisors. The skillful travel health provider will be able to help the traveler run this gauntlet of conflicting advice by knowing more about why guidelines differ.

HOW ARE GUIDELINES CREATED?

Most guidelines of interest to travel health providers and travelers focus on recommendations for immunizations, prophylactic medications, and self-treatment regimens (such as those for travelers' diarrhea). Guidelines come from many sources. A regulatory agency in each country must review and approve an application from the sponsor of a product in order for the product to be commercially distributed. Regulatory authorities review data from prelicensure clinical trials and also assess the manufacturing process. International organizations such as the World Health Organization (WHO) promote their own sets of guidelines. At national levels, agencies such as CDC make recommendations for the use of approved vaccines and medications for travelers. In addition, professional organizations may create consensus clinical practice guidelines based on published medical literature and expert opinion. Travel medicine–specific subscription services use experts to organize and present travel medicine recommendations for clinicians. However, these services can use information and sources that may not be fully validated by national and international authorities. Finally, vast quantities of unregulated opinions are published on the Internet. People new to travel medicine may not be aware of the decision-making process or the source information that results in formal recommendations from these organizations.

Regulatory Authorities

Countries typically have a national regulatory authority which acts as the government body that approves vaccines and drugs. In the United States, this is the Food and Drug Administration (FDA). For the vaccines and medications commonly prescribed in a pre-travel consultation, providers are expected to use the products in accordance with the product label as approved by the FDA. The product label is a valuable source of information that is accurate at the time it is published. Manufacturers submit a detailed application that undergoes rigorous, multidisciplinary review. The approved product label reflects the information provided by the manufacturer in response to the requirements specified by a large body of regulatory law developed over many years. Since each country has different laws and requirements, approved products and their product labels may differ from country to country. This difference is then reflected in the national guidelines that relate to that product.

International Organizations

Travelers' health information is provided by WHO's publication, *International Travel and Health* (the "Green Book") and also in the WHO International Health

Regulations 2005. Countries with less-developed or nonexistent regulatory agencies often default to the WHO guidelines, while more-developed countries with resources devoted to travelers' health may be aware of the WHO recommendations but may not be able to reconcile WHO recommendations with their own country's recommendations in every situation.

US National Organizations

CDC provides recommendations for travel health and publishes those recommendations in this book. Subject-matter experts at CDC review information in their area of expertise and formulate recommendations. For vaccines, the Advisory Committee on Immunization Practices (ACIP) develops written recommendations for the administration of vaccines, including travelers' vaccines, to children and adults in the civilian population. Recommendations include age for vaccine administration, number of doses and dosing interval, and precautions and contraindications. ACIP, which is the only entity appointed by the federal government to make such recommendations, consists of 15 experts in fields associated with immunization who have been selected to provide advice and guidance to the Department of Health and Human Services and CDC on the control of vaccine-preventable diseases (Box 2-1).

Professional Organizations

Professional organizations often develop, write, and publish practice guidelines using committees of experts from their membership. These practice guidelines typically follow an evidence-based medicine approach that links recommendations to the strength and quality of the evidence as assessed by the committee members. The Infectious Disease Society of America has published a travel medicine practice guideline that many find useful.

Peer-Reviewed Medical Literature and Open Sources

As experience with a vaccine or a drug is acquired over the years, these results are often published in the peer-reviewed medical literature. In addition, people who use these products gain experience over time and develop their own opinions ("experience-based medicine"). The data that would be most useful in deciding how to use a vaccine or medication may not be available in published reports, so expert opinion attempts to interpret available information or provide background perspective.

WHY DO GUIDELINES DIFFER?

Guidelines in different countries and organizations may differ in substantial ways. Some of the reasons why guidelines differ include availability of products in different countries, a different cultural perception of risk, lack of evidence (or differing interpretations of the same evidence), and sometimes just honest differences in opinion among experts. Occasionally, public opinion may influence recommendations (for example, the widespread adverse publicity about mefloquine that was reported in the media).

Availability of Products

Travel health providers can only use the products that are available to them. Availability is determined by the regulatory approval status of the product and, to a lesser extent, the marketing and distribution plan of the manufacturer.

Among the various vaccines and antimalarial drugs commercially available worldwide, the process for regulatory approvals varies greatly. For example, registering a new vaccine or antimalarial drug in the United States is a costly and rigorous process. If the market is insufficient to justify the expense of registration, then a commercial company may not seek registration in a particular country. The standards for licensure vary, and what may be sufficient for one regulatory authority may not suffice for another. For example, primaquine, an option for malaria chemoprophylaxis in the United States, is not registered or commercially available in Switzerland. Atovaquone-proguanil was available for malaria chemoprophylaxis in the United States before many other countries. On the other hand, an oral vaccine against cholera is approved for use and widely available in many countries, but is not approved by the FDA; therefore, CDC and ACIP guidelines do not include any recommendations for the use of this vaccine.

Even when the same products are available, the recommendations for their use may differ. The injectable capsular polysaccharide typhoid vaccine and the oral typhoid vaccine are examples. In the United States, a booster of the polysaccharide vaccine is recommended after 2 years, but in most European countries, a booster is recommended after 3 years. In the United States, a packet of 4 oral typhoid capsules is dispensed, whereas in Europe, 3 doses are considered adequate. The regulatory agencies may have reviewed the same data and drawn different conclusions, or they may have reviewed different data at separate times and reached different conclusions. Regulatory submissions to various agencies rarely are ready and occur at the same time; therefore, the data available for review by each agency may not be the same, for legitimate reasons.

Perception of Risk

People from varying backgrounds can view the same risk data and come to different conclusions as to the cost and benefit of preventing that risk. For example, national-level recommendations to prevent malaria while traveling to India vary widely. Germany does not recommend using standard prophylaxis for any travel to an Indian destination; standby emergency treatment (SBET or self-treatment) is the recommendation for identified risk destinations. The guidelines in the United Kingdom recommend only awareness and mosquito bite prevention as the default recommendation for more than half the Indian subcontinent, including large cities and popular tourist destinations in the north and south, while recommending an individual risk assessment that is based on activities and types of travel for consideration of chemoprophylaxis. For some defined higher-risk areas, the recommendation is for standard chemoprophylaxis for most, with the option to consider mosquito avoidance for low-risk travelers. However, CDC recommends malaria chemoprophylaxis for any Indian destination except for some mountainous areas of northern states above 2,000 m (6,561 ft) as the default recommendation for most travelers, with consideration of individual risk and benefit. Is one of these recommendations better than the others? Not necessarily, as the recommendations may be based on the national experience with different types of travelers and the risk assessment approach of the organization formulating the national guidelines. For example, in 2011, CDC reported 223 malaria cases acquired in India by returning US travelers, the highest known absolute number of cases from any destination. However, when viewed as estimated relative case rates (the number of cases among US travelers attributable to each country divided by the estimated travel volume for US travelers to that country), countries in sub-Saharan Africa remain well above the median estimated risk, and India falls below the median estimated risk because of the much higher volume of travel to India. India reports active transmission in all provinces in the country. Based on the extremely large population of India, some of these provinces have high absolute numbers of cases but low case rates. Some countries base their recommendations on these relatively low case rates, but other countries believe that the high absolute numbers of cases results in large numbers of infective mosquitoes that can, in turn, infect travelers. In any case, travelers to India are likely to encounter diverse recommendations for malaria prevention from different sources, the Internet, or other travelers.

The best available data should always balance the risk of the intervention— and the costs—against the risk of the disease so that the decision to recommend a vaccine or prophylactic medicine may be understood by the clinician and the traveler.

Lack of Evidence

In many cases, limited or no data are available to inform an evidence-based assessment. In this setting, travel health providers defer to expert opinion or an extrapolation from limited data in conjunction with expert opinion. In travel medicine, it is rare to have actual prospective numerator and denominator data on the risk of any vaccine-preventable diseases in travelers. For example, any data on the risk of hepatitis A in travelers would have to account for the immunization rate with hepatitis A vaccine. These data are rarely available, and therefore, we often rely on historical data that captured few actual cases.

CAN WE HARMONIZE GUIDELINES?

The complex nature of how we obtain, evaluate, and verify data, combined with the fundamental differences in risk perception, makes it likely that multiple, overlapping, and at times conflicting guidelines will continue to exist. However, given the international nature of travel medicine and the existence of the International Society of Travel Medicine, conflicting guidelines have decreased in the past decade. In one example of an effort to harmonize guidelines, from 2008 through 2010, WHO convened an international group of yellow fever and travel medicine experts to review available data on yellow fever virus transmission. The product of this collaboration was a country-specific list of yellow fever vaccine recommendations based on the geographic distribution of risk (see Chapter 3, Yellow Fever & Malaria Information, by Country).

In summary, the role of the travel health provider is to become more sophisticated in his or her understanding of the various differences in guidelines, in interpreting this information, and in conveying it in an assured and comforting manner to travelers.

BIBLIOGRAPHY

1. CDC. Advisory Committee on Immunization Practices (ACIP). Atlanta: CDC; 2014 [cited 2014 Sep 10]. Available from: http://www.cdc.gov/vaccines/acip/.

2. CDC. Malaria surveillance—United States, 2011. MMWR Surveill Summ. 2013 Nov 1;62(5):1–17.

3. Chiodini PL, Field VK, Whitty CJM, Lalloo DG. Guidelines for malaria prevention

in travellers from the United Kingdom. London: Public Health England; 2014 [cited 2014 Sep 16]. Available from: https://www.gov.uk/government/uploads/system/uploads/attachment_data/file/337761/Guidelines_for_malaria_prevention_in_travellers_UK_PC.pdf.

4. Committee to Advise on Tropical Medicine and Travel (CATMAT). Canadian recommendations for the prevention and treatment of malaria. Ottawa: Public Health Agency of Canada; 2014 [cited 2014 Sep 10]. Available from: http://publications.gc.ca/collections/collection_2014/aspc-phac/HP40-102-2014-eng.pdf.

5. German Society for Tropical Medicine and International Health Association (DTG). [Recommendations for malaria prevention]. 2014 [cited 2014 Sep 10].

Available from: http://www.dtg.org/malaria.html. German.

6. Hill DR, Ericsson CD, Pearson RD, Keystone JS, Freedman DO, Kozarsky PE, et al. The practice of travel medicine: guidelines by the Infectious Diseases Society of America. Clin Infect Dis. 2006 Dec 15;43(12): 1499–539.

7. World Health Organization. International Health Regulations (2005). Geneva: World Health Organization; 2008 [cited 2014 Sep 10]. Available from: http://www.who.int/ihr/9789241596664/en/index.html.

8. World Health Organization. International Travel and Health. Geneva: World Health Organization; 2012 (with 2014 updates) [cited 2014 Sep 10]. Available from: http://www.who.int/ith/en/.

The Pre-Travel Consultation

THE PRE-TRAVEL CONSULTATION

Lin H. Chen, Natasha S. Hochberg, Alan J. Magill

The pre-travel consultation offers a dedicated time to prepare travelers for the health concerns that might arise during their trips. The objectives of the pre-travel consultation are to assess the traveler's trip plans and determine potential health hazards; to educate the traveler regarding anticipated risks and methods for prevention; to provide immunizations for vaccine-preventable diseases and medications for prophylaxis, self-treatment, or both; and to educate and empower the traveler to manage his or her health during the trip through counseling and prevention messages.

QUALIFICATIONS FOR PROVIDING A PRE-TRAVEL CONSULTATION

Much evidence has accumulated relevant to travelers' health and forms the basis of pre-travel advice. Providers of pre-travel consultations should possess a general knowledge of the evidence base, understand disease epidemiology as well as routes of transmission and preventive measures, and be able to discuss the risks clearly with travelers.

The outcome of a pre-travel consultation likely depends on the expertise and communication skills of the provider, as well as the health beliefs of the traveler. In-person counseling by trained staff can effectively deliver some messages, in particular with regard to malaria risk and prevention. Familiarity with the traveler's destination, its culture, infrastructure, and disease patterns can assist the travel health advisor in providing targeted messages.

Various health care providers may be asked to provide pre-travel consultation, including primary care providers and specialists who see their patients regularly (such as transplant surgeons or oncologists). These clinicians are familiar with the traveler's medical history but may not have detailed knowledge of travel medicine. Travel medicine specialists have in-depth knowledge regarding immunizations, risks associated with specific destinations, and the implications of traveling with underlying conditions. Therefore, a comprehensive consultation with a travel medicine expert is indicated for any traveler with a complicated health history, special risks, or exotic or complicated itineraries.

COMPONENTS OF A PRE-TRAVEL CONSULTATION

Effective pre-travel consultations require attention to the health background of the traveler and incorporate the itinerary, trip duration, travel purpose, and activities, all of which determine health risks (Table 2-1). Advice

Table 2-1. Information necessary for a risk assessment during pre-travel consultations

Health Background

Past medical history	• Age • Sex • Underlying conditions • Allergies (especially any pertaining to vaccines, eggs, or latex) • Medications
Special conditions	• Pregnancy • Breastfeeding • Disability or handicap • Immunocompromised state • Older age • Psychiatric condition • Seizure disorder • Recent surgery • Recent cardiopulmonary event • Recent cerebrovascular event
Immunization history	• Routine vaccines • Travel vaccines
Prior travel experience	• Experience with malaria chemoprophylaxis • Experience with altitude • Illnesses related to prior travel

Trip Details

Itinerary	• Countries and specific regions, including order of countries if >1 country • Rural or urban
Timing	• Trip duration • Season of travel • Time to departure
Reason for travel	• Tourism • Business • Visiting friends and relatives • Volunteer, missionary, or aid work • Research or education • Adventure • Pilgrimage • Adoption • Seeking health care (medical tourism)

continued

TABLE 2-1. INFORMATION NECESSARY FOR A RISK ASSESSMENT DURING PRE-TRAVEL CONSULTATIONS (continued)

Travel style	• Independent travel or package tour • Propensity for "adventurous" eating • Traveler risk tolerance • General hygiene standards at destination • Modes of transportation • Accommodations (such as tourist or luxury hotel, guest house, hostel or budget hotel, dormitory, local home or host family, or tent)
Special activities	• Disaster relief • Medical care (providing or receiving) • High altitude or climbing • Diving • Cruise ship • Rafting • Cycling • Extreme sports

should be personalized, highlighting the likely exposures and also reminding the traveler of ubiquitous risks such as injury, foodborne and waterborne infections, respiratory tract infections, and bloodborne and sexually transmitted infections. Written information is essential to supplement the discussion and highlight key advice for travelers. Balancing the cautions with an appreciation of the positive aspects of the journey leads to a more meaningful pre-travel consultation. Attention to the cost of recommended interventions may be critical. Some travelers may not be able to afford all of the recommended immunizations and medications, a situation that requires prioritizing interventions. (See *Perspectives: Prioritizing for the Resource-Limited Traveler* later in this chapter.)

Assess Individual Risk

Many elements merit consideration in assessing a traveler's health risks (Table 2-1). Certain travelers may confront special risks. Recent hospitalization for serious problems may even lead the advisor to recommend delaying travel. Air travel is contraindicated for certain conditions, and the travel health provider and traveler should consult with the relevant health care providers most familiar with the underlying illnesses. Other traveler characteristics that are associated with specific risks

include travelers who are visiting friends and relatives, long-term travelers, travelers with chronic illnesses, immunocompromised travelers, pregnant travelers, and travelers with small children. More comprehensive discussion on advising travelers with specific needs is available in Chapter 8.

In addition to recognizing the traveler's characteristics, health background, and destination-specific risks, the exposures related to special activities also merit discussion. For example, river rafting could expose a traveler to schistosomiasis or leptospirosis, and spelunking in Central America could put the traveler at risk of histoplasmosis. Flying from lowlands to high-altitude areas and trekking or climbing in mountainous regions introduces the risk of altitude illness. Therefore, the provider should inquire about plans for specific activities.

Manage Risk

Immunizations are a crucial component of pre-travel consultations, and the risk assessment forms the basis of recommendations for travel vaccines. At the same time, the pre-travel consultation presents an opportunity to update routine vaccines (Table 2-2). In considering travel immunizations, the approach to address "aggregate travel" or cumulative risk over years of travel, rather than risk associated

Table 2-2. Vaccines to update or consider during pre-travel consultations

VACCINE	TRAVEL-RELATED OCCURRENCES AND RECOMMENDATIONS
Routine Vaccines	
Haemophilus influenzae type b	No report of travel-related infection, although organism is ubiquitous.
Hepatitis B	Recommended for travelers visiting countries where HBsAg prevalence is ≥2% as well as screening for chronic hepatitis B in people from countries with HBsAg prevalence ≥2% (see Map 3-4). Vaccination may be considered for all international travelers, regardless of destination, depending upon the traveler's behavioral risk as determined by the provider and traveler.
Human papillomavirus (HPV)	No report of travel-acquired infection; however, sexual activity during travel may lead to HPV and other sexually transmitted infections.
Influenza	Outbreaks have occurred on cruise ships, and 2009 influenza A (H1N1) illustrated the rapidity of spread via travel. Novel influenza viruses such as avian influenza H5N1 and H7N9 can also be transmitted to travelers visiting areas with circulation of these viruses.
Measles, mumps, rubella	Infections are common in countries and communities that do not immunize children routinely, including Europe. Outbreaks have occurred in the United States as a result of infection in returning travelers.
Meningococcal	Outbreaks occur regularly in sub-Saharan Africa in the "meningitis belt" during the dry season, generally December through June. Outbreaks occurred with Hajj pilgrimage, and the Kingdom of Saudi Arabia requires the quadrivalent vaccine for pilgrims.
Pneumococcal	Organism is ubiquitous, and causal relationship to travel is difficult to establish.
Polio	Unimmunized or underimmunized travelers can acquire poliovirus, as occurred in a case reported in association with a stay with a host family in a Latin American country that had been declared polio-free.
Rotavirus	Common in developing countries, although not a common cause of travelers' diarrhea in adults. The vaccine is only recommended in young children.
Tetanus, diphtheria, pertussis	Rare cases of diphtheria have been attributed to travel. Pertussis has occurred in travelers, recently in adults whose immunity has waned.
Varicella	Infections are common in countries that do not immunize children routinely, as in most developing countries. Naturally occurring disease also occurs later in tropical countries.

continued

TABLE 2-2. VACCINES TO UPDATE OR CONSIDER DURING PRE-TRAVEL CONSULTATIONS (continued)

VACCINE	TRAVEL-RELATED OCCURRENCES AND RECOMMENDATIONS
Zoster	Travel (a form of stress) may trigger varicella zoster reactivation, but causal relationship is difficult to establish.
Travel Vaccines	
Cholera (not available in the United States)	Cases in travelers have occurred recently in association with travel to the Dominican Republic and Haiti.
Hepatitis A	Prevaccination incidence was 3–20 cases/1,000 person-months of travel, but recent surveillance indicated a decline to 3–11 cases/100,000 person-months of travel. Prevalence patterns of hepatitis A virus infection may vary among regions within a country, and missing or obsolete data present a challenge. Serologic testing may be considered in travelers from highly endemic countries since they may already be immune. Some expert travel clinicians advise people traveling outside the United States to consider hepatitis A vaccination regardless of their country of destination.
Japanese encephalitis	Rare cases have occurred, estimated at <1 case/1 million travelers to endemic countries.
Rabies	Rabies preexposure immunization simplifies postexposure immunoprophylaxis, as immunoglobulin in particular may be difficult to obtain in many destinations.
Tickborne encephalitis (not available in the United States)	Cases have been identified in travelers with an estimated risk of 1/10,000 person-months in travelers. Endemic areas are expanding in Europe.
Typhoid	UK surveillance found the highest risk to be travel to India (6 cases/100,000 visits), Pakistan (9 cases/100,000 visits), and Bangladesh (21 cases/100,000 visits), although risk is substantial in many destinations.
Yellow fever	Risk occurs mainly in defined areas of sub-Saharan Africa and the Amazonian regions of South America. Some countries require proof of vaccination for entry. For travelers visiting multiple countries, order of travel may make a difference in the requirements.

Abbreviation: HBsAg, hepatitis B surface antigen.

with a single trip, allows travelers to prepare for multiple trips. Travelers should receive a record of immunizations administered.

Another major focus of pre-travel consultations for many destinations is the prevention of malaria. Malaria continues to cause substantial morbidity and mortality in travelers. In 2011, the number of US malaria cases reported to CDC was the highest since 1971; therefore, pre-travel consultation must carefully assess travelers' risk for malaria and recommend preventive measures. For travelers going to malaria-endemic countries, it is imperative to discuss malaria transmission, ways to reduce risk, and recommendations for chemoprophylaxis.

Travelers with underlying health conditions require attention to their health issues as they relate to the destination and activities. For example, a traveler with a history of cardiac disease should carry medical reports, including a recent electrocardiogram. Asthma may flare in a traveler visiting a polluted city or from physical exertion during a hike; planning for treatment in case of asthma exacerbation can be lifesaving. Travelers should be counseled on how they can find reputable medical facilities at their destination. Any allergies or serious medical conditions should be identified on a bracelet or a card to expedite medical care in emergency situations.

The pre-travel consultation also provides the ideal setting to review wellness strategies with travelers and to remind them of healthy practices during travel. Topics to be explored are numerous and could be organized into a checklist, placing priority on the most serious and frequently encountered issues (Table 2-3). General issues such as preventing injury and sunburn also deserve mention. Written information is essential to supplement the oral advice and enable travelers to review the abundant instructions from their clinic visits. Advice on self-treatable conditions may minimize the need for travelers to seek medical care while abroad and possibly lead to faster return to good health.

Self-Treatable Conditions

Despite providers' best efforts, some travelers will become ill. Obtaining reliable and timely medical care during travel can be problematic in many destinations. As a result, prescribing certain medications in advance can empower the traveler to self-diagnose and treat common health problems. With some activities in remote settings, such as trekking, the only alternative to self-treatment would be no treatment. Pre-travel counseling may actually result in a more accurate self-diagnosis and treatment than relying on local medical care in some areas. In addition, the increasing awareness of substandard and counterfeit drugs in pharmacies in the developing world (as many as 50% of the drugs on the shelves) makes it more important for travelers to bring quality manufactured drugs with them from a reliable supplier in their own country

(see *Perspectives*: Pharmaceutical Quality & Counterfeit Drugs later in this chapter).

Travel health providers need to recognize the conditions for which the traveler may be at risk and educate the traveler about the diagnosis and treatment of those particular conditions. The keys to successful self-treatment strategies are providing a simple disease or condition definition, providing a treatment, and educating the traveler about the expected outcome of treatment. Using travelers' diarrhea as an example, a practitioner could provide the following advice:

- "Travelers' diarrhea" is the sudden onset of abnormally loose, frequent stools.
- The treatment is ciprofloxacin 500 mg, every 12 hours, for 1 day (2 doses).
- The traveler should feel better within 6–24 hours.
- If symptoms persist for 24–36 hours despite self-treatment, it may be necessary to seek medical attention.

To minimize the potential negative effects of a self-treatment strategy, the recommendations should follow a few key points:

- Drugs recommended must be safe, well tolerated, and effective for use as self-treatment.
- A drug's toxicity or potential for harm, if used incorrectly or in an overdose situation, should be minimal.
- Simple and clear directions are critical. Consider providing handouts describing how to use the drugs. Keeping the directions simple will increase the effectiveness of the strategy.

The following are some of the most common situations in which people would find self-treatment useful. The extent of self-treatment recommendations offered to the traveler should reflect the remoteness and difficulty of travel and the availability of reliable medical care at the particular destination. The recommended self-treatment options for each disease are provided in the designated section of the Yellow Book or discussed below.

- Travelers' diarrhea (see section in this chapter)

 THE PRE-TRAVEL CONSULTATION | 33

Table 2-3. Major topics for discussion during pre-travel consultations

Immunizations	• Review routine immunizations and those travel immunizations indicated for the specific itinerary. • Discuss utility of titers when records are unavailable or unreliable, particularly for measles, mumps, rubella. • Screen for chronic hepatitis B for people born in countries with HBsAg prevalence ≥2%. • Discuss indications for, effectiveness of, and adverse reactions to immunizations.
Malaria chemoprophylaxis	• Determine if there is a risk of malaria. • Discuss personal protective measures. • Discuss risks and benefits of chemoprophylaxis and recommended choices of chemoprophylaxis for the itinerary.
Travelers' diarrhea	• Recommend strategies to minimize diarrhea. • Discuss antibiotics for self-treatment and adjunct medications such as loperamide.
Respiratory illnesses	• Discuss areas of particular concern (such as avian influenza in Asia or MERS in the Arabian Peninsula). • Consider influenza treatment for high-risk travelers.
Other vectorborne diseases	• Define risk of disease in specific itinerary and insect precautions needed.
Altitude illness	• Determine if the itinerary puts the traveler at risk of altitude illness. • Discuss preventive measures such as gradual ascent, adequate hydration, and medications to prevent and treat.
Other environmental hazards	• Caution travelers to avoid contact with animals to reduce the potential for bites and scratches that can transmit rabies. • Advise travelers to avoid walking barefoot, as parasites can enter intact or damaged skin. • Advise travelers to avoid wading or swimming in freshwater where there is risk for schistosomiasis or leptospirosis. • Remind travelers to apply sunscreen to skin exposed to the sun.
Personal safety	• Discuss precautions travelers can take to minimize risks specific to the trip, such as traffic accidents, alcohol excess, personal assault, robbery, or drowning. • Provide information on travel health and medical evacuation insurance.
Sexual health and bloodborne pathogens	• Caution the traveler to avoid activities that can lead to sexually transmitted infections, unwanted pregnancy, or bloodborne infections. • Remind travelers to use condoms if they do have sex.
Disease-specific counseling	• Remind travelers to hand carry medications and supplies. • Advise travelers to prepare for exacerbations or complications from underlying disease.

Abbreviations: HBsAg, hepatitis B surface antigen; MERS, Middle East respiratory syndrome.

- Altitude illness (see section in this chapter)
- Jet lag (see section in this chapter)
- Motion sickness (see section in this chapter)
- Respiratory infections (see section in this chapter)
- Skin conditions: skin reactions due to allergic or irritant triggers usually respond to topical steroids; discomfort from superficial fungal infections respond to antifungal creams. See also Chapter 5, Skin and Soft Tissue Infections in Returned Travelers.
- Urinary tract infections: common among many women; carrying an antibiotic for empiric treatment may be valuable.
- Vaginal yeast infections: self-treatment course of patient's preferred antifungal medication can be prescribed for women who are prone to infections, sexually active, or who may be receiving antibiotics for other reasons (including doxycycline for malaria chemoprophylaxis).
- Occupational exposure to HIV (see Chapter 8, Health Care Workers)
- Malaria self-treatment (see Chapter 3, Malaria)

In sum, travelers should be encouraged to carry a travel health kit with prescription and nonprescription medications. Typical medications include malaria chemoprophylaxis, self-management of travelers' diarrhea, and prophylaxis or treatment for acute mountain sickness. If a traveler anticipates the need to treat motion sickness, jet lag, or severe allergic reactions, consider medications for self-management, such as motion sickness therapy, a sleep aid, and epinephrine. Prescribing multiple medications, particularly for travelers already taking medications, warrants a review for possible drug interactions. More detailed information for providers and travelers is given in Chapter 2, Travel Health Kits; Chapter 8, Travelers with Chronic Illnesses; and Chapter 8, Humanitarian Aid Workers.

BIBLIOGRAPHY

1. Chen LH, Hill DR, Wilder-Smith A. Vaccination of travelers: how far have we come and where are we going? Expert Rev Vaccines. 2011 Nov;10(11):1609–20.
2. DuPont HL, Ericsson CD, Farthing MJ, Gorbach S, Pickering LK, Rombo L, et al. Expert review of the evidence base for self-therapy of travelers' diarrhea. J Travel Med. 2009 May–Jun;16(3):161–71.
3. Freedman DO. Clinical practice. Malaria prevention in short-term travelers. N Engl J Med. 2008 Aug 7;359(6):603–12.
4. Hatz CFR, Chen LH. Pre-travel consultation. In: Keystone JS, Freedman DO, Kozarsky PE, Connor BA, Nothdurft HD, editors. Travel Medicine. 3rd ed. Philadelphia: Saunders Elsevier; 2013. p. 31–6.
5. Hill DR, Ericsson CD, Pearson RD, Keystone JS, Freedman DO, Kozarsky PE, et al. The practice of travel medicine: guidelines by the Infectious Diseases Society of America. Clin Infect Dis. 2006 Dec 15;43(12):1499–539.
6. International Society of Travel Medicine. Body of knowledge for the practice of travel medicine—2012.

Atlanta: International Society of Travel Medicine; 2012 [cited 2014 Oct 1]. Available from: http://www.istm.org/bodyofknowledge.
7. LaRocque RC, Rao SR, Lee J, Ansdell V, Yates JA, Schwartz BS, et al. Global TravEpiNet: a national consortium of clinics providing care to international travelers—analysis of demographic characteristics, travel destinations, and pretravel healthcare of high-risk US international travelers, 2009–2011. Clin Infect Dis. 2012 Feb 15;54(4):455–62.
8. Leder K, Chen LH, Wilson ME. Aggregate travel vs. single trip assessment: arguments for cumulative risk analysis. Vaccine. 2012 Mar 28;30(15):2600–4.
9. Leder K, Torresi J, Libman MD, Cramer JP, Castelli F, Schlagenhauf P, et al. GeoSentinel surveillance of illness in returned travelers, 2007–2011. Ann Intern Med. 2013 Mar 19;158(6):456–68.
10. Schwartz BS, Larocque RC, Ryan ET. In the clinic. Travel medicine. Ann Intern Med. 2012 Jun 5;156(11):ITC6-1–16.

Perspectives

TRAVELERS' PERCEPTION OF RISK

David R. Shlim

Travel medicine is based on the concept of the reduction of risk. In the context of travel medicine, "risk" refers to the possibility of harm during the course of a planned trip. Some risks may be avoidable, and others may not. Vaccine-preventable diseases may be mostly avoidable, depending on the risk of the disease and the protective efficacy of the vaccine. Non-disease risks, such as motor vehicle accidents or drowning, account for a much higher percentage of deaths among travelers than infectious diseases.

For many years, travel medicine practitioners have felt that if they knew the statistics for a given risk, they could objectively advise travelers about that risk. However, it has become clear that the perception and tolerance of risk are subjective factors that must be considered when addressing risks of travel. Travel health providers may know statistics for a given risk, but whether the risk is considered high or low depends on the perception of the traveler or the travel medicine provider. For example, the risk of dying while trekking in Nepal is 15 deaths per 100,000 trekkers, but there is no objective way to determine whether this risk is high or low. When the manuscript that reported this risk of dying while trekking was peer-reviewed, one reviewer wrote, "You need to emphasize that these data show how dangerous trekking actually is." The other reviewer wrote, "You should make a point of stating that these data show how safe trekking is."

The subjective sense of risk is based on one's perception of risk ("15 per 100,000 means it's dangerous") and one's tolerance for risk ("it may be 15 per 100,000, but it's worth it"). This subjective sense of risk suffuses the field of travel medicine, but it is rarely discussed. Some travelers canceled travel plans to Asia because of their fear of H5N1 avian influenza, even though the actual risk to travelers was virtually zero. Other travelers plan to ascend Mount Everest, even though the risk of dying during an Everest climb is 1 in 40.

Regardless of the perception and tolerance of risk, the hazards associated with travel cannot be eliminated, just as the risks of staying home are not zero. Even the act of trying to prevent a risk—such as yellow fever—can lead to a fatal reaction to the vaccine in very rare cases. Therefore, the goal in travel and in travel medicine should be skillfully managing risk, rather than trying to eliminate risk. The pre-travel consultation is an opportunity to discuss risks and develop plans that minimize these risks. Each traveler may have individual concepts about the risks and benefits of vaccines, prophylaxis, and behavior modification.

Travelers should also consider the psychological and emotional aspects of foreign travel. Culture shock can occur on either end of a journey: on arrival when one encounters an entirely strange new world, and on return when one's

Perspectives sections are written as editorial discussions aiming to add depth and clinical perspective to the official recommendations contained in the book. The views and opinions expressed in this section are those of the author and do not necessarily represent the official position of CDC.

own world may temporarily appear unfamiliar. Travelers with underlying psychiatric conditions should be cautious when heading out to a stressful new environment, particularly if they are traveling alone.

Travel medicine providers should promote the understanding of the concept of commitment, the idea that certain parts of a journey cannot easily be reversed. A person trekking into a remote area may need to accept that rescue, if available at all, may be delayed for days. A person who has a myocardial infarction in a country with no advanced cardiac services may have a difficult time getting to definitive medical care. If the traveler has already contemplated these concerns and accepted them, it will be easier to deal with them if they come to pass.

Travel medicine practitioners should explore their own perception and tolerance of risk, so that they can help travelers find their individual comfort level when making decisions about destinations, activities, and prophylactic measures.

Perspectives

PRIORITIZING CARE FOR THE RESOURCE-LIMITED TRAVELER
Zoon Wangu, Elizabeth D. Barnett

Travelers seen in pre-travel clinic consultations often have financial constraints. Prioritizing immunizations and prophylactic medications should be part of an individualized assessment based on the travel itinerary, efficacy and safety of vaccines and medications, and associated costs. Travelers must often pay out of pocket for pre-travel care, as many health insurance plans do not cover travel immunizations or prophylaxis. As an example, the estimated cost of a US pre-travel consultation for a backpacker planning a 4-week trip to West Africa may be as high as $1,400 for the initial consultation and vaccinations, excluding malaria chemoprophylaxis. However, travelers with limited budgets tend to be at higher risk for travel-associated infections, as they often visit remote areas, stay in lower-grade accommodations, and are more likely to eat local street food. Therefore, the cost of disease (such as malaria) may, in many cases, outweigh costs of vaccination and prophylaxis. The financial benefits of obtaining travel health insurance and evacuation insurance before travel must also be considered (see Travel Insurance, Travel Health Insurance, & Medical Evacuation Insurance later in this chapter). Clinicians need to understand

Perspectives sections are written as editorial discussions aiming to add depth and clinical perspective to the official recommendations contained in the book. The views and opinions expressed in this section are those of the authors and do not necessarily represent the official position of CDC.

travelers' financial constraints in order to provide realistic recommendations. The variety of insurance plans, number of travelers without adequate insurance coverage, and number of student and budget travelers challenges even the most savvy travel medicine clinicians. This section provides guidance for busy practitioners in prioritizing vaccine and prophylaxis choices.

VACCINES
Required Vaccines
Only 2 vaccines are categorically required for some travelers: meningococcal vaccine for pilgrims traveling to Mecca during the Hajj and yellow fever vaccine for travelers to certain countries in Africa and South America (see Chapter 3, Yellow Fever & Malaria Information, by Country). If either of these vaccines is required for an itinerary, prioritize it since the traveler may be denied entry to the country without proof of vaccination. Note that travelers who may only be staying in a yellow fever–endemic country briefly (such as during an airport layover) may still need evidence of vaccination to enter other countries on their itinerary. In a few specific circumstances, travelers to countries that are exporting polio may be asked to show proof of polio vaccination before they are allowed to leave those countries if they have spent >4 weeks in the country (see Chapter 3, Poliomyelitis).

Routine Vaccines
CDC recommends that all travelers should be up-to-date with routine vaccines before international travel, regardless of destination. The benefits of vaccine administration extend beyond the travel period, and in many cases lifelong immunity is achieved. Routine vaccines are generally associated with lower costs, since they are mass-produced as part of the scheduled national childhood and adult vaccination programs. Moreover, many health insurance plans will reimburse the patient for the cost of vaccine administration. If cost of routine vaccines is a limitation, a traveler can explore opportunities for obtaining them in a health department or primary care setting, where cost may be lower than in a travel clinic. Prioritize the routine vaccines that protect against diseases for which the traveler is most likely to be at general risk. At this time, top priorities for most destinations would include vaccines against influenza, measles, and hepatitis A and B.

Recommended Vaccines
Review the itinerary to determine the need for specific vaccines based on destination or purpose of travel, such as rabies vaccine for adventure travelers going to endemic countries or Japanese encephalitis vaccine for travelers to rural areas of Asia during the local transmission season. In addition, availability of postexposure rabies prophylaxis in the destination country should be considered. Recent surveys of US embassy medical staff show that in up to 37% of locations worldwide, rabies vaccine or immune globulin were available only "sometimes" to "never."

In some cases, the patient may be immune to the disease for which immunization is being considered. Testing for antibody concentrations may be covered by insurance while vaccines are not. Specifically, hepatitis A and B vaccines should be considered for most travelers, especially those with underlying liver disease. Testing for immunity to these infections may determine whether vaccination is warranted.

Also consider time until departure, risk of disease at the destination, effectiveness and safety of vaccine, and likelihood of repeat travel. For example, parenteral typhoid vaccine may be less cost-effective for certain travelers (especially when departures are imminent and trip duration is short) because of the relatively low efficacy, short duration of protection, and time needed for onset of protection.

Educate about alternative ways to reduce risk. For example, advise travelers to avoid animal bites and seek care for such bites should they occur, use insect precautions, and observe food and water precautions at all times. All travelers should practice these preventive behaviors, but they are critical for travelers who elect not to receive recommended vaccinations for any reason.

MALARIA CHEMOPROPHYLAXIS

Malaria chemoprophylaxis can be a financial burden for the traveler. The risk of acquiring malaria in a traveler staying in air-conditioned hotels and commuting in a rented car is much lower than that assumed by the backpacker staying in a rural guesthouse or the traveler returning to his or her native land staying with friends or relatives. Tailoring advice to the traveler's financial needs in addition to his or her medical needs can improve compliance with prophylaxis and protect those who are at highest risk.

Every pre-travel consultation should include detailed advice about preventing mosquito bites (see Protection against Mosquitoes, Ticks, & Other Arthropods later in this chapter). Malaria chemoprophylaxis, if needed, should be offered based on the risk profile of the traveler.

Costs associated with the different regimens vary widely. For example, based on current prices in the United States, a prophylactic treatment course for a 3-week trip to a malaria-endemic destination would cost $100–$250 for doxycycline, $50–$70 for chloroquine, $100 for mefloquine, and $200–$250 for atovaquone-proguanil (depending on health insurance and other factors). Atovaquone-proguanil cost may be equivalent to that of mefloquine for short trips, but mefloquine (or chloroquine, in the few regions where malaria remains susceptible) will be more cost-effective for trips lasting 2 weeks or more. Travelers who raise the question of purchasing antimalarial drugs at their destination must be advised about the risk of inappropriate, substandard, and counterfeit medications (see *Perspectives*: Pharmaceutical Quality & Counterfeit Drugs later in this chapter).

PREVENTIVE BEHAVIORS

Budget travelers and those who cannot afford costly travel vaccines will continue to challenge travel medicine practitioners. Such travelers will benefit from additional strategies to safeguard their health during travel. These strategies include following safety (especially road traffic safety) and security guidelines and observing sun protection, following insect precautions, avoiding food hazards, and following safe sexual practices. Travelers can be reassured that the actions they take to avoid these hazards may, in the long run, be more beneficial than obtaining vaccines or prophylaxis for diseases of low prevalence.

BIBLIOGRAPHY

1. Adachi K, Coleman MS, Khan N, Jentes ES, Arguin P, Rao SR, et al. Economics of malaria prevention in US travelers to West Africa. Clin Infect Dis. 2014 Jan;58(1):11–21.

2. Jentes ES, Blanton JD, Johnson KJ, Petersen BW, Lamias MJ, Robertson K, et al. The global availability of rabies immune globulin and rabies vaccine in clinics

providing indirect care to travelers. J Travel Med. 2014 Jan–Feb;21(1):62–6.

3. Johnson DF, Leder K, Torresi J. Hepatitis B and C infection in international travelers. J Travel Med. 2013 May–Jun;20(3):194–202.

4. Mangtani P, Roberts JA. Economic evaluations of travelers' vaccinations. In: Zuckerman JN, Jong EC, editors. Travelers' Vaccines. 2nd ed. Shelton,

CT: People's Medical Publishing House; 2010. p. 553–67.

5. Steffen R, Connor BA. Vaccines in travel health: from risk assessment to priorities. J Travel Med. 2005 Jan–Feb;12(1):26–35.

6. Wu D, Guo CY. Epidemiology and prevention of hepatitis A in travelers. J Travel Med. 2013 Nov–Dec;20(6):394–9.

Perspectives

COST ANALYSIS OF TRAVEL MEDICINE

Edward T. Ryan

What are the resource and financial implications of a pre-travel medical encounter, and from whose perspective are we addressing the issue: society's, the traveler's, the insurance carrier's? The encounter requires specific resources and incurs specific costs, including a consultation (whether as part of a primary care or specialist visit), costs of administered vaccines and prescribed drugs, and costs associated with missed work and missed opportunities. The economic benefit of this encounter reflects the likelihood of preventing or reducing the risk of an illness and incorporates all the expenses of a travel-related illness. However, no unified economic analysis of these factors in travel medicine has yet been done.

We should first acknowledge what we know and do not know about the clinical benefit of a pre-travel medical encounter. We know that vaccination and chemoprophylaxis can be medically effective (although much vaccine efficacy data is extrapolated from studies unrelated to travel). We also know that benefits may be long term (such as long-term immunity after vaccination) and that such benefits may be particularly pertinent for people who travel frequently. We have fewer data on the impact of pre-travel education and advice; for example, educating travelers on ways to limit foodborne and waterborne diseases has not had a demonstrable effect on the risk of travelers' diarrhea. We also need to recognize that the risk of acquiring a travel-related illness (and therefore potential benefit) is hard to assess, relating not just to destination but also to itinerary, duration and timing of travel, and behavior of the traveler at the destination. Moreover, the consequences (and therefore potential benefits and expenses) of becoming ill will vary by the type of traveler (such as immunocompromised,

Perspectives sections are written as editorial discussions aiming to add depth and clinical perspective to the official recommendations contained in the book. The views and opinions expressed in this section are those of the author and do not necessarily represent the official position of CDC.

elderly, pediatric, or pregnant), as well as where the traveler becomes ill. Many travel-related risks are also not fixed: risks will change as destination infrastructure and economy change, disease control programs advance, or new or emerging infections evolve or spread into new zones. Further confounding the issue is the reality that what data we do have for generating our best estimates of disease risk at a destination often reflect disease prevalence among a local population and may not correlate with the real risk to travelers.

Perhaps the most overlooked economic aspect of the pre-travel medical encounter, however, is its potential effect on the many travel-related illnesses that have public health implications. For instance, if a traveler introduced measles or hepatitis A into a community, it would prompt extensive contact tracing, intervention, and follow-up. Travelers also spread influenza; Middle East respiratory syndrome coronavirus; a range of arboviruses including West Nile, dengue, and chikungunya; and highly drug-resistant pathogens such as NDM-1–expressing bacteria and multidrug-resistant *Mycobacterium tuberculosis*. The public health and infection control costs associated with responses to these pathogens can be staggering. Right now, such costs are largely borne by the public health sector and by society in general and do not appear in the financial calculus of the individual traveler or the insurance carrier.

COMPLEX MODELING AND OUTCOMES ANALYSIS FOR TRAVEL MEDICINE

Economic outcome analyses relating to travel medicine will need to be complex. Travel medicine models should reflect the true mix of travelers (visiting friends and relatives, business, leisure, service) and should incorporate the fact that many travelers do not seek pre-travel medical care, which may dilute the benefit generated by those who do. Travel medicine models should also take into account a wide range of illnesses, recognize that some diseases may present late (such as with tuberculosis), and that many of these illnesses may lead to chronic sequelae (such as neurologic damage from cerebral malaria, encephalitis, or traumatic brain injury). The models should also incorporate accurate assessments of risk, potential interactions of risk (for instance, travelers at higher risk of one illness may be at a lower risk of another), and accurate assessments of the effect of the pre-travel encounter on mitigating any risks. Importantly, the models should incorporate public health–related resources and expenditures relating to the importation of pathogens, not only to trace and limit ongoing disease transmission but also to mitigate the risk of establishing environmental or animal reservoirs in home communities. Since disease risk at destinations is constantly evolving, the models should be constructed as sensitivity analyses.

Perhaps the most logical way forward is to begin by focusing initial analyses around a number of core areas. For instance, a recent analysis of data from the GlobalTravEpiNet (GTEN) program (see Chapter 1, Travel Epidemiology) evaluated the economic aspects of a health consultation on malaria prevention among US travelers bound for West Africa. A reasonable approach might be to perform similar analyses for each major group of travel-related illness, with the goal of using such analyses to define core metrics and their dependencies and to incorporate these into a single integrated analysis. Although possible, such an approach will not be easy.

BIBLIOGRAPHY

1. Adachi K, Coleman MS, Khan N, Jentes ES, Arguin P, Rao SR, et al. Economics of malaria prevention in US travelers to West Africa. Clin Infect Dis. 2014 Jan;58(1):11–21.

GENERAL RECOMMENDATIONS FOR VACCINATION & IMMUNOPROPHYLAXIS

Andrew T. Kroger, Raymond A. Strikas

Recommendations for the use of vaccines and other biologic products (such as immune globulin [IG] products) in the United States are developed by the Advisory Committee on Immunization Practices (ACIP) and are harmonized with ACIP liaison organizations including the American Academy of Pediatrics, the American Academy of Family Physicians, the American College of Physicians, the American College of Obstetricians and Gynecologists, and others. Recommendations voted on by the ACIP are reviewed by the CDC director and, if adopted, become official recommendations of the Department of Health and Human Services/CDC upon publication in CDC's *Morbidity and Mortality Weekly Report* (MMWR). ACIP recommendations are based on scientific evidence of benefits (disease immunity) and risks (vaccine adverse reactions) and, where few or no data are available, on expert opinion. Recommendations include information on general immunization issues and the use of specific vaccines. Box 2-1 provides more information about ACIP. This section is based primarily on the ACIP General Recommendations on Immunization.

Evaluation of people before travel should include a review and provision of routine vaccines recommended based on age and other individual characteristics. Additionally, some routine vaccines are recommended at earlier ages for international travelers. For example, MMR (measles-mumps-rubella) vaccine is recommended for infants aged 6–11 months who travel abroad to protect them from measles. Recommendations for specific vaccines related to travel will depend on itinerary, duration of travel, and host factors. Vaccinations against diphtheria, tetanus, pertussis, measles, mumps, rubella, varicella, poliomyelitis, hepatitis A, hepatitis B, *Haemophilus influenzae* type b (Hib), rotavirus, human papillomavirus (HPV), and pneumococcal and meningococcal invasive disease are routinely administered in the United States, usually in childhood or adolescence. Influenza vaccine is routinely recommended for all people aged ≥6 months, each year. A dose of herpes zoster (shingles) vaccine is recommended for adults aged ≥60 years. If a person does not have a history of adequate protection against these diseases, immunizations appropriate to age and previous immunization status should be obtained, whether or not international travel is planned. A visit to a clinician for travel-related immunizations should be seen as an opportunity to bring an incompletely vaccinated person up-to-date on his or her routine vaccinations.

Both the child and adolescent vaccination schedules, and an adult vaccination schedule, are published annually. Clinicians should obtain the most current schedules from the CDC Vaccines and Immunization website (www.cdc.gov/vaccines/schedules). The text and many tables of this publication present recommendations for the use, number of doses, dose intervals, adverse reactions, precautions, and contraindications for vaccines and toxoids that may be indicated for travelers. Recommendations for travelers are not always the same as routine recommendations. For instance, most adults born after 1956 are recommended to receive 1 dose of MMR vaccine; however, international travelers of this age are recommended to receive 2 doses. For specific vaccines and toxoids, additional details on background, adverse reactions, precautions, and contraindications, refer to the respective ACIP recommendations (www.cdc.gov/vaccines/acip/index.html).

SPACING OF IMMUNOBIOLOGICS
Simultaneous Administration
With some exceptions (such as PCV13 and PPSV23, as well as PCV13 and MenACWY-D [Menactra]), all commonly used vaccines

2

BOX 2-1. THE ADVISORY COMMITTEE ON IMMUNIZATION PRACTICES (ACIP)

In 1964, the Department of Health, Education, and Welfare chartered the Advisory Committee on Immunization Practices (ACIP) to provide guidance to CDC for making immunization policy. Guidance includes scheduling of vaccine doses, specific risk groups for whom vaccination is recommended, and vaccine contraindications and precautions.

ACIP is composed of 15 voting members selected by the Secretary of Health and Human Services. The ACIP chair, a consumer representative, and 13 members are balanced among various sectors, including academic immunology, medicine, and public health. In addition to the 15 voting members, the committee includes 8 ex officio members representing federal agencies and 35 nonvoting representatives of liaison organizations with broad responsibilities for vaccine development, administration of vaccines to various segments of the population, and operation of immunization programs. ACIP is subdivided into 4 permanent workgroups that address child/adolescent immunization schedules, adult immunization schedules, influenza vaccine, and general immunization issues. In addition to the 4 permanent workgroups, 10 additional workgroups focus on particular vaccines. Input into the development of immunization schedules is shared with professional organizations, including the American Academy of Pediatrics, American College of Physicians, American Academy of Family Physicians, American College of Obstetricians and Gynecologists, and American College of Nurse-Midwives.

ACIP workgroups are led by a member of ACIP who works in close collaboration with a CDC workgroup lead staff member. Members of the vaccine pharmaceutical industry may not serve as workgroup members. The workgroup develops consensus on various policy points, then the CDC workgroup lead writes specific content for presentation to the ACIP at large. When it is difficult to achieve consensus, options with plans are developed and presented to the ACIP at large for a vote.

ACIP holds 3 public meetings a year during which the various workgroups present content that has been developed and is ready for discussion or voting. Sometimes ACIP members are involved in academic vaccine research supported by the pharmaceutical industry. These members must state these conflicts and must recuse themselves from votes regarding vaccines manufactured by companies from which they receive support. The result of various discussions and votes is an ACIP document published in CDC's *Morbidity and Mortality Weekly Report* (www.cdc.gov/mmwr), representing the official policy of the Department of Health and Human Services.

can safely and effectively be given simultaneously (on the same day) at separate sites without impairing antibody responses or increasing rates of adverse reactions. This knowledge is particularly helpful for international travelers, for whom exposure to several infectious diseases might be imminent. Simultaneous administration of all indicated vaccines is encouraged for people who are the recommended age to receive these vaccines and for whom no contraindications exist. If not administered on the same day, an inactivated vaccine may be given at any time before or after a different inactivated vaccine or a live-virus vaccine.

The immune response to an injected or intranasal live-virus vaccine (such as MMR, varicella, yellow fever, or live attenuated influenza vaccines) might be impaired if administered within 28 days of another live-virus vaccine (within 30 days for yellow fever vaccine). Whenever possible, injected live-virus vaccines administered on different days should be given ≥28 days apart (≥30 days for yellow fever vaccine). If 2 injected or intranasal live-virus vaccines are not administered on the same day but <28 days apart (<30 days for yellow fever vaccine), the second vaccine should be repeated in ≥28 days (≥30 days for yellow fever vaccine).

Measles and other live-virus vaccines may interfere with the response to tuberculin skin testing and the interferon-γ release assay. Tuberculin testing, if otherwise indicated, can be done either on the day that live-virus vaccines are administered or 4–6 weeks later. Tuberculin skin testing is not a prerequisite for administration of any vaccine. Oral typhoid vaccine, a live attenuated bacterial vaccine, has not been associated with suppressing the response to tuberculosis testing.

Missed Doses and Boosters

All vaccines require a primary dose or series to ensure immunity, and some require periodic repeat, or booster, doses to maintain immunity. Occasionally, the demand for a vaccine may exceed its supply, and providers may have difficulty obtaining vaccines. Information on vaccine shortages and recommendations can be found on the CDC Vaccines and Immunization website at www.cdc.gov/vaccines/vac-gen/shortages/default.htm.

In some cases, a scheduled dose of vaccine may not be given on time. If this occurs, the dose should be given at the next visit. However, travelers may forget to return to complete a series or for a booster at the specified time. Available data indicate that intervals between doses longer than those routinely recommended do not affect seroconversion rate or titer when the schedule is completed. Consequently, it is not necessary to restart the series or add doses of any vaccine because of an extended interval between doses. The only exception to this rule is oral typhoid vaccine in some circumstances. Some experts recommend repeating the series of oral typhoid vaccine if the 4-dose series is extended to more than 3 weeks.

Antibody-Containing Blood Products

Antibody-containing blood products from the United States, such as immune globulin (IG) products, do not interfere with the immune response to yellow fever vaccine and are not believed to interfere with the response to live typhoid, live attenuated influenza, rotavirus, or zoster vaccines. When MMR and varicella vaccines are given shortly before, simultaneously with, or after an antibody-containing blood product, response to the vaccine can be diminished. The duration of inhibition of MMR and varicella vaccines is related to the dose of IG in the product. MMR and varicella vaccines either should be administered ≥2 weeks before receipt of a blood product or should be delayed 3–11 months after receipt of the blood product, depending on the vaccine (Table 2-4).

IG administration may become necessary for another indication after MMR or varicella vaccines have been given. In such a situation, the IG may interfere with the immune response to the MMR or varicella vaccines. Vaccine virus replication and stimulation of immunity usually occur 2–3 weeks after vaccination. If the interval between administration of one of these vaccines and the subsequent administration of an IG preparation is ≥14 days, the vaccine need not be readministered. If the interval is <14 days, the vaccine should be readministered after the interval shown in Table 2-4, unless serologic testing indicates that antibodies have been produced. Such testing should be performed after the interval shown in Table 2-4, to avoid detecting antibodies from the IG preparation.

If administration of IG becomes necessary, MMR or varicella vaccines can be administered simultaneously with IG, with the recognition that vaccine-induced immunity can be compromised. The vaccine should be administered at a body site different from that chosen for the IG injection. Vaccination should be repeated after the interval noted in Table 2-4, unless serologic testing indicates antibodies have been produced.

When IG is given with the first dose of hepatitis A vaccine, the proportion of recipients who develop a protective level of antibody is not affected, but antibody concentrations are lower. Because the final concentrations of antibody are many times higher than those considered protective, this reduced immunogenicity is not expected to be clinically relevant.

IG preparations interact minimally with other inactivated vaccines and toxoids. Other inactivated vaccines may be given simultaneously, or at any time interval before or after an antibody-containing blood product is used. However, such vaccines should be administered at different sites from the IG.

VACCINATION OF PEOPLE WITH ACUTE ILLNESSES

Every opportunity should be taken to provide needed vaccinations. The decision to delay vaccination because of a current or recent acute illness depends on the severity of the symptoms and their cause. Although a moderate or severe acute illness is sufficient reason to postpone vaccination, minor illnesses (such as diarrhea, mild upper respiratory infection with or without low-grade fever, other low-grade febrile illness) are not contraindications to vaccination.

Table 2-4. Recommended intervals between administration of antibody-containing products and measles-containing vaccine or varicella-containing vaccine[1]

INDICATION	DOSE AND ROUTE	RECOMMENDED INTERVAL BEFORE MEASLES OR VARICELLA VACCINATION
Blood transfusion		
Red blood cells (RBCs), washed	10 mL/kg (negligible IgG/kg) IV	None
RBCs, adenine-saline added	10 mL/kg (10 mg IgG/kg) IV	3 months
Packed RBCs (hematocrit 65%)[2]	10 mL/kg (60 mg IgG/kg) IV	6 months
Whole blood (hematocrit 35%–50%)[2]	10 mL/kg (80–100 mg IgG/kg) IV	6 months
Plasma/platelet products	10 mL/kg (160 mg IgG/kg) IV	7 months
Botulism immune globulin, intravenous	1.5 mL/kg (75 mg IgG/kg) IV	6 months
Cytomegalovirus prophylaxis (CMV IGIV)	150 mg/kg IV (maximum)	6 months
Hepatitis A (IG), duration of international travel		
<3-month stay	0.02 mL/kg (3.3 mg IgG/kg) IM	3 months
≥3-month stay	0.06 mL/kg (10 mg IgG/kg) IM	3 months
Hepatitis B prophylaxis (HBIG)	0.06 mL/kg (10 mg IgG/kg) IM	3 months
Intravenous immune globulin (IVIG)		
Replacement therapy	300–400 mg/kg IV	8 months
Immune thrombocytopenic purpura (ITP)	400 mg/kg IV	8 months
	1 g/kg IV	10 months
Postexposure measles prophylaxis (includes immunocompromised people)	400mg/kg IV	8 months
Postexposure varicella prophylaxis[3]	400 mg/kg IV	8 months
Kawasaki disease	2 gm/kg IV	11 months
Measles prophylaxis (IG)		
Immunocompetent contact	0.5 mL/kg (80 mg IgG/kg) IM	6 months
Monoclonal antibody to respiratory syncytial virus (RSV) F protein (Synagis [MedImmune])[4]	15 mg/kg IM	None
Rabies prophylaxis (HRIG)	20 IU/kg (22 mg IgG/kg) IM	4 months

continued

TABLE 2-4. RECOMMENDED INTERVALS BETWEEN ADMINISTRATION OF ANTIBODY-CONTAINING PRODUCTS AND MEASLES-CONTAINING VACCINE OR VARICELLA-CONTAINING VACCINE[1] (continued)

INDICATION	DOSE AND ROUTE	RECOMMENDED INTERVAL BEFORE MEASLES OR VARICELLA VACCINATION
Tetanus (TIG)	250 units (10 mg IgG/kg) IM	3 months
Varicella zoster immune globulin[3]	125 units/10 kg (60–200 mg IgG/kg) IM (maximum 625 units)	5 months

Abbreviations: IG, immune globulin; IM, intramuscular; IV, intravenous.

[1] Adapted from Table 5, CDC. General recommendations on immunization: recommendations of the Advisory Committee on Immunization Practices (ACIP). MMWR Recomm Rep. 2011 Jan 28;60(RR-2):1–61. Updated with information from CDC. Prevention of measles, rubella, congenital rubella syndrome, and mumps, 2013: summary recommendations of the Advisory Committee on Immunization Practices (ACIP). MMWR Recomm Rep. 2013 Jun 14; 62(RR-04):1–34. This table is not intended for determining the correct indications and dosage for the use of IG preparations. Unvaccinated people may not be fully protected against measles during the entire recommended interval, and additional doses of IG or measles vaccine may be indicated after measles exposure. Concentrations of measles antibody in an IG preparation can vary by manufacturer's lot. For example, more than a 4-fold variation in the amount of measles antibody titers has been demonstrated in different IG preparations. Rates of antibody clearance after receipt of an IG preparation can also vary. Recommended intervals are extrapolated from an estimated half-life of 30 days for passively acquired antibody and an observed interference with the immune response to measles vaccine for 5 months after a dose of 80 mg IgG/kg. Does not include zoster vaccine. Zoster vaccine may be given with antibody-containing products.

[2] Assumes a serum IgG concentration of 16 mg/mL.

[3] If varicella zoster immune globulin is not available, IVIG can be used. The recommendation for use of IVIG is based on best judgment of experts and is supported by reports comparing varicella IgG titers measured in both IVIG and varicella zoster immune globulin preparations and patients given IVIG and varicella zoster immune globulin. Although licensed IVIG preparations contain antivaricella antibodies, the titer of any specific lot of IVIG is uncertain, because IVIG is not tested routinely for antivaricella antibodies. No clinical data demonstrating effectiveness of IVIG for postexposure prophylaxis of varicella are available. The recommended IVIG dose for postexposure prophylaxis of varicella is one dose of 400 mg/kg, intravenously (see http://aapredbook.aappublications.org/content/1/SEC131/SEC289.body).

[4] Contains only antibody to respiratory syncytial virus.

People with moderate or severe acute illness, with or without fever, should be vaccinated as soon as the condition improves. This precaution is to avoid superimposing adverse effects from the vaccine on underlying illness, or mistakenly attributing a manifestation of underlying illness to the vaccine. Antimicrobial therapy is not a contraindication to vaccination, with 3 exceptions:

- Antibacterial agents may interfere with the response to oral typhoid vaccine.
- Antiviral agents active against herpesviruses (such as acyclovir) may interfere with the response to varicella-containing vaccines.
- Antiviral agents active against influenza virus (such as zanamivir and oseltamivir) may interfere with the response to live attenuated influenza vaccine.

A physical examination or temperature measurement is not a prerequisite for vaccinating a person who appears to be in good health. Asking if a person is ill, postponing a vaccination for someone with moderate or severe acute illness, and vaccinating someone who does not have contraindications are appropriate procedures for clinic immunizations.

ALTERED IMMUNOCOMPETENCE

Altered immunocompetence is a general term that is often used interchangeably with the terms immunosuppression, immunodeficiency, and a weakened immune system. It can be caused either by a disease (leukemia,

HIV infection) or by drugs or other therapies (cancer chemotherapy, radiation therapy, prolonged high-dose corticosteroids). It can also include conditions such as asplenia and chronic renal disease.

Determination of altered immunocompetence is important because the incidence or severity of some vaccine-preventable diseases is higher in people with altered immunocompetence. Therefore, certain vaccines (such as inactivated influenza vaccine, pneumococcal vaccines) are recommended specifically for people with altered immunocompetence. Inactivated vaccines may be safely administered to a person with altered immunocompetence, although response to such vaccines may be suboptimal. These vaccines may need to be repeated after immune function has improved.

People with altered immunocompetence may be at increased risk for an adverse reaction after administration of live attenuated vaccines because of reduced ability to mount an effective immune response. Live vaccines should generally be deferred until immune function has improved. This is particularly important when planning to give yellow fever vaccine (see Chapter 3, Yellow Fever). For HIV-infected people with mild or moderate immunosuppression, MMR vaccine is recommended and varicella vaccine can be considered.

For an in-depth discussion, see Chapter 8, Immunocompromised Travelers.

VACCINATION SCHEDULING FOR LAST-MINUTE TRAVELERS

As noted, for people anticipating imminent travel, most vaccine products can be given during the same visit. Unless the vaccines given are booster doses of those typically given during childhood, vaccines may require a month or more to induce a sufficient immune response, depending on the vaccine and the number of doses in the series. Some vaccines require more than 1 dose for best protection. Recommended spacing should be maintained between doses (Table 2-5). Doses given at less than minimum intervals can lessen the antibody response. It is important to note that if a traveler needs yellow fever vaccination to meet a country requirement under the International Health Regulations, the yellow fever vaccine is not considered valid until 10 days after administration. Intervals between doses longer than those routinely recommended do not affect the immune response when the schedule is completed. Consequently, it is not necessary to restart the series or add doses of any vaccine because of an extended interval between doses.

Administration of a vaccine earlier than the recommended minimum age or at an interval shorter than the recommended minimum is discouraged. Table 2-5 lists the minimum age and minimum interval between doses for vaccines routinely recommended in the United States.

Because some travelers visit their health care providers at the last minute, studies have been performed to determine whether accelerated scheduling is adequate. This concern is primarily the case for hepatitis B vaccine or the combined hepatitis A and B vaccine. An accelerated schedule for combined hepatitis A and B vaccine has been approved by the Food and Drug Administration (FDA). It is unclear what level of protection any given traveler will have if he or she does not complete a full series of multidose vaccination.

ALLERGY TO VACCINE COMPONENTS

Vaccine components can cause allergic reactions in some recipients. These reactions can be local or systemic and can include anaphylaxis or anaphylactic-like responses. The vaccine components responsible can include the vaccine antigen, animal proteins, antibiotics, preservatives (such as thimerosal), or stabilizers (such as gelatin). The most common animal protein allergen is egg protein in vaccines prepared by using embryonated chicken eggs (influenza and yellow fever vaccines). Generally, people who can eat eggs or egg products safely may receive these vaccines, while those with histories of anaphylactic allergy (swelling of the mouth and throat, difficulty breathing, hypotension, shock) to eggs or egg proteins ordinarily should not. Screening people by asking whether they can eat eggs without adverse effects is a reasonable way to identify those who might be at risk from receiving yellow fever and influenza vaccines. Protocols have been developed for testing and vaccinating people with anaphylactic reactions to egg ingestion. The available

Table 2-5. Recommended and minimum ages and intervals between vaccine doses[1,2]

VACCINE AND DOSE NUMBER	RECOMMENDED AGE FOR THIS DOSE	MINIMUM AGE FOR THIS DOSE	MINIMUM INTERVAL TO NEXT DOSE[3]
Diphtheria and tetanus toxoids and acellular pertussis vaccine, pediatric (6 weeks through 6 years) (DTaP)-1[4]	2 months	6 weeks	4 weeks
DTaP-2	4 months	10 weeks	4 weeks
DTaP-3	6 months	14 weeks	6 months[5]
DTaP-4	15–18 months	12 months	6 months[5]
DTaP-5	4–6 years	4 years	NA
Haemophilus influenzae type b (Hib)-1[4,6]	2 months	6 weeks	4 weeks
Hib-2	4 months	10 weeks	4 weeks
Hib-3[7]	6 months	14 weeks	8 weeks
Hib-4	12–15 months	12 months	NA
Hepatitis A (HepA)-1	12–23 months	12 months	6 months[5]
HepA-2	≥18 months	18 months	NA
Hepatitis B (HepB)-1[4]	Birth	Birth	4 weeks
HepB-2	1–2 months	4 weeks	8 weeks
HepB-3[8]	6–18 months	24 weeks	NA
Herpes zoster[9]	≥60 years	60 years	NA
Human papillomavirus (HPV)-1[10]	11–12 years	9 years	4 weeks
HPV-2	2 months after dose 1	9 years, 4 weeks	12 weeks
HPV-3[11]	6 months after dose 1	9 years, 24 weeks	NA

continued

TABLE 2-5. RECOMMENDED AND MINIMUM AGES AND INTERVALS BETWEEN VACCINE DOSES[1, 2] (continued)

VACCINE AND DOSE NUMBER	RECOMMENDED AGE FOR THIS DOSE	MINIMUM AGE FOR THIS DOSE	MINIMUM INTERVAL TO NEXT DOSE[3]
Inactivated poliovirus (IPV)-1[4]	2 months	6 weeks	4 weeks
IPV-2	4 months	10 weeks	4 weeks
IPV-3	6–18 months	14 weeks	6 months[5]
IPV-4[12]	4–6 years	4 years	NA
Influenza, inactivated[13]	≥6 months	6 months[14]	4 weeks
Influenza, live attenuated[13]	2–49 years	2 years	4 weeks
Japanese encephalitis, Vero cell (Ixiaro)-1[15]	≥2 years	≥2 years	28 days
Ixiaro-2	28 days after dose 1	≥2 years, 28 days	NA
Measles, mumps, and rubella (MMR)-1[16]	12–15 months	12 months	4 weeks
MMR-2[16]	4–6 years	13 months	NA
Meningococcal conjugate (MenACWY-1)[17]	11–12 years	2 months (Menveo) or 9 months (Menactra)	8 weeks[18]
MenACWY-2	16 years	4 months (Menveo) or 11 months (Menactra)	3–5 years if at increased risk of disease[18]
Meningococcal polysaccharide (MPSV4)-1[17]	NA	2 years	5 years
MPSV4–2	NA	7 years	NA
Pneumococcal conjugate (PCV)-1[6]	2 months	6 weeks	4 weeks
PCV-2	4 months	10 weeks	4 weeks

continued

TABLE 2-5. RECOMMENDED AND MINIMUM AGES AND INTERVALS BETWEEN VACCINE DOSES[1, 2] (continued)

VACCINE AND DOSE NUMBER	RECOMMENDED AGE FOR THIS DOSE	MINIMUM AGE FOR THIS DOSE	MINIMUM INTERVAL TO NEXT DOSE[3]
PCV-3	6 months	14 weeks	8 weeks
PCV-4	12–15 months	12 months	NA
Pneumococcal polysaccharide (PPSV)-1	NA	2 years	5 years
PPSV-2[19]	NA	7 years	NA
Rabies-1 (preexposure)	See footnote 20	See footnote 20	7 days
Rabies-2	7 days after dose 1	7 days after dose 1	14 days
Rabies-3	21 days after dose 1	21 days after dose 1	NA
Rotavirus (RV)-1[21]	2 months	6 weeks	4 weeks
RV-2[21]	4 months	10 weeks	4 weeks
RV-3[21]	6 months	14 weeks	NA
Tetanus and reduced diphtheria toxoids (Td)	11–12 years	7 years	5 years
Tetanus toxoid, reduced diphtheria toxoid, and reduced acellular pertussis vaccine (Tdap)[22]	≥11 years	7 years	NA
Typhoid, inactivated (ViCPS)	≥2 years	≥2 years	NA
Typhoid, live attenuated (Ty21a)	≥6 years	≥6 years	See footnote 23
Varicella (Var)-1[16]	12–15 months	12 months	12 weeks[24]
Varicella (Var)-2	4–6 years	15 months	NA
Yellow fever	≥9 months[25]	≥9 months[25]	10 years

continued

TABLE 2-5. RECOMMENDED AND MINIMUM AGES AND INTERVALS BETWEEN VACCINE DOSES[1,2] (continued)

[1] Adapted from Table 1, CDC. General recommendations on immunization: recommendations of the Advisory Committee on Immunization Practices (ACIP). MMWR Recomm Rep. 2011 Jan 28;60(RR-2):1–61.

[2] Combination vaccines are available. Use of licensed combination vaccines is generally preferred over separate injections of their equivalent component vaccines (CDC. Combination vaccines for childhood immunization. MMWR Recomm Rep. 1999 May 14;48(RR-5):1–14.). When administering combination vaccines, the minimum age for administration is the oldest age for any of the individual components (exception: the minimum age for the first dose of MenHibrix is 6 weeks); the minimum interval between doses is equal to the largest interval of any of the individual components.

[3] See www.cdc.gov/vaccines/schedules/ for recommended revaccination (booster) schedules.

[4] Combination vaccines containing the HepB component are available (HepB-Hib, DTaP-HepB-IPV, HepA-HepB). These vaccines should not be administered to infants aged <6 weeks because of the other components (Hib, DTaP, IPV). HepA-HepB is not licensed for children aged <18 years in the United States.

[5] Calendar months.

[6] For Hib and PCV, children receiving the first dose of vaccine at ≥7 months of age require fewer doses to complete the series (see the current childhood and adolescent immunization schedule at www.cdc.gov/vaccines).

[7] If PRP-OMP (Pedvax-Hib, Merck Vaccine Division) was administered at 2 and 4 months of age, a dose at 6 months of age is not indicated. The final dose has a minimum age of 12 months.

[8] HepB-3 should be administered ≥8 weeks after Hep B-2 and ≥16 weeks after Hep B-1; it should not be administered before age 24 weeks.

[9] Herpes zoster (shingles) vaccine is recommended as a single dose for people aged ≥60 years.

[10] Bivalent HPV vaccine is approved for girls/women aged 10–26 years. It is recommended to prevent cervical and other anogenital cancers and precursors for girls/women aged 11–26 years. Quadrivalent HPV vaccine is approved for boys/men and girls/women aged 9–26 years. It is recommended to prevent cervical and other anogenital cancers, precursors, and genital warts for girls/women aged 11–26 years. It is recommended for boys/men aged 11–21 years and high-risk boys or men (men who have sex with men, HIV-positive men, or immunocompromised men) aged 22–26 years. It may be given to girls aged 9–10 years to prevent the same diseases, and to boys/men aged 9–10 years and 22–26 years to prevent genital warts.

[11] The third dose of HPV should be administered ≥12 weeks after the second and ≥24 weeks after the first. Dose 3 need not be repeated if administered ≥16 weeks after dose 1, as long as a minimum interval of 4 weeks is maintained between dose 1 and dose 2 and as long as a minimum interval of 12 weeks is maintained between dose 2 and dose 3.

[12] For people receiving an all-IPV or all-OPV series, if the third dose is given after the fourth birthday, a fourth dose is not needed. For IPV, the next-to-last and the last dose must be spaced by 6 months.

[13] Two doses of influenza vaccine are recommended for children aged <9 years who are receiving the vaccine for the first time, and for certain incompletely vaccinated children (see reference 2).

[14] The minimum age for inactivated influenza vaccine varies by vaccine manufacturer. See package insert for vaccine-specific minimum ages.

[15] Ixiaro is approved by the Food and Drug Administration for people aged ≥2 years.

[16] Combination MMR-varicella (MMRV) can be used for children aged 12 months through 12 years

[17] **Infants aged 2–18 months.** Routine vaccination with HibMenCY – TT (MenHibrix) or Menveo (4-dose primary series) is recommended for infants aged 2–18 months who are at increased risk for meningococcal disease. The first dose of either vaccine may be administered as early as age 6 weeks. The fourth dose may be administered as late as age 18 months. Infants and children who received Hib-MenCY-TT and are traveling to areas with high endemic rates of meningococcal disease such as the African "meningitis belt" are not protected against serogroups A and W-135 and should receive a quadrivalent meningococcal vaccination before travel.

People aged 9 months through 55 years. People aged 9 months through 55 years at increased risk for meningococcal disease should receive Menveo or Menactra. Infants aged 9–23 months are recommended to receive a 2-dose primary series with a dosing interval of 12 weeks.

People aged ≥56 years. Menomune is the only licensed meningococcal vaccine for adults aged ≥56 years and is immunogenic in older adults. For adults who have received a conjugate meningococcal vaccine previously, limited data demonstrate a higher antibody response after a subsequent dose of a conjugate vaccine compared with a subsequent dose of Menomune. For meningococcal vaccine-naïve people aged ≥56 years who anticipate requiring a single dose of meningococcal vaccine (such as travelers and people at risk as a result of a community outbreak), Menomune is preferred. For people now aged ≥56 years who were vaccinated previously with a meningococcal conjugate vaccine and are recommended for revaccination or for whom multiple doses are anticipated (such as people with asplenia and microbiologists), a conjugate vaccine is preferred.

[18] Revaccination with meningococcal vaccine is recommended for people previously vaccinated who remain at high risk for meningococcal disease. MenACWY is preferred for revaccinating people aged 2–55 years (CDC. Prevention and control of meningococcal disease. Recommendations of the Advisory Committee on Immunization Practices [ACIP]. MMWR Recomm Rep. 2013 March 22;62(RR-2):1–28.).

[19] A second dose of PPSV is recommended for people aged ≥65 years who received a first dose at an age <65 years and at a 5-year minimum interval. A second dose is also recommended for people aged <65 years at highest risk for serious pneumococcal infection and those who are likely to have a rapid decline in pneumococcal antibody concentration (CDC. Updated recommendations for prevention of invasive pneumococcal disease among adults using the 23-valent pneumococcal polysaccharide vaccine [PPSV23]. MMWR Recomm Rep. 2010;59[34]:1102–6.).

[20] There is no minimum age for preexposure immunization for rabies (CDC. Human rabies prevention—United States, 2008: recommendations of the Advisory Committee on Immunization Practices. MMWR Recomm Rep. 2008 May 23;57[RR-3]:1–28.).

continued

GENERAL RECOMMENDATIONS FOR VACCINATION & IMMUNOPROPHYLAXIS

[21] The first dose of RV must be administered by 14 weeks and 6 days of age. The vaccine series should not be started at ≥15 weeks of age. The final dose in the series should be administered by age 8 months, 0 days. If Rotarix rotavirus vaccine is administered at 2 and 4 months of age, a dose at 6 months of age is not indicated.

[22] Only 1 dose of Tdap is recommended. Subsequent doses should be given as Td. Children aged 7–10 years who are not fully vaccinated against pertussis and for whom no contraindication to pertussis vaccine exists should receive a single dose of Tdap. If additional doses of tetanus and diphtheria toxoid-containing vaccines are needed, then children aged 7–10 years should be vaccinated according to catch-up guidance, with Tdap preferred as the first dose. Tdap vaccine, when indicated, should be administered regardless of the interval since the last dose of Td vaccine. For management of a tetanus-prone wound, the minimum interval after a previous dose of any tetanus-containing vaccine is 5 years. A dose of Tdap is recommended for pregnant women, preferably at 27–36 weeks' gestation, regardless of history of previous Tdap vaccination.

[23] Oral typhoid vaccine is recommended to be administered 1 hour before a meal with a cold or lukewarm drink (temperature not to exceed body temperature—98.6°F [37°C]) on alternate days, for a total of 4 doses.

[24] The minimum interval from Var-1 to Var-2 for people beginning the series at ≥13 years of age is 4 weeks.

[25] Yellow fever vaccine may be administered to children aged <9 months in certain situations (CDC. Yellow fever vaccine: recommendations of the Advisory Committee on Immunization Practices [ACIP]. MMWR Recomm Rep. 2010 Jul 30;59[RR-7]:1–27.).

recombinant influenza vaccine, Flublok, is manufactured without the use of eggs and does not carry a contraindication for egg allergy. Therefore, Flublok can be administered to people with egg allergy of any severity who are aged 18–49 years and do not have other contraindications. Recent studies have indicated that other components in vaccines in addition to egg proteins (such as gelatin) may cause allergic reactions, including anaphylaxis in rare instances.

Some vaccines contain a preservative or trace amounts of antibiotics to which people might be allergic. Providers administering the vaccines should carefully review the prescribing information before deciding if the rare person with such an allergy should receive the vaccine. No recommended vaccine contains penicillin or penicillin derivatives. Some vaccines (MMR vaccine, inactivated polio vaccine [IPV], hepatitis A vaccine, some hepatitis B vaccines, some influenza vaccines, rabies vaccine, varicella vaccine, and smallpox vaccine) contain trace amounts of neomycin or other antibiotics; the amount is less than would normally be used for the skin test to determine hypersensitivity. However, people who have experienced anaphylactic reactions to this antibiotic generally should not receive these vaccines. Most often, neomycin allergy is a contact dermatitis—a manifestation of a delayed-type (cell-mediated) immune response rather than anaphylaxis.

A history of delayed-type reactions to neomycin is not a contraindication to receiving these vaccines.

Thimerosal, an organic mercurial compound in use since the 1930s, has been added to certain immunobiologic products as a preservative. Thimerosal is present at preservative concentrations in multidose vials of some brands of vaccine. Receiving thimerosal-containing vaccines has been postulated to lead to induction of allergy. However, there is limited scientific evidence for this assertion. Allergy to thimerosal usually consists of local delayed-type hypersensitivity reactions. Thimerosal elicits positive delayed-type hypersensitivity patch tests in 1%–18% of people tested, but these tests have limited or no clinical relevance. Most people do not experience reactions to thimerosal administered as a component of vaccines, even when patch or intradermal tests for thimerosal indicate hypersensitivity. A localized or delayed-type hypersensitivity reaction to thimerosal is not a contraindication to receipt of a vaccine that contains thimerosal.

Since mid-2001, vaccines routinely recommended for infants have been manufactured without thimerosal as a preservative. Additional information about thimerosal and the thimerosal content of vaccines is available on the FDA website (www.fda.gov/cber/vaccine/thimerosal.htm).

REPORTING ADVERSE EVENTS AFTER IMMUNIZATION

Modern vaccines are extremely safe and effective. Benefits and risks are associated with the use of all immunobiologics—no vaccine is completely effective or completely safe for all recipients. Adverse events after immunization have been reported with all vaccines, ranging from frequent, minor, local reactions to extremely rare, severe, systemic illness, such as that associated with yellow fever vaccine. Adverse events following specific vaccines and toxoids are discussed in detail in each ACIP statement. In the United States, clinicians are required by law to report selected adverse events occurring after vaccination with any vaccine in the recommended childhood series (see www.hrsa.gov/vaccinecompensation/authoringleg.pdf). In addition, CDC strongly recommends that all vaccine adverse events be reported to the Vaccine Adverse Event Reporting System (VAERS), even if a causal relation to vaccination is not certain. VAERS reporting forms and information are available electronically at www.vaers.hhs.gov, or they may be requested by telephone: 800-822-7967 (toll-free). Clinicians are encouraged to report electronically at https://vaers.hhs.gov/esub/step1.

INJECTION ROUTE AND INJECTION SITE

Injectable vaccines are administered by intramuscular, intradermal, and subcutaneous routes. The method of administration of injectable vaccines depends in part on the presence of an adjuvant in some vaccines. The term *adjuvant* refers to a vaccine component distinct from the antigen, which enhances the immune response to the antigen. Vaccines containing an adjuvant (DTaP, DT, HPV, Td, Tdap, pneumococcal conjugate, Hib, hepatitis A, hepatitis B) should be injected into a muscle mass, because administration subcutaneously or intradermally can cause local irritation, induration, skin discoloration, inflammation, and granuloma formation.

Routes of administration are recommended by the manufacturer for each immunobiologic. Deviation from the recommended route of administration may reduce vaccine efficacy or increase local adverse reactions. Detailed recommendations on the route and site for all vaccines have been published in ACIP recommendations; a compiled list of these publications is available on the CDC website at www.cdc.gov/vaccines/hcp/acip-recs (also see Table B-1 in Appendix B).

BIBLIOGRAPHY

1. CDC. General recommendations on immunization: recommendations of the Advisory Committee on Immunization Practices (ACIP). MMWR Recomm Rep. 2011 Jan 28;60(RR-2):1–64.

2. CDC. Human rabies prevention—United States, 2008: recommendations of the Advisory Committee on Immunization Practices. MMWR Recomm Rep. 2008 May 23;57(RR-3):1–28.

3. CDC. Prevention and control of meningococcal disease: recommendations of the Advisory Committee on Immunization Practices (ACIP). MMWR Recomm Rep. 2013 Mar 22;62(RR-2):1–28.

4. CDC. Prevention and control of seasonal influenza with vaccines: recommendations of the Advisory Committee on Immunization Practices—United States, 2013–2014. MMWR Recomm Rep. 2013 Sep 20;62(RR-07):1–43.

5. CDC. Prevention of measles, rubella, congenital rubella syndrome, and mumps, 2013: summary recommendations of the Advisory Committee on Immunization Practices (ACIP). MMWR Recomm Rep. 2013 Jun 14;62(RR-04):1–34.

6. CDC. Prevention of pneumococcal disease among infants and children—use of 13-valent pneumococcal conjugate vaccine and 23-valent pneumococcal polysaccharide vaccine: recommendations of the Advisory Committee on Immunization Practices (ACIP). MMWR Recomm Rep. 2010 Dec 10;59(RR-11):1–18.

7. CDC. Updated recommendations for prevention of invasive pneumococcal disease among adults using the 23-valent pneumococcal polysaccharide vaccine (PPSV23). MMWR Morb Mortal Wkly Rep. 2010 Sep 3;59(34):1102–6.

8. CDC. Updated recommendations for use of tetanus toxoid, reduced diphtheria toxoid, and acellular pertussis (Tdap) vaccine in adults aged 65 years and older—Advisory Committee on Immunization Practices (ACIP), 2012. MMWR Morb Mortal Wkly Rep. 2012 Jun 29;61(25):468–70.

9. CDC. Yellow fever vaccine: recommendations of the Advisory Committee on Immunization Practices (ACIP). MMWR Recomm Rep. 2010 Jul 30;59(RR-7):1–27.

10. Varricchio F, Iskander J, Destefano F, Ball R, Pless R, Braun MM, et al. Understanding vaccine safety information from the Vaccine Adverse Event Reporting System. Pediatr Infect Dis J. 2004 Apr;23(4):287–94.

INTERACTIONS AMONG TRAVEL VACCINES & DRUGS

Ilan Youngster, Elizabeth D. Barnett

Vaccines and medications are prescribed frequently in pre-travel consultations, and potential interactions between vaccines and medications, including those already taken by the traveler, must be considered. Although a comprehensive list of interactions is beyond the scope of this section, some of the more serious interactions of commonly used travel-related vaccines and medications are discussed here.

INTERACTIONS BETWEEN VACCINES

In general, concomitant administration of multiple vaccines, including live attenuated immunizations, is safe and effective. Administering a live-virus vaccine within 4 weeks after administration of another live-virus vaccine can decrease immunogenicity to the second administered vaccine. This observation has given rise to the recommendation that live-virus vaccines should be administered the same day or ≥4 weeks apart. If the 4-week span is not achievable, the second vaccine may be administered sooner to afford some protection, but it should be readministered ≥4 weeks later if the traveler is at continued risk. A study examining concurrent administration of the yellow fever vaccine with the measles-mumps-rubella (MMR) vaccine in 12-month-old children showed slightly reduced immunogenicity to yellow fever and mumps components, compared with responses following separate vaccination with MMR and yellow fever vaccines 30 days apart. The clinical significance of this finding is uncertain. Similarly, a single study suggested that in adults, concomitant administration of the 13-valent pneumococcal conjugate vaccine with the trivalent inactivated influenza vaccine results in lower immunogenicity to the PCV13 components. However, the clinical significance of this observation is uncertain, as responses still met FDA criteria of noninferiority. In infants given PCV13 and inactivated influenza vaccine concomitantly,

the risk of fever and febrile seizure is slightly increased. However, this risk must be weighed against the need for both vaccines before travel and the time available to separate them.

INTERACTIONS BETWEEN TRAVEL VACCINES AND DRUGS

Oral Typhoid Vaccine

Live attenuated vaccines should generally be avoided in immunocompromised travelers, including those who are taking immunomodulators, calcineurin inhibitors, cytotoxic agents, antimetabolites, and high-dose steroids (see Table 8-8).

Antimicrobial agents may be active against the vaccine strain in the oral typhoid vaccine and may prevent an adequate immune response to the vaccine. Therefore, oral typhoid vaccine should not be given to people taking antibacterial agents. Vaccination with oral typhoid vaccine should be delayed for >72 hours after the administration of any such agent. Parenteral typhoid vaccine may be a more appropriate choice for these people.

Chloroquine and atovaquone-proguanil at doses used for malaria chemoprophylaxis may be given concurrently with the oral typhoid vaccine.

Rabies Vaccine

Concomitant use of chloroquine may reduce the antibody response to intradermal rabies vaccine administered for preexposure vaccination. The intramuscular route should be used for people taking chloroquine concurrently. (Currently, intradermal administration of rabies vaccine is not approved in the United States.)

INTERACTIONS BETWEEN ANTIMALARIALS AND SELECTED OTHER DRUGS

This section describes some of the more commonly encountered drug interactions. Any time a new medication is prescribed, clinicians should check for any interactions and inform the traveler of the potential risk.

Mefloquine

Mefloquine may interact with several categories of drugs, including other antimalarial drugs, drugs that alter cardiac conduction, and anticonvulsants. Mefloquine is associated with increased toxicities of the antimalarial drug lumefantrine (available in the United States in fixed combination to treat people with uncomplicated *Plasmodium falciparum* malaria), potentially causing fatal prolongation of the QTc interval. Lumefantrine should therefore be avoided or used with caution in patients taking mefloquine prophylaxis. Although no conclusive data are available with regard to coadministration of mefloquine and other drugs that may affect cardiac conduction, mefloquine should be used with caution or avoided in patients taking antiarrhythmic or β-blocking agents, calcium-channel blockers, antihistamines, H_1-blocking agents, tricyclic antidepressants, or phenothiazines. In general, mefloquine should also be avoided in travelers with a history of seizures. Mefloquine may also lower plasma levels of a number of anticonvulsants, such as valproic acid, carbamazepine, phenobarbital, and phenytoin; concurrent use of mefloquine with these agents should be avoided. Mefloquine can also lead to increased levels of calcineurin inhibitors and mTOR inhibitors (tacrolimus, cyclosporine A, and sirolimus) (see Table 8-10). Potent CYP3A4 inhibitors such as macrolides (clarithromycin, erythromycin), azole antifungals (ketoconazole, voriconazole, and itraconazole), antiretroviral protease inhibitors (ritonavir, lopinavir, darunavir, atazanavir), and cobicistat (available in a combination with elvitegravir) may increase the levels of mefloquine, increasing the risk for QT prolongation. CYP3A4 inducers such as efavirenz, nevirapine, etravirine, rifampin, and rifabutin may reduce plasma concentrations of mefloquine, and concurrent use should be avoided. Concurrent use of mefloquine with the new direct-acting protease inhibitors boceprevir and telaprevir used to treat hepatitis C should also be avoided.

Chloroquine

Chloroquine may increase risk of prolonged QTc interval when given with other QT-prolonging agents (such as sotalol, amiodarone, and lumefantrine), and the combination should be avoided. The antiretroviral rilpivirine has also been shown to prolong QTc, and coadministration should be avoided. Chloroquine inhibits CYP2D6; when given concomitantly with substrates of this enzyme (such as metoprolol, propranolol, fluoxetine, paroxetine, flecainide), increased monitoring for side effects may be warranted. Chloroquine absorption may be reduced by antacids or kaolin; ≥4 hours should elapse between doses of these medications. Concomitant use of cimetidine and chloroquine should be avoided, as cimetidine can inhibit the metabolism of chloroquine and may increase drug levels. CYP3A4 inhibitors such as ritonavir, ketoconazole, and erythromycin may also increase chloroquine levels, and concomitant use should be avoided. Chloroquine inhibits bioavailability of ampicillin, and 2 hours should elapse between doses. Chloroquine is also reported to decrease the bioavailability of ciprofloxacin and methotrexate. Chloroquine may increase digoxin levels; increased digoxin monitoring is warranted. Use of chloroquine could possibly also lead to increased levels of calcineurin inhibitors and should be used with caution.

Atovaquone-Proguanil

Tetracycline, rifampin, and rifabutin may reduce plasma concentrations of atovaquone and should not be used concurrently with atovaquone-proguanil. Metoclopramide may reduce bioavailability of atovaquone; unless no other antiemetics are available, this antiemetic should not be used to treat the vomiting that may accompany use of atovaquone at treatment doses. Atovaquone-proguanil should not be used with other medications that contain proguanil. Patients on anticoagulants may need to reduce their anticoagulant dose or monitor their prothrombin time more closely while taking atovaquone-proguanil, although coadministration of these drugs is not contraindicated. Atovaquone-proguanil may interact with the antiretroviral protease inhibitors ritonavir, darunavir, atazanavir, indinavir, and lopinavir, in addition to the nonnucleoside reverse transcriptase inhibitors nevirapine, etravirine, and efavirenz. Despite the potential for interactions, atovaquone-proguanil is well tolerated in most patients receiving these antivirals and is the preferred antimalarial for short-term travel. Cimetidine and fluvoxamine interfere with the metabolism of proguanil and should therefore be avoided.

Doxycycline

Phenytoin, carbamazepine, and barbiturates may decrease the half-life of doxycycline. Patients on anticoagulants may need to reduce their anticoagulant dose while taking doxycycline because of its ability to depress plasma prothrombin activity. Absorption of tetracyclines may be impaired by bismuth subsalicylate, preparations containing iron, and antacids containing calcium, magnesium, or aluminum; these preparations should not be taken within 3 hours of taking doxycycline. Doxycycline may interfere with the bactericidal activity of penicillin, so these drugs, in general, should not be taken together. Doxycycline has no known interaction with antiretroviral agents, but concurrent use may lead to increased levels of calcineurin inhibitors and mTOR inhibitors (sirolimus).

INTERACTIONS WITH DRUGS FOR TREATMENT OF TRAVELERS' DIARRHEA

Fluoroquinolones

Increase in the international normalized ratio has been reported when levofloxacin and warfarin are used concurrently. Concurrent administration of ciprofloxacin and antacids that contain magnesium or aluminum hydroxide may reduce bioavailability of ciprofloxacin. Ciprofloxacin decreases clearance of theophylline and caffeine; theophylline levels should be monitored when ciprofloxacin is used concurrently. Ciprofloxacin and other fluoroquinolones should not be used with tizanidine. Sildenafil should not be used in patients on ciprofloxacin, as concomitant use is associated with increased rates of adverse effects. Fluoroquinolones have no known interaction with antiretroviral agents, but concurrent use may increase levels of calcineurin inhibitors and fluoroquinolone levels, and use should reflect renal function.

Azithromycin

Close monitoring for side effects of azithromycin is recommended when azithromycin is used with nelfinavir. Increased anticoagulant effects have been noted when azithromycin is used with warfarin; monitoring prothrombin time is recommended for people taking these drugs concomitantly. Additive QTc prolongation may occur when azithromycin is used with the antimalarial artemether, and concomitant therapy should be avoided. Drug interactions have been reported with macrolides and antiretroviral protease inhibitors, as well as efavirenz and nevirapine, and can increase risk of QTc prolongation, though a short treatment course is not contraindicated for those without an underlying cardiac abnormality. Concurrent use with macrolides may lead to increased levels of calcineurin inhibitors.

Rifaximin

Rifaximin is not absorbed in appreciable amounts by intact bowel, and no clinically significant drug interactions have been reported to date with rifaximin.

INTERACTIONS WITH DRUGS USED FOR TRAVEL TO HIGH ALTITUDES

Acetazolamide

Acetazolamide produces alkaline urine that can increase the rate of excretion of barbiturates and salicylates and may potentiate salicylate toxicity, particularly if taking a high dose of aspirin. Decreased excretion of dextroamphetamine, anticholinergics, mecamylamine, ephedrine, mexiletine, or quinidine may also occur. Hypokalemia caused by corticosteroids may be potentiated by concurrent use of acetazolamide. Acetazolamide should not be given to patients taking the anticonvulsant topiramate, as concurrent use is associated with increased toxicity. Increased monitoring of cyclosporine, tacrolimus, and sirolimus is warranted if these drugs are given with acetazolamide. Concurrent administration of metformin and acetazolamide should be done with caution as there may be an additive risk for lactic acidosis. Acetaminophen and diclofenac sodium form complex bonds with acetazolamide in the stomach's acidic environment, impairing absorption. These agents should not be taken within 30 minutes of acetazolamide.

Dexamethasone

Dexamethasone interacts with multiple classes of drugs. Using this drug to treat altitude illness may, however, be life-saving. Interactions may occur with dexamethasone and the following drugs and drug classes: macrolide antibiotics, anticholinesterases, anticoagulants, hypoglycemic agents, isoniazid, digitalis preparations, oral contraceptives, and phenytoin.

DRUG INTERACTIONS IN PATIENTS ON HIV MEDICATIONS

Patients with HIV can be a challenge in the pre-travel consultation (See Chapter 8, Immunocompromised Travelers). A recent study in Europe showed that as many as 29% of HIV-positive travelers do not disclose their disease and medication status when seeking pre-travel advice. Antiretroviral medications have multiple drug interactions, especially through activation or inhibition of CYP3A4 and CYP2D6. There are several reports of antimalarial treatment failure and prophylaxis failure in patients on protease inhibitors and both nucleoside or nonnucleoside reverse transcriptase inhibitors. A number of the potential interactions are listed above, and 2 excellent resources for HIV medication interactions can be found at www.hiv-druginteractions.org and at www.aidsinfo.nih.gov.

BIBLIOGRAPHY

1. Bouchaud O, Imbert P, Touze JE, Dodoo AN, Danis M, Legros F. Fatal cardiotoxicity related to halofantrine: a review based on a worldwide safety data base. Malar J. 2009;8:289.

2. Frenck RW Jr, Gurtman A, Rubino J, Smith W, van Cleeff M, Jayawardene D, et al. Randomized, controlled trial of a 13-valent pneumococcal conjugate vaccine administered concomitantly with an influenza vaccine in healthy adults. Clin Vaccine Immunol. 2012 Aug;19(8):1296–303.

3. Hoey LL, Lake KD. Does ciprofloxacin interact with cyclosporine? Ann Pharmacother. 1994 Jan;28(1):93–6.

4. Horowitz H, Carbonaro CA. Inhibition of the *Salmonella typhi* oral vaccine strain, Ty21a, by mefloquine and chloroquine. J Infect Dis. 1992 Dec;166(6):1462–4.

5. Jabeen E, Qureshi R, Shah A. Interaction of antihypertensive acetazolamide with nonsteroidal anti-inflammatory drugs. J Photochem Photobiol B. 2013 Aug 5;125:155–63.

6. Kolawole JA, Mustapha A, Abdul-Aguye I, Ochekpe N, Taylor RB. Effects of cimetidine on the pharmacokinetics of proguanil in healthy subjects and in peptic ulcer patients. J Pharm Biomed Anal. 1999 Sep;20(5):737–43.

7. Kollaritsch H, Que JU, Kunz C, Wiedermann G, Herzog C, Cryz SJ Jr. Safety and immunogenicity of live oral cholera and typhoid vaccines administered alone or in combination with antimalarial drugs, oral polio vaccine, or yellow fever vaccine. J Infect Dis. 1997 Apr;175(4):871–5.

8. Nascimento Silva JR, Camacho LA, Siqueira MM, FreireMde S, Castro YP, Maia Mde L, et al. Mutual interference on the immune response to yellow fever vaccine and a combined vaccine against measles, mumps and rubella. Vaccine. 2011 Aug 26;29(37):6327–34.

9. Nielsen US, Jensen-Fangel S, Pedersen G, Lohse N, Pedersen C, Kronborg G, et al. Travelling with HIV: a cross sectional analysis of Danish HIV-infected patients. Travel Med Infect Dis. 2014 Jan–Feb;12(1):72–8.

10. Pappaioanou M, Fishbein DB, Dreesen DW, Schwartz IK, Campbell GH, Sumner JW, et al. Antibody response to preexposure human diploid-cell rabies vaccine given concurrently with chloroquine. N Engl J Med. 1986 Jan 30;314(5):280–4.

11. Ridtitid W, Wongnawa M, Mahatthanatrakul W, Raungsri N, Sunbhanich M. Ketoconazole increases plasma concentrations of antimalarial mefloquine in healthy human volunteers. J Clin Pharm Ther. 2005 Jun;30(3):285–90.

12. Uriel A, Lewthwaite P. Malaria therapy in HIV: drug interactions between nevirapine and quinine. Int J STD AIDS. 2011 Dec;22(12):768.

Perspectives

2

FEAR OF VACCINES
Paul Offit

Pre-travel consultations often provide the opportunity to update routine vaccinations for both children and adults. One of the first topics covered in such sessions is whether the traveler is immune to diseases such as measles and varicella. Unfortunately, in some circumstances, providers may be surprised to find that travelers have no interest in being vaccinated or in having their children vaccinated, whether for measles or other potentially life-threatening, travel-related infections, such as yellow fever.

Although travel-related vaccines may not have implications for community health, such as providing herd immunity, they can protect people against severe and occasionally fatal illness. For these vaccines, the discussion between clinicians and patients is one of weighing the risks and benefits of travel-related vaccines for particular destinations. Travelers are often at a higher risk of exposure to diseases for which routine vaccines provide protection, even when traveling to countries in Europe. For example, measles outbreaks of 27,134 cases were reported in the World Health Organization's European Region in 2012, and an additional 31,520 cases were reported in 2013. The European measles outbreak belied a common belief that severe and occasionally fatal vaccine-preventable diseases are the province of the developing world.

Because so much is at stake, the travel health provider should educate all travelers, and especially parents, about the use of vaccines. Those providing travel health advice should familiarize themselves with the literature on the safety of both routine and travel-related vaccines, so they can address any concerns that their patients may have.

The history of the development of vaccination complacency and avoidance is a curious one. During the 1940s, parents in the United States did not hesitate to get the diphtheria, tetanus, and pertussis vaccines; they knew that diphtheria and pertussis were common killers of young children, and they had watched tetanus claim the lives of soldiers in World Wars I and II. During the 1950s, the polio vaccine was a godsend; everyone knew what poliovirus could do. During the 1960s, parents gladly accepted the measles, mumps, and rubella vaccines. They knew that measles caused tens of thousands of hospitalizations and hundreds of deaths every year, mostly from pneumonia; that mumps was a common cause of deafness and a rare cause of sterility; and that rubella caused thousands of children to suffer severe birth defects of the eyes, ears, and heart.

The widespread use of vaccines caused a dramatic decrease—and in some cases a virtual elimination—of several diseases. Parents, no longer compelled by fear of the diseases around them, became complacent. Immunization rates

Perspectives sections are written as editorial discussions aiming to add depth and clinical perspective to the official recommendations contained in the book. The views and opinions expressed in this section are those of the author and do not necessarily represent the official position of CDC.

plateaued. Now, the United States (as well as many European countries) finds itself in a situation where vaccine safety issues, real or imagined, are a primary concern. Parents confront a flood of misinformation from radio and television programs, magazine and newspaper articles, antivaccine blogs, YouTube, and Twitter. Vaccines—considered mankind's greatest lifesaver—are now feared by some to cause a variety of chronic diseases, including autism, diabetes, allergies, asthma, learning disabilities, multiple sclerosis, and attention deficit disorder. As a consequence, some parents are choosing not to immunize their children according to recommended schedules. Travel health providers must be aware of these issues and arm themselves with accurate information to properly educate their patients.

In addition to protecting the health of the vaccine recipient, vaccination safeguards the health of entire communities, both at home and possibly at travel destinations. Predictably, in communities with clusters of underimmunized children, there is increased risk of vaccine-preventable diseases. Some of the outbreaks in these communities have been linked to international travel to the United States. More measles cases were reported in the United States in 2014 than in any year since 1994. Many of the cases in 2014 were associated with people returning to the United States from the Philippines. Pertussis outbreaks have swept the nation, fueled in part by inadequately vaccinated children. *Haemophilus influenzae* type b meningitis has claimed the lives of several children in Minnesota and Pennsylvania, deaths that could have easily been avoided if parents had not feared vaccines more than the diseases they prevent.

So, where do we go from here? How do we again inspire people to vaccinate themselves and their children? One way would be to make parents aware of the impact of vaccine-preventable diseases and to provide the science that supports the safety of vaccines in a manner that is compelling and easily understood. Some of this information is available from CDC (www.cdc.gov/vaccines/hcp/patient-ed/conversations/index.html), the American Academy of Pediatrics (www.aap.org), the Immunization Action Coalition (www.immunize.org), the Vaccine Education Center at the Children's Hospital of Philadelphia (www.vaccine.chop.edu), Every Child By Two (www.ecbt.org), the National Network for Immunization Information (www.immunizationinfo.org), the Institute for Vaccine Safety at Johns Hopkins Hospital (www.vaccinesafety.edu), and Parents of Kids with Infectious Diseases (www.pkids.org), among other groups.

But is it enough? As providers whose job it is to protect people against vaccine-preventable diseases, travel-related or otherwise, we need to enhance our efforts to educate ourselves and our patients, so that we will not once again be compelled to vaccinate after witnessing the suffering, hospitalization, and death caused by vaccine-preventable diseases—an unwanted return to an earlier and darker phase in history.

BIBLIOGRAPHY

1. Atwell JE, Van Otterloo J, Zipprich J, Winter K, Harriman K, Salmon DA, et al. Nonmedical vaccine exemptions and pertussis in California, 2010. Pediatrics. 2013 Oct;132(4):624–30.
2. CDC. Invasive *Haemophilus influenzae* type b disease in five young children—Minnesota, 2008. MMWR Morb Mortal Wkly Rep. 2009 Jan 30;58(3):58–60.
3. CDC. Measles—United States, January 1–May 23, 2014. MMWR Morb Mortal Wkly Rep. 2014 Jun 6;63(22):496–9.
4. CDC. Notes from the field: outbreak of pertussis in a school and religious community averse to health care and vaccinations—Columbia county, Florida, 2013. MMWR Morb Mortal Wkly Rep. 2014 Aug 1;63(30):655.

5. Chen RT, Mootrey G, DeStefano F. Safety of routine childhood vaccinations. An epidemiological review. Paediatr Drugs. 2000 Jul–Aug;2(4):273–90.

6. Muscat M, Shefer A, Ben Mamou M, Spataru R, Jankovic D, Deshevoy S, et al. The state of measles and rubella in the WHO European Region, 2013. Clin Microbiol Infect. 2014 May;20 Suppl 5:12–8.

Self-Treatable Conditions

TRAVELERS' DIARRHEA

Bradley A. Connor

Travelers' diarrhea (TD) is the most predictable travel-related illness. Attack rates range from 30% to 70% of travelers, depending on the destination and season of travel. Traditionally, it was thought that TD could be prevented by following simple recommendations such as "boil it, cook it, peel, it, or forget it," but studies have found that people who follow these rules may still become ill. Poor hygiene practice in local restaurants is likely the largest contributor to the risk for TD.

TD is a clinical syndrome that can result from a variety of intestinal pathogens. Bacterial pathogens are the predominant risk, thought to account for 80%–90% of TD. Intestinal viruses usually account for 5%–8% of illnesses, although increasing use of improved diagnostics may increase recognition of norovirus infections in the future. Infections with protozoal pathogens are slower to manifest symptoms and collectively account for approximately 10% of diagnoses in longer-term travelers. What is commonly known as "food poisoning" involves the ingestion of preformed toxins in food. In this syndrome, vomiting and diarrhea may both be present, but symptoms usually resolve spontaneously within 12 hours.

INFECTIOUS AGENTS

Bacteria are the most common cause of TD. Overall, the most common pathogen is enterotoxigenic *Escherichia coli*, followed by *Campylobacter jejuni, Shigella* spp., and *Salmonella* spp. Enteroadherent and other *E. coli* pathotypes are also common pathogens in TD. There is increasing discussion of *Aeromonas* spp. and *Plesiomonas* spp. as potential causes of TD as well. Viral diarrhea can be caused by a number of pathogens, including norovirus, rotavirus, and astrovirus.

Giardia is the main protozoal pathogen found in TD. *Entamoeba histolytica* is a relatively uncommon pathogen in travelers. *Cryptosporidium* is also relatively uncommon. The risk for *Cyclospora* is highly geographic and seasonal: the most well-known risks are in Nepal, Peru, Haiti, and Guatemala. *Dientamoeba fragilis* is a low-grade but persistent pathogen that is occasionally diagnosed in travelers. The individual pathogens are each discussed in their own sections in Chapter 3, and persistent diarrhea in returned travelers is discussed in Chapter 5.

OCCURRENCE

The most important determinant of risk is travel destination, and there are regional differences in both the risk for and etiology of diarrhea. The world is generally divided into 3 grades of risk: low, intermediate, and high.

- Low-risk countries include the United States, Canada, Australia, New Zealand, Japan, and countries in Northern and Western Europe.

- Intermediate-risk countries include those in Eastern Europe, South Africa, and some of the Caribbean islands.
- High-risk areas include most of Asia, the Middle East, Africa, Mexico, and Central and South America.

RISK FOR TRAVELERS

TD occurs equally in male and female travelers and is more common in young adult travelers than in older travelers. In short-term travelers, bouts of TD do not appear to protect against future attacks, and >1 episode of TD may occur during a single trip. A cohort of expatriates residing in Kathmandu, Nepal, experienced an average of 3.2 episodes of TD per person in their first year. In more temperate regions, there may be seasonal variations in diarrhea risk. In south Asia, for example, much higher TD attack rates are reported during the hot months preceding the monsoon.

In environments where large numbers of people do not have access to plumbing or latrines, the amount of stool contamination in the environment will be higher and more accessible to flies. Inadequate electrical capacity may lead to frequent blackouts or poorly functioning refrigeration, which can result in unsafe food storage and an increased risk for disease. Lack of safe water may lead to contaminated foods and drinks prepared with such water; inadequate water supply may lead to shortcuts in cleaning hands, surfaces, utensils, and foods such as fruits and vegetables. In addition, handwashing may not be a social norm and could be an extra expense, thus there may be no handwashing stations in food preparation areas. In destinations in which effective food handling courses have been provided, the risk for TD has been demonstrated to decrease. However, even in developed countries, pathogens such as *Shigella sonnei* have caused TD linked to handling and preparation of food in restaurants.

CLINICAL PRESENTATION

Bacterial and viral TD presents with the sudden onset of bothersome symptoms that can range from mild cramps and urgent loose stools to severe abdominal pain, fever, vomiting, and bloody diarrhea, although with norovirus vomiting may be more prominent. Protozoal diarrhea, such as that caused by *Giardia intestinalis* or *E. histolytica*, generally has a more gradual onset of low-grade symptoms, with 2–5 loose stools per day. The incubation period of the pathogens can be a clue to the etiology of TD:

- Bacterial and viral pathogens have an incubation period of 6–72 hours.
- Protozoal pathogens generally have an incubation period of 1–2 weeks and rarely present in the first few weeks of travel. An exception can be *Cyclospora cayetanensis*, which can present quickly in areas of high risk.

Untreated bacterial diarrhea lasts 3–7 days. Viral diarrhea generally lasts 2–3 days. Protozoal diarrhea can persist for weeks to months without treatment. An acute bout of gastroenteritis can lead to persistent gastrointestinal symptoms, even in the absence of continued infection (see Chapter 5, Persistent Travelers' Diarrhea). Other postinfectious sequelae may include reactive arthritis and Guillain-Barré syndrome.

PREVENTION

For travelers to high-risk areas, several approaches may be recommended that can reduce, but never completely eliminate, the risk for TD. These include instruction regarding food and beverage selection, use of agents other than antimicrobial drugs for prophylaxis, and use of prophylactic antibiotics. Carrying small containers of alcohol-based hand sanitizers (containing ≥60% alcohol) may make it easier for travelers to clean their hands before eating. No vaccines are available for most pathogens that cause TD, but travelers should refer to the Hepatitis A and Typhoid & Paratyphoid Fever sections in Chapter 3 regarding vaccines that can prevent other foodborne or waterborne infections to which travelers are prone.

Food and Beverage Selection

Care in selecting food and beverages for consumption helps to minimize the risk for acquiring TD. See the Food & Water Precautions section later in this chapter for CDC's detailed food and beverage recommendations. Although food and water precautions continue to be recommended, travelers may not always be able to adhere to the advice. Furthermore, many of the factors that ensure

 TRAVELERS' DIARRHEA |

food safety, such as restaurant hygiene, are out of the traveler's control.

Nonantimicrobial Drugs for Prophylaxis

The primary agent studied for prevention of TD, other than antimicrobial drugs, is bismuth subsalicylate (BSS), which is the active ingredient in Pepto-Bismol. Studies from Mexico have shown that this agent (taken daily as either 2 oz of liquid or 2 chewable tablets 4 times per day) reduces the incidence of TD by approximately 50%. BSS commonly causes blackening of the tongue and stool and may cause nausea, constipation, and rarely tinnitus. BSS should be avoided by travelers with aspirin allergy, renal insufficiency, and gout and by those taking anticoagulants, probenecid, or methotrexate. In travelers taking aspirin or salicylates for other reasons, the use of BSS may result in salicylate toxicity. BSS is not generally recommended for children aged <12 years; however, some clinicians use it off-label with caution in certain circumstances. Caution should be taken in administering BSS to children with viral infections, such as varicella or influenza, because of the risk for Reye syndrome. BSS is not recommended for children aged <3 years. Studies have not established the safety of BSS use for periods >3 weeks. Because of the number of tablets required and the inconvenient dosing, BSS is not commonly used as prophylaxis for TD.

The use of probiotics, such as *Lactobacillus* GG and *Saccharomyces boulardii*, has been studied in the prevention of TD in small numbers of people. Results are inconclusive, partially because standardized preparations of these bacteria are not reliably available. Some people report beneficial outcomes using bovine colostrum as a daily prophylaxis agent for TD. However, commercially sold preparations of bovine colostrum are marketed as dietary supplements that are not Food and Drug Administration (FDA) approved for medical indications. Because no data from rigorous clinical trials demonstrate efficacy in controlled trials, there is insufficient information to recommend the use of bovine colostrum to prevent TD.

Although not available in the United States, a cholera vaccine that provides partial protection against enterotoxigenic E. *coli* is available in some other countries. Several clinical trials of new vaccines against TD pathogens are in progress.

Prophylactic Antibiotics

Prophylactic antibiotics are effective in the prevention of some TD. Controlled studies have shown that diarrhea attack rates are reduced by 90% or more by the use of antibiotics. The prophylactic antibiotic of choice has changed over the past few decades as resistance patterns have evolved. Agents such as trimethoprim-sulfamethoxazole and doxycycline are no longer considered effective antimicrobial agents against enteric bacterial pathogens. The fluoroquinolones have been the most effective antibiotics for the prophylaxis and treatment of bacterial TD pathogens, but increasing resistance to these agents, mainly among *Campylobacter* and *Shigella* species, may limit their benefit in the future. A nonabsorbable antibiotic, rifaximin, is being investigated but is not currently approved by the FDA for its potential use in TD prophylaxis. In one study, rifaximin reduced the risk for TD in travelers to Mexico by 77%.

At this time, prophylactic antibiotics should not be recommended for most travelers. Prophylactic antibiotics afford no protection against nonbacterial pathogens and can remove normally protective microflora from the bowel, which could make a traveler more susceptible to infection with resistant bacterial pathogens. A traveler relying on prophylactic antibiotics will need to carry an alternative antibiotic to use in case diarrhea develops despite prophylaxis. Additionally, the use of antibiotics may be associated with allergic or adverse reactions in a certain percentage of travelers and may potentially contribute to drug resistance. The use of prophylactic antibiotics should be weighed against the result of using prompt, early self-treatment with antibiotics when TD occurs, which can limit the duration of illness to 6–24 hours in most cases. Prophylactic antibiotics may be considered for short-term travelers who are high-risk hosts (such as those who are immunosuppressed) or who are taking critical trips (such as engaging in a sporting event) during which even a short bout of diarrhea could affect the trip.

TREATMENT

Antibiotics are the principal element in the treatment of TD and are effective in cases caused by bacterial pathogens that are susceptible to the particular antibiotic prescribed.

Adjunctive agents used for symptomatic control may also be recommended.

Antibiotics

As bacterial causes of TD far outnumber other microbial causes, empiric treatment with an antibiotic directed at enteric bacterial pathogens remains the best therapy for TD. The benefit of treating TD with antibiotics has been proven in numerous studies. The effectiveness of a particular antimicrobial depends on the etiologic agent and its antibiotic sensitivity. Both as empiric therapy or for treatment of a specific bacterial pathogen, first-line antibiotics include fluoroquinolones, such as ciprofloxacin or levofloxacin. Increasing microbial resistance to the fluoroquinolones, especially among *Campylobacter* isolates, may limit their usefulness in some destinations, such as Thailand, where *Campylobacter* is prevalent. Increasing cases of fluoroquinolone resistance have been reported from other destinations and in other bacterial pathogens, including *Shigella* and *Salmonella*. A potential alternative to the fluoroquinolones in these situations is azithromycin, although enteropathogens with decreased azithromycin susceptibility have been documented in several countries. Rifaximin has been approved to treat TD caused by noninvasive strains of E. coli. However, since it is often difficult for travelers to distinguish between invasive and noninvasive diarrhea, and since they would have to carry a back-up drug in the event of invasive diarrhea, the overall usefulness of rifaximin as empiric self-treatment remains to be determined.

Single-dose or 1-day therapy for TD with a fluoroquinolone is well established, both by clinical trials and clinical experience. The best regimen for azithromycin treatment is not yet established. One study used a single dose of 1,000 mg, but side effects (mainly nausea) may limit the acceptability of this large dose. Azithromycin, 500 mg per day for 1–3 days, appears to be effective in most cases of TD.

Antimotility Agents

Antimotility agents provide symptomatic relief and serve as useful adjuncts to antibiotic therapy in TD. Synthetic opiates, such as loperamide and diphenoxylate, can reduce frequency of bowel movements and enable travelers to ride on an airplane or bus while awaiting the effects of antibiotics. Loperamide appears to have antisecretory properties as well. The safety of loperamide when used along with an antibiotic has been well established, even in cases of invasive pathogens. Antimotility agents are not generally recommended for patients with bloody diarrhea or those who have diarrhea and fever. Loperamide can be used in children, and liquid formulations are available. In practice, however, these drugs are rarely given to small children (aged <6 years).

Oral Rehydration Therapy

Fluids and electrolytes are lost during TD, and replenishment is important, especially in young children or adults with chronic medical illness. In adult travelers who are otherwise healthy, severe dehydration resulting from TD is unusual unless vomiting is prolonged. Nonetheless, replacement of fluid losses remains an adjunct to other therapy and helps the traveler feel better more quickly. Travelers should remember to use only beverages that are sealed, treated with chlorine, boiled, or are otherwise known to be purified. For severe fluid loss, replacement is best accomplished with oral rehydration solution (ORS), prepared from packaged oral rehydration salts, such as those provided by the World Health Organization. ORS is widely available at stores and pharmacies in most developing countries. ORS is prepared by adding 1 packet to the indicated volume of boiled or treated water—generally 1 liter. Travelers may find most ORS formulations to be relatively unpalatable, due to their saltiness. In mild cases, rehydration can be maintained with any palatable liquid (including sports drinks), although overly sweet drinks, such as sodas, can cause osmotic diarrhea if consumed in quantity.

Treatment of TD Caused by Protozoa

The most common parasitic cause of TD is *Giardia intestinalis*, and treatment options include metronidazole, tinidazole, and nitazoxanide (see Chapter 3, Giardiasis). Although cryptosporidiosis is usually a self-limited illness in immunocompetent people, nitazoxanide can be considered as a treatment option. Cyclosporiasis is treated with trimethoprim-sulfamethoxazole. Treatment of amebiasis is with metronidazole or tini-dazole, followed by treatment with a luminal agent such as iodoquinol or paromomycin.

Treatment for Children

Children who accompany their parents on trips to high-risk destinations can contract TD as well. There is no reason to withhold antibiotics from children who contract TD unless they have drug allergies, are taking medications that may interact with the antibiotic, or there is a strong suspicion that the illness is viral. In older children and teenagers, treatment recommendations for TD follow those for adults, with possible adjustments in the dose of medication. Among younger children, macrolides such as azithromycin are considered first-line antibiotic therapy, although some experts now use short-course fluoroquinolone therapy (despite its not being FDA-approved for this indication in children) for travelers aged <18 years. Rifaximin is approved for use in children aged ≥12 years.

Infants and younger children with TD are at higher risk for developing dehydration, which is best prevented by the early initiation of oral rehydration. Breastfed infants should continue to nurse on demand, and bottle-fed infants can continue to drink formula. Older infants and children should be encouraged to eat and may consume a regular diet. Children in diapers are at risk for developing diaper rash on their buttocks in response to the liquid stool. Barrier creams, such as zinc oxide or petrolatum, could be applied at the onset of diarrhea to help prevent and treat rash. More information about diarrhea and dehydration is discussed in Chapter 7, Traveling Safely with Infants & Children.

TROPICAL SPRUE

Tropical sprue is a syndrome of persistent TD often associated with malabsorption, steatorrhea, and folate and vitamin B12 deficiency. Tropical sprue is rare in short-term travelers, and recent surveys of returned travelers suggest that it is occurring less frequently worldwide. Although exhaustive searches to identify the etiologic agent of tropical sprue have been futile, it bears all the hallmarks of an infectious disease. Exclusion of other diarrheal etiologies is required for diagnosis. Treatment with tetracycline 250 mg 4 times daily and folate 5 mg daily for at least 6 weeks is generally successful. Patients with concomitant vitamin B12 deficiency may require parenteral vitamin B12.

BIBLIOGRAPHY

1. Adachi JA, Jiang ZD, Mathewson JJ, Verenkar MP, Thompson S, Martinez-Sandoval F, et al. Enteroaggregative Escherichia coli as a major etiologic agent in traveler's diarrhea in 3 regions of the world. Clin Infect Dis. 2001 Jun 15;32(12):1706–9.
2. Behrens RH, Cramer JP, Jelinek T, Shaw H, von Sonnenburg F, Wilbraham D, et al. Efficacy and safety of a patch vaccine containing heat-labile toxin from Escherichia coli against travellers' diarrhoea: a phase 3, randomised, double-blind, placebo-controlled field trial in travellers from Europe to Mexico and Guatemala. Lancet Infect Dis. 2014 Mar;14(3):197–204.
3. Black RE. Epidemiology of travelers' diarrhea and relative importance of various pathogens. Rev Infect Dis. 1990 Jan–Feb;12 Suppl 1:S73–9.
4. Connor BA. Sequelae of traveler's diarrhea: focus on postinfectious irritable bowel syndrome. Clin Infect Dis. 2005 Dec 1;41 Suppl 8:S577–86.
5. DuPont HL, Ericsson CD. Prevention and treatment of traveler's diarrhea. N Engl J Med. 1993 Jun 24;328(25):1821–7.
6. Greenwood Z, Black J, Weld L, O'Brien D, Leder K, Von Sonnenburg F, et al. Gastrointestinal infection among international travelers globally. J Travel Med. 2008 Jul–Aug;15(4):221–8.
7. Kendall ME, Crim S, Fullerton K, Han PV, Cronquist AB, Shiferaw B, et al. Travel-associated enteric infections diagnosed after return to the United States, Foodborne Diseases Active Surveillance Network (FoodNet), 2004–2009. Clin Infect Dis. 2012 Jun;54 Suppl 5:S480–7.
8. Shah N, DuPont HL, Ramsey DJ. Global etiology of travelers' diarrhea: systematic review from 1973 to the present. Am J Trop Med Hyg. 2009 Apr;80(4):609–14.
9. Shlim DR. Update in traveler's diarrhea. Infect Dis Clin North Am. 2005 Mar;19(1):137–49.
10. Swaminathan A, Torresi J, Schlagenhauf P, Thursky K, Wilder-Smith A, Connor BA, et al. A global study of pathogens and host risk factors associated with infectious gastrointestinal disease in returned international travellers. J Infect. 2009 Jul;59(1):19–27.

A HISTORY OF THE DEFINITION & MANAGEMENT OF TRAVELERS' DIARRHEA

Herbert L. DuPont

Travelers' diarrhea (TD) is defined as the passage of ≥3 unformed stools per day plus ≥1 associated enteric symptoms, such as abdominal pain or cramps, occurring in a traveler after arrival, usually in a resource-limited destination. Many colorful terms have been used for the condition according to the places where diarrhea commonly occurred, such as Aztec Two-Step, Delhi Belly, Hong Kong Dog, Montezuma's Revenge, and the Pharaoh's Curse.

While it was known for centuries that diarrhea and dysentery complicated armed conflicts in international settings, it wasn't until the 1940s that diarrhea was closely correlated with international travel and relocation in tropical regions. In the 1950s, B. H. Kean from Cornell University increased awareness of the problem by studying travelers and students from the United States in Mexico. The field mushroomed in later years, when groups studied international students and travelers, expatriates, and military populations. The history of TD can be viewed in 3 time blocks based on the nature of the research conducted, focusing first on the magnitude of the problem, then with studies of etiology and specific therapy and prevention, followed by a better understanding of the consequences of the illness.

THE 1950s THROUGH THE 1960s—IDENTIFICATION OF THE PROBLEM AND SUCCESSFUL CHEMOPROPHYLAXIS

Kean and Waters studied the risk of TD among students and travelers to Mexico, finding rates of illness in international travelers of 40%—a rate that persists in many areas of the developing world. They described low rates of TD when international visitors from one developing region visited another suggesting that immunity developed secondary to exposure to common etiologic agents. This group also demonstrated successful disease prevention with antibiotic chemoprophylaxis, which provided the first evidence, albeit indirect, that bacterial pathogens were responsible for most TD. Chemoprophylaxis was used in a little more than one-third of US visitors to Mexico in the 1950s and 1960s and was used by the US, Australian, and British athletes competing in the Olympics in Mexico City in 1968.

THE 1970s THROUGH THE 1990s—EPIDEMIOLOGY, ETIOLOGY, AND THERAPY

Clinical and epidemiologic features of TD were described. Microbiologic studies were carried out to determine the etiology of the illness, beginning with a study published in 1970 describing a single strain of *Escherichia coli* as the cause of TD in British troops stationed in Aden on the Red Sea. The next year, 2 strains of *E. coli* isolated from American soldiers with diarrhea acquired in Vietnam were shown to be enterotoxigenic in animals and adult volunteers, and 4 years later enterotoxigenic E. coli (ETEC) was found in most cases of TD among US students studying in a language school in Mexico.

The first clear evidence that antibiotics were effective in treating TD was in 1981 when trimethoprim-sulfamethoxazole was shown to reduce the duration of the illness in a group of travelers with TD caused by different etiologies. Placebo-controlled clinical trials then demonstrated the value of fluoroquinolones in treating TD. Regions of the tropical and semitropical world were studied, allowing scientists to categorize areas according to risk that international visitors would face of acquiring TD.

Although oral fluid electrolyte therapy had been shown to prevent dehydration-associated deaths in children, otherwise healthy travelers were able to keep up with fluids and salt requirements through diet and available drinks.

Although prophylactic antibiotics were used by international travelers at the time, in 1985 chemoprophylaxis with systemic antibiotics was strongly discouraged because of concerns about adverse drug events and development of drug resistance. The Consensus Development Panel favored self-treatment with short-course (single-dose or 3 days) antibiotics. Bismuth subsalicylate, a commonly used over-the-counter drug, was shown during this time period to prevent TD, giving hope that prevention strategies without stimulation of resistance might be achievable.

2000 AND BEYOND—ANTIBIOTIC RESISTANCE AND CHRONIC COMPLICATIONS

During this phase, the fluoroquinolones, particularly ciprofloxacin, became the mainstay of therapy for TD. The poorly absorbed (<0.4%) rifamycin antibiotic, rifaximin, was found to be as effective as ciprofloxacin for the most common TD syndrome, watery diarrhea. After more than a decade of use of fluoroquinolones for a variety of infectious disease conditions, resistance to this class of drugs has become more common among some bacterial causes of TD, particularly Campylobacter jejuni. The emergence of resistance encouraged the wider use of azithromycin, either single-dose or 3-day courses, to treat TD, particularly that associated with fever or bloody stools.

Chemoprophylaxis was once more examined with rifaximin, having a more acceptable safety profile and fewer concerns about resistance compared with the absorbed antibiotics. Currently, there are no general recommendations for this approach.

With the knowledge that bacterial diarrhea may be associated with the development of postinfectious irritable bowel syndrome and that bacterial enteropathogens caused most cases of TD, studies of travelers were undertaken. These small studies found that 5%–10% of people developed new-onset irritable bowel syndrome after experiencing TD in Mexico or Asia, although in most of these people no bacterial pathogen was identified. Studies are needed to further analyze this possible association and to develop and analyze methods of prevention, which could include early therapy (with passage of the first unformed stool), antibiotic chemoprophylaxis, or a vaccine. Studies are also needed to assess the effect of TD and its chemoprophylaxis and treatment on the intestinal microbiome. Rates of TD seem to be decreasing in many regions, and some areas that were previously considered high risk (such as Thailand) appear to currently have lower rates of the disease.

BIBLIOGRAPHY

1. DuPont HL, Ericsson CD, Farthing MJ, Gorbach S, Pickering LK, Rombo L, et al. Expert review of the evidence base for prevention of travelers' diarrhea. J Travel Med. 2009 May–Jun;16(3):149–60.

2. DuPont HL, Formal SB, Hornick RB, Snyder MJ, Libonati JP, Sheahan DG, et al. Pathogenesis of Escherichia coli diarrhea. N Engl J Med. 1971 Jul 1;285(1):1–9.

3. DuPont HL, Jiang ZD, Ericsson CD, Adachi JA, Mathewson JJ, DuPont MW, et al. Rifaximin versus ciprofloxacin for the treatment of traveler's diarrhea: a randomized, double-blind clinical trial. Clin Infect Dis. 2001 Dec 1;33(11):1807–15.

4. Gorbach SL, Edelman R. Travelers' diarrhea: National Institutes of Health Consensus Development Conference. Bethesda, Maryland, January 28–30, 1985. Rev Infect Dis. 1986 May–Jun;8 Suppl 2:S109–233.

5. Kean BH, Waters SR. The diarrhea of travelers. III. Drug prophylaxis in Mexico. N Engl J Med. 1959 Jul 9;261(2):71–4.

6. Kuschner RA, Trofa AF, Thomas RJ, Hoge CW, Pitarangsi C, Amato S, et al. Use of azithromycin for the treatment of Campylobacter enteritis in travelers to Thailand, an area where ciprofloxacin resistance is prevalent. Clin Infect Dis. 1995 Sep;21(3):536–41.

7. Okhuysen PC, Jiang ZD, Carlin L, Forbes C, DuPont HL. Post-diarrhea chronic intestinal symptoms and irritable bowel syndrome in North American travelers to Mexico. Am J Gastroenterol. 2004 Sep;99(9):1774–8.

8. Owen JR. Diarrhoea at the Olympics. Br Med J. 1968 Dec 7;4(5631):645.

9. Rowe B, Taylor J, Bettelheim KA. An investigation of traveller's diarrhoea. Lancet. 1970 Jan 3;1(7636):1–5.

10. Tribble DR, Sanders JW, Pang LW, Mason C, Pitarangsi C, Baqar S, et al. Traveler's diarrhea in Thailand: randomized, double-blind trial comparing single-dose and 3-day azithromycin-based regimens with a 3-day levofloxacin regimen. Clin Infect Dis. 2007 Feb 1;44(3):338–46.

ALTITUDE ILLNESS

Peter H. Hackett, David R. Shlim

The high-altitude environment exposes travelers to cold, low humidity, increased ultraviolet radiation, and decreased air pressure, all of which can cause problems. The biggest concern, however, is hypoxia. At 10,000 ft (3,000 m), for example, the inspired PO_2 is only 69% of sea-level value. The magnitude of hypoxic stress depends on altitude, rate of ascent, and duration of exposure. Sleeping at high altitude produces the most hypoxemia; day trips to high altitude with return to low altitude are much less stressful on the body. Typical high-altitude destinations include Cusco (11,000 ft; 3,300 m), La Paz (12,000 ft; 3,640 m), Lhasa (12,100 ft; 3,650 m), Everest Base Camp (17,700 ft; 5,400 m), and Kilimanjaro (19,341 ft; 5,895 m).

The human body adjusts very well to moderate hypoxia, but requires time to do so (Box 2-2). The process of acute acclimatization to high altitude takes 3–5 days; therefore, acclimatizing for a few days at 8,000–9,000 ft before proceeding to a higher altitude is ideal. Acclimatization prevents altitude illness, improves sleep, and increases comfort and well-being, although exercise performance will always be reduced compared with low altitude. Increase in ventilation is the most important factor in acute acclimatization; therefore, respiratory depressants must be avoided. Increased red-cell production does not play a role in acute acclimatization.

BOX 2-2. TIPS FOR ACCLIMATIZATION

- Ascend gradually, if possible. Avoid going directly from low altitude to more than 9,000 ft (2,750 m) sleeping altitude in 1 day. Once above 9,000 ft (2,750 m), move sleeping altitude no higher than 1,600 ft (500 m) per day, and plan an extra day for acclimatization every 3,300 ft (1,000 m).
- Consider using acetazolamide to speed acclimatization, if abrupt ascent is unavoidable.
- Avoid alcohol for the first 48 hours.
- Participate in only mild exercise for the first 48 hours.
- Having a high-altitude exposure at more than 9,000 ft (2,750 m) for 2 nights or more, within 30 days before the trip, is useful.

RISK FOR TRAVELERS

Inadequate acclimatization may lead to altitude illness in any traveler going to 8,000 ft (2,500 m) or higher, and sometimes even at lower altitude. Susceptibility and resistance to altitude illness are genetic traits, and no simple screening tests are available to predict risk. Risk is not affected by training or physical fitness. Children are equally susceptible as adults; people aged >50 years have slightly lower risk. How a traveler has responded to high altitude previously is the most reliable guide for future trips, but is not infallible. However, given certain baseline susceptibility, risk is largely influenced by rate of ascent and exertion (see Table 2-6). Determining an itinerary that will avoid any occurrence of altitude illness is difficult because of variations in individual susceptibility, as well as in starting points and terrain. The goal for the traveler may not be to avoid all symptoms of altitude illness but to have no more than mild illness.

CLINICAL PRESENTATION

Altitude illness is divided into 3 syndromes: acute mountain sickness (AMS), high-altitude cerebral edema (HACE), and high-altitude pulmonary edema (HAPE).

Acute Mountain Sickness

AMS is the most common form of altitude illness, affecting, for example, 25% of all visitors sleeping above 8,000 ft (2,500 m) in Colorado. Symptoms are those of an alcohol hangover: headache is the cardinal symptom, sometimes accompanied by fatigue, loss of appetite, nausea, and occasionally vomiting. Headache onset is usually 2–12 hours after arrival at a higher altitude and often during or after the first night. Preverbal children may develop loss of appetite, irritability, and pallor. AMS generally resolves with 24–72 hours of acclimatization.

High-Altitude Cerebral Edema

HACE is a severe progression of AMS and is rare; it is most often associated with HAPE. In addition to AMS symptoms, lethargy becomes profound, with drowsiness, confusion, and ataxia on tandem gait test. A person with HACE requires immediate descent; death from HACE can ensue within 24 hours of developing ataxia, if the person fails to descend.

High-Altitude Pulmonary Edema

HAPE can occur by itself or in conjunction with AMS and HACE; incidence is 1 per 10,000 skiers in Colorado and up to 1 per 100 climbers at more than 14,000 ft (4,270 m). Initial symptoms are increased breathlessness with exertion, and eventually increased breathlessness at rest, associated with weakness and cough. Oxygen or descent is life-saving. HAPE can be more rapidly fatal than HACE.

Preexisting Medical Problems

Travelers with medical conditions, such as heart failure, myocardial ischemia (angina), sickle cell disease, or any form of pulmonary insufficiency, should be advised to consult a physician familiar with high-altitude medical issues before undertaking high-altitude travel. The risk for new ischemic heart disease in previously healthy travelers does not appear to be increased at high altitudes. People with diabetes can travel safely to high altitudes, but they must be accustomed to exercise and carefully monitor their blood glucose. Diabetic ketoacidosis may be triggered by altitude illness and

Table 2-6. Risk categories for acute mountain sickness

RISK CATEGORY	DESCRIPTION	PROPHYLAXIS RECOMMENDATIONS
Low	• People with no prior history of altitude illness and ascending to less than 9,000 ft (2,750 m) • People taking more than 2 days to arrive at 8,200–9,800 ft (2,500–3,000 m), with subsequent increases in sleeping elevation less than 1,600 ft (500 m) per day, and an extra day for acclimatization every 3,300 ft (1,000 m)	Acetazolamide prophylaxis generally not indicated.
Moderate	• People with prior history of AMS and ascending to 8,200–9,100 ft (2,500–2,800 m) or higher in 1 day • No history of AMS and ascending to more than 9,100 ft (2,800 m) in 1 day • All people ascending more than 1,600 ft (500 m) per day (increase in sleeping elevation) at altitudes above 9,900 ft (3,000 m), but with an extra day for acclimatization every 3,300 ft (1,000 m)	Acetazolamide prophylaxis would be beneficial and should be considered.
High	• History of AMS and ascending to more than 9,100 ft (2,800 m) in 1 day • All people with a prior history of HAPE or HACE • All people ascending to more than 11,400 ft (3,500 m) in 1 day • All people ascending more than 1,600 ft (500 m) per day (increase in sleeping elevation) above 9,800 ft (3,000 m), without extra days for acclimatization • Very rapid ascents (such as less than 7-day ascents of Mount Kilimanjaro)	Acetazolamide prophylaxis strongly recommended.

Abbreviations: AMS, acute mountain sickness; HACE, high-altitude cerebral edema; HAPE, high-altitude pulmonary edema.

may be more difficult to treat in those on acetazolamide. Not all glucose meters read accurately at high altitudes.

Most people do not have visual problems at high altitudes. However, at very high altitudes some people who have had radial keratotomy may develop acute farsightedness and be unable to care for themselves. LASIK and other newer procedures may produce only minor visual disturbances at high altitudes.

There are no studies or case reports of harm to a fetus if the mother travels briefly to high altitudes during pregnancy. However, it may be prudent to recommend that pregnant women do not stay at sleeping altitudes higher than 12,000 ft (3,658 m), if possible. The dangers of having a pregnancy complication in remote, mountainous terrain should also be discussed.

DIAGNOSIS AND TREATMENT
Acute Mountain Sickness/High-Altitude Cerebral Edema

The differential diagnosis of AMS/HACE includes dehydration, exhaustion, hypoglycemia, hypothermia, or hyponatremia. Focal neurologic symptoms, or seizures, are rare in HACE and should lead to suspicion of an intracranial lesion or seizure disorder. Patients with AMS can descend ≥300 m, and symptoms will rapidly abate. Alternatively, supplemental oxygen at 2 L per minute will relieve headache quickly and resolve AMS over hours, but it is rarely available. People with AMS can also safely remain at their current altitude and treat symptoms with nonopiate analgesics and antiemetics, such as ondansetron. They may also take acetazolamide, which speeds acclimatization and effectively treats AMS, but is better for prophylaxis than treatment. Dexamethasone is more effective than acetazolamide at rapidly relieving the symptoms of moderate to severe AMS. If symptoms are getting worse while the traveler is resting at the same altitude, he or she must descend.

HACE is an extension of AMS characterized by neurologic findings, particularly ataxia, confusion, or altered mental status. HACE may also occur in the presence of HAPE. People developing HACE in populated areas with access to medical care can be treated at altitude with supplemental oxygen and dexamethasone. In remote areas, descent should be initiated in any person suspected of having HACE. If descent is not feasible because of logistical issues, supplemental oxygen or a portable hyperbaric chamber can be lifesaving.

High-Altitude Pulmonary Edema

Although the progression of decreased exercise tolerance, increased breathlessness, and breathlessness at rest is almost always recognizable as HAPE, the differential diagnosis includes pneumonia, bronchospasm, myocardial infarction, or pulmonary embolism. Descent in this situation is urgent and mandatory, and should be accomplished with as little exertion as is feasible for the patient. If descent is not immediately possible, supplemental oxygen or a portable hyperbaric chamber is critical. Patients with mild HAPE who have access to oxygen (at a hospital or high-altitude medical clinic, for example) may not need to descend to lower elevation and can be treated with oxygen at the current elevation. In the field setting, where resources are limited and there is a lower margin for error, nifedipine can be used as an adjunct to descent, oxygen, or portable hyperbaric therapy. A phosphodiesterase inhibitor may be used if nifedipine is not available, but concurrent use of multiple pulmonary vasodilators is not recommended.

Medications

In addition to the discussion below, recommendations for the usage and dosing of medications to prevent and treat altitude illness are outlined in Table 2-7.

Acetazolamide

Acetazolamide prevents AMS when taken before ascent and can speed recovery if taken after symptoms have developed. The drug works by acidifying the blood, which causes an increase in respiration and arterial oxygenation and thus aids acclimatization. An effective dose that minimizes the common side effects of increased urination and paresthesias of the fingers and toes is 125 mg every 12 hours, beginning the day before ascent and continuing the first 2 days at altitude, or longer if ascent continues. Allergic reactions to acetazolamide are uncommon. As a nonantimicrobial sulfonamide, it does not cross-react with antimicrobial sulfonamides. However, it is best avoided by people with history of anaphylaxis to any sulfa. People with history of severe penicillin allergy have occasionally had allergic reactions to acetazolamide. The pediatric dose is 5 mg/kg/day in divided doses, up to 125 mg twice a day.

Dexamethasone

Dexamethasone is effective for preventing and treating AMS and HACE, and perhaps HAPE as well. Unlike acetazolamide, if the drug is discontinued at altitude before acclimatization, rebound can occur. Acetazolamide is preferable to prevent AMS while ascending, with dexamethasone reserved for treatment, as an adjunct to descent. The adult dose is 4 mg every 6 hours. An increasing trend is to use dexamethasone for "summit day" on high peaks such as Kilimanjaro and Aconcagua, in order to prevent abrupt altitude illness.

Nifedipine

Nifedipine prevents HAPE and ameliorates it as well. For prevention, it is generally reserved for people who are particularly susceptible to the condition. The adult dose for prevention or treatment is 30 mg of extended release every 12 hours, or 20 mg every 8 hours.

Other Medications

Phosphodiesterase-5 inhibitors can also selectively lower pulmonary artery pressure, with less effect on systemic blood pressure. Tadalafil, 10 mg twice a day, during ascent can prevent HAPE and is being studied for treatment. When taken before ascent, gingko biloba, 100–120 mg twice a day, was shown to reduce AMS in adults in some trials, but it was not effective in others, probably due to variation in ingredients. Ibuprofen 600 mg every 8 hours was recently found to help prevent AMS, although it was not as effective as acetazolamide. However, it is over-the-counter, inexpensive, and well-tolerated.

Table 2-7. Recommended medication doses to prevent and treat altitude illness

MEDICATION	INDICATION	ROUTE	DOSE
Acetazolamide	AMS, HACE prevention	Oral	125 mg twice a day; 250 mg twice a day if >100 kg Pediatrics: 2.5 mg/kg every 12 h
	AMS treatment[1]	Oral	250 mg twice a day Pediatrics: 2.5 mg/kg every 12 h
Dexamethasone	AMS, HACE prevention	Oral	2 mg every 6 h or 4 mg every 12 h Pediatrics: should not be used for prophylaxis
	AMS, HACE treatment	Oral, IV, IM	AMS: 4 mg every 6 h HACE: 8 mg once, then 4 mg every 6 h Pediatrics: 0.15 mg/kg/dose every 6 h up to 4 mg
Nifedipine	HAPE prevention	Oral	30 mg SR version every 12 h, or 20 mg SR version every 8 h
	HAPE treatment	Oral	30 mg SR version every 12 h, or 20 mg SR version every 8 h
Tadalafil	HAPE prevention	Oral	10 mg twice a day
Sildenafil	HAPE prevention	Oral	50 mg every 8 h
Salmeterol	HAPE prevention	Inhaled	125 µg twice a day[2]

Abbreviations: AMS, acute mountain sickness; HACE, high-altitude cerebral edema; HAPE, high-altitude pulmonary edema; IM, intramuscular; IV, intravenous; SR, sustained release.
[1] Acetazolamide can also be used at this dose as an *adjunct* to dexamethasone in HACE treatment, but dexamethasone remains the primary treatment for that disorder.
[2] Should not be used as monotherapy and should only be used in conjunction with oral medications.

PREVENTION OF SEVERE ALTITUDE ILLNESS OR DEATH

The main point of instructing travelers about altitude illness is not to eliminate the possibility, but to prevent death or evacuation due to altitude illness. Since the onset of symptoms and the clinical course are sufficiently slow and predictable, there is no reason for anyone to die from altitude illness, unless trapped by weather or geography in a situation in which descent is impossible. Three rules can prevent death or serious consequences from altitude illness:

- Know the early symptoms of altitude illness, and be willing to acknowledge when they are present.
- Never ascend to sleep at a higher altitude when experiencing symptoms of altitude illness, no matter how minor they seem.
- Descend if the symptoms become worse while resting at the same altitude.

For trekking groups and expeditions going into remote high-altitude areas, where descent to a lower altitude could be problematic, a pressurization bag (such as the Gamow bag) can be beneficial. A foot pump produces an increased pressure of 2 lb/in^2, mimicking a descent of 5,000–6,000 ft (1,500–1,800 m) depending on the starting altitude. The total packed weight of bag and pump is about 14 lb (6.5 kg).

BIBLIOGRAPHY

1. Bartsch P, Swenson ER. Acute high-altitude illnesses. N Engl J Med. 2013 Oct 24;369(17):1666–7.
2. Hackett P. High altitude and common medical conditions. In: Hornbein TF, Schoene RB, editors. High Altitude: an Exploration of Human Adaptation. New York: Marcel Dekker; 2001. p. 839–85.
3. Hackett PH, Roach RC. High altitude cerebral edema. High Alt Med Biol. 2004 Summer;5(2):136–46.
4. Hackett PH, Roach RC. High-altitude medicine and physiology. In: Auerbach PS, editor. Wilderness Medicine. 6th ed. Philadelphia: Mosby Elsevier; 2012. p. 2–32.
5. Johnson TS, Rock PB, Fulco CS, Trad LA, Spark RF, Maher JT. Prevention of acute mountain sickness by dexamethasone. N Engl J Med. 1984 Mar 15;310(11):683–6.
6. Luks AM, McIntosh SE, Grissom CK, Auerbach PS, Rodway GW, Schoene RB, et al. Wilderness Medical Society consensus guidelines for the prevention and treatment of acute altitude illness. Wilderness Environ Med. 2010 Jun;21(2):146–55.
7. Luks AM, Swenson ER. Medication and dosage considerations in the prophylaxis and treatment of high-altitude illness. Chest. 2008 Mar;133(3):744–55.
8. Maggiorini M, Brunner-La Rocca HP, Peth S, Fischler M, Bohm T, Bernheim A, et al. Both tadalafil and dexamethasone may reduce the incidence of high-altitude pulmonary edema: a randomized trial. Ann Intern Med. 2006 Oct 3;145(7):497–506.
9. Pollard A, Murdoch D. The High Altitude Medicine Handbook. 3rd ed. Abingdon, UK: Radcliffe Medical Press; 2003.
10. Pollard AJ, Niermeyer S, Barry P, Bartsch P, Berghold F, Bishop RA, et al. Children at high altitude: an international consensus statement by an ad hoc committee of the International Society for Mountain Medicine, March 12, 2001. High Alt Med Biol. 2001 Fall;2(3):389–403.

For the Record

A HISTORY OF THE DEFINITION & MANAGEMENT OF ALTITUDE ILLNESS
David R. Shlim

As explorers began to challenge the higher parts of the Earth, first in Europe in 1786 with the ascent of Mont Blanc and later in Asia and South America, the high-altitude environment occasionally proved unexpectedly fatal. Deaths in otherwise healthy young men were attributed to "heart failure" or "pneumonia," and a specific syndrome associated with rapid ascent was not suspected. The first detailed clinical descriptions of high-altitude pulmonary edema (HAPE) and high-altitude cerebral edema (HACE) were published in 1913 by Thomas Ravenhill, based on his work with high-altitude miners in Chile. Scottish physiologist A. M. Kellas also provided detailed descriptions of "mountain sickness" in papers that were a prelude to the British attempts on Mount Everest in the 1920s.

These early descriptions were overlooked until the syndromes of altitude illness were rediscovered in the early 1960s. Herbert Hultgren, a Stanford cardiologist, documented HAPE in the Andes in 1959. A year later, Charles Houston, a physician and mountain climber noted for an epic attempt on K2 in 1953, documented a case of pulmonary edema in a healthy 21-year-old backcountry skier in Aspen, Colorado, in which a cardiac cause was definitively ruled out. The first modern description of HACE is credited to Fitch in 1964. Originally, the spectrum of altitude illness was thought to include 3 syndromes: acute mountain sickness (AMS), along with HAPE and HACE. In recent times, however, AMS is understood to represent early HACE, although the term is still used. All the syndromes are classified under the term "altitude illness."

China, having annexed Tibet in the 1950s, invaded a remote corner of northern India in 1962 at altitudes of 15,000–18,000 ft. Chinese troops, attacking from the Tibetan plateau, had no problems with the altitude, but the Indian troops transported rapidly to those heights experienced considerable rates of altitude illness. The Indian physician treating these troops, Inder Singh, reported on almost 2,000 cases of altitude illness during the brief war. One of his key observations was that the severity of illness was not related to the altitude at which the symptoms began. Illness could be just as severe at 11,000 ft as at 18,000 ft. His insightful 1969 paper in the *New England Journal of Medicine* is well worth reading today.

The advent of high-altitude trekking in Nepal in the late 1960s and early 1970s opened up a new group of people—nonmountaineers—to the risk of altitude illness. The trekking route to Mount Everest involves walking on trails that range in altitude from 5,000 to 18,000 ft (1,525 to 5,500 m). The technical ease encouraged trekkers to ascend faster than they could acclimatize, and an estimated 5–10 people per year died of altitude illness in the Everest region in the early 1970s. In 1974, Dr. Peter Hackett trekked to Mount Everest and stayed to run an aid post at 14,000 ft on the way to Everest Base Camp. He remained in Nepal for 18 months and brought back detailed correlations between the risk of altitude illness and the rate of ascent.

At that time, trekkers had the choice of walking over several high passes on the way to Everest Base Camp, starting from close to Kathmandu, or flying into Lukla, an airstrip located at 9,000 ft. The trekkers who walked experienced altitude illness at a rate of 42%, while those who flew were ill at a rate of 60%. Dr. Hackett recommended 2 extra acclimatization days in the upper portions of the trek, which decreased the rate of altitude illness to <40%. His recommendations are still the basis of the itineraries for trekking to Everest Base Camp, even though the rate of altitude illness on this schedule remains approximately 35%.

In addition to trekkers walking into high-altitude destinations, travelers increasingly fly to a number of cities where they risk altitude illness, including Cusco, Peru (11,150 ft, 3,400 m); Lhasa, Tibet (12,000 ft, 3,660 m); and La Paz, Bolivia (12,400 ft, 3,780 m). Tourists who fly from a low altitude to any of these destinations should consider taking acetazolamide to help prevent altitude illness.

In the 1930s, the antibiotic sulphanilamide was noted to cause metabolic acidosis and compensatory hyperventilation, an effect later attributed to inhibition of renal carbonic anhydrase. Another sulfonamide, acetazolamide, was a more potent carbonic anhydrase inhibitor. Inducing healthy people to breathe more was postulated to improve acclimatization to altitude, and in an article published in 1968, acetazolamide was shown to prevent altitude illness. To this day, acetazolamide remains the best drug to prevent altitude illness.

Because of variations in individual susceptibility and the modern tendency to take short trips that do not permit gradual acclimatization, altitude illness will continue to occur in travelers. However, there is no longer any reason why high-altitude sojourners should die of altitude illness. Education on acclimatization, recognition of symptoms, and appropriate response can ensure that an otherwise inconvenient and uncomfortable illness does not turn into a tragedy.

BIBLIOGRAPHY

1. Forwand SA, Landowne M, Follansbee JN, Hansen JE. Effect of acetazolamide on acute mountain sickness. N Engl J Med. 1968 Oct 17;279(16):839–45.

2. Hackett PH, Rennie D, Levine HD. The incidence, importance, and prophylaxis of acute mountain sickness. Lancet. 1976 Nov 27;2(7996):1149–55.

3. Singh I, Khanna PK, Srivastava MC, Lal M, Roy SB, Subramanyam CS. Acute mountain sickness. N Engl J Med. 1969 Jan 23;280(4):175–84.

4. Swenson ER. Carbonic anhydrase inhibitors and ventilation: a complex interplay of stimulation and suppression. Eur Res J. 1998 Dec;12(6):1242–7.

5. West JB. High life: a history of high-altitude physiology and medicine. New York: Oxford University Press; 1998.

JET LAG
Ronnie Henry

Jet lag is a temporary sleep disorder among air travelers who rapidly travel across ≥3 time zones. Jet lag occurs as a result of the slow adjustment of the body clock to the destination time. Consequently, the daily rhythms and the internal drive for sleep and wakefulness are out of synchronization with the new environment.

The secretion of melatonin by the pineal gland is responsible for setting our sleep–wake cycle. Its synthesis and release are stimulated by darkness and suppressed by light.

RISK FOR TRAVELERS
Eastward travel is associated with difficulty falling asleep at the destination bedtime and difficulty arising in the morning. Westward travel is associated with early evening sleepiness and predawn awakening at the travel destination. Travelers flying within the same time zone typically experience the fewest problems, such as nonspecific travel fatigue. Crossing more time zones or traveling eastward generally increases the time required for adaptation. After eastward flights, jet lag lasts for the number of days roughly equal to two-thirds the number of time zones crossed; after westward flights, the number of days is roughly half the number of time zones.

Individual responses to crossing time zones and ability to adapt to a new time zone vary. Increased age may contribute to a longer recovery period. The intensity and duration of jet lag are related to the number of time zones crossed, the direction of travel, the ability to sleep while traveling, the availability and intensity of local circadian time cues at the destination, and individual differences in phase tolerance.

CLINICAL PRESENTATION
Jet-lagged travelers may experience the following symptoms:

- Poor sleep, including delayed sleep onset (after eastward flight), early awakening

(after westward flight), and fractionated sleep (after flights in either direction)
- Poor performance in physical and mental tasks during the new daytime
- Negative subjective changes such as fatigue, headache, irritability, stress, inability to concentrate, and depression
- Gastrointestinal disturbances and decreased interest in and enjoyment of meals

PREVENTION

Travelers can minimize jet lag by doing the following before travel:

- Exercise, eat a healthful diet, and get plenty of rest.
- Begin to reset the body clock by shifting the timing of sleep to 1–2 hours later for a few days before traveling westward and shifting the timing of sleep to 1–2 hours earlier for a few days before traveling eastward. It can also be helpful to shift mealtimes to hours that coincide with these changes.
- Seek exposure to bright light in the evening if traveling westward, in the morning if traveling eastward. Mobile apps, such as Jet Lag Rooster and Entrain, are available to help travelers calculate and adhere to a light/dark schedule.
- Break up a long journey with a stopover, if possible.

Travelers should do the following during travel:

- Avoid large meals, alcohol, and caffeine.
- Drink plenty of water to remain hydrated.
- Move around on the plane to promote mental and physical acuity, as well as protect against deep vein thrombosis.
- Wear comfortable shoes and clothing.
- Sleep, if possible, during long flights.

Travelers should do the following on arrival at the destination:

- Avoid situations requiring critical decision making, such as important meetings, for the first day after arrival.
- Adapt to the local schedule as soon as possible.
- Depending on the number of time zones crossed, people with diabetes may need to adjust their insulin schedule during

travel and on arrival at their destination. Providers should work with their patients to arrange schedule changes before travel.
- Optimize exposure to sunlight after arrival from either direction. Exposure to bright light in the morning moves the stage of circadian rhythm forward, while exposure to light in the evening delays the stage and encourages later sleep.
- Eat meals appropriate to the local time, drink plenty of water, and avoid excess caffeine or alcohol. Eat a balanced diet, including carbohydrates.
- Take short naps (20–30 minutes) to increase energy but not undermine nighttime sleep.

The use of the nutritional supplement melatonin is controversial for preventing jet lag. Some clinicians advocate the use of 0.5–5.0 mg of melatonin during the first few days of travel, and data suggest its efficacy. However, its production is not regulated by the Food and Drug Administration, and contaminants have been found in commercially available products. Current information also does not support the use of special diets to ameliorate jet lag.

TREATMENT

The 2008 American Academy of Sleep Medicine recommendations include the following:

- Remain on home time if the travel period is ≤2 days.
- Promote sleep with hypnotic medication, although the effects of hypnotics on daytime symptoms of jet lag have not been well studied.
- Nonaddictive sedative hypnotics (non-benzodiazepines), such as zolpidem, have been shown in some studies to promote longer periods of high-quality sleep. If a benzodiazepine is preferred, a short-acting one, such as temazepam, is recommended to minimize oversedation the following day. Because alcohol intake is often high during international travel, the risk of interaction with hypnotics should be emphasized with patients.
- If necessary, promote daytime alertness with a stimulant such as caffeine in limited quantities. Avoid caffeine after midday.
- Take short naps (20–30 minutes), shower, and spend time in the afternoon sun.

BIBLIOGRAPHY

1. Barion A, Zee PC. A clinical approach to circadian rhythm sleep disorders. Sleep Med. 2007 Sep;8(6):566–77.

2. Daurat A, Benoit O, Buguet A. Effects of zopiclone on the rest/activity rhythm after a westward flight across five time zones. Psychopharmacology (Berl). 2000 Apr;149(3):241–5.

3. Dubocovich ML, Markowska M. Functional MT1 and MT2 melatonin receptors in mammals. Endocrine. 2005 Jul;27(2):101–10.

4. Herxheimer A. Jet lag. Clin Evid. 2005 Jun;(13):2178–83.

5. Jamieson AO, Zammit GK, Rosenberg RS, Davis JR, Walsh JK. Zolpidem reduces the sleep disturbance of jet lag. Sleep Med. 2001 Sep;2(5):423–30.

6. Reid KJ, Chang AM, Zee PC. Circadian rhythm sleep disorders. Med Clin North Am. 2004 May;88(3):631–51, viii.

7. Reilly T, Waterhouse J, Edwards B. Jet lag and air travel: implications for performance. Clin Sports Med. 2005 Apr;24(2):367–80, xii.

8. Sack RL. Clinical practice. Jet lag. N Engl J Med. 2010 Feb 4;362(5):440–7.

9. Sack RL, Auckley D, Auger RR, Carskadon MA, Wright KP Jr, Vitiello MV, et al. Circadian rhythm sleep disorders: part I, basic principles, shift work and jet lag disorders. An American Academy of Sleep Medicine review. Sleep. 2007 Nov 1;30(11):1460–83.

10. Waterhouse J, Reilly T, Atkinson G, Edwards B. Jet lag: trends and coping strategies. Lancet. 2007 Mar 31;369(9567):1117–29.

MOTION SICKNESS

Stefanie K. Erskine

RISK FOR TRAVELERS

Motion sickness is the term attributed to physiologic responses of the body to motion by sea, car, train or air. Given sufficient stimulus all people with functional vestibular systems can develop motion sickness. However, people vary in their susceptibility. Risk factors include the following:

- Age—children aged 2–12 years are especially susceptible, but infants and toddlers are generally immune.
- Sex—women are more likely to have motion sickness, especially when pregnant, menstruating, or on hormones.
- Migraines—people who get migraine headaches are more prone to motion sickness, especially during a migraine.
- Medication—some prescriptions can worsen the nausea of motion sickness (Table 2-8).

TREATMENT

Nonpharmacologic treatments for preventing and treating motion sickness can be effective with few adverse side effects (see Prevention below). However, these measures can be time-consuming and unpleasant for travelers. Many patients will prefer medication. A primary side effect of most efficacious medications used for motion sickness is drowsiness, along with other drug-specific side effects. Some medications may interfere with or delay acclimation to the offending movement. Because gastric stasis can occur with motion sickness, parenteral delivery may be advantageous.

Antihistamines are the most frequently used and widely available medications for motion sickness; non-sedating ones appear to be less effective. Antihistamines commonly used for motion sickness include cinnarizine (not currently available in the United States), cyclizine, dimenhydrinate, meclizine, and promethazine (oral and suppository). Other common medications used to treat motion sickness are scopolamine (hyoscine, oral and transdermal), antidopaminergic drugs (such as prochlorperazine), metoclopramide, sympathomimetics, and benzodiazepines. Clinical trials have not shown that ondansetron, a drug commonly used as an antiemetic in cancer patients, is effective in the prevention of nausea associated with motion sickness.

Table 2-8. Medications that may increase nausea

MEDICATION CLASS	EXAMPLES
Antibiotics	Azithromycin, metronidazole, erythromycin, trimethoprim-sulfamethoxazole
Antiparasitics	Albendazole, thiabendazole, iodoquinol, chloroquine, mefloquine
Estrogens	Oral contraceptives, estradiol
Cardiovascular	Digoxin, levodopa
Narcotic analgesics	Codeine, morphine, meperidine
Nonsteroidal analgesics	Ibuprofen, naproxen, indomethacin
Antidepressants	Fluoxetine, paroxetine, sertraline
Asthma medication	Aminophylline
Bisphosphonates	Alendronate sodium, ibandronate sodium, risedronate sodium

When recommending any of these medications to travelers, providers should make sure that patients understand the risks and benefits, possible undesirable side effects, and potential drug interactions. Travelers may consider trying the medication before travel to see what effect it has on them.

Medications in Children

For children aged 2–12 years, dimenhydrinate (Dramamine), 1–1.5 mg/kg per dose, or diphenhydramine (Benadryl), 0.5–1 mg/kg per dose up to 25 mg, can be given 1 hour before travel and every 6 hours during the trip. Because some children have paradoxical agitation with these medicines, a test dose should be given at home before departure.

Antihistamines are not approved by the Food and Drug Administration to treat motion sickness in children. Caregivers should be reminded to always ask a physician, pharmacist, or other clinician if they have any questions about how to use or dose antihistamines in children before they administer the medication. Oversedation of young children with antihistamines can be life-threatening.

Scopolamine can cause dangerous adverse effects in children and should not be used; prochlorperazine and metoclopramide should be used with caution in children.

Medications in Pregnancy

Drugs with the most safety data regarding the treatment of the nausea of pregnancy are the logical first choice. Alphabetical scoring of the safety of medications in pregnancy may not be helpful, and clinicians should review the actual safety data or call the patient's obstetric provider for suggestions. Web-based information may be found at the websites www.Motherisk.org and www.Reprotox.org.

PREVENTION

Nonpharmacologic interventions to prevent or treat motion sickness include the following:

- Being aware of and avoiding situations that tend to trigger symptoms.

- Optimizing position to reduce motion or motion perception—for example, driving a vehicle instead of riding in it, sitting in the front seat of a car or bus, or sitting over the wing of an aircraft.
- Reducing sensory input—lying prone, shutting eyes, or looking at the horizon.
- Maintaining hydration by drinking water, eating small meals frequently, and limiting alcoholic and caffeinated beverages.

- Adding distractions—listening to music or using aromatherapy scents such as mint or lavender. Flavored lozenges may also help, in particular ginger-flavored. Lozenges may also function as distractions or, in the case of ginger, may hasten gastric emptying.
- Using acupressure or magnets is advocated by some to prevent or treat nausea, although scientific data on efficacy of these interventions for preventing motion sickness are equivocal.

BIBLIOGRAPHY

1. Murdin L, Golding J, Bronstein A. Managing motion sickness. BMJ. 2011;343:d7430.
2. Priesol AJ. Motion Sickness. Deschler DG, editor. Waltham MA: UpToDate; 2012.
3. Shupak A, Gordon CR. Motion sickness: advances in pathogenesis, prediction, prevention, and treatment. Aviat Space Environ Med. 2006 Dec;77(12):1213–23.
4. Takeda N, Morita M, Horii A, Nishiike S, Kitahara T, Uno A. Neural mechanisms of motion sickness. J Med Invest. 2001 Feb;48(1–2):44–59.

RESPIRATORY INFECTIONS
Regina C. LaRocque, Edward T. Ryan

Respiratory infection is a leading cause of seeking medical care in returning travelers. Respiratory infections occur in up to 20% of all travelers, which is almost as common as travelers' diarrhea. Upper respiratory infection is more common than lower respiratory infection. In general, the types of respiratory infections that affect travelers are similar to those in nontravelers, and exotic causes are rare. Clinicians must inquire about history of travel when evaluating a patient for respiratory infections.

INFECTIOUS AGENT
Viral pathogens are the most common cause of respiratory infection in travelers; causative agents include rhinovirus, respiratory syncytial virus, influenza virus, parainfluenza virus, human metapneumovirus, measles, mumps, adenovirus, and coronavirus. Clinicians also need to consider novel viral causes of respiratory infection in travelers, including Middle East respiratory syndrome (MERS) coronavirus, avian influenza H5N1 (referred to as H5N1), and avian influenza H7N9 (referred to as H7N9). Respiratory infection due to viral pathogens may lead to bacterial sinusitis, bronchitis, or pneumonia. Bacterial pathogens are less common but can include Streptococcus pneumoniae, Mycoplasma pneumoniae, Haemophilus influenzae, and Chlamydophila pneumoniae. Coxiella burnetii and Legionella pneumophila can also cause outbreaks and sporadic cases of respiratory illness.

RISK FOR TRAVELERS
Reported outbreaks are usually associated with common exposure in hotels and cruise ships or among tour groups. A few pathogens have been associated with outbreaks in travelers, including influenza virus, L. pneumophila, and Histoplasma capsulatum. The peak influenza season in the temperate Northern Hemisphere is December through February. In the temperate Southern Hemisphere, the peak influenza season is June through August. Travelers to tropical zones are at risk all year. Exposure to an infected person from another hemisphere, such as on a cruise ship

or package tour, can lead to an outbreak of influenza at any time or place.

Air-pressure changes during ascent and descent of aircraft can facilitate the development of sinusitis and otitis media. Direct airborne transmission aboard commercial aircraft is unusual because of frequent air recirculation and filtration, although influenza, tuberculosis, measles, and other diseases have resulted from transmission in modern aircraft. Transmission may occur between passengers who are seated near one another, usually through direct contact or droplets. Intermingling of large numbers of people in locations such as airports, cruise ships, and hotels can also facilitate transmission of respiratory pathogens.

The air quality at many travel destinations may not be optimal, and exposure to sulfur dioxide, nitrogen dioxide, carbon monoxide, ozone, and particulate matter is associated with a number of health risks, including respiratory tract inflammation, exacerbations of asthma and chronic obstructive pulmonary disease, impaired lung function, bronchitis, and pneumonia. Certain travelers have a higher risk for respiratory tract infection, including children, the elderly, and people with comorbid pulmonary conditions, such as asthma and chronic obstructive pulmonary disease (COPD).

The risk for tuberculosis among most travelers is low (see Chapter 3, Tuberculosis).

DIAGNOSIS

Identifying a specific etiologic agent, especially in the absence of pneumonia or serious disease, is not always clinically necessary. If indicated, the following methods of diagnosis can be used:

- Molecular methods are available to detect a number of respiratory viruses, including influenza virus, parainfluenza virus, adenovirus, human metapneumovirus, and respiratory syncytial virus, and for certain nonviral pathogens.
- Rapid tests are also available to detect some pathogens such as respiratory syncytial virus, influenza virus, *L. pneumophila*, and group A *Streptococcus*.
- Microbiologic culturing of sputum and blood, although insensitive, can help identify a causative respiratory pathogen.

- Special consideration should be given to diagnosing patients with suspected MERS (www.cdc.gov/coronavirus/mers/guidelines-clinical-specimens.html), H5N1 (www.cdc.gov/flu/avianflu/h5n1/testing.htm), or H7N9 (www.cdc.gov/flu/avianflu/h7n9/testing.htm).

CLINICAL PRESENTATION

Most respiratory tract infections, especially those of the upper respiratory tract, are mild and not incapacitating. Upper respiratory tract infections often cause rhinorrhea or pharyngitis. Lower respiratory tract infections, particularly pneumonia, can be more severe. Lower respiratory tract infections are more likely to cause fever, dyspnea, or chest pain than upper respiratory tract infections. Cough is often present in either upper or lower tract infections. People with influenza commonly have acute onset of fever, myalgia, headache, and cough. At present, MERS should be considered in travelers who develop fever and pneumonia within 14 days after traveling from countries in or near the Arabian Peninsula or who have close contact with such travelers. Practitioners should be aware that regions associated with MERS may expand or change (www.cdc.gov/coronavirus/MERS/about/index.html). H5N1 and H7N9 should be considered in patients with new-onset severe acute respiratory illness requiring hospitalization when no alternative etiology has been identified and if the patient has recently (within 10 days) been to a country with recently confirmed human or animal cases of H5N1 (www.cdc.gov/flu/avianflu/h5n1-virus.htm) or H7N9 (www.cdc.gov/flu/avianflu/h7n9-virus.htm) or has had close contact with an ill person who has traveled to these areas in the last 10 days. Pulmonary embolism should be considered in the differential diagnosis of travelers who present with dyspnea, cough, or pleurisy and fever, especially those who have recently been on long car or plane rides.

TREATMENT

Affected travelers are usually managed similarly to nontravelers, although travelers with progressive or severe illness should be evaluated for illnesses specific to their travel destinations and exposure history. Most respiratory infections are due to viruses, are mild, and do not require specific treatment

 RESPIRATORY INFECTIONS | 79

or antibiotics. Self-treatment with antibiotics during travel can be considered for higher-risk travelers with symptoms of lower respiratory tract infection. A respiratory-spectrum fluoroquinolone such as levofloxacin or a macrolide such as azithromycin may be prescribed to the traveler for this purpose before travel.

The rate of influenza among travelers is not known. The difficulty in self-diagnosing influenza makes it problematic to decide whether to prescribe travelers a neuraminidase inhibitor for self-treatment. This practice should probably be limited to travelers with a specific underlying condition that may predispose them to severe influenza.

Specific situations that may require medical intervention include the following:

- Pharyngitis without rhinorrhea, cough, or other symptoms that may indicate infection with group A *Streptococcus*.
- Sudden onset of cough, chest pain, and fever that may indicate pneumonia (or pulmonary embolism), resulting in a situation where the traveler may be sick enough to seek medical care right away.
- Travelers with underlying medical conditions, such as asthma, pulmonary disease, or heart disease, who may need to seek medical care earlier than otherwise healthy travelers.

PREVENTION

Vaccines are available to prevent a number of respiratory diseases, including influenza, *S. pneumoniae* infection, *H. influenzae* type B infection (in young children), pertussis, diphtheria, varicella, and measles. Unless contraindicated, travelers should be vaccinated against influenza and be up-to-date on other routine immunizations. Preventing respiratory illness while traveling may not be possible, but common-sense preventive measures include the following:

- Minimizing close contact with people who are coughing and sneezing.
- Frequent handwashing, either with soap and water or alcohol-based hand sanitizers (containing ≥60% alcohol) when soap and water are not available.
- Using a vasoconstricting nasal spray immediately before air travel, if the traveler has a preexisting eustachian tube dysfunction, may help lessen the likelihood of otitis or barotrauma.

BIBLIOGRAPHY

1. Camps M, Vilella A, Marcos MA, Letang E, Muñoz J, Salvado E, et al. Incidence of respiratory viruses among travelers with a febrile syndrome returning from tropical and subtropical areas. J Med Virol. 2008 Apr;80(4):711–5.
2. Cobelens FG, van Deutekom H, Draayer-Jansen IW, Schepp-Beelen AC, van Gerven PJ, van Kessel RP, et al. Risk of infection with Mycobacterium tuberculosis in travellers to areas of high tuberculosis endemicity. Lancet. 2000 Aug 5;356(9228):461–5.
3. Foxwell AR, Roberts L, Lokuge K, Kelly PM. Transmission of influenza on international flights, May 2009. Emerg Infect Dis. 2011 Jul;17(7):1188–94.
4. Freedman DO, Weld LH, Kozarsky PE, Fisk T, Robins R, von Sonnenburg F, et al. Spectrum of disease and relation to place of exposure among ill returned travelers. N Engl J Med. 2006 Jan 12;354(2):119–30.
5. Jauréguiberry S, Boutolleau D, Grandsire E, Kofman T, Deback C, Aït-Arkoub Z, et al. Clinical and microbiological evaluation of travel-associated respiratory tract infections in travelers returning from countries affected by pandemic A(H1N1) 2009 influenza. J Travel Med. 2012 Jan–Feb; 19(1):22–7.
6. Leder K, Newman D. Respiratory infections during air travel. Intern Med J. 2005 Jan;35(1):50–5.
7. Leder K, Sundararajan V, Weld L, Pandey P, Brown G, Torresi J. Respiratory tract infections in travelers: a review of the GeoSentinel surveillance network. Clin Infect Dis. 2003 Feb 15;36(4):399–406.
8. Leder K, Torresi J, Libman MD, Cramer JP, Castelli F, Schlagenhauf P, et al. GeoSentinel surveillance of illness in returned travelers, 2007–2011. Ann Intern Med. 2013 Mar 19;158(6):456–68.
9. Luna LK, Panning M, Grywna K, Pfefferle S, Drosten C. Spectrum of viruses and atypical bacteria in intercontinental air travelers with symptoms of acute respiratory infection. J Infect Dis. 2007 Mar 1;195(5):675–9.
10. Zaki AM, van Boheemen S, Bestebroer TM, Osterhaus AD, Fouchier RA. Isolation of a novel coronavirus from a man with pneumonia in Saudi Arabia. N Engl J Med. 2012 Nov 8;367(19):1814–20.

Counseling & Advice for Travelers

FOOD & WATER PRECAUTIONS
John C. Watson, Michele C. Hlavsa, Patricia M. Griffin

Contaminated food and water often pose a risk for travelers. Among the infectious diseases that travelers can acquire from contaminated food and water are *Escherichia coli* infections, shigellosis or bacillary dysentery, giardiasis, cryptosporidiosis, norovirus infection, hepatitis A, and salmonelloses, including typhoid fever. Contaminated food and water can also pose a risk of cholera and a variety of conditions caused by protozoan and helminthic parasites. Many of the infectious diseases associated with contaminated food and water are caused by pathogens transmitted via the fecal-oral route. Swallowing, inhaling aerosols of, or coming in contact with contaminated water, including natural saltwater or freshwater or the water in inadequately treated swimming pools, interactive fountains (splash parks or splash pads), or hot tubs or spas can transmit these and other pathogens that can cause diarrhea, vomiting, or infection of the ears, eyes, skin, or the respiratory or nervous system (see Chapter 3 for specific infectious diseases).

FOOD

To avoid illness, travelers should be advised to select food with care. All raw food is subject to contamination. Raw or undercooked meat, fish, and shellfish can carry various intestinal pathogens. In areas where hygiene and sanitation are inadequate or unknown, travelers should be advised to avoid eating salads, uncooked vegetables, unpasteurized fruit juices, and unpasteurized milk and milk products, such as cheese and yogurt. In these areas, travelers should be advised to eat only food that is fully cooked and served hot and fruit that has been washed in clean water and then peeled by the traveler. Raw fruits that are eaten unpeeled (such as strawberries) or cut should be avoided, and fruits that are eaten peeled (such as bananas) should be peeled by the person who eats them. Always refrigerate perishable cooked food within 2 hours (1 hour at temperatures >90°F [32°C]). Cooked food that has been stored should be thoroughly reheated before serving. These recommendations also apply to eggs, which should be thoroughly cooked, whether they are served alone or used in sauces. Consumption of food and beverages obtained from street vendors has been associated with an increased risk of illness.

Travelers should wash their hands with soap and water before eating, after using the bathroom or changing diapers, after caring for someone who is ill, and after direct contact with preschool-age children, animals, or feces. If soap and water are not available, use an alcohol-based hand sanitizer (with ≥60% alcohol) and wash hands with soap and water as soon as they become available. Alcohol-based hand sanitizers are not very effective against *Cryptosporidium* and norovirus and may not work well when hands are heavily soiled.

The safest way to feed an infant aged <6 months is to breastfeed exclusively. If the infant is fed formula prepared from commercial powder, the powder should be reconstituted with hot water at a temperature of ≥158°F (≥70°C). This precaution will kill most pathogens with which the infant formula may have been contaminated during manufacturing or through handling after opening. To ensure that the water is hot enough (≥158°F; ≥70°C), travelers should prepare formula within 30 minutes after boiling the water for ≥1 minute (see the Water Disinfection for Travelers section later in this chapter). The prepared formula should be cooled to a safe temperature for feeding (for example, by placing the bottle upright in a bath of safe water and safe ice [see below], keeping the bath water below the nipple ring and using within

2 hours of preparation. Bottles and nipples should be washed and then sterilized (in boiling water or in an electric sterilizer). Travelers may wish to pack enough formula for their trip, because manufacturing standards vary widely around the world.

Travelers should be advised not to bring perishable seafood from high-risk areas back to the United States. Cholera has occurred in people who ate crab that had been brought into the United States from Latin America by travelers. Moreover, travelers should not assume that food and water aboard commercial aircraft are safe, because food and water may be obtained in the country of departure, where hygiene and sanitation may be inadequate.

WATER
Drinking Water and Other Beverages
In many parts of the world, particularly where water treatment, sanitation, and hygiene are inadequate, tap water may contain disease-causing contaminants, including viruses, bacteria, and parasites. As a result, tap water in some places may be unsafe for drinking, preparing food and beverages, making ice, cooking, and brushing teeth. Contaminated tap water, including droplets and aerosols, may also cause illness if inadvertently swallowed or inhaled, as can occur during showering or bathing. Infants, young children, pregnant women, the elderly, and people whose immune systems are compromised because of AIDS, chemotherapy, or transplant medications may be especially susceptible to illness from some disease-causing organisms (such as *Cryptosporidium* and *Legionella*).

Travelers should avoid drinking or otherwise ingesting tap water unless they are reasonably certain it is not contaminated. Many people choose to disinfect or filter their water when traveling to destinations where safe tap water may not be available (see the Water Disinfection for Travelers section later in this chapter). Tap water is not sterile and should not be used for sinus or nasal irrigation or rinsing, including use in neti pots and for ritual ablution (see Chapter 4, Saudi Arabia: Hajj Pilgrimage) unless it is disinfected for these purposes (see www.cdc.gov/parasites/naegleria/ritual-ablution.html and www.cdc.gov/parasites/naegleria/sinus-rinsing.html). Tap water should never be used to clean or rinse contact lenses. Water contaminated with fuels or toxic chemicals will not be made safe by boiling or disinfection; travelers should use a different source of water if they suspect this type of contamination.

In areas where tap water may be contaminated, only commercially bottled water from an unopened, factory-sealed container or water that has been adequately disinfected should be used for drinking, preparing food and beverages, making ice, cooking, and carrying out oral hygiene, including brushing teeth. (See Water Disinfection for Travelers later in this chapter for proper disinfection techniques.)

Beverages made with boiled water and served steaming hot (such as tea and coffee) are generally safe to drink. When served in unopened, factory-sealed cans or bottles, carbonated beverages, commercially prepared fruit drinks, water, alcoholic beverages, and pasteurized drinks generally can be considered safe. Because water on the outside of cans and bottles may be contaminated, they should be wiped clean and dried before opening or drinking directly from the container.

Beverages that may not be safe for consumption include fountain drinks, fruit drinks made with tap water, iced tea, and iced coffee. Because ice might be made from contaminated water, travelers in areas with unsafe tap water should request that beverages be served without ice.

Recreational Water
Pathogens that cause gastrointestinal, respiratory, skin, ear, eye, and neurologic illnesses can be transmitted by contaminated water during swimming, wading, or participating in other activities in saltwater or freshwater or the water in inadequately treated pools, interactive fountains (splash pads or spray parks), or hot tubs and spas. Water contaminated by sewage, animal waste, wastewater runoff, or human feces from swimmers can appear clear but still contain disease-causing pathogens or chemicals. Ingesting even small amounts of such water can cause illness. Pathogens, such as *Cryptosporidium*, can survive for days even in well-maintained pools and interactive fountains. Travelers should avoid ingesting any water in which they are swimming, wading, or participating in other

recreational activities. They also should not swim when they have open cuts, abrasions, or other wounds that could serve as entry points for pathogens. To protect other swimmers, children and adults with diarrhea should *not* enter the water to avoid contaminating it.

Maintaining proper chlorine or bromine levels and pH is necessary to prevent transmission of most infectious pathogens in water in pools and interactive fountains. Travelers should avoid pools and interactive fountains if the water is cloudy. Additional pool user tips can be found at www.cdc.gov/healthywater/pdf/swimming/resources/pool-user-tips-factsheet.pdf.

Maintaining proper chlorine or bromine levels in hot tubs and spas may be especially difficult, because the high water temperature depletes their concentration. *Pseudomonas*, which can cause "hot tub rash" and "swimmer's ear," and *Legionella* (see Chapter 3, Legionellosis) can multiply in hot tubs and spas in which chlorine or bromine levels are not properly maintained. Travelers should avoid hot tubs and spas where bather limits are not enforced or where the water is visibly cloudy. Additional tips can be found at www.cdc.gov/healthywater/pdf/swimming/resources/hot-tub-user-tips-factsheet.pdf. Travelers at increased risk for legionellosis, such as the elderly or those with immuno-compromising conditions such as cancer or diabetes, may choose to avoid high-risk areas such hot tubs or spas (see Chapter 3, Legionellosis).

To protect their health in oceans, lakes, and rivers, travelers should try not to swim or wade 1) in water that may be contaminated with sewage, human or animal feces, or wastewater runoff; 2) near storm drains; 3) after heavy rainfall; 4) in freshwater streams, canals, and lakes in schistosomiasis-endemic areas of the Caribbean, South America, Africa, and Asia (see Chapter 3, Schistosomiasis); 5) in water that may be contaminated with urine from animals infected with *Leptospira* (see Chapter 3, Leptospirosis); or 6) in warm seawater when they have cuts, abrasions, or other wounds. To help prevent a rare but fatal infection caused by *Naegleria fowleri* (www.cdc.gov/parasites/naegleria), a parasite found in warm freshwater around the world, travelers should prevent water from entering the nose by holding the nose shut or wearing a nose clip when swimming, diving, or participating in similar activities in warm freshwater (including lakes, rivers, ponds, hot springs, or locations with water warmed by discharge from power plants and industrial complexes), and avoid digging in or stirring up the sediment, especially during periods of high water temperature. Although *Naegleria fowleri* infection is typically associated with exposure to recreational water, infection has also been associated with use of tap water for sinus and nasal irrigation or rinsing.

BIBLIOGRAPHY

1. Cartwright R, Colbourne J. Cryptosporidiosis and hotel swimming pools—a multifaceted challenge. Water Science and Technology: Water Supply. 2002;2(3):47–54.

2. CDC. Drinking water: camping, hiking, travel. Atlanta: CDC; 2012 [cited 2014 Sep 12]. Available from: http://www.cdc.gov/healthywater/drinking/travel/index.html.

3. CDC. *Legionella* (Legionnaires' disease and Pontiac fever) [Internet]. Atlanta: CDC; 2013 [cited 2014 Sep 12]. Available from: http://www.cdc.gov/legionella/ index.html.

4. CDC. *Naegleria fowleri*—Primary amebic meningoencephalitis (PAM). Atlanta: CDC; 2012 [cited 2014 Sep 12]. Available from: http://www.cdc.gov/ parasites/naegleria/.

5. CDC. Notes from the field: primary amebic meningoencephalitis associated with ritual nasal rinsing—St. Thomas, US Virgin Islands, 2012. MMWR Morb Mortal Wkly Rep. 2013 Nov 15;62(45):903.

6. CDC. Swimmer protection. Atlanta: CDC; 2013 [cited 2014 Sep 12]. Available from: http://www.cdc.gov/healthywater/swimming/protection/ index.html.

7. Eberhart-Phillips J, Besser RE, Tormey MP, Koo D, Feikin D, Araneta MR, et al. An outbreak of cholera from food served on an international aircraft. Epidemiol Infect. 1996 Feb;116(1):9–13.

8. Finelli L, Swerdlow D, Mertz K, Ragazzoni H, Spitalny K. Outbreak of cholera associated with crab brought from an area with epidemic disease. J Infect Dis. 1992 Dec;166(6):1433–5.

9. Yoder JS, Straif-Bourgeois S, Roy SL, Moore TA, Visvesvara GS, Ratard RC, et al. Primary amebic meningoencephalitis deaths associated with sinus irrigation using contaminated tap water. Clin Infect Dis. 2012 Nov; 55(9):e79–85.

Perspectives

PREVENTION OF TRAVELERS' DIARRHEA—IT'S NOT ONLY WHAT YOU EAT & DRINK

David R. Shlim

Travel health providers in the 1980s seemed certain that travelers' diarrhea (TD) could be avoided by observing sensible food precautions. A consensus statement published in 1985 concluded, "Data indicate that meticulous attention to food and beverage preparation can decrease the likelihood of developing TD." The experts in the consensus group had 7 studies available to them at that time. In retrospect, it is surprising to note that 6 of the studies concluded that there was no relationship between recommended food and water precautions and the likelihood of developing TD. The seventh article showed a small correlation between eating "mistakes" and the likelihood of developing TD in the first 3 days of a journey.

Overall, the risk of acquiring TD in many countries has not decreased in the >50 years since the syndrome was first characterized in Mexico, despite decades of messages urging travelers to follow food and water precautions. The earliest study that addressed the question of food and water precautions was published in 1973; it concluded that "drinking bottled liquids, and avoiding salads, raw vegetables, and unpeeled fruits failed to prevent illness." In a study of returning travelers from Mexico and Peru published in 1978, in which >70% of travelers reported TD, the author noted that "avoidance of tap water, uncooked foods, and ice cubes did not make a difference in the outcome." In a famous study in 1983, a survey of >10,000 travelers worldwide found not only that observing food and water precautions failed to prevent TD, but also that people who claimed that they exercised more caution were at increased risk of acquiring TD: "Diarrhea seemed to occur more frequently the more a person tried to elude it!" Although careful travelers are unlikely to have more diarrhea than careless eaters, the authors were not able to confirm what seemed logical—that careful travelers will have *less* diarrhea.

Although these studies do not appear to support the traditional guidance, travelers should not abandon common sense in regard to being careful with food and water. However, the question remains as to why travelers do not measurably decrease their risk of diarrhea even when trying to be scrupulous with food and water precautions.

Since the 1980s, studies have suggested that *where* travelers eat makes more difference than *what* they eat. At least 3 studies have shown that people who eat in restaurants have a significantly higher risk of TD than expatriates who eat in their own homes. Investigation into the state of restaurant hygiene in several developing countries has demonstrated that many basic health precautions are violated. Some restaurants fail to provide sinks for employees to wash their hands after going to the toilet. Cutting boards may not be washed between cutting raw meat and peeling and cutting vegetables. Foods are cooked, but then may be left to sit at ambient temperatures for extended periods of time because of a paucity of refrigerator space or power cuts. Windows may not be screened to keep out flies. Defrosting meat can sit on a refrigerator shelf and drip juices on cooked foods. In tourist destinations where these restaurant violations were corrected, the rate of TD among the tourists visiting those sites decreased substantially.

How should this information be used in the pre-travel consultation? A few rules have been proven to help. Food that is served hot is almost always safe to eat. However, eating local foods is for some a major activity associated with travel, and travelers who eat only food that is cooked and "steaming," may feel as if they are missing an essential part of the travel experience. Foods that are cooked earlier in the day and sit out for long periods of time, such as on a buffet, can be unsafe. Dry foods such as cakes, cookies, and bread are usually safe. Beverages that come in factory-sealed containers are safe. All carbonated beverages that come in sealed bottles or cans should be safe because of their high acidity.

Because the risk of TD is not 100% avoidable by taking food and water precautions, travelers should always be counseled on self-diagnosis and treatment strategies. Future reductions in the rate of TD are more likely to be attributable to improved restaurant hygiene in developing countries than strategies applied by travelers themselves. Expatriates can control food preparation in their own kitchens, but poor restaurant hygiene in developing countries will continue to pose a risk for a high percentage of travelers.

BIBLIOGRAPHY

1. Ashley DV, Walters C, Dockery-Brown C, McNab A, Ashley DE. Interventions to prevent and control food-borne diseases associated with a reduction in traveler's diarrhea in tourists to Jamaica. J Travel Med. 2004 Nov–Dec;11(6):364–7.

2. Blaser MJ. Environmental interventions for the prevention of travelers' diarrhea. Rev Infect Dis. 1986 May–Jun;8 Suppl 2:S142–50.

3. Ericsson CD, Pickering LK, Sullivan P, DuPont HL. The role of location of food consumption in the prevention of travelers' diarrhea in Mexico. Gastroenterology. 1980 Nov;79(5 Pt 1):812–6.

4. NIH Consensus Development Conference. Travelers' diarrhea. JAMA. 1985 May 10;253(18):2700–4.

5. Shlim DR. Looking for evidence that personal hygiene precautions prevent traveler's diarrhea. Clin Infect Dis. 2005 Dec 1;41 Suppl 8:S531–5.

6. Shlim DR. Update in traveler's diarrhea. Infect Dis Clin North Am. 2005 Mar;19(1):137–49.

7. Tjoa WS, DuPont HL, Sullivan P, Pickering LK, Holguin AH, Olarte J, et al. Location of food consumption and travelers' diarrhea. Am J Epidemiol. 1977 Jul;106(1):61–6.

WATER DISINFECTION FOR TRAVELERS

Howard D. Backer

RISK FOR TRAVELERS

Waterborne disease is a risk for international travelers who visit countries that have poor hygiene and inadequate sanitation, and for wilderness visitors who rely on surface water in any country, including the United States. The list of potential waterborne pathogens is extensive and includes bacteria, viruses, protozoa, and parasitic helminths. Most of the organisms that can cause travelers' diarrhea can be waterborne. Where treated tap water is available, most travelers' intestinal infections are probably transmitted by food, but aging or inadequate water treatment infrastructure may not effectively disinfect water or maintain water quality during distribution. Where untreated surface or well water is used and there is no sanitation infrastructure, the risk of waterborne infection is high. Microorganisms with small infectious doses (such as *Giardia*, *Cryptosporidium*, *Shigella*, *Escherichia coli* O157:H7, and norovirus) can even cause illness through recreational water exposure, via inadvertent water ingestion.

Bottled water has become the convenient solution for most travelers, but in some places it may not be superior to tap water. Moreover, the plastic bottles create an ecological problem, since most developing countries do not recycle plastic bottles. All international travelers, especially long-term travelers or expatriates, should become familiar with and use simple methods to ensure safe drinking water. Several methods are scalable and some can be improvised from local resources, allowing adaptation to disaster relief and refugee situations. Table 2-9 compares benefits and limitations of different methods.

FIELD TECHNIQUES FOR WATER TREATMENT

Heat

Common intestinal pathogens are readily inactivated by heat. Microorganisms are killed in a shorter time at higher temperatures, whereas temperatures as low as 140°F (60°C) are effective with a longer contact time. Pasteurization uses this principle to kill foodborne enteric pathogens and spoilage-causing organisms at temperatures between 140°F (60°C) and 158°F (70°C), well below the boiling point of water (212°F [100°C]).

Although boiling is not necessary to kill common intestinal pathogens, it is the only easily recognizable end point that does not require a thermometer. All organisms except bacterial spores, which are rarely waterborne enteric pathogens, are killed in seconds at boiling temperature. In addition, the time required to heat the water from 60°C to boiling works toward heat disinfection. Although any water that is brought to a boil should be adequately disinfected, to allow for a margin of safety, boil for 1 minute. Although the boiling point decreases with altitude, at common terrestrial travel elevations it is still above temperatures required to inactivate enteric pathogens. To conserve fuel, the same results can be obtained by bringing water to a boil and then turning off the stove but keeping the container covered for several minutes.

If no other means of water treatment is available, a potential alternative to boiling is to use tap water that is too hot to touch, which is probably at a temperature between 131°F (55°C) and 140°F (60°C). This temperature may be adequate to kill pathogens if the water has been kept hot in the tank for some time. Travelers with access to electricity can bring a small electric heating coil or a lightweight beverage warmer to boil water.

Filtration and Clarification

Portable hand-pump or gravity-drip filters with various designs and types of filter media are commercially available to international travelers. Filter pore size is the primary determinant of a filter's effectiveness, but microorganisms also adhere to filter media by electrochemical reactions. Microfilters with

Table 2-9. Comparison of water disinfection techniques

TECHNIQUE	ADVANTAGES	DISADVANTAGES
Heat	• Does not impart additional taste or color • Single step that inactivates all enteric pathogens • Efficacy is not compromised by contaminants or particles in the water as for halogenation and filtration	• Does not improve taste, smell, or appearance of source water • Fuel sources may be scarce, expensive, or unavailable • Does not prevent recontamination during storage
Filtration	• Simple to operate • Requires no holding time for treatment • Large choice of commercial product designs • Adds no unpleasant taste and often improves taste and appearance of water • Can be combined with halogens to remove or kill all pathogenic waterborne microbes	• Adds bulk and weight to baggage • Many filters do not reliably remove viruses • Channeling of water or high pressure can force microorganisms through the filter • More expensive than chemical treatment • Eventually clogs from suspended particulate matter and may require some field maintenance or repair • Does not prevent recontamination during storage
Halogens (chlorine, iodine)	• Inexpensive and widely available in liquid or tablet form • Taste can be removed by simple techniques • Flexible dosing • Equally easy to treat large and small volumes • Will preserve microbiologic quality of stored water	• Impart taste and odor to water • Flexible dosing requires understanding of principles • Iodine is physiologically active, with potential adverse effects • Not readily effective against *Cryptosporidium* oocysts • Efficacy decreases with low water temperature and decreasing water clarity • Corrosive and stain clothing
Chlorine dioxide	• Low doses have no taste or color • Simple to use and available in liquid or tablet form • More potent than equivalent doses of chlorine • Effective against all waterborne pathogens	• Volatile and sensitive to sunlight: do not expose tablets to air, and use generated solutions rapidly • No persistent residual concentration, so does not prevent recontamination during storage
Ultraviolet (UV)	• Imparts no taste • Portable devices now available • Effective against all waterborne pathogens • Extra doses of UV can be used for added assurance and with no side effects • Solar UV exposure (SODIS) also provides substantial benefit	• Requires clear water • Does not improve taste or appearance of water • Relatively expensive (except solar) • Requires batteries or power source • Difficult to know if devices are delivering required UV doses • No persistent residual concentration, so does not prevent recontamination during storage

"absolute" pore sizes of 0.1–0.4 µm are usually effective to remove cysts and bacteria but may not adequately remove viruses, which are a major concern in water with high levels of fecal contamination (Table 2-10). Filters that claim Environmental Protection Agency (EPA) designation of water "purifier" undergo company-sponsored testing that has demonstrated removal of 10^6 bacteria, 10^4 (9,999 of 10,000) viruses, and 10^3 *Cryptosporidium* oocysts or *Giardia* cysts. (EPA does not independently test the validity of these claims.)

Progressively finer levels of filtration known as ultrafiltration, nanofiltration, and reverse osmosis filter water under pressure through semipermeable membranes and can physically remove particles smaller than 0.1 µm, including viruses, proteins, metal ions, and even salt molecules. One new portable filter design incorporates hollow fiber technology, which is a cluster of tiny tubules with variable pore sizes that can remove virus-size particles. Reverse-osmosis filters achieve nanofiltration levels that can remove all microbiologic contamination and desalinate water. The high price and slow output of small hand-pump reverse-osmosis units prohibit use by land-based travelers; however, they are important survival aids for ocean voyagers, and larger powered devices are used for military and refugee situations.

Filters made from ceramic clay or simple sand and gravel (slow sand or biosand) filters are successfully used for households in developing countries. Gravel and sand filters can be improvised in remote or austere situations when no other means of disinfection is available.

Coagulation-flocculation (CF) removes suspended particles that cause a cloudy appearance and bad taste and do not settle by gravity; this process removes many but not all microorganisms. CF is easily applied in the field. Alum, an aluminum salt that is widely used in food, cosmetic, and medical applications, or one of several other natural substances is added to the water and stirred. The clumped particulates that form are allowed to settle, then poured through a coffee filter or fine cloth to remove the sediment. Tablets or packets of powder that combine flocculent and hypochlorite disinfection are available (products include Chlor-floc and PUR Purifier of Water [Proctor and Gamble—for humanitarian use, not sold commercially]).

Granular-activated carbon (GAC) purifies water by adsorbing organic and inorganic chemicals and most heavy metals, thereby improving odor, taste, and safety. GAC is a common component of household and field filters. It may trap but does not kill organisms. In field water treatment, GAC is best

Table 2-10. Microorganism size and susceptibility to filtration

ORGANISM	AVERAGE SIZE (µm)	MAXIMUM RECOMMENDED FILTER RATING (µm ABSOLUTE)
Viruses	0.03	Not specified (optimally 0.01, ultrafiltration)
Enteric bacteria (*Escherichia coli*)	0.5 × 3.0–8.0	0.2–0.4 (microfiltration)
Cryptosporidium oocyst	4–6	1 (microfiltration)
Giardia cyst	6.0–10.0 × 8.0–15.0	3.0–5.0 (microfiltration)
Nematode eggs	30 × 60	Not specified; any microfilter
Schistosome larvae	50 × 100	Not specified; any microfilter

used after chemical disinfection to remove disinfection byproducts as well as the taste of iodine and chlorine (see Halogens below).

Chemical Disinfection

Halogens

The most common chemical water disinfectants are halogens, mainly chlorine and iodine, although bromine has similar qualities. Worldwide, chemical disinfection with chlorine is the most commonly used method for improving and maintaining the microbiologic quality of drinking water, though boiling may be more common than chemical disinfection in low- and middle-income countries. Sodium hypochlorite, the active ingredient in common household bleach, is the primary disinfectant promoted by CDC and the World Health Organization Safe Water System at a 1.5% concentration for household use in the developing world. Other chlorine-containing compounds, such as calcium hypochlorite and sodium dichloroisocyanurate, available in granular or tablet formulation, are also effective for household water treatment.

Given adequate concentrations and length of exposure (contact time), chlorine and iodine have similar activity and are effective against bacteria and viruses (www.cdc.gov/safewater/effectiveness-on-pathogens.html). *Giardia* cysts are more resistant to halogens; however, field-level concentrations are effective with longer contact times. For this reason, dosing and concentrations of halogen products are targeted to the cysts. Some common waterborne parasites, such as *Cryptosporidium*, are poorly inactivated by halogen disinfection at practical concentrations, even with extended contact times.

Since many factors for halogen disinfection in the field are uncontrolled, extending the contact time when feasible is always recommended to add a margin of safety. Chemical disinfection may be supplemented with filtration to remove resistant oocysts from drinking water. Cloudy water contains substances that will neutralize disinfectant, so it will require higher concentrations or contact times or, preferably, clarification through settling, CF, or filtration before disinfectant is added.

Both chlorine and iodine are available in liquid and tablet form. Because iodine has physiologic activity, WHO recommends limiting iodine water disinfection to a few weeks of emergency use. Iodine use is not recommended for people with unstable thyroid disease or known iodine allergy. In addition, iodine should not be used by pregnant women because of the potential effect on the fetal thyroid.

The taste of halogens in water can be improved by several means:

- Reduce concentration and increase contact time proportionally.
- After the required contact time, run water through a filter that contains activated carbon.
- After the required contact time, add a 25-mg tablet of vitamin C (or a "tiny pinch" of powdered ascorbic acid), which reduces the disinfectant to tasteless and colorless forms of chloride or iodide.

Iodine Resins

Iodine resins transfer iodine to microorganisms that come into contact with the resin, but leave little iodine dissolved in the water. The resins have been incorporated into many different filter designs available for field use. Most contain a 1-μm cyst filter, which should effectively remove protozoan cysts. Few models are sold in the United States because of inconsistent test results, but some models are still available for international use.

Salt (Sodium Chloride) Electrolysis

Passing a current through a simple brine salt solution generates oxidants, including hypochlorite, which can be used to disinfect microbes. This technique has been engineered into a pocket-sized, battery-powered product, which is commercially available.

Chlorine Dioxide

Chlorine dioxide (ClO_2) can kill most waterborne pathogens, including *Cryptosporidium* oocysts, at practical doses and contact times. Tablets and liquid formulations are available to generate chlorine dioxide in the field for small-quantity water treatment.

Ultraviolet (UV) Light

UV light kills bacteria, viruses, and *Cryptosporidium* oocysts in water. The effect depends on UV dose and exposure time. Portable battery-operated units that deliver a metered, timed dose of UV are an effective way to disinfect small quantities of clear water in the field. Larger units with higher output are available where a power source is available. These units have limited effectiveness in water with high levels of suspended solids and turbidity, because suspended particles can shield microorganisms from UV rays.

Solar Irradiation and Heating

UV irradiation by sunlight in the UVA range can substantially improve the microbiologic quality of water and may be used in austere emergency situations. Recent work has confirmed the efficacy and optimal procedures of the solar disinfection (SODIS) technique. Transparent bottles (such as clear plastic PET beverage bottles), preferably lying on a reflective surface, are exposed to sunlight for a minimum of 6 hours. UV and thermal inactivation are synergistic for solar disinfection of drinking water. Use of a simple reflector or solar cooker can achieve temperatures of 149°F (65°C), which will pasteurize the water after 4 hours. Solar disinfection is not effective on turbid water. If the headlines in a newspaper cannot be read through the bottle of water, then the water must be clarified before solar irradiation is used. Under cloudy conditions, water must be placed in the sun for 2 consecutive days.

Photocatalytic Disinfection

Advanced oxidation processes use UV light or natural sunlight to catalyze the production of potent oxidizers that are excellent disinfectants for microorganisms and can break down complex organic contaminants and even most heavy metals into nontoxic forms. Titanium dioxide (TiO_2) is the most effective substance. For field water disinfection, a product is commercially available that uses nanoparticles coated with TiO_2 that are integrated into a plastic bag and remain active for hundreds of uses.

Silver and Other Products

Silver ion has bactericidal effects in low doses and some attractive features, including absence of color, taste, and odor. The use of silver as a drinking water disinfectant is popular in Europe, but it is not approved for this purpose in the United States, because silver concentration in water is strongly affected by adsorption onto the surface of the container and there has been limited testing on viruses and cysts. In the United States, silver is approved for maintaining microbiologic quality of stored water.

Several other common products, including hydrogen peroxide, citrus juice, and potassium permanganate have antibacterial effects in water and are marketed in commercial

Table 2-11. Summary of field water disinfection techniques

	BACTERIA	VIRUSES	*GIARDIA/ AMEBAS*	CRYPTOSPORIDIA	NEMATODES/ CERCARIAE
Heat	+	+	+	+	+
Filtration	+	+/−[1]	+	+	+
Halogens	+	+	+[2]	−	+/−[3]
Chlorine dioxide and photocatalytic	+	+	+	+	+

[1] Most filters make no claims for viruses. Reverse osmosis is effective. Virus removal is based on company claims of electrostatic attraction between viruses and filter media.
[2] Require higher concentrations and contact time.
[3] Eggs are not very susceptible to halogens but risk of waterborne transmission is very low.

products for travelers. None have sufficient data to recommend them for primary water disinfection at low doses in the field.

THE PREFERRED TECHNIQUE

Table 2-11 summarizes field water disinfection techniques. The optimal technique for a person or group depends on personal preference, size of the group, water source, and the style of travel. Boiling is the most reliable single-step treatment, but certain filters,

UV, and chlorine dioxide are also effective in most situations. Optimal treatment of highly contaminated or cloudy water may require CF followed by chemical disinfection. On long-distance, ocean-going boats where water must be desalinated during the voyage, only reverse-osmosis membrane filters are adequate. Halogens are used to maintain microbiological quality of stored water because of their capacity to maintain a persistent residual concentration.

BIBLIOGRAPHY

1. Backer H. Field water disinfection. In: Auerbach PS, editor. Wilderness medicine. 6th ed. Philadelphia: Elsevier Mosby; 2012. p. 1324–59.
2. Backer H, Hollowell J. Use of iodine for water disinfection: iodine toxicity and maximum recommended dose. Environ Health Perspect. 2000 Aug;108(8):679–84.
3. CDC. Safe water systems for the developing world: a handbook for implementing household-based water treatment and safe storage projects. Atlanta: CDC; 2001 [cited 2014 Sep 19]. Available from: http://www.cdc.gov/safewater/pdf/sws-for-the-developing-world-manual.pdf.
4. Center for Affordable Water and Sanitation Technology. Biosand filter. Alberta, Canada: Center for Affordable Water and Sanitation Technology; 2012 [cited 2014 Sep 12]. Available from: http://www.cawst.org/en/resources/biosand-filter.
5. Clasen T, Roberts I, Rabie T, Schmidt W, Cairncross S. Interventions to improve water quality for preventing diarrhoea. Cochrane Database Syst Rev. 2006(3):CD004794.
6. Departments of the Army, Navy, and Air Force. TB MED 577 Technical bulletin: sanitary control and surveillance of field water supplies. Washington, DC: US Army Medical Department; 2010 [cited 2014 Sep 12]. Available from: http://armypubs.army.mil/med/DR_pubs/dr_a/pdf/tbmed577.pdf.
7. Lantagne DS. Sodium hypochlorite dosage for household and emergency water treatment. Journal of American Water Works Association. 2008;100(8):106–19.
8. McGuigan KG, Conroy RM, Mosler HJ, du Preez M, Ubomba-Jaswa E, Fernandez-Ibanez P. Solar water disinfection (SODIS): a review from bench-top to roof-top. J Hazard Mater. 2012 Oct 15;235–6:29–46.
9. Sobsey MD, Stauber CE, Casanova LM, Brown JM, Elliott MA. Point of use household drinking water filtration: A practical, effective solution for providing sustained access to safe drinking water in the developing world. Environ Sci Technol. 2008 Jun 15;42(12):4261–7.
10. Swiss Federal Institute of Aquatic Science and Technology. SODIS method. Dübendorf, Switzerland: Swiss Federal Institute of Aquatic Science and Technology; 2012 [cited 2014 Sep 12]. Available from: http://www.sodis.ch/methode/index_EN.

FOOD POISONING FROM MARINE TOXINS

Vernon E. Ansdell

Seafood poisoning from marine toxins is an under-recognized hazard for travelers, particularly in the tropics and subtropics. Furthermore, the risk is increasing because of factors such as climate change, coral reef damage, and spread of toxic algal blooms.

CIGUATERA FISH POISONING

Ciguatera fish poisoning occurs after eating reef fish contaminated with toxins such as ciguatoxin or maitotoxin. These potent toxins originate from *Gambierdiscus toxicus*, a small marine organism (dinoflagellate)

that grows on and around coral reefs. Dinoflagellates are ingested by herbivorous fish. The toxins produced by G. *toxicus* (gambiertoxins) are then modified and concentrated as they pass up the food chain to carnivorous fish and finally to humans. Ciguatoxins are concentrated in fish liver, intestines, roe, and heads.

G. *toxicus* may proliferate on dead coral reefs more effectively than other dinoflagellates. The risk of ciguatera is likely to increase as more coral reefs deteriorate because of climate change, ocean acidification, construction, and nutrient runoff.

Risk for Travelers

More than 50,000 cases of ciguatera poisoning occur globally every year. The incidence in travelers to highly endemic areas has been estimated as high as 3 per 100. Ciguatera is widespread in tropical and subtropical waters, usually between the latitudes of 35°N and 35°S; it is particularly common in the Pacific and Indian Oceans and the Caribbean Sea. The incidence and geographic distribution of ciguatera poisoning are increasing. Newly recognized areas of risk include the Canary Islands, the eastern Mediterranean, and the western Gulf of Mexico.

Fish that are most likely to cause ciguatera poisoning are carnivorous reef fish, including barracuda, grouper, moray eel, amberjack, sea bass, or sturgeon. Omnivorous and herbivorous fish such as parrot fish, surgeonfish, and red snapper can also be a risk.

Clinical Presentation

Typical ciguatera poisoning results in a gastrointestinal illness and may also cause neurologic symptoms. Although very rare, cardiovascular collapse may result. The first symptoms generally include nausea, vomiting, diarrhea, and abdominal pain, followed by neurologic symptoms such as paresthesias, pain in the teeth or the sensation that the teeth are loose, itching, metallic taste, blurred vision, or even transient blindness. Cold allodynia (abnormal sensation when touching cold water or objects) has historically been reported as characteristic, though new studies have found that there can be acute sensitivity to both hot and cold. Neurologic symptoms usually last a few days to several weeks.

The overall death rate from ciguatera poisoning is <0.1% but varies according to the toxin dose and availability of medical care to deal with complications. The diagnosis of ciguatera poisoning is based on the clinical signs and symptoms and a history of eating species of fish that are known to carry ciguatera toxin. Fish testing can be done by the Food and Drug Administration (FDA) in their laboratory at Dauphin Island. There is no easily available test for ciguatera toxins in human clinical specimens.

Prevention

Travelers can take the following precautions to prevent ciguatera fish poisoning:

- Avoid or limit consumption of the reef fish listed above, especially if the fish weighed >6 lb (2.7 kg).
- Never eat high-risk fish such as barracuda or moray eel.
- Avoid the parts of the fish that concentrate ciguatera toxin: liver, intestines, roe, and head

Remember that ciguatera toxins do not affect the texture, taste, or smell of fish, and they are not destroyed by gastric acid, cooking, smoking, freezing, canning, salting, or pickling.

Treatment

There is no specific antidote for ciguatoxin or maitotoxin poisonings. Treatment is generally for specific symptoms and includes supportive care. Intravenous mannitol has been reported in uncontrolled studies to reduce the severity and duration of neurologic symptoms, particularly if given within 48 hours of the appearance of symptoms.

SCOMBROID

Scombroid, one of the most common fish poisonings, occurs worldwide in both temperate and tropical waters. The illness occurs after eating improperly refrigerated or preserved fish containing high levels of histamine, and often resembles a moderate to severe allergic reaction.

Fish typically associated with scombroid have naturally high levels of histidine in the flesh and include tuna, mackerel, mahimahi (dolphin fish), sardine, anchovy, herring, bluefish, amberjack, and marlin.

Histidine is converted to histamine by bacterial overgrowth in fish that has been improperly stored after capture. Histamine and other scombrotoxins are resistant to cooking, smoking, canning, or freezing.

Clinical Presentation

Symptoms of scombroid poisoning resemble an acute allergic reaction and usually appear 10–60 minutes after eating contaminated fish. They include flushing of the face and upper body (resembling sunburn), severe headache, palpitations, itching, blurred vision, abdominal cramps, and diarrhea. Untreated, symptoms usually resolve within 12 hours. Rarely, there may be respiratory compromise, malignant arrhythmias, and hypotension requiring hospitalization. Diagnosis is usually clinical. A clustering of cases helps exclude the possibility of true fish allergy.

Prevention

Fish contaminated with histamine may have a peppery, sharp, salty, taste or "bubbly" feel but may also look, smell, and taste normal. The key to prevention is to make sure that the fish is properly iced or refrigerated at temperatures <38°F (<3.3°C), or immediately frozen after it is caught. Cooking, smoking, canning, or freezing will not destroy histamine in contaminated fish.

Treatment

Scombroid poisoning usually responds well to antihistamines (H_1-receptor blockers, although H_2-receptor blockers may also be of benefit).

SHELLFISH POISONING

Several forms of shellfish poisoning may occur after ingesting filter-feeding bivalve mollusks (such as mussels, oysters, clams, scallops, and cockles) that contain potent toxins. The toxins originate in small marine organisms (dinoflagellates or diatoms) that are ingested and are concentrated by shellfish.

Risk for Travelers

Contaminated shellfish may be found in temperate and tropical waters, typically during or after dinoflagellate blooms called harmful algal blooms (HABs). One example of a HAB is the Florida red tide caused by *Karenia brevis*.

Clinical Presentation

Poisoning results in gastrointestinal and neurologic illness of varying severity. Symptoms typically appear 30–60 minutes after ingesting toxic shellfish but can be delayed for several hours. Diagnosis is usually one of exclusion and is usually made clinically in patients who recently ate shellfish.

Paralytic Shellfish Poisoning

Paralytic shellfish poisoning (PSP) is the most common and most severe form of shellfish poisoning. PSP is caused by eating shellfish contaminated with saxitoxins produced by dinoflagellates from *Aelxandrium, Pyrodinium,* and *Gymnodinium* genera. Symptoms usually appear 30–60 minutes after eating toxic shellfish and include numbness and tingling of the face, lips, tongue, arms, and legs. There may be headache, nausea, vomiting, and diarrhea. Severe cases are associated with ingestion of large doses of toxin and clinical features such as ataxia, dysphagia, mental status changes, flaccid paralysis, and respiratory failure. The case-fatality ratio is dependent on the availability of modern medical care, including mechanical ventilation. The death rate may be particularly high in children.

Neurotoxic Shellfish Poisoning

Neurotoxin shellfish poisoning is caused by eating shellfish contaminated with brevetoxins produced by the dinoflagellate *K. brevis.* Neurotoxic shellfish poisoning usually presents as gastroenteritis accompanied by minor neurologic symptoms resembling mild ciguatera poisoning or mild paralytic shellfish poisoning. Inhalation of aerosolized toxin in the sea spray associated with a Florida red tide (*K. brevis* bloom) can induce bronchoconstriction and may cause acute, temporary respiratory discomfort in healthy people. People with asthma may experience more severe and prolonged respiratory effects.

Diarrheic Shellfish Poisoning

Diarrheic shellfish poisoning (DSP) is caused by eating shellfish contaminated with a group of toxins that include polyether molecules (such as okadaic acid) produced by dinoflagellates from the genera *Dinophysis* and *Prorocentrum lima.* DSP produces chills, nausea, vomiting, abdominal cramps, and diarrhea. No deaths have been reported.

Amnesic Shellfish Poisoning

Amnesic shellfish poisoning (ASP) is a rare form of shellfish poisoning caused by eating shellfish, particularly blue mussels, contaminated with domoic acid produced by the diatom *Nitzchia pungens*. The first cases of ASP were reported after an outbreak associated with eating contaminated cultivated mussels. These cases were reported to have severe gastroenteric and neurologic symptoms. More recently, domoic acid exposure via the food web was implicated in die-off of marine mammals along the US Pacific Coast.

Prevention

Shellfish poisoning can be prevented by avoiding potentially contaminated bivalve mollusks. This is particularly important in areas during or shortly after algal blooms, which may be locally referred to as "red tides" or "brown tides." Travelers to developing countries should avoid eating all shellfish, because they carry a high risk of viral and bacterial infections. Marine shellfish toxins cannot be destroyed by cooking or freezing.

Treatment

Treatment is symptomatic and supportive. Severe cases of paralytic shellfish poisoning may require mechanical ventilation.

BIBLIOGRAPHY

1. Ansdell V. Food-borne illness. In: Keystone JS, Freedman DO, Kozarsky PE, Connor BA, Nothdurft HD, editors. Travel Medicine. 3rd ed. Philadelphia: Saunders Elsevier; 2013. p. 425–32.
2. Backer L, Fleming L, Rowan A, Baden D. Epidemiology and public health of human illnesses associated with harmful marine algae. In: Hallegraeff GM, Anderson DM, Cembella A, editors. Manual on Harmful Marine Microalgae. Paris: UNESCO; 2003. p. 723–49.
3. Backer LC, Schurz-Rogers H, Fleming LE, Kirkpatrick B, Benson J. Marine phycotoxins in seafood. In: Dąbrowski WM, Sikorski ZE, editors. Toxins in Food. Boca Raton, FL: CRC Press; 2005. p. 144–74.
4. Hungerford JM. Scombroid poisoning: a review. Toxicon. 2010 Aug 15;56(2):231–43.
5. Isbister GK, Kiernan MC. Neurotoxic marine poisoning. Lancet Neurol. 2005 Apr;4(4):219–28.
6. Palafox NA, Buenoconsejo-Lum LE. Ciguatera fish poisoning: review of clinical manifestations. J Toxicol Toxin Rev. 2001;20(2):141–60.
7. Perl TM, Bedard L, Kosatsky T, Hockin JC, Todd EC, Remis RS. An outbreak of toxic encephalopathy caused by eating mussels contaminated with domoic acid. N Engl J Med. 1990 Jun 21;322(25):1775–80.
8. Schnorf H, Taurarii M, Cundy T. Ciguatera fish poisoning: a double-blind randomized trial of mannitol therapy. Neurology. 2002 Mar 26;58(6):873–80.
9. Sobel J, Painter J. Illnesses caused by marine toxins. Clin Infect Dis. 2005 Nov 1;41(9):1290–6.
10. Stewart I, Lewis RJ, Eaglesham GK, Graham GC, Poole S, Craig SB. Emerging tropical diseases in Australia. Part 2. Ciguatera fish poisoning. Ann Trop Med Parasitol. 2010 Oct;104(7):557–71.

PROTECTION AGAINST MOSQUITOES, TICKS, & OTHER ARTHROPODS

Roger S. Nasci, Robert A. Wirtz, William G. Brogdon

Vaccines or chemoprophylactic drugs are available to protect against some vector-borne diseases such as yellow fever, Japanese encephalitis, and malaria; however, travel health practitioners should advise travelers to use repellents and other general protective measures against biting arthropods. The effectiveness of malaria chemoprophylaxis is variable, depending on patterns of drug resistance, bioavailability, and compliance with medication, and no similar preventive measures exist for other mosquitoborne diseases such as dengue, chikungunya, Zika, and West Nile encephalitis or tickborne diseases such as Lyme borreliosis, tickborne encephalitis, and relapsing fever.

The Environmental Protection Agency (EPA) regulates repellent products in the United States. CDC recommends that consumers use repellent products that have been registered by EPA. EPA registration indicates the materials have been reviewed and approved for both efficacy and human safety when applied according to the instructions on the label.

GENERAL PROTECTIVE MEASURES

Avoid outbreaks. To the extent possible, travelers should avoid known foci of epidemic disease transmission. The CDC Travelers' Health website provides updates on regional disease transmission patterns and outbreaks (www.cdc.gov/travel).

Be aware of peak exposure times and places. Exposure to arthropod bites may be reduced if travelers modify their patterns or locations of activity. Although mosquitoes may bite at any time of day, peak biting activity for vectors of some diseases (such as dengue and chikungunya) is during daylight hours. Vectors of other diseases (such as malaria) are most active in twilight periods (dawn and dusk) or in the evening after dark. Avoiding the outdoors or taking preventive actions (such as using repellent) during peak biting hours may reduce risk. Place also matters; ticks and chiggers are often found in grasses, woodlands, or other vegetated areas. Local health officials or guides may be able to point out areas with increased arthropod activity.

Wear appropriate clothing. Travelers can minimize areas of exposed skin by wearing long-sleeved shirts, long pants, boots, and hats. Tucking in shirts, tucking pants into socks, and wearing closed shoes instead of sandals may reduce risk. Repellents or insecticides, such as permethrin, can be applied to clothing and gear for added protection. (Additional information on clothing is below.)

Check for ticks. Travelers should inspect themselves and their clothing for ticks during outdoor activity and at the end of the day. Prompt removal of attached ticks can prevent some infections. Showering within 2 hours of being in a tick-infested area reduces the risk of some tickborne diseases.

Bed nets. When accommodations are not adequately screened or air conditioned, bed nets are essential in providing protection and reducing discomfort caused by biting insects. If bed nets do not reach the floor, they should be tucked under mattresses. Bed nets are most effective when they are treated with a pyrethroid insecticide. Pretreated, long-lasting bed nets can be purchased before traveling, or nets can be treated after purchase. Effective, treated nets may also be available in destination countries. Nets treated with a pyrethroid insecticide will be effective for several months if they are not washed. Long-lasting pretreated nets may be effective for much longer.

Insecticides and spatial repellents. More spatial repellent products are becoming commercially available. These products, containing active ingredients such as metofluthrin and allethrin, augment aerosol insecticide sprays, vaporizing mats, and mosquito coils that have been available for some time. Such products can help to clear rooms or areas of mosquitoes (spray aerosols) or repel mosquitoes from a circumscribed area (coils, spatial repellents). Although many of these products appear to have repellent or insecticidal activity under particular conditions, they have not yet been adequately evaluated in peer-reviewed studies for their efficacy in preventing vectorborne disease. Travelers should supplement the use of these products with repellent on skin or clothing and using bed nets in areas where vectorborne diseases are a risk or biting arthropods are noted. Since some products available internationally may contain pesticides that are not registered in the United States, it may be preferable for travelers to bring their own. Insecticides and repellent products should always be used with caution, avoiding direct inhalation of spray or smoke.

Optimum protection can be provided by applying the repellents described in the following sections to clothing and to exposed skin (Box 2-3).

REPELLENTS FOR USE ON SKIN AND CLOTHING

CDC has evaluated information published in peer-reviewed scientific literature and data available from EPA to identify several types of EPA-registered products that provide repellent activity sufficient to help people reduce the bites of disease-carrying mosquitoes.

Products containing the following active ingredients typically provide reasonably long-lasting protection:

- **DEET** (chemical name: N,N-diethyl-m-toluamide or N,N-diethyl-3-methyl-benzamide). Products containing DEET include, but are not limited to, Off!, Cutter, Sawyer, and Ultrathon.
- **Picaridin** (KBR 3023 [Bayrepel] and icaridin outside the United States; chemical name: 2-(2-hydroxyethyl)-1-piperidinecarboxylic acid 1-methylpropyl ester). Products containing picaridin include, but are not limited to, Cutter Advanced, Skin So Soft Bug Guard Plus, and Autan (outside the United States).
- **Oil of lemon eucalyptus (OLE) or PMD** (chemical name: para-menthane-3,8-diol), the synthesized version of OLE. Products containing OLE and PMD include, but are not limited to, Repel and Off! Botanicals. This recommendation refers to EPA-registered repellent products containing the active ingredient OLE (or PMD). "Pure" oil of lemon eucalyptus (essential oil not formulated as a repellent) is not recommended; it has not undergone similar, validated testing for safety and efficacy, is not registered with EPA as an insect repellent, and is not covered by this recommendation.
- **IR3535** (chemical name: 3-[N-butyl-N-acetyl]-aminopropionic acid, ethyl ester). Products containing IR3535 include, but are not limited to, Skin So Soft Bug Guard Plus Expedition and SkinSmart.

EPA characterizes the active ingredients DEET and picaridin as "conventional repellents" and OLE, PMD, and IR3535 as "biopesticide repellents," which are either derived from or are synthetic versions of natural materials.

Repellent Efficacy

Published data indicate that repellent efficacy and duration of protection vary considerably among products and among mosquito and tick species. Product efficacy and duration of protection are also markedly affected by ambient temperature, level of activity, amount of perspiration, exposure to water, abrasive removal, and other factors. In general, higher concentrations of active ingredient provide longer duration of protection, regardless of the active ingredient. Products with <10% active ingredient may offer only limited protection, often 1–2 hours. Products that offer sustained-release or controlled-release (microencapsulated) formulations, even with lower active ingredient concentrations, may provide longer protection times. Studies suggest that concentrations of DEET above approximately 50% do not offer a marked increase in protection time against mosquitoes; DEET efficacy tends to plateau at a concentration of approximately 50%. CDC recommends using products with ≥20% DEET on exposed skin to reduce biting by ticks that may spread disease.

Recommendations are based on peer-reviewed journal articles and scientific studies and data submitted to regulatory agencies. People may experience some variation in protection from different products. Regardless of what product is used, if travelers start to get insect bites they should reapply the repellent according to the label instructions, try a different product, or, if possible, leave the area with biting insects.

Ideally, repellents should be purchased before traveling and can be found online or in hardware stores, drug stores, and supermarkets. A wide variety of repellents can be found in camping, sporting goods, and military surplus stores. When purchasing repellents overseas, look for the active ingredients specified above on the product labels; some names of products available internationally have been specified in the list above.

Repellency Awareness Graphic

The Environmental Protection Agency (EPA) allows companies to apply for permission to include a new repellency awareness graphic on the labels of insect repellents that are applied to the skin (Figure 2-1). The graphic helps consumers easily identify the time a repellent is effective against mosquitoes and ticks. EPA reviews products that apply to use the graphic to ensure that their data meet current testing protocols and standard evaluation practices. Use of this graphic by manufacturers is voluntary. For more information, visit www2.epa.gov/insect-repellents/repellency-awareness-graphic.

Repellents and Sunscreen

Repellents that are applied according to label instructions may be used with sunscreen with no reduction in repellent activity; however, limited data show a one-third decrease in the sun protection factor (SPF) of sunscreens when DEET-containing insect repellents are used after a sunscreen is applied. Products that combine sunscreen

FIGURE 2-1. SAMPLE REPELLENCY AWARENESS GRAPHIC FOR SKIN-APPLIED INSECT REPELLENTS[1]

[1] Image from: www2.epa.gov/insect-repellents/repellency-awareness-graphic

and repellent are not recommended, because sunscreen may need to be reapplied more often and in larger amounts than needed for the repellent component to provide protection from biting insects. In general, the recommendation is to use separate products, applying sunscreen first and then applying the repellent. Due to the decrease in SPF when using a DEET-containing insect repellent after applying sunscreen, travelers may need to reapply the sunscreen more frequently.

Repellents and Insecticides for Use on Clothing

Clothing, hats, shoes, bed nets, jackets, and camping gear can be treated with permethrin for added protection. Products such as Permanone and Sawyer, Permethrin, Repel, and Ultrathon Permethrin Clothing Treatment are registered with EPA specifically for use by consumers to treat clothing and gear. Alternatively, clothing pretreated with permethrin is commercially available, marketed to consumers in the United States as Insect Shield, BugsAway, or Insect Blocker.

Permethrin is a highly effective insecticide-acaricide and repellent.

Permethrin-treated clothing repels and kills ticks, chiggers, mosquitoes, and other biting and nuisance arthropods. Clothing and other items must be treated 24–48 hours in advance of travel to allow them to dry. As with all pesticides, follow the label instructions when using permethrin clothing treatments.

Permethrin-treated materials retain repellency or insecticidal activity after repeated laundering but should be retreated, as described on the product label, to provide continued protection. Clothing that is treated before purchase is labeled for efficacy through 70 launderings. Clothing treated with the other repellent products described above (such as DEET) provides protection from biting arthropods but will not last through washing and will require more frequent reapplications.

Precautions when Using Insect Repellents

Travelers should take the following precautions:

- Apply repellents only to exposed skin or clothing, as directed on the product label. Do not apply repellents under clothing.
- Never use repellents over cuts, wounds, or irritated skin.
- When using sprays, do not spray directly on face—spray on hands first and then apply to face. Do not apply repellents to eyes or mouth, and apply sparingly around ears.
- Wash hands after application to avoid accidental exposure to eyes or ingestion.
- Children should not handle repellents. Instead, adults should apply repellents to their own hands first, and then gently spread on the child's exposed skin. Avoid applying directly to children's hands. After returning indoors, wash your child's treated skin and clothing with soap and water or give the child a bath.
- Use just enough repellent to cover exposed skin or clothing. Heavy application and saturation are generally unnecessary for effectiveness. If biting insects do not respond to a thin film of repellent, apply a bit more.
- After returning indoors, wash repellent-treated skin with soap and water or bathe.

Wash treated clothing before wearing it again. This precaution may vary with different repellents—check the product label.

If a traveler experiences a rash or other reaction, such as itching or swelling, from an insect repellent, the repellent should be washed off with mild soap and water and its use discontinued. If a severe reaction has occurred, a local poison-control center should be called for further guidance, if feasible. Travelers seeking health care because of the repellent should take the repellent to the doctor's office and show the doctor. Permethrin should *never* be applied to skin but only to clothing, bed nets, or other fabrics as directed on the product label.

Children and Pregnant Women

Most repellents can be used on children aged >2 months. Protect infants aged <2 months from mosquitoes by using an infant carrier draped with mosquito netting with an elastic edge for a tight fit. Products containing OLE specify that they should not be used on children aged <3 years. Other than the safety tips listed above, EPA does not recommend any additional precautions for using registered repellents on children or on pregnant or lactating women.

Useful Links

- Insect Repellents: Use and Effectiveness (EPA): http://cfpub.epa.gov/oppref/insect/
- Using Insect Repellents Safely (EPA): http://epa.gov/pesticides/insect/safe.htm
- FAQ: Insect Repellent Use and Safety (CDC): www.cdc.gov/westnile/faq/repellent.html
- Choosing and Using Insect Repellents (National Pesticide Information Center): http://npic.orst.edu/ingred/ptype/repel.html

BEDBUGS

There has been a recent resurgence in bedbug infestations worldwide, particularly in developed countries. Although bedbugs do not transmit diseases, their bites may be a nuisance. Travelers can take measures to avoid bedbug bites and avoid transporting them in luggage and clothing (Box 2-4).

BOX 2-4. BEDBUGS AND INTERNATIONAL TRAVEL

A recent resurgence in bedbug infestations worldwide, particularly in developed countries, is thought to be related to the increase in international travel, pest control strategy changes in travel lodgings, and insecticide resistance. Bedbug infestations have been increasingly reported in hotels, theaters, and any locations where people congregate, even in the workplace, dormitories, and schools. Bedbugs may be transported in luggage and on clothing. Transport of personal belongings in contaminated transport vehicles is another means of spread of these insects.

Bedbugs are small, flat insects that are reddish-brown in color, wingless, and range from 1 to 7 mm in length. Although bedbugs have not been shown to transmit disease, their bites can produce strong allergic reactions and considerable emotional stress.

Protective Measures against Bedbugs

Travelers should be encouraged to take the following precautions to avoid or reduce their exposure to bedbugs:

- Inspect the premises of hotels or other sleeping locations for bedbugs on mattresses, box springs, bedding, and furniture, particularly built-in furniture with the bed, desk, and closets as a continuous structural unit. Travelers who observe evidence of bedbug activity—whether it be the bugs themselves or physical signs such as blood-spotting on linens—should seek alternative lodging.
- Keep suitcases closed when they are not in use and try to keep them off the floor.
- Remove clothing and personal items (such as toiletry bags and shaving kits) from the suitcase only when they are in use.
- Carefully inspect clothing and personal items before returning them to the suitcase.
- Keep in mind that bedbug eggs and nymphs are very small and can be easily overlooked.

Prevention is by far the most effective and inexpensive way to protect oneself from these pests. The costs of ridding a personal residence of these insects are considerable, and efforts at control are often not immediately successful even when conducted by professionals.

BIBLIOGRAPHY

1. Barnard DR, Xue RD. Laboratory evaluation of mosquito repellents against *Aedes albopictus, Culex nigripalpus*, and *Ochlerotatus triseriatus* (Diptera: Culicidae). J Med Entomol. 2004 Jul;41(4):726–30.

2. Fradin MS, Day JF. Comparative efficacy of insect repellents against mosquito bites. N Engl J Med. 2002 Jul 4;347(1):13–8.

3. Goodyer LI, Croft AM, Frances SP, Hill N, Moore SJ, Onyango SP, et al. Expert review of the evidence base for arthropod bite avoidance. J Travel Med. 2010 May–Jun;17(3):182–92.

4. Lupi E, Hatz C, Schlagenhauf P. The efficacy of repellents against *Aedes, Anopheles, Culex* and *Ixodes* spp.—a literature review. Travel Med Infect Dis. 2013 Nov–Dec;11(6):374–411.

5. Montemarano AD, Gupta RK, Burge JR, Klein K. Insect repellents and the efficacy of sunscreens. Lancet. 1997 Jun 7;349(9066):1670–1.

6. Murphy ME, Montemarano AD, Debboun M, Gupta R. The effect of sunscreen on the efficacy of insect repellent: a clinical trial. J Am Acad Dermatol. 2000 Aug;43(2 Pt 1):219–22.

7. Pages F, Dautel H, Duvallet G, Kahl O, de Gentile L, Boulanger N. Tick repellents for human use: prevention of tick bites and tick-borne diseases. Vector Borne Zoonotic Dis. 2014 Feb;14(2):85–93.

SUN EXPOSURE

Vernon E. Ansdell, Amy K. Reisenauer

Increased exposure to ultraviolet (UV) radiation occurs near the equator, during summer months, at high elevation, and between 10 AM and 4 PM. Reflection from the snow, sand, and water increases exposure, a particularly important consideration for snow skiing, beach activities, swimming, and sailing. In addition, several common medications may cause photosensitivity reactions in travelers:

- Acetazolamide
- Amiodarone
- Antibiotics (fluoroquinolones, sulfonamides, and tetracyclines, especially demeclocycline and doxycycline)
- Furosemide
- Nonsteroidal anti-inflammatory drugs
- Phenothiazines
- Sulfonylureas
- Thiazide diuretics
- Voriconazole

Medical conditions such as connective tissue diseases, polymorphous light eruption, rosacea, and vitiligo can increase sun sensitivity, and alcohol consumption can lead to behavioral changes that increase the risk of sunburn.

Both UVA rays (320–400 nm) and UVB rays (290–320 nm) are carcinogenic. UVA rays are present throughout the day and can pass through window glass. UVA rays cause premature aging of the skin and are primarily responsible for drug-related phototoxicity and photoallergic reactions. UVB rays are most intense from 10 AM to 4 PM, are blocked by window glass, and are most responsible for sunburn. Serious burns are painful, and the skin may be red, tender, swollen, and blistered. These sunburns may be accompanied by fever, headache, itching, and malaise. Cumulative overexposure to the sun leads to premature aging of the skin, including wrinkling and age spots and an increased risk for skin cancer, including basal cell carcinoma, squamous cell carcinoma, and melanoma. Repeated exposure to sunlight in the eyes can also result in ocular pterygium formation, cataracts, and macular degeneration.

PREVENTION

Avoid Overexposure to the Sun

Sun exposure is the most preventable risk factor for skin cancer, including melanoma. Staying indoors or seeking shade between 10 AM and 4 PM is very important in limiting exposure to UV rays, particularly UVB rays. Be aware that sunburn and sun damage can occur even on cloudy days. Sunburn can occur after as little as 10–15 minutes of unprotected sun exposure in a fair-skinned person. Tanning beds and sun lamps are also carcinogenic and should be avoided.

Protective Clothing

Wide-brimmed hats, long sleeves, and long pants protect against UV rays. Tightly woven clothing and darker fabrics provide additional protection. High-UPF (ultraviolet protection factor >30) clothing is recommended for travelers at increased risk of sunburn or with a history of skin cancer. This type of clothing contains colorless compounds, fluorescent brighteners, or treated resins that absorb UV rays. Sunglasses that provide 100% protection against both UVA and UVB radiation are strongly recommended.

Sunscreens

Sun protection factor (SPF) defines the extra protection against UVB rays that a person receives by using a sunscreen. Although higher-SPF sunscreens provide more protection than lower-SPF sunscreens, SPF is not linear. An SPF 30 sunscreen does not offer twice the protection of SPF 15. Sunscreens that offer protection from both UVA and UVB rays are labeled "broad-spectrum SPF" and are recommended for best protection.

Physical sunscreens contain titanium dioxide or zinc oxide, inorganic molecules that are confined to the stratum corneum and reflect and scatter both visible and UV light. They are effective, broad-spectrum sunscreens that protect against both UVA and UVB radiation. With the advent of nanotechnology, these products no longer cause an opaque white film on the skin and have become cosmetically acceptable for widespread use. They are recommended for people who burn easily or who take medications that may cause photosensitivity reactions.

Chemical sunscreens absorb rather than reflect UV radiation. A combination of chemical agents is recommended to provide broad-spectrum protection against UVA and UVB rays. Although the Food and Drug Administration (FDA) recommends using sunscreen with ≥15 SPF, the American Academy of Dermatology recommends using sunscreen with ≥30 SPF. A debate exists as to the value of additional protection provided by sunscreens with SPFs >15. In a controlled environment, the marginal protection provided by these high-SPF sunscreens is only 2%–4%. However, since most people underapply sunscreen, the higher-SPF sunscreens may have a margin of safety and give the user at least an SPF 15 level of protection. Travelers should consider the following key points regarding sunscreens:

- Choose a broad-spectrum sunscreen with ≥15 SPF to ensure adequate UVA and UVB protection.
- For UVA protection, look for the following active ingredients: zinc oxide, titanium dioxide, avobenzone, ecamsule, oxybenzone, dioxybenzone, or sulisobenzone.
- Use broad-spectrum products that contain both UVA and UVB protection.
- Select a waterproof or water-resistant product. Waterproof sunscreens confer approximately 80 minutes of protection in the water, and water-resistant products offer 40 minutes of protection.
- Apply to dry skin 15 minutes before exposure to the sun.
- At least 1 oz (2 tablespoons or enough to fill a shot glass) of sunscreen is needed to cover the exposed areas of the body. Most people only apply 25%–50% of the recommended amount of sunscreen, which decreases the achieved SPF.
- Apply to all exposed areas, especially the ears, scalp, back of the neck, tops of the feet, and backs of the hands.

- Reapply every 2 hours and after sweating, swimming, or towel-drying (even on cloudy days).
- Use a lip balm or lipstick with broad-spectrum SPF of ≥15.
- The FDA requires that all sunscreens retain their original strength for at least 3 years. Always check the expiration date and discard all expired product.
- Sunscreens should be applied to the skin before insect repellents. (Note: DEET-containing insect repellents may decrease the SPF of sunscreens by one-third. Sunscreens may increase absorption of DEET through the skin.)
- Avoid products that contain both sunscreens and insect repellents, because sunscreen may need to be reapplied more often and in larger amounts than the repellent.

TREATMENT

Travelers with sunburn should maintain hydration and stay in a cool, shaded, or indoor environment. Topical and oral nonsteroidal anti-inflammatory drugs decrease skin redness if used before or soon after exposure to the sun and may relieve symptoms such as headache, fever, and local pain. The pain of sunburn is usually most intense 6–48 hours after sun exposure, and skin usually peels 4–7 days later. Topical steroids are of limited benefit, and systemic steroids appear to be ineffective in alleviating pain. Cool compresses, colloidal oatmeal baths, moisturizing creams, and topical aloe vera gel may relieve symptoms. Oral diphenhydramine may relieve itching. If blisters occur, they should be left intact to promote faster healing. Open erosions should be coated with petrolatum jelly and covered with sterile gauze to decrease the risk of infection. If infection occurs, oral antibiotics may be necessary. In severe cases of sunburn, dehydration and hypovolemia may occur, presenting with severely inflamed or reddened skin, disorientation, dizziness or fainting, nausea, chills, high fever, and headache. Hospitalization for intravenous rehydration and narcotic analgesics for pain relief may be required in these extreme cases.

BIBLIOGRAPHY

1. Diffey BL, Grice J. The influence of sunscreen type on photoprotection. Br J Dermatol. 1997 Jul;137(1):103–5.
2. Gu X, Wang T, Collins DM, Kasichayanula S, Burczynski FJ. In vitro evaluation of concurrent use of commercially available insect repellent and sunscreen preparations. Br J Dermatol. 2005 Jun;152(6):1263–7.
3. Han A, Maibach HI. Management of acute sunburn. Am J Clin Dermatol. 2004;5(1):39–47.
4. Krakowski AC, Kaplan LA. Exposure to radiation from the sun. In: Auerbach PS, editor. Wilderness Medicine. 6th ed. Philadelphia: Mosby Elsevier; 2012. p. 294–313.
5. McLean DI, Gallagher R. Sunscreens. Use and misuse. Dermatol Clin. 1998 Apr;16(2):219–26.
6. Murphy ME, Montemarano AD, Debboun M, Gupta R. The effect of sunscreen on the efficacy of insect repellent: a clinical trial. J Am Acad Dermatol. 2000 Aug;43(2 Pt 1):219–22.
7. Wang SQ, Stanfield JW, Osterwalder U. In vitro assessments of UVA protection by popular sunscreens available in the United States. J Am Acad Dermatol. 2008 Dec;59(6):934–42.
8. Wang SQ, Tooley IR. Photoprotection in the era of nanotechnology. Seminars in cutaneous medicine and surgery. 2011 Dec;30(4):210–3.

PROBLEMS WITH HEAT & COLD
Howard D. Backer, David R. Shlim

International travelers encounter environments that may include extremes of climate to which the traveler is not accustomed. Exposure to heat and cold can result in serious injury or death. Travelers should investigate climate extremes that they will face during their journey and prepare with proper clothing, knowledge, and equipment.

PROBLEMS ASSOCIATED WITH A HOT CLIMATE
Risk for Travelers
Many of the most popular travel destinations are tropical or desert areas. Travelers who sit on the beach or by the pool and do only short walking tours incur minimal risk of heat illness. Those who do strenuous hiking, biking, or work in the heat are at risk, especially travelers coming from cool or temperate climates who are not in good physical condition and are not acclimatized to the heat.

Clinical Presentations
Physiology of Heat Injuries
Tolerance to heat depends largely on physiologic factors, unlike cold environments where adaptive behaviors are more important. The major means of heat dissipation are radiation while at rest and evaporation of sweat during exercise, both of which become minimal with air temperatures above 95°F (35°C) and high humidity.

The major organs involved in temperature regulation are the skin, where sweating and heat exchange take place, and the cardiovascular system, which must increase blood flow to shunt heat from the core to the surface, while meeting the metabolic demands of exercise. Cardiovascular status and conditioning are the major physiologic variables affecting the response to heat stress at all ages. In addition to environmental conditions and intensity of exercise, dehydration is the most important predisposing factor in heat illness. Dehydration also reduces exercise performance, decreases time to exhaustion, and increases internal heat load; temperature and heart rate increase in direct proportion to the level of dehydration. Sweat is a hypotonic fluid containing sodium and chloride. Sweat rates commonly reach 1 L per hour and may exceed this level, which results in substantial fluid and sodium loss.

Minor Heat Disorders
Heat cramps are painful muscle contractions following exercise in heat. They begin an hour or more after stopping exercise and most often involve heavily used muscles in the calves, thighs, and abdomen. Rest and passive

stretching of the muscle, supplemented by fluids and salt, will rapidly relieve symptoms. Water with a salty snack is sufficient; an oral salt solution, as in rehydration solutions, can be made by adding one-fourth to one-half teaspoon of table salt (or two 1-g salt tablets) to 1 L of water. To improve taste, add a few teaspoons of sugar and/or orange juice or lemon juice.

Heat syncope is sudden fainting in heat that occurs in unacclimatized people while standing in the heat or after 15–20 minutes of exercise. Consciousness rapidly returns to normal when the patient is supine. Rest, relief from heat, and oral fluids are sufficient treatment.

Heat edema is mild swelling of the hands and feet, more frequent in women during the first few days of heat exposure. It resolves spontaneously and should not be treated with diuretics, which may delay heat acclimatization and cause dehydration.

Prickly heat (miliaria or heat rash) manifests as small, red, raised itchy bumps on the skin caused by obstruction of the sweat ducts. It resolves spontaneously, aided by avoiding continued sweating and relief from heat. It is best prevented by wearing light, loose clothing and avoiding heavy, continuous sweating.

Major Heat Disorders
Heat exhaustion
Most people who experience acute collapse or other symptoms associated with exercise in the heat are suffering from heat exhaustion, simply defined as the inability to continue exertion in the heat. The presumed cause of heat exhaustion is loss of fluid and electrolytes, but there are no objective markers to define the syndrome, which is a spectrum ranging from minor complaints to a vague boundary shared with heat stroke. Transient mental changes, such as irritability, confusion, or irrational behavior may be present in heat exhaustion, but major neurologic signs, such as seizures or coma, indicate heat stroke or hyponatremia. Body temperature may be normal or mildly elevated.

Most cases can be treated with supine rest in the shade or other cool place, and oral water or fluids containing glucose and salt; subsequently, spontaneous cooling occurs, and patients recover within hours without progression to more serious illness. An oral solution for treating heat exhaustion can be made by adding one-fourth to one-half teaspoon of table salt (or two 1-g salt tablets) to 1 L of water plus 4–6 teaspoons of sugar. To further improve taste, add one-quarter cup of orange juice or 2 teaspoons of lemon juice. Commercial sports-electrolyte drinks or water with snacks are also effective. Plain water plus salty snacks may be more palatable and equally effective. Subacute heat exhaustion may develop over several days and is often misdiagnosed as "summer flu" because of findings of weakness, fatigue, headache, dizziness, anorexia, nausea, vomiting, and diarrhea. Treatment is as described for acute heat exhaustion.

Exercise-associated hyponatremia
Hyponatremia (low sodium [salt] levels in the blood) occurs in both endurance athletes and recreational hikers, likely due to loss of sodium through sweating and replacement of fluids with excessive amounts of plain water. The kidney fails to correct the excess water because of inappropriate influence of a hormone (antidiuretic hormone) that results in retention of water and loss of sodium.

In the field setting, altered mental status with normal body temperature and a history of large volumes of water intake suggest hyponatremia. The vague and nonspecific symptoms are the same as those described for hyponatremia in other settings (for example, anorexia, nausea, emesis, headache, muscle weakness, lethargy, confusion, and seizures). Symptoms of heat exhaustion and early hyponatremia are similar. Hyponatremia can be distinguished by persistent alteration of mental status without elevated temperature. Delay in onset of major neurologic symptoms (confusion, seizures, or coma) or deterioration after cessation of exercise and removal from heat point to hyponatremia.

The recommendation to force fluid intake during prolonged exercise and the attitude that "you can't drink too much" are major contributors to exercise-associated hyponatremia. Prevention includes drinking only enough to relieve thirst and to maintain dilute urine output. During prolonged exercise or heat exposure, supplemental sodium should be taken. Most sports-electrolyte drinks do not contain sufficient amounts of sodium to prevent hyponatremia; however, salt tablets often cause nausea and vomiting. For hikers, food is the most efficient vehicle for salt replacement. Trail snacks should include salty foods (such as trail mix, crackers, pretzels, and jerky) and not just sweets.

Heat stroke

Heat stroke is an extreme medical emergency requiring aggressive cooling measures and hospitalization for support. Heat stroke is the only form of heat illness in which the mechanisms for thermal homeostasis have failed, and the body does not spontaneously restore the temperature to normal. As a result of uncontrolled fever and circulatory collapse, organ damage can occur in the brain, liver, kidneys, and heart. Damage is related to duration, as well as peak elevation of body temperature. The onset of heat stroke may be acute (exertional heat stroke), which can affect healthy people who are exercising in the heat, or gradual (nonexertional heat stroke, also referred to as classic or epidemic), which occurs in those with chronic illness from passive heat exposure.

Early symptoms are similar to those of heat exhaustion, with confusion or change in personality, loss of coordination, dizziness, headache, and nausea that progress to more severe symptoms. A presumptive diagnosis of heat stroke is made in the field when people have elevation of body temperature (hyperpyrexia) and marked alteration of mental status, including delirium, convulsions, and coma. Body temperatures in excess of 106°F (41°C) can occur in heat stroke; even without a thermometer, people will feel hot to the touch. If a thermometer is available, a rectal temperature is the safest and most reliable way to check the temperature of someone who may have heat stroke.

In the field, immediately institute cooling measures by one of several simple methods:

- Use evaporative cooling by maximizing skin exposure, spraying tepid water on the skin, and maintaining air movement over the body by fanning. Alternatively, place cool or cold wet towels over the body and fan to promote evaporation.
- Apply ice or cold packs to the neck, axillas, and groin. Vigorously massage the skin to prevent constriction of blood vessels and try to avoid shivering, which will increase body temperature.
- Immerse the person in cool water, such as a nearby pool or natural body of water or bath. (Always attend and hold the person while in the water.)

Heat stroke is life threatening, and many complications may occur in the first 24–48 hours, such as liver or kidney damage and abnormal bleeding. Most victims require hospital intensive care management. If recovery to normal mental status is rapid and evacuation to a hospital is not feasible, encourage rehydration for those able to take oral fluids and monitor closely for several hours for temperature swings.

Prevention of Heat Disorders
Heat Acclimatization

Heat acclimatization is a process of physiologic adaptation to a hot environment that occurs in both residents and visitors. The result of acclimatization is an increase in sweating with less salt content, and decreased energy expenditure with lower rise in body temperature for a given workload. Only partial adaptation occurs by passive exposure to heat. Full acclimatization, especially cardiovascular response, requires 1–2 hours of exercise in the heat each day. Most acclimatization changes occur within 10 days, provided a suitable amount of exercise is taken each day in the heat. After this time, only increased physical fitness will result in further exercise tolerance. Decay of acclimatization occurs within days to weeks if there is no heat exposure.

Physical Conditioning and Acclimatization

Higher levels of physical fitness improve exercise tolerance and capacity in heat, but not as much as acclimatization. If possible, travelers should acclimatize before leaving by exercising ≥1 hour daily in the heat. If this is not possible before departing, exercise during the first week of travel in a hot climate should be limited in intensity and duration. It is a good idea to conform to the local practice in most hot regions and avoid strenuous activity during the hottest part of the day.

2

Clothing

Clothing should be lightweight, loose, and light-colored to allow maximum air circulation for evaporation yet give protection from the sun. A wide-brimmed hat markedly reduces radiant heat exposure.

Fluid and Electrolyte Replacement

During exertion, fluid intake improves performance and decreases the likelihood of illness. Reliance on thirst alone is not sufficient to prevent mild dehydration, but forcing a person who is not thirsty to drink water creates the potential danger of hyponatremia. During mild to moderate exertion, electrolyte replacement offers no advantage over plain water. However, for those exercising many hours in heat, salt replacement is recommended. Eating salty snacks or lightly salting mealtime food or fluids is the most efficient way to replace salt losses. Salt tablets, when swallowed whole, may cause gastrointestinal irritation and vomiting, but 2 tablets can be dissolved in 1 L of water. Urine volume and color are a reasonable means to monitor fluid needs.

PROBLEMS ASSOCIATED WITH A COLD CLIMATE
Risk for Travelers

Travelers do not have to be in an arctic or high-altitude environment to encounter problems with the cold. Humidity, rain, and wind can produce hypothermia even with temperatures around 50°F (10°C). Reports of severe hypothermia in international travelers are rare. Many high-altitude destinations are not wilderness areas, and villages offer an escape from extreme weather. In Nepal, trekkers almost never experience hypothermia, except in the rare instance in which they get lost in a storm. Even in a temperate climate, a traveler in a small boat that overturns in very cold water can rapidly become hypothermic.

Clinical Presentations
Hypothermia

Hypothermia can be defined, in general terms, as having a core body temperature below 95°F (35°C). When people are faced with an environment in which they cannot keep warm, they first feel chilled, then begin to shiver, and eventually stop shivering as their metabolic reserves are exhausted. At that point, body temperature continues to decrease, depending on the ambient temperatures. As the core temperature falls, neurologic functioning decreases until almost all hypothermic people with a core temperature of 86°F (30°C) or lower are comatose. The record low core body temperature in an adult who survived is 56°F (13°C). Travelers headed to a cold climate should be encouraged to ask questions and research clothing and equipment. Modern clothing, gloves, and particularly footwear have greatly decreased the chances of suffering cold injury in extreme climates. Cold injuries occur more often after accidents, such as avalanches or unexpected nights outside, than during normal recreational activities.

Travelers who will be engaging in recreational activities or working around cold water face a different sort of risk. Immersion hypothermia can render a person unable to swim or keep floating in <15 minutes. In these cases, a personal flotation device is critical, as is knowledge about self-rescue and righting a capsized boat.

The other medical conditions associated with cold affect mainly the skin and the extremities. These can be divided into nonfreezing cold injuries and freezing injuries (frostbite).

Nonfreezing Cold Injury

The nonfreezing cold injuries are trench foot, pernio (chilblains), and cold urticaria. Trench foot (immersion foot) is caused by prolonged immersion of the feet in cold water (32°F–59°F; 0°C–15°C). The damage is mainly to nerves and blood vessels, and the result is pain that is aggravated by heat and a dependent position of the limb. Severe cases can take months to resolve. Unlike the treatment for frostbite, immersion foot should not be rapidly rewarmed, which can make the damage much worse.

Pernio are localized, inflammatory lesions that occur mainly on the hands of susceptible people. They can occur with exposure to only moderately cold weather. The bluish-red lesions are thought to be caused by prolonged, cold-induced vasoconstriction. As with trench foot, rapid rewarming should be avoided, as it makes the pain worse. Nifedipine may be an effective treatment.

Cold urticaria involves the formation of localized or general wheals and itching after

 PROBLEMS WITH HEAT & COLD |

exposure to cold. It is not the absolute temperature that induces this form of urticaria but the rate of change of temperature in the skin.

Freezing Cold Injury
Categories of frostbite

Frostbite is the term that is used to describe tissue damage from direct freezing of the skin. Modern equipment and clothing have decreased the risk of frostbite resulting from adventure tourism, and frostbite occurs mainly during an accident, severe unexpected weather, or as a result of poor planning.

Once frostbite injury has occurred, little can be done to reverse the changes. Therefore, taking great care to prevent frostbite is crucial. Frostbite is usually graded like burns. First-degree frostbite involves reddening of the skin without deeper damage. The prognosis for complete healing is virtually 100%. Second-degree frostbite involves blister formation. Blisters filled with clear fluid have a better prognosis than blood-tinged blisters. Third-degree frostbite represents full-thickness injury to the skin and possibly the underlying tissues. No blister forms, the skin darkens over time and may turn black, and if the tissue is completely devascularized, amputation will be necessary.

Management of frostbite

Frostbitten skin is numb and appears whitish or waxy. The generally accepted method for treating a frozen digit or limb is through rapid rewarming in water heated to 104°F–108°F (40°C–42°C). The frozen area should be completely immersed in the warm water. A thermometer is needed to ensure the water is kept at the correct temperature. Rewarming can be associated with severe pain, and analgesics can be given if needed. Once the area is rewarmed, it must be safeguarded against freezing again. It is thought to be better to keep digits frozen a little longer and rapidly rewarm them, than to allow them to thaw

out slowly or to thaw and refreeze. A cycle of freeze-thaw-refreeze is devastating to tissue and leads more directly to the need for amputation.

Once the area has rewarmed, it can be examined. If blisters are present, note whether they extend to the end of the digit. Proximal blisters usually mean that the tissue distal to the blister has suffered full-thickness damage. Treatment consists of avoiding further mechanical trauma to the area and preventing infection. Reasonable field treatment consists of washing the area thoroughly with a disinfectant such as povidone-iodine, putting dressings between the toes or fingers to prevent maceration, using fluffs (expanded gauze sponges) for padding, and covering with a roller gauze bandage. These dressings can safely be left on for up to 3 days at a time. By leaving the dressings on longer, the traveler can preserve what may be limited supplies of bandages. Prophylactic antibiotics are not needed in most situations.

In the rare situation in which a foreign traveler suffers frostbite and can be evacuated to an advanced medical setting within 24 hours, there may be a role for thrombolytics, such as prostacyclin and recombinant tissue plasminogen activator. If you are managing frostbite in the first 24 hours, you should consult someone with expertise in frostbite as soon as possible. The risks and benefits of using these drugs should be carefully considered in each patient. Beyond 24 hours after thawing, these interventions are probably not beneficial.

Once the patient has reached a definitive medical setting, there should be no rush to do surgery. The usual time from injury to surgery is 4–5 weeks. Technetium (Tc)-99 scintigraphy and magnetic resonance imaging can be used to help define the extent of the damage. Once the delineation between dead tissue and viable becomes clear, surgery that preserves the remaining digits can be planned.

BIBLIOGRAPHY

1. Armstrong LE, Casa DJ, Millard-Stafford M, Moran DS, Pyne SW, Roberts WO. American College of Sports Medicine position stand. Exertional heat illness during training and competition. Med Sci Sports Exerc. 2007 Mar;39(3):556–72.

2. Cauchy E, Cheguillaume B, Chetaille E. A controlled trial of a prostacyclin and rt-PA in the treatment of severe frostbite. N Engl J Med. 2011 Jan 13;364(2):189–90.

3. Epstein Y, Moran DS. Extremes of temperature and hydration. In: Keystone JS, Freedman DO, Kozarsky PE, Connor BA, Nothdurft HD, editors. Travel Medicine. 3rd ed. Philadelphia: Saunders Elsevier; 2013. p. 381–90.

4. Freer L, Imray CHE. Frostbite. In: Auerbach PS, editor. Wilderness Medicine. 6th ed. Philadelphia: Mosby Elsevier; 2012. p. 181–201.

5. Hadad E, Rav-Acha M, Heled Y, Epstein Y, Moran DS. Heat stroke: a review of cooling methods. Sports Med. 2004;34(8):501–11.

6. O'Brien KK, Leon LR, Kenefick RW. Clinical management of heat-related illnesses. In: Auerbach

PS, editor. Wilderness Medicine. 6th ed. Philadelphia: Mosby Elsevier; 2012. p. 232–8.

7. Rogers IR, Hew-Butler T. Exercise-associated hyponatremia: overzealous fluid consumption. Wilderness Environ Med. 2009 Summer; 20(2): 139–43.

INJURY PREVENTION

David A. Sleet, David J. Ederer, Michael F. Ballesteros

According to the World Health Organization (WHO), injuries are among the leading causes of death and disability in the world, and they are the leading cause of preventable death in travelers. Among travelers, data show that injuries are one of the leading causes for consulting a physician, hospitalization, repatriation, and death. Worldwide, injuries are the leading cause of death for young people aged 15–29 years. Estimates have reported that 18%–24% of deaths among travelers in foreign countries are caused by injuries. Infectious diseases accounted for only 2% of deaths to travelers abroad. Contributing to the injury toll while traveling are exposure to unfamiliar and perhaps risky environments, differences in language and communications, less stringent product safety and vehicle standards, unfamiliar rules and regulations, a carefree holiday or vacation spirit leading to more risk-taking behavior, and overreliance on travel and tour operators to protect one's safety and security.

From 2011 through 2013, an estimated 2,466 US citizens died from non-natural causes, such as injuries and violence, while in foreign countries (excluding deaths occurring in the wars in Iraq and Afghanistan). Motor vehicle crashes—not crime or terrorism—are the number 1 killer of healthy US citizens living, working, or traveling in foreign countries. From 2011 through 2013, 621 Americans died in road traffic crashes abroad (25% of all non-natural deaths to US citizens abroad). Another 555 were victims of homicide (23%), 392 committed suicide (16%), and 309 were victims of drowning (13%) (Figure 2-2). Other

less common but serious injuries are related to natural disasters, aviation accidents, drugs, terrorism, falls, burns, and poisoning.

If a traveler is seriously injured, emergency care may not be available or acceptable by US standards. Trauma centers capable of providing optimal care for serious injuries are uncommon outside urban areas in many foreign destinations. Travelers should be aware of the increased risk of certain injuries while traveling or residing abroad, particularly in developing countries, and be prepared to take preventive steps.

ROAD TRAFFIC INJURIES

Globally, an estimated 3,300 people are killed each day, including 720 children, in road traffic crashes involving cars, buses, motorcycles, bicycles, trucks, and pedestrians. Annually, 1.24 million are killed and 20–50 million are injured in traffic crashes—a number likely to double by 2030. Although only 53% of the world's vehicles are in developing countries, >90% of road traffic casualties occur in these countries.

International efforts to combat road deaths command a tiny fraction of the resources deployed to fight diseases such as malaria and tuberculosis, yet the burden of road traffic injuries is comparable. In response to this crisis, in March 2010 the 64th General Assembly of the United Nations described the global road safety crisis as "a major public health problem" and proclaimed 2011–2020 as "The Decade of Action for Road Safety." On April 19, 2012, the United Nations

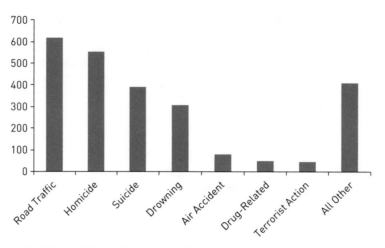

FIGURE 2-2. LEADING CAUSES OF INJURY DEATH FOR US CITIZENS IN FOREIGN COUNTRIES, 2011–2013[1,2]

[1] Data from US Department of State. Death of US citizens abroad by non-natural causes. Washington, DC: US Department of State; 2014 [cited 2014 March 26]. Available from: http://travel.state.gov/content/travel/english/statistics/deaths.html.

[2] Excludes deaths of US citizens fighting wars in Afghanistan or Iraq, and deaths that were not reported to the nearest US embassy or consulate.

General Assembly adopted a new resolution (A/66/PV.106) to improve global road safety by implementing plans for the decade, setting ambitious targets, and monitoring global road traffic fatalities.

According to Department of State data, road traffic crashes are the leading cause of injury deaths to US citizens while abroad (Figure 2-2). Of the 621 US citizens killed in road traffic crashes from 2011 through 2013, approximately 110 (18%) deaths involved motorcycles. Unlike in the United States, in many countries, 2- and 3-wheeled vehicles outnumber cars, and travelers unfamiliar with driving or riding motorcycles may be at higher risk of crashing. Most non-natural American deaths in Thailand and Vietnam, popular travel destinations, were related to motorcycle use. Motorcycle use is also dangerous for travelers in countries where motorcycles are not the primary mode of transportation. The reported rate of motorbike injuries in Bermuda is much higher in tourists than in the local population, and the rate is highest in people aged 50–59 years. Motor vehicle rentals in Bermuda and some other small Caribbean islands are typically limited to motorbikes for tourists, possibly contributing to the higher rates of motorbike injuries. Loss of vehicular control, unfamiliar equipment, and inexperience with motorized 2-wheelers contributed to crashes and injuries, even at speeds <30 miles per hour.

Road traffic crashes are common among foreign travelers for a number of reasons: lack of familiarity with the roads, driving on the opposite side of the road, lack of seat belt use, the influence of alcohol, poorly made or maintained vehicles, travel fatigue, poor road surfaces without shoulders, unprotected curves and cliffs, and poor visibility due to lack of adequate lighting. In many developing countries, unsafe roads and vehicles and an inadequate transportation infrastructure contribute to the traffic injury problem. In many of these countries, motor vehicles often share the road with vulnerable road users, such as pedestrians, bicyclists, and motorcycle users. The mix of traffic involving cars, buses, taxis, rickshaws, large trucks, and even animals increases the risk for crashes and injuries.

Millions of US citizens travel to Mexico each year, and >150,000 people cross the US–Mexico border daily. Travelers should be particularly cautious in Mexico; from 2011 through 2013, 27% of all deaths of US citizens abroad occurred in that country, where >200 Americans died in road traffic crashes.

Strategies to reduce the risk of traffic injury are shown in Table 2-12. The Association for International Road Travel (www.asirt.org) and Make Roads Safe

Table 2-12. Recommended strategies to reduce injuries while abroad

HAZARD	PREVENTION STRATEGIES
Road Traffic Crashes	
Lack of seat belts and child safety seats	Always use safety belts and child safety seats. Rent vehicles with seat belts; when possible, ride in taxis with seat belts and sit in the rear seat; bring child safety seats and booster seats from home for children to ride properly restrained.
Driving hazards	When possible, avoid driving at night in developing countries; always pay close attention to the correct side of the road when driving in countries that drive on the left.
Country-specific driving hazards	Check the Association for Safe International Road Travel website for driving hazards or risks by country (www.asirt.org).
Motorcycles, motor bikes, and bicycles	Always wear helmets (bring a helmet from home, if needed). When possible, avoid driving or riding on motorcycles or motorbikes, including motorcycle and motorbike taxis. Traveling overseas is a bad time to learn to drive a motorcycle or motorbike.
Alcohol-impaired driving	Alcohol increases the risk for all causes of injury. Do not drive after consuming alcohol, and avoid riding with someone who has been drinking.
Cellular telephones	Do not use a cellular telephone or text while driving. Many countries have enacted laws banning cellular telephone use while driving, and some countries have made using any kind of telephone, including hands-free, illegal while driving.
Taxis or hired drivers	Ride only in marked taxis, and try to ride in those that have safety belts accessible. Hire drivers familiar with the area.
Bus travel	Avoid riding in overcrowded, overweight, or top-heavy buses or minivans.
Pedestrian hazards	Be alert when crossing streets, especially in countries where motorists drive on the left side of the road. Walk with a companion or someone from the host country.
Other Tips	
Airplane travel	Avoid using local, unscheduled aircraft. If possible, fly on larger planes (>30 seats), in good weather, during the daylight hours, and with experienced pilots. Children <2 years should sit in a child safety seat, not on a parent's lap. Whenever possible, parents should travel with a safety seat for use before, during, and after a plane ride.
Drowning	Avoid swimming alone or in unfamiliar waters. Wear life jackets while boating or during water recreation activities.
Burns	In hotels, stay below the sixth floor to maximize the likelihood of being rescued in a fire. Bring your own smoke alarm.

(www.makeroadssafe.org) have useful safety information for international travelers, including road safety checklists and country-specific driving risks. The Department of State has safety information useful to international travelers, including road safety and security alerts, international driving permits, and travel insurance (www.travel.state.gov).

WATER AND AQUATIC INJURIES

Drowning accounts for 13% of all deaths of US citizens abroad. Although risk factors have not been clearly defined, these deaths are most likely related to unfamiliarity with local water currents and conditions, inability to swim, and the absence of lifeguards on duty. Rip currents can be especially dangerous, as are sea animals such as urchins, jellyfish, coral, and sea lice. Alcohol also contributes to drowning and boating mishaps.

Drowning was the leading cause of injury death to US citizens visiting countries where water recreation is a major activity, such as Fiji, the Bahamas, Jamaica, and Costa Rica. Young men are particularly at risk of head and spinal cord injuries from diving into shallow water, and alcohol is a factor in some cases.

Boating can be a hazard, especially if boaters are unfamiliar with the boat, do not know proper boating etiquette or rules for watercraft navigation, or are new to the water environment in a foreign country. From 2011 through 2013, maritime accidents accounted for 8% of deaths to healthy Americans abroad. Many boating fatalities result from inexperience or failure to wear lifejackets.

Scuba diving is a frequent pursuit of travelers in coastal destinations. The death rate among all divers worldwide is thought to be 15–20 deaths per 100,000 divers per year. Travelers should either be experienced divers or dive with a reliable dive shop and instructors. See the Scuba Diving section later in this chapter for a more detailed discussion about diving risks and preventive measures.

OTHER INJURIES

From 2011 through 2013, aviation incidents, drug-related incidents, and deaths classified as "other unintentional injuries" accounted for 22% of deaths to healthy US citizens abroad (Figure 2-2). Fires can be a substantial risk in developing countries where building codes do not exist or are not enforced, there

are no smoke alarms, there is no access to emergency services, and the fire department's focus is on putting out fires rather than on fire prevention or victim rescue.

Travel by local, lightweight aircraft in many countries can be risky. From 2011 through 2013, an estimated 82 US citizens abroad were killed in aircraft crashes. Travel on unscheduled flights, in small aircraft, at night, in inclement weather, and with inexperienced pilots carries the highest risk.

Before flying with children, parents and caregivers should check to make sure that their child restraint system is approved for use on an aircraft. This approval should be printed on the system's information label or on the device itself. The Federal Aviation Administration (FAA) recommends that a child weighing <20 lb use a rear-facing child restraint system. A forward-facing child safety seat should be used for children weighing 20–40 lb. FAA has also approved a harness-type device for children weighing 22–44 lb.

Travel health providers, vendors of travel services, and travelers themselves should consider the following:

- Purchasing special travel health and medical evacuation insurance if their destinations include countries where there may not be access to good medical care (see the Travel Insurance, Travel Health Insurance, & Medical Evacuation Insurance section later in this chapter).
- Because trauma care is poor in many countries, victims of injuries and violence can die before reaching a hospital, and there may be no coordinated ambulance service available. In remote areas, medical assistance and modern drugs may be unavailable, and travel to the nearest medical facility can take a long time.
- Adventure activities, such as mountain climbing, skydiving, whitewater rafting, dune-buggying, and kayaking, are popular with travelers. The lack of rapid emergency trauma response, inadequate trauma care in remote locations, and sudden, unexpected weather changes that compromise safety and hamper rescue efforts can delay access to care.
- Travelers should avoid using local, unscheduled, small aircraft. If available, choose larger aircraft (>30 seats), as they

are more likely to have undergone more strict and regular safety inspections. Larger aircraft also provide more protection in the event of a crash. For country-specific airline crash events, see www.airsafe.com.

- When traveling by air with young children, consider bringing a child safety seat approved for use on an aircraft.
- To prevent fire-related injuries, travelers should select accommodations no higher than the sixth floor. (Fire ladders generally cannot reach higher than the sixth floor.) Hotels should be checked for smoke alarms and preferably sprinkler systems. Travelers may want to bring their own smoke alarm. Two escape routes from buildings should always be identified. Crawling low under smoke and covering one's mouth with a wet cloth are helpful in escaping a fire. Families should agree on a meeting place outside the building in case a fire erupts.
- Improperly vented heating devices may cause poisoning from carbon monoxide.

Carbon monoxide at the back of boats near the engine can be especially dangerous. Travelers may want to carry a personal detector that can sound an alert in the presence of this lethal gas.

- Travelers should consider learning basic first aid and CPR before travel overseas with another person. Travelers should bring a travel health kit, which should be customized to the anticipated itinerary and activities (see the Travel Health Kits section later in this chapter).
- Suicide is the third-leading cause of injury death to US citizens abroad, accounting for 16% of non-natural deaths. For longer-term travelers (such as missionaries and volunteers), social isolation and substance abuse, particularly while living in areas of poverty and rigid gender roles, may increase the risk of depression and suicide. See the Mental Health section later in this chapter for more detailed information.

BIBLIOGRAPHY

1. Ball DJ, Machin N. Foreign travel and the risk of harm. Int J Inj Contr Saf Promot. 2006 Jun;13(2):107–15.
2. Cortes LM, Hargarten SW, Hennes HM. Recommendations for water safety and drowning prevention for travelers. J Travel Med. 2006 Jan–Feb;13(1):21–34.
3. FIA Foundation for the Automobile and Society. Make roads safe report: a decade of action for road safety. FIA Foundation for the Automobile and Society; 2009 [cited 2014 Aug 8]. Available from: http://www.fiafoundation.org/publications/Pages/PublicationHome.aspx.
4. Guse CE, Cortes LM, Hargarten SW, Hennes HM. Fatal injuries of US citizens abroad. J Travel Med. 2007 Sep–Oct;14(5):279–87.
5. Krug EG, Mercy JA, Dahlberg LL, Zwi AB. The world report on violence and health. Lancet. 2002 Oct 5;360(9339):1083–8.
6. Lawson CJ, Dykewicz CA, Molinari NA, Lipman H, Alvarado-Ramy F. Deaths in international travelers arriving in the United States, July 1, 2005 to June 30, 2008. J Travel Med. 2012 Mar–Apr;19(2):96–103.
7. Leggat PA, Fischer PR. Accidents and repatriation. Travel Med Infect Dis. 2006 May–Jul;4(3–4):135–46.
8. McInnes RJ, Williamson LM, Morrison A. Unintentional injury during foreign travel: a review. J Travel Med. 2002 Nov–Dec;9(6):297–307.
9. Sleet DA, Balaban V. Travel medicine: preventing injuries to children. Am J Lifestyle Med. 2013 Mar 10;7(2):121–9.
10. World Health Organization. WHO global status report on road safety 2013: supporting a decade of action Geneva: World Health Organization; 2013 [cited 2014 Sep 19]. Available from: http://www.who.int/violence_injury_prevention/road_safety_status/2013/en/.

SAFETY & SECURITY
Ronnie Henry

In 2010, approximately 338,000 people around the world died from interpersonal violence. Violence is a leading worldwide public health problem and a growing concern of US citizens traveling, working, or residing abroad. Rates of violent deaths in developing countries are

>3 times those in industrialized countries, although there are variations within countries. Homicide is the second-leading cause of injury death among US citizens abroad; it accounted for 22.5% of all injury deaths, or >500 deaths from 2011 through 2013 (see Figure 2-2 in the previous section, Injury Prevention).

International terrorism and crime are risks anywhere in the world, but international travelers operating in an unfamiliar environment face particular hurdles. Travelers may not have access to networks of friends or family to assist them. Local government responses to problems may be different from what US residents expect, or an effective local government may not exist to respond at all. Language barriers, unexpected costs, or different cultural mores can also complicate what happens in an emergency. The best way for US residents going overseas to manage their risk is to prepare before they travel. Travelers should research conditions in their destination to learn what risks they are likely to face and the context of those risks. They should then plan what they will need to do to mitigate those risks while they are abroad.

RESEARCH AND PREPARATION

Travelers need information to make good decisions about risks while traveling and to make plans to deal with those risks. The Department of State's Bureau of Consular Affairs publishes comprehensive information on safety and security concerns for every independent nation, along with basic advice for safe travel anywhere at http://travel.state.gov. More information can also be found at individual embassy and consulate websites, all of which can be found at www.usembassy.gov. The Department of State also publishes travel alerts that focus on emergent or chronic safety issues in countries around the world. They encourage all US citizens to avoid travel to areas with major threats to safety and security. Travelers should take these warnings seriously as they cover areas where security threats and instability severely limit the help the US government can offer to its citizens in those areas.

Travelers should enroll with the Department of State's Smart Traveler Enrollment Program (STEP) before leaving on their trip. This will allow them to receive updated information about safety and security conditions and messages about emergent threats while they are abroad. The governments of the United Kingdom, Canada, and Australia also have excellent websites with safety and security information for travelers.

CRIME

By far the most common threat to the safety of US citizens abroad comes from criminal activity. Travelers to foreign countries are viewed by many criminals as wealthy, naïve targets, who are inexperienced, unfamiliar with the culture, and inept at seeking assistance once victimized. Traveling in high-poverty areas or regions of civil unrest, using alcohol or drugs, and traveling in unfamiliar environments at night increase the likelihood that a traveler will be the victim of crime.

Travelers should take the time to research crime trends and patterns at their destination through the Overseas Security Advisory Council at www.osac.gov. Strategies for avoiding becoming the victim of a crime overseas are, for the most part, the same common-sense habits that people should follow everywhere, but the following actions should be stressed with international travelers:

- Limit travel at night, travel with a companion, and vary routine travel habits.
- Do not wear expensive clothing or accessories.
- Criminals are less likely to victimize upper floors of buildings, so avoid accommodations on the ground floor or immediately next to the stairs.
- Lock all doors and windows and consider carrying and using a door intruder alarm and a rubber doorstop that can be used as a supplemental lock.
- Take only well-marked modes of local transportation and check taxi drivers' names and licenses. When renting a car, select one that is similar to local models and rent from an established company.
- If confronted, give up all valuables and do not resist attackers.

Victims of a crime overseas should contact the nearest US embassy, consulate, or consular agency. US federal and state governments can offer guidance and assistance in most situations, but they do not have the legal authority to conduct a criminal investigation and prosecution.

TERRORISM

International terrorism is also a threat to US citizens abroad. The Department of State maintains a worldwide caution addressing this threat on its consular affairs website. Terrorist groups continue to plan attacks against Western interests in multiple regions, including Europe, Asia, Africa, and the Middle East. These attacks may employ a wide variety of tactics, including suicide operations, assassinations, kidnappings, hijackings, and bombings. Possible targets include high-profile sporting events, public transportation systems, residential areas, business offices, hotels, clubs, restaurants, places of worship, schools, public areas, shopping malls, and other tourist destinations where US citizens gather in large numbers.

Although terrorism is a worldwide threat and can be a major cause of concern to travelers, it should be seen in context. In 2013, 17 private US citizens were killed in terrorist attacks, 7 were injured, and 12 were held as hostages. All of these incidents took place in 8 nations, 5 of which have ongoing civil wars or major insurgencies. Although threats of this type cannot be totally eliminated, travelers can lower the chance they will be a victim through knowledge and planning:

- Look out for unattended packages or bags in public places and other crowded areas.
- Be cautious of unexpected packages.
- When packing, choose clothing that does not identify one as a tourist (such as T-shirts emblazoned with the US flag or logos of the traveler's local sports team).
- Try to blend in with the locals.

These strategies incorporate the same defensive alertness and good judgment that people should use to keep safe from crime at home or abroad. Awareness is key—taking precautions to be aware of surroundings and adopting protective measures.

OTHER ISSUES

Just as important as learning about safety and security conditions at a traveler's destination country is to learn about legal differences that may cause problems for US citizens. Many countries have weapons laws that are much stricter than those in the United States, such that a single loose bullet in a suitcase can lead to arrest and possible jail time. Some countries prohibit certain religious activities or the possession of religious literature. Prescription medications that are commonly used in the United States may be illegal in another country. Some countries do not have the same free speech protections as those in the United States, and statements made in public or online can lead to arrest or detention. These and other legal differences can be researched online at the Department of State website.

Since travelers may become the victim of a crime, regardless of the precautions they take, they should have plans for what they will do in an emergency. Many medical insurance programs, including Medicare and Medicaid, will not pay for medical treatment overseas. Travelers should ensure they have adequate medical coverage before going overseas. They should also consider insurance that can help return them to the United States if that becomes necessary. For more information, see Travel Insurance, Travel Health Insurance, & Medical Evacuation Insurance in this chapter.

USEFUL WEBSITES
Department of State Consular Affairs

- Know Before You Go: http://travel.state.gov/content/passports/english/go.html
- Alerts and Warnings: http://travel.state.gov/content/passports/english/alertswarnings.html
- Country Information: http://travel.state.gov/content/passports/english/country.html
- US Citizen Deaths Overseas: http://travel.state.gov/content/travel/english/statistics/deaths.html

Federal Bureau of Investigation, Crime Statistics: www.fbi.gov/stats-services/crimestats

Overseas Security Advisory Council: www.osac.gov

 SAFETY & SECURITY | 113

ACKNOWLEDGMENT

The author thanks Tom Simon in the Division of Violence Prevention at the National Center for Injury Prevention and Control at CDC for reviewing the information on interpersonal violence and homicide.

ANIMAL-ASSOCIATED HAZARDS

Nina Marano, G. Gale Galland

HUMAN INTERACTION WITH ANIMALS: A RISK FACTOR FOR INJURY AND ILLNESS

Animals, even those in close association with humans, such as dogs, can attack if they perceive threat, are protecting their young or territory, or are injured or ill. Although attacks by wild animals are more dramatic, attacks by domestic animals are far more common, and secondary infections of wounds may result in serious systemic disease. This section will cover the most common routes of transmission of illness and injury from animals and insects. However, most animals can transmit disease by more than one route. This section provides examples of high-priority diseases and injuries from animals and refers the reader to other sections for more detailed descriptions of the specific diseases.

BITES AND SCRATCHES

Bites from certain mammals, such as monkeys, dogs, bats, and rodents, present a risk for rabies, tetanus, pasteurellosis, bartonellosis, and other infections. These animals' saliva can be so heavily contaminated with bacteria that a bite may not even be necessary to cause infection if the animal licks a preexisting cut or scratch. Young children are more likely to be bitten by animals and to sustain more severe injuries from animal bites.

Prevention

Before departure, travelers should have a current tetanus vaccination or documentation of a booster vaccination in the previous 5–10 years. Travel health providers should assess a traveler's need for preexposure rabies immunization (see Chapter 3, Rabies). While traveling, people should never try to pet, handle, or feed unfamiliar animals (whether domestic or wild, even in captive settings such as game ranches or petting zoos), particularly in areas where rabies is endemic. Travelers should never attempt to feed, pet, or handle any animal such as monkeys, bats, or rodents while traveling. To mitigate the risk of exposure to rabies, stray dogs should be avoided, and travelers should avoid the temptation to adopt a stray dog from abroad.

Management

To prevent infection, all bite and scratch wounds should be promptly cleaned with soap and water, and the wound should be promptly debrided if necrotic tissue, dirt, or other foreign materials are present. Often times, a course of antibiotics is appropriate after dog or cat bites or scratches as these can lead to local or systemic infections. Wound care is especially important for tetanus- or rabies-prone wounds (see the Rabies and Tetanus sections in Chapter 3). Travelers who might have been exposed to rabies should contact a health care provider as soon as possible for advice about rabies postexposure prophylaxis (PEP). Travelers who received their most recent tetanus toxoid–containing vaccine >5 years previously, or who have not received ≥3 doses of tetanus toxoid–containing vaccines, may require a dose of tetanus toxoid–containing vaccine (Tdap, Td, or DTaP).

Bats

If a bite occurs or if infectious material (such as saliva) from a bat gets into the eyes, nose, mouth, or a wound, the traveler should wash the affected area thoroughly and seek medical advice immediately. Any suspected or documented bite or scratch from a bat anywhere in the world should be considered a risk, and the traveler should be evaluated for rabies PEP. It is not possible to tell if a bat has rabies without laboratory confirmation; however, any bat that is active by day, is found where bats are not usually seen (for example, indoors or outdoors in areas near humans), or is unable to fly is far more likely to be rabid. People usually know when they have been bitten by a bat, but bats have tiny teeth, and not all wounds may be apparent. Travelers should seek medical advice even in the absence of an obvious bite wound if they wake up to find a bat in the room or see a bat in the room of an unattended child.

Monkeys

After a monkey bite or scratch, travelers should be advised to thoroughly clean the wound and seek medical care immediately to be evaluated for possible rabies and herpes B PEP. Macaque bites can transmit herpes B virus, a virus related to the herpes simplex viruses (see Chapter 3, B virus). Additional information and photos of macaques can be found at the website for the National B Virus Resource Center at the Georgia State University Viral Immunology Center (www2. gsu.edu/~wwwvir).

Rodents

Wild rodents are unlikely to have rabies; however, each exposure needs to be evaluated. If the bite was provoked (such as through feeding, petting, or playing with the animal) and the animal appeared healthy, the animal was probably not rabid at the time of the bite. Most experts would not recommend postexposure prophylaxis in this situation. If the bite was unprovoked or the animal appeared unhealthy and is unavailable for testing, rabies PEP should be considered.

STINGS AND ENVENOMATIONS
Snakes

Poisonous snakes are hazards in many locations, although deaths from snakebites are rare. Snakebites usually occur in areas where dense human populations coexist with dense snake populations, such as Southeast Asia, sub-Saharan Africa, and tropical areas in the Americas.

Prevention

Common sense is the best precaution. Most snakebites result from startling, handling, or harassing snakes. Therefore, all snakes should be left alone. Travelers should be aware of their surroundings, especially at night and during warm weather when snakes tend to be more active. For extra precaution, when practical, travelers should wear heavy, ankle-high or higher boots and long pants when walking outdoors in areas possibly inhabited by venomous snakes.

Management

Travelers should be advised to seek immediate medical attention any time a bite wound breaks the skin or when snake venom is ejected into their eyes or mucous membranes. Immobilization of the affected limb and application of a pressure bandage that does not restrict blood flow are recommended first aid measures while the victim is moved as quickly as possible to a medical facility. Incision of the bite site and tourniquets that restrict blood flow to the affected limb are not recommended. Specific therapy for snakebites is controversial and should be left to the judgment of local emergency medical personnel. Specific antivenoms are available for some snakes in some areas, so trying to ascertain the species of snake that bit the victim may be critical.

Insects and other Arthropods

Bites and stings from spiders and scorpions can be painful and can result in illness and death, particularly among infants and children. Other insects and arthropods, such as mosquitoes and ticks, can transmit infections. See the Protection against Mosquitoes, Ticks, & Other Arthropods section earlier in this chapter.

Marine Animals

Most marine animals are generally harmless unless threatened. Most injuries are the result of chance encounters or defensive maneuvers. Resulting wounds have many common characteristics: bacterial contamination, foreign bodies, and occasionally venom. Venomous injuries from marine fish and invertebrates are increasing with the popularity of surfing, scuba diving, and snorkeling. Most species responsible for human injuries, including stingrays, jellyfish, stone-fish, sea urchins, and scorpionfish, live in tropical coastal waters.

Prevention

Travelers should be advised to maintain vigilance while engaging in recreational water activities. Prevention is the best defense:

- Avoid contact. This may be difficult in conditions of poor visibility, rough water, currents, and confined areas.
- Do not attempt to feed, handle, tease, or annoy marine animals.
- Wear protective clothing, such as protective footwear.
- Make an effort to find out which animals may be encountered at the destination and learn about their characteristics and habitats before engaging in recreational water activities.

Management

In case of injury, identifying the species involved can help determine the best course of treatment. Signs and symptoms may not appear for hours after contact, or the animal may not have been seen or recognized at the time of injury. In such cases, treatment is based on the injury. Symptoms of venomous injuries can range from mild swelling and redness at the site to more severe symptoms, such as difficulty breathing or swallowing, chest pain, or intense pain at the site of the sting, for which immediate medical treatment should be sought. Management will vary according to the severity of symptoms and can include medications, such as diphenhydramine, steroids, pain medication, and antibiotics.

OTHER HAZARDS

Bats

Viral infections such as rabies and viral hemorrhagic fevers can be transmitted from bats to people. A recent example of an indirect exposure is an imported case of Marburg fever in a tourist who had visited a "python cave" inhabited by bats in western Uganda. This case illustrates the risk of acquiring diseases from indirect contact with cave-dwelling bats. This same cave was the source of a fatal case of Marburg hemorrhagic fever in a Dutch tourist in 2008.

Exposure to bats can occur during adventure activities, such as caving or spelunking, and can include bites, scratches, and mucosal or cutaneous exposure to bat saliva. Like any other wild animal, bats, whether sick or healthy, will bite in self-defense if handled.

Bats should never be handled. Travelers should be discouraged from going into caves or mines that have large bat infestations. Depending on the country being visited, rabies vaccination may be recommended for people engaged in activities such as caving.

Rodents

Rodents carry a variety of viral, bacterial, and parasitic agents that may pose a threat to human health. Human exposure can occur directly by a bite or scratch, or indirectly by exposure to surfaces or water contaminated with urine or feces.

Rodents should never be handled. Travelers should avoid places that have evidence of infestation with rodents and should avoid contact with rodent feces. Travelers should not eat or drink anything that is suspected to be contaminated by rodent feces or urine.

Travelers who were exposed to rodents and who develop febrile illness shortly thereafter should be evaluated by a clinician. Depending on the history and symptoms, diseases such as yersiniosis, plague, leptospirosis, hantavirus, rickettsial infections, Lyme disease, Lassa fever, tickborne encephalitis, poxvirus, and bartonellosis (all discussed in further detail in Chapter 3) should be included in the list of possible diagnoses.

Birds

Ill and asymptomatic birds have been associated with cases of highly pathogenic avian influenza in humans. When traveling in an area where outbreaks of avian influenza have been reported, travelers should avoid contact with live poultry (such as chickens, ducks, geese, pigeons, turkeys, and quail) or any wild birds and should avoid settings where avian influenza A (H5N1)–infected poultry may be present, such as commercial or backyard poultry farms and live poultry markets. Travelers should not eat uncooked or undercooked poultry or poultry products, including dishes that contain uncooked eggs or poultry blood. Other pathogens from birds may infect humans through infected feces or by aerosol. These cause diseases such as histoplasmosis (see Chapter 3, Histoplasmosis), salmonellosis (see Chapter 3, Salmonellosis [Nontyphoidal]), psittacosis, and avian mycobacteriosis. Travelers should wash their hands if they come in contact with bird feces.

BIBLIOGRAPHY

1. Callahan M. Bites, stings and envenoming injuries. In: Keystone JS, Freedman DO, Kozarsky PE, Connor BA, Nothdurft HD, editors. Travel Medicine. 3rd ed. Philadelphia: Saunders Elsevier; 2013. p. 413–24.
2. Cohen JI, Davenport DS, Stewart JA, Deitchman S, Hilliard JK, Chapman LE. Recommendations for prevention of and therapy for exposure to B virus (cercopithecine herpesvirus 1). Clin Infect Dis. 2002 Nov 15;35(10):1191–203.
3. Diaz JH. The global epidemiology, syndromic classification, management, and prevention of spider bites. Am J Trop Med Hyg. 2004 Aug;71(2):239–50.
4. Gibbons RV. Cryptogenic rabies, bats, and the question of aerosol transmission. Ann Emerg Med. 2002 May;39(5):528–36.
5. Gold BS, Dart RC, Barish RA. Bites of venomous snakes. N Engl J Med. 2002 Aug 1;347(5):347–56.
6. Lankau EW, Cohen NJ, Jentes ES, Adams LE, Bell TR, Blanton JD, et al. Prevention and control of rabies in an age of global travel: a review of travel- and trade-associated rabies events—United States, 1986–2012. Zoonoses Public Health. 2014 Aug;61(5):305–16.
7. Meerburg BG, Singleton GR, Kijlstra A. Rodent-borne diseases and their risks for public health. Crit Rev Microbiol. 2009;35(3):221–70.
8. Pan American Health Organization. Rabies. In: Acha PN, Szyfres B, editors. Zoonoses and Communicable Diseases Common to Man and Animals. 3rd ed. Washington, DC: Pan American Health Organization; 2003. p. 246–76.
9. World Health Organization. WHO Expert Consultation on rabies. World Health Organ Tech Rep Ser. 2005;931:1–88.

NATURAL DISASTERS

Amy F. Wolkin, Josephine Malilay

Travelers should be aware of the potential for natural disasters such as hurricanes, floods, tsunamis, tornadoes, or earthquakes. Natural disasters can contribute to the transmission of some diseases, especially since water supplies and sewage systems may be disrupted; sanitation and hygiene may be compromised by population displacement and overcrowding; and normal public health services may be interrupted.

DISASTER PREPAREDNESS

Travelers can better prepare themselves for disasters by staying well informed and planning ahead. Travelers should know how to recognize impending hazards and know what to do to protect themselves before the disaster occurs. When arriving at a destination, travelers should be familiar with local risks for earthquakes, floods, landslides, tsunamis, and other hazards, as well as warning systems, evacuation routes, and shelters in areas of high risk. Travelers can find information on travel alerts and disaster threats from the Department of State website (http://travel.state.gov/content/passports/english/alertswarnings.html), as well as CDC's Travelers Health website (wwwnc.cdc.gov/travel/notices). Recommendations from these sites may include specific immunizations or cautions about unique hazards in the area. The Department of State's Smart Traveler Enrollment Program offers a free service to US travelers to register upcoming trips abroad so that the Department of State can send alerts (https://step.state.gov/step/).

Travelers should have access to a first aid kit and an adequate supply of prescription medication in the event of an emergency. They also should develop a family emergency plan (see www.fema.gov for more information), which should include how travelers will locate separated family members or contact family members back at home during a disaster. Domestic or overseas travelers can connect to missing family members through American Red Cross Family Linking Services (www.redcross.org/find-help/contact-family).

HEALTH RISKS

During a disaster and when recovering from a disaster, travelers should consider safety as well as mental and physical well-being. The risk for outbreaks of an infectious disease is minimal unless a disease is endemic in an area before the disaster. Although typhoid can be endemic in developing countries, natural disasters have seldom led to epidemic levels of disease. Floods can prompt outbreaks of leptospirosis and cholera in endemic areas.

When water and sewage systems have been disrupted, safe water and food supplies are necessary to prevent enteric disease transmission. If contamination is suspected, water should be boiled or disinfected (see Water Disinfection for Travelers in this chapter). Travelers who are injured during a natural disaster should have a medical evaluation to determine what additional care may be required for wounds potentially contaminated with feces, soil, or saliva, or that have been exposed to fresh or sea water that may contain parasites or bacteria. Tetanus booster status always should be kept current.

During a natural disaster, deaths are rarely due to infectious diseases. Rather, they are most often due to blunt trauma, crush-related injuries, or drowning. Therefore, travelers should be aware of the risks for injury during and after a natural disaster. In floods, people should avoid driving through swiftly moving water. Travelers should exercise caution during clean-up, particularly when encountering downed power lines, water-affected electrical outlets, interrupted gas lines, and stray or frightened animals. Travelers should also be aware of hazards from alternative sources of fuel and electricity for heating or cooking during power outages (such as carbon monoxide poisoning from an improperly used generator). During natural disasters, technological malfunctions may release hazardous materials (such as release of toxic chemicals from a point source displaced by strong winds, seismic motion, or rapidly moving water).

Natural disasters can lead to wide-ranging air pollution. For example, wildfires have caused widespread pollution over vast expanses, worsening symptoms of chronic heart and lung diseases and other respiratory conditions (such as asthma). Natural disasters resulting in massive structural collapse or dust clouds can release chemical or biologic contaminants (such as asbestos). Health risks associated with these environmental occurrences have not been fully studied. Travelers with chronic pulmonary disease, pregnant, or who are immunocompromised may be more susceptible to adverse effects from these types of exposures; if advised, travelers should evacuate the affected area.

BIBLIOGRAPHY

1. Brandt M, Brown C, Burkhart J, Burton N, Cox-Ganser J, Damon S, et al. Mold prevention strategies and possible health effects in the aftermath of hurricanes and major floods. MMWR Recomm Rep. 2006 Jun 9;55(RR-8):1–27.

2. Chin CS, Sorenson J, Harris JB, Robins WP, Charles RC, Jean-Charles RR, et al. The origin of the Haitian cholera outbreak strain. N Engl J Med. 2011 Jan 6;364(1):33–42.

3. Iqbal S, Clower JH, Hernandez SA, Damon SA, Yip FY. A review of disaster-related carbon monoxide poisoning: surveillance, epidemiology, and opportunities for prevention. Am J Public Health. 2012 Oct;102(10):1957–63.

4. Kinney PL. Climate change, air quality, and human health. Am J Prev Med. 2008 Nov;35(5):459–67.

5. Noji EK. The Public Health Consequences of Disasters. New York: Oxford University Press; 1997.

6. Nukushina J. Japanese earthquake victims are being exposed to high density of asbestos. We need protective masks desperately. Epidemiol Prev. 1995 Jun;19(63):226–7.

7. PAHO. Natural Disasters: Protecting the Public's Health. Washington, DC: PAHO Emergency Preparedness Program; 2000 [cited 2014 Sep 19]. Available from: http://www.paho.org/English/dd/ped/SP575.htm.

8. Watson JT, Gayer M, Connolly MA. Epidemics after natural disasters. Emerg Infect Dis. 2007 Jan;13(1):1–5.

9. Young S, Balluz L, Malilay J. Natural and technologic hazardous material releases during and after natural disasters: a review. Sci Total Environ. 2004 Apr 25;322(1–3):3–20.

ENVIRONMENTAL HAZARDS

Armin Ansari, Suzanne Beavers

AIR

Air pollution has decreased in many parts of the world, but it is worsening in certain industrializing countries. Polluted air can be difficult or impossible to avoid, but the risk to healthy short-term travelers is most likely low. People with preexisting heart and lung disease, children, and older adults are at higher risk.

Travelers should be familiar with the air quality at their destination. The AirNow website (http://airnow.gov/) provides information about the effects of particulate matter and ozone, as well as links to international air quality sites. Historical data on outdoor air pollution in urban areas is available from the World Health Organization at http://gamapserver.who.int/gho/interactive_charts/phe/oap_exposure/atlas.html.

Travelers should also limit exposure to indoor air pollution and carbon monoxide. Possible sources of indoor air pollutants include environmental tobacco smoke and cooking or combustion sources (such as kerosene, coal, wood, or animal dung). Major sources of indoor carbon monoxide include gas ranges and ovens, unvented gas or kerosene space heaters, and coal- or wood-burning stoves.

Travelers to countries where air pollution may be a problem should consider the following:

- For people with preexisting conditions such as asthma, chronic obstructive pulmonary disease, and heart disease, limit strenuous or prolonged outdoor activity, particularly in cities.
- For long-term travelers and expatriates, consider investing in an indoor air filtration system.
- Avoid indoor areas with high levels of indoor air pollutants such as tobacco smoke.
- As much as possible, look for lodging with working smoke and carbon monoxide detectors.

Travelers to areas where air pollution is reported to be high might inquire about the advisability of wearing face masks. CDC has no recommendations regarding the use of face masks for travelers. One small study in Beijing showed that wearing a dust respirator appeared to mitigate the effects of air pollution on blood pressure and heart rate. However, it should be noted that the respirators used in the study had better filtration than the surgical masks commonly worn in some countries. The decision to wear a mask should be left to the traveler's discretion.

MOLD CONTAMINATION

Extensive water damage after hurricanes or floods can lead to mold contamination in buildings. Travelers may visit flooded areas overseas as part of emergency, medical, or humanitarian missions. Mold is a more serious health hazard for people who are immunocompromised or have respiratory problems. To prevent exposure that could result in adverse health effects from disturbed mold, people should adhere to the following recommendations:

- Avoid areas where mold contamination is obvious.
- If the traveler will be working in a moldy environment (such as on a medical or humanitarian mission), use personal protective equipment (PPE), such as gloves, goggles, and a fit-tested N-95 respirator or higher. These travelers should take sufficient PPE with them, as these may be scarce in the countries visited.
- Keep hands, skin, and eyes clean and free from mold-contaminated dust.
- Review the CDC guidance, Mold Prevention Strategies and Possible Health Effects in the Aftermath of Hurricanes and Major Floods (www.cdc.gov/mmwr/preview/mmwrhtml/rr5508a1.htm), which provides recommendations for dealing with mold in these settings.

RADIATION

Natural background radiation levels can vary substantially from region to region, but these variations are not a health concern. Travelers should be aware of regions known to have been contaminated with radioactive materials, such as the areas surrounding the Chernobyl nuclear power plant in Ukraine and the Fukushima Daiichi nuclear power plant in Japan.

The Chernobyl plant is located 100 km (62 miles) northwest of Kiev. The 1986 accident contaminated regions in 3 republics—Ukraine, Belarus, and Russia—but the highest radioactive ground contamination is within 30 km (19 miles) of Chernobyl.

The Fukushima Daiichi plant is located 240 km (150 miles) north of Tokyo. After the accident in 2011, the area within a 20-km (32-mile) radius of the plant was evacuated, and Japanese authorities also advised evacuation from locations farther away to the northwest of the plant. As Japanese authorities continue to clean the affected areas and monitor the situation, access requirements and travel advisories change. The Department of State recommends against all unnecessary travel to areas designated by the Japanese government. For up-to-date information or any travel advisories, see the Department of State's information for Japan (http://travel.state.gov/content/passports/english/country/japan.html).

In most countries, areas of known radioactive contamination are fenced or marked with signs. Any traveler seeking long-term (more than a few months) residence near a known or suspected contaminated area should consult with staff of the nearest US embassy and inquire about any advisories regarding drinking water quality or purchase of meat, fruit, and vegetables from local farmers. Radiation emergencies are rare events. In case of such an emergency, however, travelers should follow instructions provided by local authorities. If such information is not forthcoming, US travelers should seek advice from the nearest US embassy or consulate.

Natural disasters (such as floods) may also displace industrial or clinical radioactive sources. In all circumstances, travelers should exercise caution when they encounter unknown objects or equipment, especially if they bear the basic radiation tri-foil symbol or other radiation signs (see www.remm.nlm.gov/radsign.htm for examples). Travelers who encounter a questionable object should notify local authorities.

BIBLIOGRAPHY

1. Ansari A. Radiation Threats and Your Safety: A Guide to Preparation and Response for Professionals and Community. Boca Raton, FL: Chapman & Hall/CRC; 2009.

2. Brandt M, Brown C, Burkhart J, Burton N, Cox-Ganser J, Damon S, et al. Mold prevention strategies and possible health effects in the aftermath of hurricanes and major floods. MMWR Recomm Rep. 2006 Jun 9;55(RR-8):1–27.

3. Eisenbud M, Gesell TF. Environmental Radioactivity: from Natural, Industrial, and Military Sources. 4th ed. San Diego Academic Press; 1997.

4. Langrish JP, Mills NL, Chan JK, Leseman DL, Aitken RJ, Fokkens PH, et al. Beneficial cardiovascular effects of reducing exposure to particulate air pollution with a simple facemask. Part Fibre Toxicol. 2009;6:8.

5. Nuclear Emergency Response Headquarters, Government of Japan. Report of Japanese Government to IAEA Ministerial Conference on Nuclear Safety: the accident at TEPCO's Fukushima Nuclear Power Stations. 2011 [cited 2014 Sep 19]. Available from: http://www.iaea.org/newscenter/focus/fukushima/japan-report/.

6. Scientific Committee on the Effects of Atomic Radiation. Annex J: exposure and effects of the Chernobyl accident. In: Sources and Effects of Ionizing Radiation. New York: United Nations; 2000. p. 451–556.

7. Shofer S, Chen TM, Gokhale J, Kuschner WG. Outdoor air pollution: counseling and exposure risk reduction. Am J Med Sci. 2007 Apr;333(4):257–60.

8. Trasande L, Thurston GD. The role of air pollution in asthma and other pediatric morbidities. J Allergy Clin Immunol. 2005 Apr;115(4):689–99.

SCUBA DIVING

Daniel A. Nord

Published estimates report anywhere from one-half to 4 million people who participate in recreational diving in the United States, and many travel to tropical areas of the world to dive. Traveling divers can face a variety of medical challenges, but because dive injuries are generally rare, few clinicians are trained in their diagnosis and treatment. Therefore, the recreational diver must be able to recognize the signs of injury and find qualified dive medicine help when needed.

PREPARING FOR DIVE TRAVEL

Planning for dive-related travel should take into account any recent changes in health, including injuries or surgery, and medication use. Respiratory disorders (such as asthma), disorders that affect higher function and consciousness (such as diabetes or seizures), psychological problems (such as anxiety), cardiovascular disease, and pregnancy raise special concerns about diving fitness.

Special mention must be made regarding cardiovascular fitness. Diving should be considered a potentially strenuous activity that can make substantial demands on the cardiovascular system. People with known risk factors for coronary disease who wish to either begin a dive program or continue diving should undergo a physical examination with assessment of their cardiovascular fitness. This may include an electrocardiogram and exercise treadmill test.

DIVING DISORDERS
Barotrauma
Ear and sinus

Ear barotrauma is the most common injury in divers. On descent, failure to equalize pressure changes in the middle ear space creates a pressure gradient across the eardrum. This pressure change must be controlled through proper equalization techniques to avoid bleeding or fluid accumulation in the middle

ear and avoid stretching or rupture of the eardrum and the membranes covering the windows of the inner ear. Symptoms of barotrauma include the following:

- pain
- tinnitus (ringing in the ears)
- vertigo (dizziness or sensation of spinning)
- sensation of fullness
- effusion (fluid accumulation in the ear)
- decreased hearing

Paranasal sinuses, because of their relatively narrow connecting passageways, are especially susceptible to barotrauma, generally on descent. With small changes in pressure (depth), symptoms are usually mild and subacute but can be exacerbated by continued diving. Larger pressure changes, especially with forceful attempts at equilibration (such as the Valsalva maneuver), can be more injurious. Additional risk factors for ear and sinus barotrauma include the following:

- earplugs
- medications
- ear or sinus surgery
- nasal deformity
- disease

A diver who may have sustained ear or sinus barotrauma should discontinue diving and seek medical attention.

Pulmonary

A scuba diver must reduce the risk of lung overpressure problems by breathing normally and ascending slowly when breathing compressed gas. Overinflation of the lungs can result if a scuba diver ascends toward the surface without exhaling, which may happen, for example, when a novice diver panics. During ascent, compressed gas trapped in the lung increases in volume until the expansion exceeds the elastic limit of lung tissue, causing damage and allowing gas bubbles to escape into 1 or more of 3 possible locations:

- Gas entering the pleural space can cause lung collapse or pneumothorax.
- Gas entering the space around the heart, trachea, and esophagus (the mediastinum) causes mediastinal emphysema and frequently tracks under the skin (subcutaneous emphysema) or into the tissue around the larynx, sometimes precipitating a change in voice characteristics.
- Gas rupturing the alveolar walls can enter the pulmonary capillaries and pass via the pulmonary veins to the left side of the heart, where it is distributed according to relative blood flow, resulting in arterial gas embolism (AGE).

While mediastinal or subcutaneous emphysema may resolve spontaneously, pneumothorax generally requires specific treatment to remove the air and reinflate the lung. AGE is a medical emergency, requiring intervention, which includes recompression treatment with hyperbaric oxygen.

Lung overinflation injuries from scuba diving can range from dramatic and life threatening to mild symptoms of chest pain and dyspnea. Although pulmonary barotrauma is relatively uncommon in divers, prompt medical evaluation is necessary, and evidence for this condition should always be considered in the presence of respiratory or neurologic symptoms following a dive.

Decompression Illness

Decompression illness (DCI) is an all-inclusive term that describes the dysbaric injuries(AGE) and decompression sickness (DCS). Because the 2 diseases are considered to result from separate causes, they are described here separately. However, from a clinical and practical standpoint, distinguishing between them in the field may be impossible and unnecessary, since the initial treatment is the same for both. DCI can occur even in divers who have carefully followed the standard decompression tables and the principles of safe diving. Serious permanent injury may result from either AGE or DCS.

Arterial Gas Embolism

Gas entering the arterial blood through ruptured pulmonary vessels can distribute bubbles into the body tissues, including the heart and brain, where they can disrupt circulation or damage vessel walls. AGE may cause minimal neurologic symptoms, dramatic symptoms that require immediate attention, or death. Common signs and symptoms include the following:

- numbness
- weakness
- tingling
- dizziness
- blurred vision
- chest pain
- personality change
- paralysis or seizures
- loss of consciousness

In general, any scuba diver who surfaces unconscious or loses consciousness within 10 minutes after surfacing should be suspected to have AGE. Intervention with basic life support is indicated, including the administration of the highest fraction of oxygen, followed by rapid evacuation to a hyperbaric oxygen treatment facility.

Decompression Sickness

Breathing air under pressure causes excess inert gas (usually nitrogen) to dissolve in body tissues. The amount of gas dissolved is proportional to and increases with depth and time. As the diver ascends back to the surface, the excess dissolved gas must be cleared through respiration via the bloodstream. Depending on the amount dissolved and the rate of ascent, some gas can supersaturate tissues, where it separates from solution to form bubbles, interfering with blood flow and tissue oxygenation and causing the following signs and symptoms of DCS:

- joint aches or pain
- numbness or tingling
- mottling or marbling of skin
- coughing spasms or shortness of breath
- itching
- unusual fatigue
- dizziness
- weakness
- personality changes

- loss of bowel or bladder function
- staggering, loss of coordination, or tremors
- paralysis
- collapse or unconsciousness

FLYING AFTER DIVING

The risk of developing decompression sickness is increased when divers are exposed to increased altitude too soon after a dive. The cabin pressure of commercial aircraft may be the equivalent of 6,000–8,000 ft (1,829–2,438 m). Thus, divers should avoid flying or an altitude exposure >2,000 ft (610 m) for

- ≥12 hours after surfacing from a single no-decompression dive
- ≥18 hours after repetitive dives or multiple days of diving
- substantially longer than 18 hours after dives where decompression stops were required

These recommended preflight surface intervals do not eliminate risk of DCS, and longer surface intervals will further reduce this risk.

PREVENTING DIVING DISORDERS

Recreational divers should dive conservatively and well within the no-decompression limits of their dive tables or computers. Risk factors for DCI are primarily dive depth, dive time, and rate of ascent. Additional factors such as repetitive dives, strenuous exercise, dives to depths >60 ft (18 m), altitude exposure soon after a dive, and certain physiological variables also increase risk. Divers should be cautioned to stay hydrated and rested and dive within the limits of their training. Diving is a skill that requires training and certification and should be done with a companion.

TREATMENT OF DIVING DISORDERS

Definitive treatment of DCI begins with early recognition of symptoms, followed by recompression with hyperbaric oxygen. A high concentration (100%) of supplemental oxygen is recommended. Surface-level oxygen given for first aid may relieve the signs and symptoms of DCI and should be administered as soon as possible. Divers are often dehydrated, either because of incidental causes, immersion, or DCI itself, which can cause capillary leakage. Administration of isotonic glucose-free intravenous fluid is recommended in most cases. Oral rehydration fluids may also be helpful, provided they can be safely administered (for example, if the diver is conscious). The definitive treatment of DCI is recompression and oxygen administration in a hyperbaric chamber.

Divers Alert Network (DAN) maintains 24-hour emergency consultation and evacuation assistance at 919-684-9111 (collect calls are accepted). DAN will help with managing the injured diver, help decide if recompression is needed, provide the location of the closest recompression facility, and help arrange patient transport. DAN can also be contacted for routine, non-emergency consultation by telephone at 919-684-2948, extension 222, or by accessing the DAN website (www.diversalert network.org).

Travelers who plan to scuba dive may want to ascertain whether there are recompression facilities at their destination before embarking on their trip.

HAZARDOUS MARINE LIFE

The oceans and waterways are filled with creatures and, although some are capable of wounding and poisoning, most marine animals are generally harmless unless threatened. Most injuries are the result of chance encounters or defensive maneuvers. Resulting wounds have many common characteristics: bacterial contamination, foreign bodies, and occasionally venom. See the Animal-Associated Hazards section earlier in this chapter for prevention and injury management recommendations.

BIBLIOGRAPHY

1. Brubakk AO, Neuman TS, Bennett PB, Elliott DH. Bennett and Elliott's Physiology and Medicine of Diving. 5th ed. London: Saunders; 2003.

2. Dear G, Pollock N. DAN America Dive and Travel Medical Guide. 5th ed. Durham, NC: Divers Alert Network; 2009.

3. Moon RE. Treatment of decompression illness. In: Bove AA, Davis JC, editors. Bove and Davis' Diving Medicine. 4th ed. Philadelphia: WB Saunders; 2004. p. 195–223.

4. Neuman TS, Thom SR. Physiology and medicine of hyperbaric oxygen therapy. Philadelphia, PA: Saunders; 2008.

5. Sheffield P, Vann R. Flying after recreational diving, workshop proceedings of the Divers Alert Network 2002 May 2. Durham, NC: Divers Alert Network; 2004 [cited 2014 Sep 12]. Available from: http://www.diversalertnetwork.org/research/projects/fad/workshop/FADWorkshopProceedings.pdf.

MEDICAL TOURISM

Joanna Gaines, Duc B. Nguyen

Medical tourism is the term commonly used to describe people traveling outside their home country for medical treatment. Patients may pursue medical care abroad for a variety of reasons, such as decreased cost, a preference for care from providers from a similar culture, or to receive a procedure or therapy not available in their country of residence. In the United States, medical tourism generally refers to people traveling to less-developed countries for medical care. Medical tourism is a worldwide, multibillion-dollar phenomenon that is expected to grow substantially in the next 5–10 years. Studies have estimated that hundreds of thousands of medical tourists travel from the United States annually. Little reliable epidemiologic data on medical tourism exist, but ongoing reports of disease outbreaks serve as a reminder that medical tourism is not without risks.

Common categories of procedures that US travelers pursue during medical tourism trips include orthopedic surgery, cosmetic surgery, cardiology (cardiac surgery), oncologic care, and dentistry. Common destinations include Thailand, Mexico, Singapore, India, Malaysia, Cuba, Brazil, Argentina, and Costa Rica. The type of procedure and the destination need to be considered when reviewing the risk of travel for medical care.

Most medical tourists pay for their care out of pocket and rely on private companies or medical concierge services to identify foreign health care facilities. These companies may not require accreditation of foreign providers, track patient outcome data, or maintain formal medical record security policies. Some insurers and large employers have formed alliances with overseas hospitals to control health care costs, and several major medical schools in the United States have developed joint initiatives with overseas providers, such as the Harvard Medical School Dubai Center, the Johns Hopkins Singapore International Medical Center, and the Duke-National University of Singapore.

RISKS ASSOCIATED WITH MEDICAL TOURISM

Medical tourism has been associated with complications, including infections caused by antibiotic-resistant strains of bacteria not previously seen in the United States. Patients who are considering seeking medical care overseas should be aware of this risk. Health care providers should be vigilant for the possibility of resistant infections among patients who have traveled for medical procedures.

Several outbreaks of infectious disease have been documented among medical tourists after their return to the United States. Although patients who experience complications after receiving medical care overseas should inform their providers of their travel history and their medical history, such patients may be reluctant to divulge their travel history or may lack adequate documentation of the care they received; both can complicate treatment.

PRE-TRAVEL ADVICE FOR MEDICAL TOURISTS

Patients who elect to travel for medical reasons should consult a travel health provider for advice tailored to individual health needs, preferably ≥4–6 weeks before travel. In addition to regular considerations for healthy travel related to their destination, medical tourists should consider the additional risks associated with surgery and travel, either while being treated or while recovering from treatment. Flying and surgery both increase the risk of blood clots and pulmonary emboli. Air pressure in an aircraft is equivalent to the pressure at an altitude of approximately 6,000–8,000 ft (1,829–2,438 m). Patients should not travel for 10 days after chest or abdominal surgery to avoid risks associated with this change in pressure. The American Society of Plastic Surgeons advises people who have had cosmetic procedures of the face, eyelids, or nose, or who have had laser treatments, to wait 7–10 days before flying. Patients are also advised to avoid "vacation" activities such as sunbathing, drinking alcohol, swimming, taking long tours, and engaging in strenuous activities or exercise after surgery. The Aerospace Medical Association has published medical guidelines for airline travel that provide useful information on the risks of travel with certain medical conditions (www.asma.org/asma/media/asma/Travel-Publications/paxguidelines.pdf).

GUIDANCE FOR TRAVELERS SEEKING MEDICAL CARE ABROAD

Several professional organizations have developed guidance that includes questions useful for travelers when discussing medical or dental care abroad, either with the facility providing the care or with the group facilitating the trip. When considering a trip overseas for medical care, travelers should be aware of the guiding principles developed by the American Medical Association (Box 2-5). The American College of Surgeons (ACS) issued a similar statement on medical and surgical tourism with the additional recommendation that travelers obtain a complete set of medical records before returning home to ensure that details of their care are available

---

BOX 2-5. GUIDING PRINCIPLES ON MEDICAL TOURISM[1]

The American Medical Association advocates that employers, insurance companies, and other entities that facilitate or promote medical care outside the United States adhere to the following principles:

(a) Medical care outside the United States must be voluntary.

(b) Financial incentives to travel outside the United States for medical care should not limit the diagnostic and therapeutic alternatives that are offered to patients or restrict treatment or referral options.

(c) Patients should be referred for medical care only to institutions that have been accredited by recognized international accrediting bodies (such as the Joint Commission International or the International Society for Quality in Health Care).

(d) Before travel, local follow-up care should be coordinated and financing should be arranged to ensure continuity of care when patients return from medical care outside the United States.

(e) Coverage for travel outside the United States for medical care must include the costs of necessary follow-up care upon return to the United States.

(f) Patients should be informed of their rights and legal recourse before agreeing to travel outside the United States for medical care.

(g) Access to physician licensing and outcome data, as well as facility accreditation and outcomes data, should be arranged for patients seeking medical care outside the United States.

(h) The transfer of patient medical records to and from facilities outside the United States should be consistent with Health Insurance Portability and Accountability Action (HIPAA) guidelines.

(i) Patients choosing to travel outside the United States for medical care should be provided with information about the potential risks of combining surgical procedures with long flights and vacation activities.

---

[1] From American Medical Association. New AMA Guidelines on Medical Tourism. Chicago: AMA; 2008.

to providers in the United States. ACS also recommends that prospective medical tourists use facilities that are internationally accredited. Examples of accrediting entities include Joint Commission International, DNV International Accreditation for Hospitals, or the International Society for Quality in Healthcare, although using a facility that is accredited provides no guarantee of a satisfactory outcome. Similarly, the American Dental Association provides informational documents, including "Traveler's Guide to Safe Dental Care," through the Global Dental Safety Organization for Safety and Asepsis Procedures (Box 2-6). Although this guidance was not developed for medical tourists, it provides useful information for travelers to consider when selecting a facility or planning a trip for medical or dental care. These guides indicate the types of questions that people considering travel for medical care should discuss with their regular health care provider. Additional resources exist to assist both providers and prospective medical tourists (Box 2-7).

Many websites that market directly to travelers provide information on medical tourism. These sites may not include comprehensive details on the qualifications or certifications of a facility or provider. Furthermore, local standards for facility accreditation and provider certification can vary. The ACS recommends that patients considering treatment abroad seek care from providers certified

---

BOX 2-6. PATIENT CHECKLIST FOR OBTAINING SAFE DENTAL CARE DURING INTERNATIONAL TRAVEL[1]

Before you leave:

- Visit your dentist for a check-up to reduce the chances you will have a dental emergency.
- See a health care provider to receive any needed vaccinations, medications, and advice related to your travel destination.

When seeking treatment for a dental emergency during your trip:

- Consult hotel staff or the American Embassy or consulate for assistance in finding a dentist.
- If possible, consider recommendations from Americans living in the area or from other trusted sources.

If the answers to any of the asterisked (*) items below are "No," you should have reservations about the office's infection control standards. If the answer to a two-star item (**) is "No," consider making a swift but gracious exit.

When making the appointment, ask the following:

- Do you use new gloves for each patient?*
- Do you use an autoclave (steam sterilizer) or dry heat oven to sterilize your instruments between patients?**
- Do you sterilize your handpieces (drills)?* (If not, do you disinfect them?)**
- Do you use new needles for each patient?**
- Is sterile (or boiled) water used for surgical procedures?** (In areas where drinking water is unsafe, the water also may cause illness if used for dental treatment.)

Upon arriving at the office, observe the following:

- Is the office clean and neat?
- Do staff wash their hands, with soap, between patients?**
- Do they wear gloves for all procedures?**
- Do they clean and disinfect or use disposable covers on surfaces touched during treatment?

---

[1] Excerpt from Organization for Safety and Asepsis Procedures. Traveler's guide to safe dental care. Annapolis, MD: Organization for Safety and Asepsis Procedures; 2001. Available from: http://www.osap.org/?page=TravelersGuide.

BOX 2-7. HELPFUL RESOURCES ON MEDICAL TOURISM

- Aerospace Medical Association guidelines for airline travel provide useful information on the risks of travel with certain medical conditions: www.asma.org/asma/media/asma/Travel-Publications/paxguidelines.pdf.
- American Academy of Orthopaedic Surgeons Bulletin, July 2007, discusses safety issues that patients should consider: www.aaos.org/news/bulletin/jul07/cover1.asp.
- American Academy of Orthopaedic Surgeons discusses liability implications of medical tourism: www.aaos.org/news/aaosnow/feb08/managing7.asp.
- American College of Surgeons. Statement on medical and surgical tourism: www.facs.org/fellows_info/statements/st-65.html.
- American Society for Aesthetic Plastic Surgery. Guidelines for patients seeking cosmetic procedures abroad: www.surgery.org/consumers/consumer-resources/consumer-tips/guidelines-for-patients-seeking-cosmetic-procedures-abroad.
- American Society of Plastic Surgeons (ASPS). The dangers of plastic surgery tourism: www.plasticsurgery.org/articles-and-galleries/dangers-of-plastic-surgery-tourism.html.
- American Society of Plastic Surgeons' Find-a-surgeon tool helps identify ASPS member surgeons in the United States and overseas: www1.plasticsurgery.org/find_a_surgeon/.
- European Commission. Cross-border care policy: http://ec.europa.eu/health/cross_border_care/policy/index_en.htm.
- International Society for Aesthetic Plastic Surgery's Find-a-surgeon tool helps identify a surgeon: www.isaps.org/find-a-surgeon/.
- Joint Commission International list of its accredited facilities outside of the United States: www.jointcommissioninternational.org/JCI-Accredited-Organizations/.
- Organization for Safety and Asepsis Procedures. Traveler's guide to safe dental care: www.osap.org/?page=TravelersGuide.
- World Health Organization. Guiding principles on human cell, tissue and organ transplantation: www.who.int/transplantation/Guiding_PrinciplesTransplantation_WHA63.22en.pdf.

in their specialties through a process that is equivalent to that established by the member boards of the American Board of Medical Specialties. ACS, American Society of Plastic Surgeons, and the International Society of Aesthetic Plastic Surgery all accredit overseas physicians. Again, however, the traveler should realize that accreditation does not ensure a good outcome, and travelers should be encouraged to thoroughly research any health care facility they are considering using.

TRANSPLANT TOURISM

One of the newer and more controversial forms of medical tourism is "transplant tourism," which is travel for the purpose of receiving an organ purchased from an unrelated donor for transplant. Several studies have identified potential problems that travelers and clinicians need to be aware of when considering transplantation overseas: the

donor and the procedures lacked documentation, most patients received fewer immunosuppressive drugs than is current practice in the United States, and most patients did not receive antibiotic prophylaxis. In 2004, the World Health Assembly Resolution 57.18 encouraged member countries to "take measures to protect the poorest and vulnerable groups from 'transplant tourism' and the sale of tissues and organs." A meeting in 2008 in Istanbul addressed the issue of transplant tourism and organ trafficking, which resulted in a call for these activities to be prohibited. In view of those events, the World Health Organization revised the Guiding Principles on Human Cell, Tissue and Organ Transplantation and released those revised principles in March 2009. These guidelines emphasize that cells, tissues, and organs should only be donated freely without any form of financial incentive.

BIBLIOGRAPHY

1. Budiani-Saberi DA, Delmonico FL. Organ trafficking and transplant tourism: a commentary on the global realities. Am J Transplant. 2008 May;8(5):925–9.

2. Chen LH, Wilson ME. The globalization of healthcare: implications of medical tourism for the infectious disease clinician. Clin Infect Dis. 2013 Dec;57(12):1752–9.

3. Horowitz MD, Rosensweig JA, Jones CA. Medical tourism: globalization of the healthcare marketplace. MedGenMed. 2007;9(4):33.

4. Keckley PH, Underwood HR. Medical Tourism: Consumers in Search of Value. Washington, DC: Deloitte Center for Health Solutions; 2008.

5. Merion RM, Barnes AD, Lin M, Ashby VB, McBride V, Ortiz-Rios E, et al. Transplants in foreign countries among patients removed from the US transplant waiting list. Am J Transplant. 2008 Apr;8(4 Pt 2):988–96.

6. Organ Procurement and Transplantation Network, Scientific Registry of Transplant Recipients. United States organ transplantation annual data report, 2011. Rockville, MD: US Department of Health and Human Services; 2012 [cited 2014 Sep 19]. Available from: http://srtr.transplant.hrsa.gov/annual_reports/2011/default.aspx.

7. Reed CM. Medical tourism. Med Clin North Am. 2008 Nov;92(6):1433–46, xi.

8. Rogers BA, Aminzadeh Z, Hayashi Y, Paterson DL. Country-to-country transfer of patients and the risk of multi-resistant bacterial infection. Clin Infect Dis. 2011 Jul 1;53(1):49–56.

9. Shimazono Y. The state of the international organ trade: a provisional picture based on integration of available information. Bull World Health Organ. 2007 Dec;85(12):955–62.

10. US Department of Health and Human Services. 2007 annual report of the US Organ Procurement and Transplantation Network and the Scientific Registry of Transplant Recipients: transplant data 1997–2006. Rockville, MD: US Department of Health and Human Services; 2007 [cited 2012 Sep 18]. Available from: http://www.ustransplant.org/annual_reports/current/ar_archives.htm.

DISCUSSING COMPLEMENTARY OR ALTERNATIVE HEALTH APPROACHES WITH TRAVELERS

Catherine Law, Tina Adler, Jack Killen

Travelers often ask their health care providers about the use of complementary or alternative health approaches for travel-related illnesses and conditions. This should come as no surprise, given that many people—approximately 1 in 3 Americans—report using products or practices that have origins outside of conventional medicine to complement treatment for a variety of medical conditions or to promote general wellness. Some of these approaches for travel-related health problems are widely promoted in advertising or discussed on the Internet. However, little of this information is supported by research evidence, and some of it is misleading or false. This section focuses on what the research says about some of the herbal remedies, dietary supplements, and other complementary health approaches frequently suggested for travel-related ailments.

TRAVEL-RELATED AILMENTS AND COMPLEMENTARY HEALTH APPROACHES
Malaria Prophylaxis and Treatment
Artemisia (Artemisia annua *L. or sweet wormwood)*

Artemisinin-containing therapies, such as artemether-lumefantrine and artesunate, are pharmaceutical drugs and drug combinations originally derived from the herbal medicine *Artemisia* and are now a standard treatment for malaria in most of the world. Consumer websites and news stories have claimed that using the herb *Artemisia* alone may prevent malaria, but studies show that it does not. The World Health Organization does not recommend using *Artemisia* plant material in any form (including tea) for treating or preventing malaria. Recommended drugs used to prevent and treat malaria are described in Chapter 3, Malaria.

Vitamin A

Limited research suggests that when children with malaria are deficient in vitamin A, supplements may help lower their fever and blood levels of the parasite that causes malaria. However, there is no evidence that vitamin A prevents malaria. Vitamin A is fat soluble, and large or frequent doses of vitamin A may accumulate in the body and cause acute or chronic toxicity. High intakes of vitamin A have been linked to birth defects. Taking beta-carotene has been linked to an increased risk of lung cancer and cardiovascular disease in some smokers.

Travelers' Diarrhea Prevention and Treatment
Probiotics

Probiotics are often suggested to help prevent travelers' diarrhea (TD). Research on their use in treating acute infectious diarrhea is generally positive. Results from studies on preventing TD are mixed but encouraging. Given current data, it must be assumed that effects of probiotics in any given study are specific to the strain or strains tested. The Food and Drug Administration (FDA) has not approved any health claims for probiotics.

In healthy people, probiotics usually have only minor side effects, if any. For more information see Nonantimicrobial Drugs for Prophylaxis in the Travelers' Diarrhea section earlier in this chapter.

Goldenseal

Goldenseal is a perennial herb that has been touted as treatment for a variety of ailments. No high-quality research on goldenseal for TD has been conducted. Studies show that goldenseal inhibits cytochrome P450 2D6, raising concerns that it may increase the toxicity or alter the effects of many commonly used drugs.

Activated charcoal

There is no solid evidence that activated charcoal helps with TD, bloating, stomach cramps, or gas. The side effects of activated charcoal have not been well documented but were mild when tested on healthy people. **Warning:** Children should **not** be given activated charcoal for diarrhea and dehydration. It may absorb nutrients, enzymes, and antibiotics in the intestine and mask the severity of fluid loss.

Grapefruit seed extract

Despite claims that grapefruit seed extract prevents bacterial foodborne illnesses if taken daily, there are no published clinical trial data on its effectiveness or safety for TD.

Altitude Illness Prevention and Treatment

There is little, if any, evidence that dietary or herbal supplements help prevent or treat altitude illness (often referred to as mountain sickness).

Coca

Coca tea has been used for altitude illness, but there is no strong evidence on whether it works or has adverse effects. It will result in a positive drug test for cocaine metabolites. For more information see Chapter 4, Peru: Cusco–Machu Picchu.

Garlic

There is no evidence supporting claims that garlic helps reduce altitude illness.

Garlic supplements appear safe for most adults but may reduce blood clotting and interfere with the effectiveness of the HIV drug saquinavir.

Ginkgo biloba

Results from several small studies of ginkgo for preventing altitude illness show conflicting, but mostly negative, results. Whether these differences relate to the different preparations used in these studies cannot be determined. Products made from standardized ginkgo leaf extracts appear to be safe when used appropriately. However, National Toxicology Program studies showed that rodents developed tumors after being given a ginkgo extract for up to 2 years.

Vitamin E

Only one small study has investigated vitamin E, in combination with other antioxidants, for altitude illness, and the results were negative. Vitamin E supplements have been linked to an increased risk of hemorrhagic stroke. They also have the potential to interact with several types of medications, including statins, niacin, and warfarin.

Motion Sickness Prevention and Treatment

Acupressure and/or magnets

Using acupressure is advocated by some to prevent or treat motion sickness. Results of studies to date are mixed. There are no published data to support use of magnets, alone or in combination with acupressure.

Ginger

Studies are conflicting on whether ginger is effective for motion sickness. Based on the research to date, ginger is probably safe but may interact with many medications. The effect of using ginger supplements with common over-the-counter drugs for motion sickness (such as dimenhydrinate [Dramamine]) is unknown.

Other dietary supplements or products

There is no evidence supporting claims that vitamin B6 and homeopathic products prevent or alleviate motion sickness. Excessive use of vitamin B6 supplements can affect nerve function.

Jet Lag/Sleep

Melatonin

Melatonin supplements may help with sleep problems caused by jet lag. In a 2007 clinical practice guideline, the American Academy of Sleep Medicine supported using melatonin to reduce jet lag symptoms and improve sleep after traveling across >1 time zone. In a 2009 systematic review, results from six small studies and two large studies suggested that melatonin may ease jet lag. Taking between 0.5 and 5 mg melatonin appears to be effective. Before recommending melatonin, consider the following:

- People with epilepsy or who take an oral anticoagulant should not use melatonin without medical supervision.
- Melatonin supplements appear to be safe for most people when used short-term; less is known about its long-term safety.
- Melatonin should not be taken early in the day, as it may cause sleepiness and delay adaptation to local time.
- The amount of melatonin in products and the dosages recommended on labels can vary.
- Side effects from melatonin are uncommon but can include drowsiness, headache, dizziness, or nausea.

See the Jet Lag section earlier in this chapter for more information.

Relaxation techniques

Relaxation techniques, such as progressive relaxation and mindfulness-based stress reduction, may help with insomnia, but it has not been established whether they are effective for jet lag.

Other herbal or dietary supplements

There is very little evidence that aromatherapy, chamomile, or valerian helps with insomnia. None have substantial side effects, but chamomile can cause allergic reactions. Kava is also advertised for sleep, but good research on kava for insomnia is lacking. More importantly, kava supplements have been linked to a risk of severe liver damage.

Colds and Influenza

Zinc supplements taken orally may reduce the length and severity of a cold. Zinc, particularly in large doses, can have side effects, including nausea and diarrhea. The intranasal use of zinc can cause anosmia (loss of sense of smell), which may be long lasting or permanent. In 2009, FDA warned consumers to stop using several intranasal zinc products because they had been linked to cases of anosmia.

Nasal saline irrigation, such as with neti pots, may be useful and safe for chronic sinusitis as long as sterile or distilled water is used. There is little research to support using nasal saline irrigation for acute upper respiratory infections.

Taking vitamin C supplements regularly may slightly reduce the length and severity of colds but does not reduce the number of colds. Even at high doses, vitamin C supplements appear safe.

There is no strong evidence to support claims promoting echinacea, probiotics, or the homeopathic product Oscillococcinum for flu.

There is no good evidence that Chinese herbs, oil of oregano, or eucalyptus essential oil prevents or treats colds and other infections.

Other Common or Travel-Related Infections

Hepatitis C

Medicinal herbs should not be used for treatment of hepatitis C outside of well-designed, randomized clinical trials. A recently published randomized clinical trial found no evidence of benefit from silymarin (an extract from milk thistle seeds) in patients with advanced hepatitis C. In addition, a systematic review of 10 randomized clinical trials found no firm evidence of efficacy of any medicinal herbs for hepatitis C virus infection. Two of the trials studied a single herb or herbal ingredient; the others studied different compounds of herbs.

Vaginal infections

Probiotics have been studied for treating vaginal infections, but there is not enough supporting evidence to suggest that they are helpful.

INSECT PROTECTION: BOTANICAL REPELLENTS

Laboratory-based studies found that botanicals, including citronella products, worked for shorter periods than products containing DEET. In addition to DEET products, CDC recommends products containing oil of lemon eucalyptus (OLE), such as the products Repel and Off! Botanicals.

There are no high-quality studies on the effectiveness or safety for people of neem oil, which is used in agricultural insecticide products and promoted on some websites for human use.

HOMEOPATHIC VACCINES

There is no credible scientific evidence, nor any plausible scientific rationale, to support claims that certain homeopathic products (sometimes called nosodes or homeopathic immunizations) are effective substitutes for conventional immunizations. For more information see General Recommendations for Vaccination & Immunoprophylaxis in this chapter.

UNTESTED THERAPIES IN OTHER COUNTRIES

CDC does not recommend traveling to other countries for untested medical interventions or to buy medications that are not approved in the United States.

TALKING TO TRAVELERS ABOUT COMPLEMENTARY HEALTH APPROACHES

Given the vast number of complementary or alternative interventions and the wealth of potentially misleading information about them that can be found on the Internet, discussing the use of these approaches with patients may seem daunting. However, it is important to be proactive, as surveys show that many patients are reluctant to raise the topic with their health care providers. Federal agencies, such as the National Center for Complementary and Integrative Health (NCCIH), offer evidence-based resources (https://nccih.nih.gov/health/providers) to help you and your patients have a meaningful discussion about complementary approaches.

ACKNOWLEDGMENTS
The authors thank Dr. John Williamson of NCCIH for his scientific review and Ms. Karen Kaplan and Ms. Patricia Andersen of Westat for their editorial assistance.

BIBLIOGRAPHY

1. Achilles N, Mosges R. Nasal saline irrigations for the symptoms of acute and chronic rhinosinusitis. Curr Allergy Asthma Rep. 2013 Apr;13(2):229–35.

2. Allen SJ, Martinez EG, Gregorio GV, Dans LF. Probiotics for treating acute infectious diarrhoea. Cochrane Database Syst Rev. 2010(11):CD003048.

3. Chow T, Browne V, Heileson HL, Wallace D, Anholm J, Green SM. Ginkgo biloba and acetazolamide prophylaxis for acute mountain sickness: a randomized, placebo-controlled trial. Arch Intern Med. 2005 Feb 14;165(3): 296–301.

4. Global Malaria Programme. WHO Position statement: effectiveness of non-pharmaceutical forms of Artemisia annua L. against malaria. Geneva: World Health Organization; 2012 [cited 2014 Sep 24]. Available from: http://www.who.int/malaria/diagnosis_treatment/position_statement_herbal_remedy_artemisia_annua_l.pdf.

5. Herxheimer A. Jet lag. Clin Evid (Online). 2008 Dec 4;2008. pii: 2303.

6. Herxheimer A, Petrie KJ. Melatonin for the prevention and treatment of jet lag. Cochrane Database Syst Rev. 2002(2):CD001520.

7. Mathie RT, Frye J, Fisher P. Homeopathic Oscillococcinum® for preventing and treating influenza and influenza-like illness. Cochrane Database Syst Rev. 2012;12:CD001957.

8. McFarland LV. Meta-analysis of probiotics for the prevention of traveler's diarrhea. Travel Med Infect Dis. 2007 Mar;5(2):97–105.

9. Morgenthaler TI, Lee-Chiong T, Alessi C, Friedman L, Aurora RN, Boehlecke B, et al. Practice parameters for the clinical evaluation and treatment of circadian rhythm sleep disorders: an American Academy of Sleep Medicine report. Sleep. 2007 Nov;30(11):1445–59.

10. Singh M, Das RR. Zinc for the common cold. Cochrane Database Syst Rev. 2013;6:CD001364.

DEEP VEIN THROMBOSIS & PULMONARY EMBOLISM

Nimia L. Reyes, Scott D. Grosse, Althea M. Grant

Deep vein thrombosis (DVT) is a condition in which a blood clot develops in the deep veins, most commonly in the lower extremities. A part of the clot can break off and travel to the lungs, causing a pulmonary embolism (PE), which can be life threatening. About 25% of calf vein DVTs, if left untreated, will extend to involve the proximal lower extremity veins (popliteal, femoral, or iliac veins); a proximal lower extremity DVT, if left untreated, has about a 50% risk of leading to a PE. Venous thromboembolism (VTE) is a term that includes both DVT and PE.

Many cases are asymptomatic and resolve spontaneously. VTE is often recurrent, and long-term complications, such as post-thrombotic syndrome after a DVT or chronic thromboembolic pulmonary hypertension after a PE, are frequent.

More than 300 million people travel on long-haul flights each year. An association between VTE and air travel was first reported in the early 1950s, and since then, long-haul air travel has become more common, leading to increased concerns about travel-related VTE.

PATHOGENESIS

Virchow's classic triad for thrombus forma-tion is venous stasis, vessel wall damage, and the hypercoagulable state. Prolonged cramped sitting during long-distance travel interferes with venous flow in the legs and causes venous stasis. Seat-edge pressure on the popliteal area may contribute to ves-sel wall damage as well as venous stasis. Coagulation activation may result from an interaction between cabin conditions (such as hypobaric hypoxia) and individual risk fac-tors for VTE. Studies of the pathophysiologic mechanisms for the increased risk of VTE after long-distance travel have not produced consistent results, but venous stasis appears to play a major role; other factors specific to air travel may increase coagulation activa-tion, particularly in passengers with individ-ual risk factors for VTE.

INCIDENCE

The annual incidence of VTE in the general population has been estimated at 0.1% but is higher in subpopulations with risk fac-tors for VTE (Box 2-9). The actual incidence of travel-related VTE is difficult to determine, since there is no consensus on the definition of travel-related VTE, particularly in regards to duration of travel and time window after travel. Estimates of travel-related VTE inci-dence vary because of differences between studies in duration of travel, measured out-come, time window after the flight, and the populations studied.

In general, the overall incidence of travel-related VTE is low. Two studies reported that the absolute risk of VTE for flights >4 hours is 1 in 4,656 flights and 1 in 6,000 flights. People who travel on long-distance flights are generally healthier and therefore are at lower risk for VTE than the general popula-tion. Five prospective studies that assessed the incidence of DVT among travelers at low to intermediate risk for VTE after travel >8 hours yielded an overall incidence of VTE of 0.5%, while the incidence of symptomatic VTE was 0.3%.

ASSOCIATION WITH TRAVEL

Numerous studies have examined the asso-ciation between travel, particularly air travel, and VTE. However, these studies had differ-ences in methods. Outcomes ranged from asymptomatic DVT to symptomatic DVT/ PE to severe or fatal PE. Asymptomatic DVT is estimated to be 5- to 20-fold more com-mon than symptomatic events. Definitions of long-distance travel ranged from flight dura-tion >3 hours to >10 hours (most >4 hours). The time window until illness after the flight ranged from hours after landing to ≥8 weeks (most 4 weeks).

Published studies have yielded varying results; some studies found that long-distance travel increased the risk of VTE, and oth-ers either found no definitive evidence that it increased the risk of VTE or found that it increased the risk only if ≥1 additional risk factors were present. Most studies found

---

BOX 2-9. VENOUS THROMBOEMBOLISM (VTE) RISK FACTORS

General risk factors for VTE include the following:

- Older age (increasing risk after age 40)
- Obesity (BMI >30 kg/m^2)
- Estrogen use (hormonal contraceptives or hormone replacement therapy)
- Pregnancy and the postpartum period
- Thrombophilia (such as factor V Leiden mutation or antiphospholipid syndrome) or a family history of VTE
- Previous VTE
- Active cancer
- Serious medical illness (such as congestive heart failure or inflammatory bowel disease)
- Recent surgery, hospitalization, or trauma
- Limited mobility
- Central venous catheterization

long-distance air travel to be a weak risk factor for VTE, and most VTE occurred as asymptomatic DVT of uncertain clinical significance in passengers with additional preexisting risk factors.

Long-distance air travel may increase the risk of VTE by 2- to 4-fold. A similar increase in risk is also seen with other modes of travel, such as car, bus, or train, implying that the increase in risk is caused mainly by prolonged limited mobility rather than by the cabin environment. The risk is the same for economy-class and business-class travel. The risk increases with increasing travel duration and with preexisting risk factors. The risk decreases with time after air travel; most air travel–related VTE occurs within the first 1–2 weeks after the flight and returns to baseline by 8 weeks.

RISK FACTORS

Most travel-related VTE occurs in passengers with risk factors for VTE (Box 2-9). Some studies have shown that 75%–99.5% of those who developed travel-related VTE had ≥1 preexisting risk factor; one study showed that 20% had ≥5 risk factors. For travelers without preexisting risk factors, the risk of travel-related VTE is low. However, a person may not be aware that he or she has a risk factor such as inherited thrombophilia. The combination of air travel with preexisting individual risk factors may have a synergistic effect on the risk for VTE.

For air travelers, height appears to be an additional risk factor. Risk of travel-related VTE increases with height <1.6 m (5 ft, 3 in). Unlike car seats, airline seats are higher and cannot be adjusted to a person's height; therefore, shorter passengers who travel by air may experience seat-edge pressure to the popliteal area. Risk of travel-related VTE also increases with height >1.9 m (6 ft, 3 in), possibly because taller passengers have less leg room.

CLINICAL PRESENTATION

Signs and symptoms of DVT/PE are nonspecific:

- Typical signs or symptoms of DVT in the extremities include pain or tenderness, swelling, increased warmth in the affected area, and redness or discoloration of the overlying skin.
- The most common signs or symptoms of acute PE include unexplained shortness of breath, pleuritic chest pain, cough or hemoptysis, and syncope.

DIAGNOSIS

Imaging studies are needed for diagnosis:

- Duplex ultrasonography is the standard imaging procedure for diagnosis of DVT. Contrast venography is the gold standard but is invasive and uses potentially harmful contrast material. Magnetic resonance venography imaging and computed axial tomography venography are less frequently used.
- Computed tomographic pulmonary angiography is the standard imaging procedure for diagnosis of PE. Ventilation-perfusion scan is the second-line imaging procedure. Pulmonary angiography is the gold standard but is invasive and uses potentially harmful contrast material. Magnetic resonance angiography can also be used.

PREVENTIVE MEASURES FOR LONG-DISTANCE TRAVELERS

The American College of Chest Physicians published the 9th edition of their Antithrombotic Therapy and Prevention of Thrombosis Evidence-Based Clinical Practice Guidelines in February 2012. Recommendations for long-distance travelers (considered grade 2C: weak recommendation, low- or very low-quality evidence) are the following:

1. For long-distance travelers at increased risk of VTE (Box 2-9), frequent ambulation, calf muscle exercise, and sitting in an aisle seat if feasible are suggested.
2. For long-distance travelers at increased risk of VTE (Box 2-9), use of properly fitted, below-knee graduated compression stockings (GCS) providing 15–30 mm Hg of pressure at the ankle during travel is suggested. For all other long-distance travelers, use of GCS is not recommended.
3. For long-distance travelers, the use of aspirin or anticoagulants to prevent VTE is not recommended.

There is no evidence for an association between dehydration and travel-related VTE and no direct evidence that drinking plenty of nonalcoholic beverages to ensure adequate hydration or avoiding alcoholic beverages has a protective effect. Therefore, while maintaining hydration is reasonable and unlikely to cause harm, it cannot be strongly recommended specifically to prevent travel-related VTE.

There is evidence that immobility while flying is a risk for VTE and indirect evidence that maintaining mobility may prevent VTE. In view of the role of venous stasis in the pathogenesis of travel-related VTE, it would be reasonable to recommend frequent ambulation and calf muscle exercises for long-distance travelers.

Compared with aisle seats, window seats in one study were reported to increase the risk 2-fold, particularly in obese passengers, who had a 6-fold increase in risk. Aisle seats are reported to have a protective effect, compared with window or middle seats, probably because passengers are freer to move around.

GCS are indicated for long-distance travelers at increased risk. GCS appear to reduce asymptomatic DVT in travelers and are generally well tolerated.

Global use of anticoagulants for long-distance travel is not indicated. Pharmacologic prophylaxis for long-distance travelers at particularly high risk should be decided on an individual basis. In cases where the potential benefits of pharmacologic prophylaxis outweigh the possible adverse effects, anticoagulants rather than antiplatelet drugs are recommended.

RECOMMENDATIONS

1. General measures for long-distance travelers:
   a. Calf muscle exercises
   b. Frequent ambulation
   c. Aisle seating when feasible
2. Additional measures for long-distance travelers at increased risk of VTE:
   a. Properly fitted below-knee GCS
   b. Anticoagulant prophylaxis only in particularly high-risk cases where the potential benefits outweigh the risks

BIBLIOGRAPHY

1. Aryal KR, Al-Khaffaf H. Venous thromboembolic complications following air travel: what's the quantitative risk? A literature review. Eur J Vasc Endovasc Surg. 2006 Feb;31(2):187–99.
2. Bartholomew JR, Schaffer JL, McCormick GF. Air travel and venous thromboembolism: minimizing the risk. Cleve Clin J Med. 2011 Feb;78(2):111–20.
3. Chandra D, Parisini E, Mozaffarian D. Meta-analysis: travel and risk for venous thromboembolism. Ann Intern Med. 2009 Aug 4;151(3):180–90.
4. Eklof B, Maksimovic D, Caprini JA, Glase C. Air travel-related venous thromboembolism. Disease-a-month: DM. 2005 Feb–Mar;51(2–3):200–7.
5. Gavish I, Brenner B. Air travel and the risk of thromboembolism. Intern Emerg Med. 2011 Apr;6(2):113–6.
6. Kahn SR, Lim W, Dunn AS, Cushman M, Dentali F, Akl EA, et al. Prevention of VTE in nonsurgical patients: antithrombotic therapy and prevention of thrombosis, 9th ed: American College of Chest Physicians evidence-based clinical practice guidelines. Chest. 2012 Feb;141(2 Suppl):e195S–226S.
7. Schobersberger W, Schobersberger B, Partsch H. Travel-related thromboembolism: mechanisms and avoidance. Expert Rev Cardiovasc Ther. 2009 Dec;7(12):1559–67.
8. Schreijer AJ, Cannegieter SC, Caramella M, Meijers JC, Krediet RT, Simons RM, et al. Fluid loss does not explain coagulation activation during air travel. Thromb Haemost. 2008 Jun;99(6):1053–9.
9. Schreijer AJ, Cannegieter SC, Doggen CJ, Rosendaal FR. The effect of flight-related behaviour on the risk of venous thrombosis after air travel. Br J Haematol. 2008 Feb;144(3):425–9.
10. Watson HG, Baglin TP. Guidelines on travel-related venous thrombosis. Br J Haematol. 2011 Jan;152(1):31–4.

MENTAL HEALTH
Thomas H. Valk

International travel is stressful. Stressors vary to some extent with the type of travel; short-term travel likely offers the least stress and frequent travel and expatriation the most. Given the stressors of travel, preexisting psychiatric disorders can recur, and latent, undiagnosed problems can become apparent for the first time.

OCCURRENCE IN TRAVELERS

Incidence data based on population surveys of travelers are nonexistent. Data from clinical populations include the following:

- Patel et al. conducted a study of urgent repatriation of British diplomats and found that 11% of medical evacuations were "nonphysical," or psychological in nature. Using the authors' data, an overall incident rate of 0.34% for psychological evacuations occurred for their population. Of these, 41% were for some form of depression.
- Another study examined psychiatric evacuations over a 5-year period in the US Foreign Service population from 1982 through 1986. Using an unpublished estimate of the population served in this study, an overall incidence rate of 0.16% for psychiatric evacuations occurred. Of these, fully 50% were for substance abuse or affective disorder. Mania and hypomanic states accounted for 2.8% of these evacuations.
- Streltzer studied psychiatric emergencies in travelers to Hawaii and estimated a rate of 0.22% for tourists and 2.25% for transient travelers (those arriving in Hawaii with no immediate plans to leave) versus a rate of 1.25% for nontravelers. In order of decreasing frequency, diagnoses in this population were schizophrenia, alcohol abuse, anxiety reactions, and depression.
- Quigley et al. studied repatriations over a 2-year period (2010–2012) comparing American-sponsored college students studying abroad with American-sponsored

corporate business travelers and expatriates. They found a 23-times higher rate of repatriation because of mental health problems for the student population. In this population of repatriated students, in order of decreasing frequency, diagnoses were mood, personality, substance abuse, eating disorders, and schizophrenia or other psychotic disorders.

THE PRE-TRAVEL CONSULTATION AND MENTAL HEALTH EVALUATION

Any pre-travel consultation should include a mental health screening, especially for those planning extended travel or residence in a foreign country. Since travel medicine specialists rarely have mental health credentials, a full mental health inquiry with mental status examination and a psychiatric review of symptoms would not be practicable. Rather, a brief inquiry aimed at eliciting previously diagnosed psychiatric disorders should be undertaken. To introduce this portion of the consultation and to elicit the most cooperation, the practitioner could enumerate the following facts:

- International travel is stressful for everyone and has been associated with the emergence or reemergence of mental health problems.
- The availability of culturally compatible mental health services varies widely.
- Laws regarding the use of illicit substances can be severe in some countries.

The practitioner can then ask about factors that might indicate a mental health problem:

- Any previously treated or diagnosed psychiatric disorders and the type of treatment involved (inpatient, outpatient, medications)
- Current treatment for any psychiatric disorders and their nature
- Current or past use of illicit substances

- Any diagnosis of substance use disorder, or suggestion from medical service providers, friends, or family that the traveler might be using alcohol or other substances to excess
- Any immediate family history of serious mental health problems

In general, any history of inpatient treatment, psychotic episode, violent or suicidal behavior, affective disorder (including mania, hypomania, or major depression), any treatment for substance use problems, and any current treatments would warrant further evaluation by a mental health professional, preferably one who has had some experience in problems relating to international travel. On occasion, the patient's mental status upon examination may be notably abnormal, which would also warrant a referral.

Other issues that may be encountered and should be addressed during the pre-travel consultation include the following:

- Customs regulations: Traveling through customs with medications for personal use can be problematic in countries where those medications are prohibited. What substances are prohibited in any given country varies. Stimulants frequently used for attention deficit disorders, such as amphetamine or methylphenidate, may be problematic, along with narcotics. This list is not exhaustive, and travelers should check with the US embassy at their destination if they have any questions. It is always wise to carry medications in their original containers, along with a letter from the prescribing physician indicating that the medications have been prescribed for medical reasons. Even with these precautions, problems may still occur at customs. A health care provider or pharmacist in the destination country may be able to provide guidance about medication restrictions.
- Psychotropic medication refills: Obtaining these medications while living overseas can be problematic, as availability or even legality of the medication varies from country to country. Again, a check with the country's embassy may be helpful, as would a check with a reputable in-country pharmacy or health care provider.
- Measuring drug levels: Locating laboratory facilities for the determination of lithium levels or for other mood-stabilizing medications may be challenging and should be investigated prior to travel. High temperatures and increased sweating could lead to toxicity, even on the same dose.
- Mefloquine: In general, patients with mental health issues should not be prescribed mefloquine for malarial chemoprophylaxis because of its potential for neuropsychiatric side effects.
- Alcoholics Anonymous (AA) and Narcotics Anonymous (NA) meetings: Currently sober patients with substance use disorders should consider seeking out AA and NA meetings, depending upon their length of stay and stability of their sobriety.
- Evacuation insurance: Travelers with mental health problems should consider travel health and medical evacuation insurance for emergencies when abroad.

POST-TRAVEL MENTAL HEALTH ISSUES

Travel health practitioners may be in a unique position to inquire about traumatic experiences a traveler might have had that may lead to posttraumatic stress disorder (PTSD). Travelers continuously exposed to high levels of stress, such as disaster relief workers, may experience a subclinical syndrome of PTSD.

If the traveler has had such an experience, clinicians should inquire about possible symptoms:

- Reexperiencing the event could include recurrent and intrusive recollections or distressing dreams of the event or feeling as if the event is happening again.
- Avoidance symptoms can include avoiding thoughts, feelings, activities, places, or people that lead to memories of the event.
- Arousal symptoms can include difficulty sleeping or concentrating, irritability, or an exaggerated startle response.

As symptoms may occur months or even years after an event, education about the possibility of having such symptoms in the future is worthwhile. If there is any doubt about a possible reaction to a traumatic event, referral to a psychiatrist is warranted.

 MENTAL HEALTH

BIBLIOGRAPHY

1. Benedek DM, Wynn GH. Clinical Manual for Management of PTSD. Arlington, VA: American Psychiatric Publishing, Inc.; 2011.
2. Liese B, Mundt KA, Dell LD, Nagy L, Demure B. Medical insurance claims associated with international business travel. Occup Environ Med. 1997 Jul;54(7):499–503.
3. Patel D, Easmon CJ, Dow C, Snashall DC, Seed PT. Medical repatriation of British diplomats resident overseas. J Travel Med. 2000 Mar–Apr;7(2):64–9.
4. Quigley RL, Copeland R. Mental health and study abroad: incidence and mitigation strategies. Oral

presentation at: 13th Conference of the International Society of Travel Medicine; 2013 May 19–23; Maastricht, The Netherlands.
5. Streltzer J. Psychiatric emergencies in travelers to Hawaii. Compr Psychiatry. 1979 Sep–Oct;20(5):463–8.
6. Valk TH. Psychiatric disorders of travel. In: Keystone JS, Freedman DO, Kozarsky PE, Connor BA, Nothdurft HO, editors. Travel Medicine. 3rd ed. Philadelphia: Saunders Elsevier; 2013. p. 439–48.
7. Valk TH. Psychiatric medical evacuations within the Foreign Service. Foreign Serv Med Bull. 1988;268:9–11.

TRAVEL HEALTH KITS

Amanda W. Lee

Regardless of the destination, all international travelers should assemble and carry a travel health kit. The contents of a travel health kit should be tailored to the traveler's needs, type and length of travel, and destinations. Kits can be assembled at home or purchased at a local store, pharmacy, or online.

A travel health kit can help to ensure travelers have supplies they need to

- Manage preexisting medical conditions and treat any exacerbations of these conditions
- Prevent illness and injury related to traveling
- Take care of minor health problems as they occur

By bringing medications from home, travelers avoid having to purchase them at their destination. See *Perspectives*: Pharmaceutical Quality & Counterfeit Drugs later in this chapter for information about the risks associated with purchasing medications abroad. Even when the quality of medications is reliable, medications people are used to taking at home may be sold under different names or with different ingredients and dosage units in other countries, presenting additional challenges.

TRAVELING WITH MEDICATIONS

All medications should be carried in their original containers with clear labels, so the contents are easily identified. The patient's name and dosing regimen should be on each container. Although many travelers prefer placing medications into small containers or packing them in daily-dose containers, officials at ports of entry may require proper identification of medications.

Travelers should carry copies of all prescriptions, including their generic names and preferably translated into the local language of the destination. For controlled substances and injectable medications, travelers should carry a note from the prescribing clinician or from the travel clinic on letterhead stationery. Translating the letter into the local language of the destination and attaching this translation to the original document may prove helpful if the document is needed during the trip. Certain medications are not permitted in some countries. If there is a question about these restrictions, particularly regarding controlled substances, travelers should contact the embassy or consulate of the destination country.

A travel health kit is useful only when it is easily accessible. It should be carried with the traveler at all times (such as in a carry-on bag), although sharp objects must remain in checked luggage. Travelers should make sure that any liquid or gel-based items packed in the carry-on bags do not exceed the size limits. Exceptions are made for certain medical reasons; check the Transportation Security Administration for US outbound and inbound travel (visit www.tsa.gov/traveler-information/medically-necessary-liquids; call toll-free at 866-289-9673 M–F 8 AM to 11 PM, weekends and holidays 9 AM to 8 PM; or e-mail TSA-ContactCenter@dhs.gov) and the embassy or consulate of the destination country for their restrictions.

SUPPLIES FOR PREEXISTING MEDICAL CONDITIONS

Travelers with preexisting medical conditions should carry enough medication for the duration of their trip and an extra supply, in case the trip is extended for any reason. If additional supplies or medications would be needed to manage exacerbations of existing medical conditions, these should be carried as well. The clinician managing a traveler's preexisting medical conditions should be consulted for the best plan of action (see Chapter 8, Travelers with Chronic Illnesses).

People with preexisting conditions, such as diabetes or allergies, should consider wearing an alert bracelet and making sure this information (in English and preferably translated into the local language of the destination) is on a card in their wallet and with their other travel documents.

GENERAL TRAVEL HEALTH KIT SUPPLIES

Although the following is not a comprehensive list, basic items that should be considered for a travel health kit are listed below. See Chapter 8 for additional suggestions that may be useful in planning the contents of a kit for travelers with specific needs.

Prescription Medications and Supplies
- ☐ Medications taken on a regular basis at home
- ☐ Antibiotic for self-treatment of moderate to severe diarrhea

- ☐ Medication to prevent malaria, if needed
- ☐ Medication to prevent or treat altitude illness, if needed
- ☐ Prescription glasses/contacts for people who wear corrective lenses (consider packing an extra pair of each in case lenses are damaged)
- ☐ Epinephrine auto-injectors* (such as an EpiPen 2-Pak), especially if history of severe allergic reaction or anaphylaxis; smaller-dose packages are available for children
- ☐ Diabetes testing supplies and insulin
- ☐ Needles or syringes, if needed, such as for people with diabetes. Needles and syringes can be difficult to purchase in some locations, so take more than what is needed for the length of the trip. (These items will require a letter from the prescribing clinician on letterhead stationery.)
- ☐ Medical alert bracelet or necklace

Over-the-Counter Medications
- ☐ Medications taken on a regular basis at home
- ☐ Treatment for pain or fever (one or more of the following, or an alternative):
  - > Acetaminophen
  - > Aspirin
  - > Ibuprofen
- ☐ Treatment for stomach upset or diarrhea:
  - > Antidiarrheal medication (such as loperamide [Imodium] or bismuth subsalicylate [Pepto-Bismol])
  - > Packets of oral rehydration salts for dehydration
  - > Mild laxative
  - > Antacid
- ☐ Treatment for upper respiratory tract discomfort:
  - > Antihistamine
  - > Decongestant, alone or in combination with antihistamine
  - > Cough suppressant or expectorant
  - > Cough drops
- ☐ Anti–motion sickness medication
- ☐ Mild sedative or sleep aid

---

* Note: Injectable epinephrine and antihistamines should always be carried on one's person, including during air, sea, and land travel, for immediate treatment of a severe allergic reaction. Travelers with a history of severe allergic reactions should consider bringing along a short course of oral steroid medication (prescription required from doctor) and antihistamines as additional treatment of a severe allergic reaction.

□ Saline eye drops
□ Saline nose drops or spray

Basic First Aid Items

□ Disposable latex-free gloves (≥2 pairs)
□ Adhesive bandages, multiple sizes
□ Gauze
□ Adhesive tape
□ Antiseptic wound cleanser
□ Cotton swabs
□ Antifungal and antibacterial spray or creams
□ 1% hydrocortisone cream
□ Anti-itch gel or cream for insect bites and stings
□ Aloe gel for sunburns
□ Moleskin or molefoam for blister prevention and treatment
□ Digital thermometer
□ Tweezers**
□ Scissors**
□ Safety pins
□ Elastic/compression bandage wrap for sprains and strains
□ Triangular bandage to wrap injuries and to make an arm or shoulder sling
□ For travel in remote areas, consider a commercial suture kit
□ First aid quick reference card

Supplies to Prevent Illness or Injury

□ Antibacterial hand wipes or an alcohol-based hand sanitizer, containing ≥60% alcohol
□ Insect repellents for skin and clothing (see the Protection against Mosquitoes, Ticks, & Other Arthropods section earlier in this chapter for recommended types)
□ Bed net (if needed, for protection against insect bites while sleeping)
□ Sunscreen (≥15 SPF with UVA and UVB protection)
□ Water purification tablets (if visiting remote areas, camping, or staying in areas where access to clean water is limited)
□ Latex condoms
□ Ear plugs

□ Personal safety equipment (such as child safety seats and bicycle helmets)

Documents

Travelers should carry the following documents and leave a copy of these documents with a family member or close contact who will remain in the United States, in case of an emergency.

□ Proof of vaccination on an International Certificate of Vaccination or Prophylaxis (ICVP) card or medical waiver (if vaccinations are required)
□ Copies of all prescriptions for medications, eye glasses/contacts, and other medical supplies (including generic names and preferably translated into the local language of the destination)
□ Documentation of preexisting conditions, such as diabetes or allergies (in English and preferably translated into the local language of the destination)
□ Health insurance, supplemental travel health insurance, medical evacuation insurance, and travel insurance information (carry contact information for all insurance providers and copies of claim forms)
□ Contact card to be carried with the traveler at all times, including street addresses, phone numbers, and e-mail addresses of the following:
  > Family member or close contact remaining in the United States
  > Health care provider(s) at home
  > Place(s) of lodging at the destination(s)
  > Hospitals or clinics (including emergency services) in your destination(s)
  > US embassy or consulate in the destination country or countries

See the Obtaining Health Care Abroad for the Ill Traveler section later in this chapter for information about how to locate local health care and embassy or consulate contacts.

** Note: If traveling by air, travelers should pack these sharp items in checked baggage, since they could be confiscated by airport or airline security if packed in carry-on bags. Small bandage scissors with rounded tips may be available for purchase in certain stores or online.

COMMERCIAL MEDICAL KITS

Commercial medical kits are available for a wide range of circumstances, from basic first aid to advanced emergency life support. For more adventurous travelers, a number of companies produce advanced medical kits and will even customize kits based on specific travel needs. In addition, specialty kits are available for managing diabetes, dealing with dental emergencies, and handling aquatic environments. Many pharmacy, grocery, retail, and outdoor sporting goods stores, as well as online retailers, sell their own basic first aid kits. Travelers who choose to purchase a pre-assembled kit should review the contents of the kit carefully to ensure that it has everything needed. Additional items may be necessary and can be added to the purchased kit.

BIBLIOGRAPHY

1. Goodyer L. Travel medical kits. In: Keystone JS, Freedman DO, Kozarsky PE, Connor BA, Nothdurft HD, editors. Travel Medicine. 3rd ed. Philadelphia: Saunders Elsevier; 2013. p. 63–6.
2. Harper LA, Bettinger J, Dismukes R, Kozarsky PE. Evaluation of the Coca-Cola company travel health kit. J Travel Med. 2002 Sep–Oct; 9(5):244–6.
3. Rose SR, Keystone JS. Chapter 2, trip preparation. In: Rose SR, Keystone JS, editors. International Travel Health Guide. 14th ed. Northampton: Travel Medicine, Inc; 2008.

Perspectives

PHARMACEUTICAL QUALITY & COUNTERFEIT DRUGS

Michael D. Green

Counterfeit and substandard drugs are an international problem contributing to illness, death, toxicity, and drug resistance. A counterfeit drug is a compound that is not made by an authorized manufacturer but is presented to the consumer as if it were. Both the packaging and pill construction of counterfeit drugs are often virtually identical to the authentic medication. Substandard drugs are medicines made by a licensed manufacturer but fail to comply with pharmaceutical regulatory standards. These drugs may not contain the proper proportion of ingredients and are consequently less effective or may cause an adverse reaction. Regulatory agencies in the United States, such as the Food and Drug Administration, protect citizens from products that are inherently unsafe. In developing countries, regulatory controls are much less effective or even nonexistent, leading to conditions that allow proliferation of counterfeit and

Perspectives sections are written as editorial discussions aiming to add depth and clinical perspective to the official recommendations contained in the book. The views and opinions expressed in this section are those of the author and do not necessarily represent the official position of CDC.

substandard drugs. Overall, global estimates of drug counterfeiting are ambiguous, depending on region, but proportions range from 1% of sales in developed countries to >10% in developing countries. In specific regions in Africa, Asia, and Latin America, chances of purchasing a counterfeit drug may be >30%.

Since counterfeit drugs are not made by the legitimate manufacturer and are produced under unlawful circumstances, toxic contaminants or lack of proper ingredients may result in serious harm. For example, the active pharmaceutical ingredient may be completely lacking, present in small quantities, or substituted by a less-effective compound. In addition, the wrong inactive ingredients (excipients) can contribute to poor drug dissolution and bioavailability. As a result, a patient may not respond to treatment or may have adverse reactions to unknown substituted or toxic ingredients.

Before international departure, travel health providers should alert travelers to the dangers of counterfeit and substandard drugs and provide suggestions on how to avoid them.

HOW TO AVOID COUNTERFEIT DRUGS WHEN TRAVELING

The best way to avoid counterfeit drugs is to reduce the need to purchase medications abroad. Anticipated amounts of medications for chronic conditions (such as hypertension, sinusitis, arthritis, and hay fever), medications for gastroenteritis (such as travelers' diarrhea), and prophylactic medications for infectious diseases (such as malaria) should all be purchased before traveling.

Before departure, travelers should do the following:

- Purchase all medicines needed for the trip in advance. Prescriptions written in the United States usually cannot be filled overseas, and over-the-counter medicines may not be available in many foreign countries. Checked baggage can get lost; therefore, travelers should pack as much as possible in a carry-on bag and bring extra medicine in case of travel delays.
- Make sure medicines are in their original containers. If the drug is a prescription, the patient's name and dose regimen should be on the container.
- Bring the "patient prescription information" sheet. This sheet provides information on common generic and brand names, use, side effects, precautions, and drug interactions.

If travelers run out and require additional medications, they should take steps to ensure the medicines they buy are safe:

- Purchase medicines from a legitimate pharmacy. Patients should not buy from open markets, street vendors, or suspicious-looking pharmacies; they should request a receipt when making the purchase. The US embassy may be able to help find a legitimate pharmacy in the area.
- Do not buy medicines that are substantially cheaper than the typical price. Although generics are usually less expensive, many counterfeited brand names are sold at prices substantially below the normal price for that particular brand.
- Make sure the medicines are in their original packages or containers. If travelers receive medicines as loose tablets or capsules supplied in a plastic bag or envelope, they should ask the pharmacist to see the container from which the medicine was originally dispensed. The traveler should record the brand, batch number, and expiration date. Sometimes a wary consumer will prompt the seller into supplying quality medicine.

- Be familiar with medications. The size, shape, color, and taste of counterfeit medicines may be different from the authentic. Discoloration, splits, cracks, spots, and stickiness of the tablets or capsules are indications of a possible counterfeit. Travelers should keep examples of authentic medications to compare if they purchase the same brand.
- Be familiar with the packaging. Different color inks, poor-quality print or packaging material, and misspelled words are clues to counterfeit drugs. Travelers should keep an example of packaging for comparison, and observe the expiration date to make sure the medicine has not expired.

USEFUL WEBSITES
General Information about Counterfeit Drugs
- CDC: wwwnc.cdc.gov/travel/page/counterfeit-medicine
- World Health Organization:
  > www.who.int/mediacentre/factsheets/fs275/en/
  > www.who.int/medicines/services/counterfeit/overview/en/
- Food and Drug Administration: www.fda.gov//Drugs/DrugSafety/ucm170314.htm
- US Pharmacopeia: www.usp.org/worldwide

Traveling and Customs Guidelines
Researching what travelers can pack and bring back into the United States, especially for travelers with disabilities and medical conditions, is helpful in preparing for travel.

- Transportation Security Administration: www.tsa.gov/traveler-information/travelers-disabilities-and-medical-conditions
- Customs and Border Protection: www.cbp.gov/travel/international-visitors/kbyg/prohibited-restricted
- Reporting Counterfeit Cases
  > World Health Organization: www.who.int/medicines/services/counterfeit/report/en/

BIBLIOGRAPHY

1. Bate R, Jin GZ, Mathur A. Does price reveal poor-quality drugs? Evidence from 17 countries. J Health Econ. 2011 Dec;30(6):1150–63.
2. Nayyar GM, Breman JG, Newton PN, Herrington J. Poor-quality antimalarial drugs in southeast Asia and sub-Saharan Africa. Lancet Infect Dis. 2012 Jun;12(6):488–96.
3. Newton P, Fernandez F, Green M. Counterfeit and substandard antimalarial drugs. In: Schlagenhauf-Lawlor P, editor. Travelers' Malaria. 2nd ed. Hamilton, ON: BC Decker; 2008. p. 331–42.
4. Newton PN, Green MD, Fernandez FM, Day NP, White NJ. Counterfeit anti-infective drugs. Lancet Infect Dis. 2006 Sep;6(9):602–13.
5. World Health Organization. Medicines: counterfeit medicines [fact sheet no. 275]. Geneva: World Health Organization; 2012 [cited 2014 Sep 12]. Available from: http://www.who.int/mediacentre/factsheets/fs275/en/.

OBTAINING HEALTH CARE ABROAD FOR THE ILL TRAVELER

Pauline V. Han

The quality and availability of medical care abroad may be variable. Before departure, travelers should consider how they would access health care during their trip should a medical problem arise. Travelers may seek medical care while abroad for a range of reasons (Box 2-10).

Many insurance plans provide coverage for emergency health care while abroad, but travelers should check with their carriers to confirm what coverage is offered and what requirements exist. At a minimum, travelers will need to provide copies of bills and invoices to initiate reimbursement. Travelers should also be aware that emergency health coverage does not usually cover emergency evacuation or the costs of altered itineraries. Travelers may purchase specific policies to cover these expenses.

LOCATING ADEQUATE HEALTH CARE PROVIDERS AND FACILITIES ABROAD

Before going abroad, travelers should identify health care providers and facilities at their destination. This is especially true for travelers with preexisting or complicated medical issues. Travelers who require regular dialysis need to arrange appointments at an adequate clinical site before arriving at their destination. Similarly, pregnant travelers should identify reliable health facilities before going abroad. More choices are generally available in urban areas than in rural or remote areas, and travelers should plan accordingly.

The following is a list of resources to help identify health care providers and facilities around the world. CDC does not endorse any particular international providers, and accreditation does not necessarily ensure a good outcome. If travelers are likely to seek health care abroad, they should be encouraged to thoroughly research health care facilities in the area.

- The Department of State (www.usembassy.gov) can help travelers locate medical services and notify friends, family, or employer of an emergency.
- The International Society of Travel Medicine maintains a directory of health care professionals with expertise in travel medicine in more than 80 countries worldwide. Search these clinics at www.istm.org.
- The International Association for Medical Assistance to Travelers maintains an international network of physicians, hospitals,

---

BOX 2-10. COMMON REASONS TRAVELERS MAY SEEK MEDICAL CARE ABROAD

- Cardiovascular event
- Gastrointestinal illness
- Respiratory distress or infection
- Neurologic event
- Fever
- Injury or trauma
- Animal bite or scratch
- Severe allergic reaction
- Dialysis
- Obstetric reasons

and clinics that have agreed to provide care to members while abroad. Membership is free, although donations are suggested. Search for clinics at www.iamat.org/doctors_clinics.cfm.

- The Joint Commission International (JCI) aims to improve patient safety through accreditation and certification of health care facilities worldwide. Facilities that are accredited through JCI are said to demonstrate a standard level of quality. A list of these facilities can be found at www.jointcommissioninternational.org/JCI-Accredited-Organizations.
- Embassies and consulates in other countries, hotel doctors, and credit card companies (especially those with special privileges) may also provide information.

Supplemental medical insurance plans acquired before travel will often enable access to local providers in many countries through a 24-hour emergency hotline. (For more information on medical insurance, see the next section in this chapter, Travel Insurance, Travel Health Insurance, & Medical Evacuation Insurance.)

In addition to identifying quality health care, travelers, especially those with chronic or complicated medical issues, should know the names of their chronic conditions and allergies, their blood type, and current medications (including generic names), ideally in the local language. Travelers should also wear medical identification jewelry (such as a MedicAlert bracelet), if appropriate.

AVOID TRAVEL WHEN SICK

Travelers should evaluate their health before travel to ensure that they are healthy enough for their itinerary and should avoid travel if they become ill before or during their trip. Some airlines check for visibly sick passengers in the waiting area and during boarding. If a passenger looks visibly ill, the airline may prohibit that person from boarding. Travelers may be reluctant to postpone or cancel a trip when ill because of their financial investment in a trip, among other factors.

Encouraging travelers, especially those with chronic or complicated health conditions, to purchase trip cancellation insurance, which will protect some or all of the investment in a trip, may increase compliance with this recommendation.

DRUGS AND OTHER PHARMACEUTICALS

The quality of drugs and medical products abroad cannot be guaranteed, as they may not meet US standards or could be counterfeit (see *Perspectives*: Pharmaceutical Quality & Counterfeit Drugs earlier in this chapter). To minimize risks associated with substandard drugs and pharmaceuticals, travelers should

- Bring with them all the medicines that they think they will need, including pain relievers and antidiarrheal medication.
- Use caution when buying medications abroad, especially those that do not require a prescription. In many developing countries, a variety of drugs can be purchased without a prescription.
- Insist that a new needle and syringe be used when receiving an injection. Travelers who know beforehand that they will require injections during their trip can bring their own injection supplies (see the Travel Health Kits section earlier in this chapter).
- Carry an epinephrine autoinjector, if needed, in carry-on luggage and include a letter from the prescribing physician that explains the allergy and a copy of the prescription.

BLOOD SAFETY

A medical emergency abroad, such as a motor vehicle accident or trauma, could result in need for a blood transfusion. Not all countries have accurate, reliable, and systematic screening of blood donations for infectious agents, which increases the risk of transfusion-related transmission of disease. Although it is difficult to ensure access to safe blood, there are a few measures travelers can take to increase their chances of having a safe blood transfusion in the event of a medical emergency:

- Avoid blood transfusions as much as possible, particularly in developing countries. Travelers should receive a blood transfusion only in life-or-death situations.
- If a blood transfusion is required, travelers should make every effort to ensure that the blood has been screened for transmissible diseases, including HIV. Although

this is difficult to do at the point of service, travelers who plan ahead, especially those with medical conditions that might require transfusions, and locate medical services before traveling will increase their chances of obtaining higher-quality care abroad.

- Travelers may consider registering with agencies such as the Blood Care Foundation that attempt to rapidly deliver reliable blood products to members while abroad (www. bloodcare.org.uk/blood-transfusions-abroad.html).

All travelers should consider being immunized against hepatitis B virus before travel, especially those who travel frequently to developing countries, those whose itinerary indicates spending a prolonged period in developing countries, and those whose activities (such as adventure travel) put them at higher risk for serious injury.

BIBLIOGRAPHY

1. Hill DR. Health problems in a large cohort of Americans traveling to developing countries. J Travel Med. 2000 Sep–Oct;7(5):259–66.
2. Kolars JC. Rules of the road: a consumer's guide for travelers seeking health care in foreign lands. J Travel Med. 2002 Jul–Aug; 9(4):198–201.
3. Rack J, Wichmann O, Kamara B, Gunther M, Cramer J, Schonfeld C, et al. Risk and spectrum of diseases in travelers to popular tourist destinations. J Travel Med. 2005 Sep–Oct;12(5):248–53.
4. World Health Organization. Blood safety [fact sheet no. 279]. Geneva: World Health Organization; 2014 [cited 2014 Sep 18]. Available from: http://www.who.int/mediacentre/factsheets/fs279/en/.
5. World Health Organization. Medicines: spurious/falsely-labelled/falsified/counterfeit (SFFC) medicines [fact sheet no. 275]. Geneva: World Health Organization; 2012 [cited 2014 Sep 18]. Available from: http://www.who.int/mediacentre/factsheets/fs275/en/.

TRAVEL INSURANCE, TRAVEL HEALTH INSURANCE, & MEDICAL EVACUATION INSURANCE

Rhett J. Stoney

Severe illness or injury abroad may result in a financial burden on travelers. Although planning for every possible contingency is impossible, travelers can reduce the cost of a medical emergency by considering the purchase of 3 types of insurance for their trip: travel insurance, travel health insurance, and medical evacuation insurance. These insurance policies can be purchased before a trip to provide coverage in the event of an illness or injury and may be of particular importance to travelers with chronic medical conditions. Basic accident or travel insurance may even be required for travelers to certain destinations.

TRAVEL INSURANCE

Travel insurance protects the financial investment in a trip, including lost baggage and trip cancellation. Travelers may be more likely to avoid travel when sick if they know their financial investment in the trip is protected. Depending on the policy, this type of insurance may or may not cover medical expenses abroad, so travelers need to carefully research the coverage offered to determine if additional travel health and medical evacuation insurance is needed.

PAYING FOR HEALTH SERVICES ABROAD

Medical care abroad usually requires cash or credit card payment at the point of service, regardless of whether the traveler has insurance coverage in their home country. This could result in a large out-of-pocket expenditure of perhaps thousands of dollars. Additionally, the existence of nationalized health care services in a given destination does not ensure that nonresidents will be given full coverage. When paying out-of-pocket for care, travelers should obtain copies of all bills and receipts and, if necessary, contact a US consular officer, who can assist US citizens with transferring funds from the United States. A discussion of insurance options is an important part of any pre-travel consultation. In addition to covering costs of treatment or medical evacuation, the travel health insurer can also assist in organizing and coordinating care and keeping relatives informed. This is especially important when the traveler is severely ill or injured and requires medical evacuation. Although all travelers should consider insurance, it is particularly important for travelers who plan extended travel outside the United States, have underlying health conditions, or plan to participate in high-risk activities on their trip, especially if the destination is remote or lacks high-quality medical facilities.

DOMESTIC HEALTH INSURANCE

Some health insurance carriers in the United States may provide coverage for emergencies that occur while traveling abroad. Travelers should examine their coverage and planned itinerary to determine which medical services, if any, will be covered abroad and the level of supplemental insurance needed. The following is a list of characteristics to consider:

- Exclusions for treating exacerbations of preexisting medical conditions
- The company's policy for "out-of-network" services
- Coverage for complications of pregnancy (or for a neonate, especially if the newborn requires intensive care)
- Exclusions for high-risk activities such as skydiving, scuba diving, and mountain climbing
- Exclusions regarding psychiatric emergencies or injuries related to terrorist attacks or acts of war
- Whether preauthorization is needed for treatment, hospital admission, or other services
- Whether a second opinion is required before obtaining emergency treatment
- Whether there is a 24-hour physician-backed support center

SUPPLEMENTAL TRAVEL HEALTH AND MEDICAL EVACUATION INSURANCE

Travel health insurance and medical evacuation insurance are both short-term supplemental policies that cover health care costs on a trip and are relatively inexpensive. Many commercial companies offer travel health insurance, which may be purchased separately or in conjunction with medical evacuation insurance. Frequent travelers may consider purchasing annual policies or even policies that will provide coverage for repatriation to one's home country.

Although travel health insurance will cover some health care costs abroad, the quality of care may be inadequate, and medical evacuation from a resource-poor area to a hospital where definitive care can be obtained may be necessary. The cost of evacuation can exceed $100,000. In such cases, medical evacuation insurance would cover the cost of transportation to a facility where adequate care can be provided. Medical evacuation companies may have better resources and experience in some parts of the world than others; travelers may want to ask about a company's resources in a given area, especially if planning a trip to remote destinations. The traveler should scrutinize all policies before purchase, looking for those that provide the following:

- Arrangements with hospitals to guarantee payments directly
- Assistance via a 24-hour physician-backed support center (critical for medical evacuation insurance)
- Emergency medical transport to facilities that are equivalent to those in the home country or to the home country itself (repatriation)
- Any specific medical services that may apply to their circumstances, such as coverage of high-risk activities

Even if an insurance provider is selected carefully, travelers should be aware that unexpected delays in care may still arise, especially in remote destinations. In special circumstances, travelers may be advised to postpone or cancel international trips if the health risks are too high.

 TRAVEL INSURANCE, TRAVEL HEALTH INSURANCE, & MEDICAL EVACUATION INSURANCE

FINDING AN INSURANCE PROVIDER

The following resources, although not all-inclusive, provide information about purchasing travel health and medical evacuation insurance:

- Department of State (www.travel.state.gov)
- International Association for Medical Assistance to Travelers (www.iamat.org)
- American Association of Retired Persons (www.aarp.org) (for information about Medicare supplement plans, see below)

SPECIAL CONSIDERATIONS FOR TRAVELERS WITH UNDERLYING MEDICAL CONDITIONS

Travelers with underlying medical conditions should discuss any concerns with the insurer before departure. In one study of international travelers with travel health insurance claims, only two-thirds of claims were fully met. Preexisting illness and poor documentation were the main reasons for refusal. Travelers with medical conditions should choose a medical assistance company that allows them to store their medical history before departure, so it can be accessed anywhere. Travelers should carry a letter from their health care provider listing their medical conditions and current medications (including their generic names), written in the local language if possible. Those with cardiac disease should carry a copy (paper or electronic) of their most recent ECG. They should also pack all medications in their original bottles, checking beforehand with the destination's embassy to ensure that none are considered illegal in the destination country.

SPECIAL CONSIDERATIONS FOR MEDICARE BENEFICIARIES

The Social Security Medicare program does not provide coverage for medical costs outside the United States, except in limited circumstances. Some Medigap plans may provide limited coverage for emergency care abroad. As with all travelers, Medicare beneficiaries should examine their coverage carefully and supplement it with additional travel health insurance, as needed.

CHECKLIST FOR DISCUSSING INSURANCE WITH TRAVELERS

The following checklist can guide an insurance discussion before travel.

Before travel:

- Consider travel, travel health, and medical evacuation insurance
- Scrutinize the traveler's domestic health insurance policy to see what medical services may or may not be covered abroad
- Locate medical services in areas that the traveler plans to visit and carry this information with them on their trip

During travel:

- Carry copies of insurance policy identity cards, including any supplemental insurance purchased for a trip, and insurance claim forms
- Retain copies of all bills and receipts for medical care received abroad

BIBLIOGRAPHY

1. American Association of Retired Persons, Education and Outreach. Overview of Medicare supplemental insurance. Washington, DC: American Association of Retired Persons; 2010 [cited 2014 Jun 17]. Available from: http://www.aarp.org/health/medicare-insurance/info-10-2008/overview_medicare_supplemental_insurance.html.

2. Centers for Medicare and Medicaid Services. Medicare coverage outside the United States. Baltimore: CMS; 2014 [cited 2014 Sep 19]. Available from: http://www.medicare.gov/Publications/Pubs/pdf/11037.pdf.

3. Leggat PA, Carne J, Kedjarune U. Travel insurance and health. J Travel Med. 1999 Dec;6(4):243–8.

4. Leggat PA, Leggat FW. Travel insurance claims made by travelers from Australia. J Travel Med. 2002 Mar–Apr;9(2):59–65.

5. Teichman PG, Donchin Y, Kot RJ. International aeromedical evacuation. N Engl J Med. 2007 Jan 18;356(3):262–70.

6. US Department of State. Travel medical insurance providers. Washington, DC: US Department of State; 2014 [cited 2014 Sep 19]. Available from: http://travel.state.gov/travel/cis_pa_tw/cis/cis_1470.html.

Infectious Diseases Related to Travel

AMEBIASIS
Sharon L. Roy

INFECTIOUS AGENT
The protozoan parasite *Entamoeba histolytica*, possibly other *Entamoeba* spp.

TRANSMISSION
Fecal-oral route, either directly by person-to-person contact (such as by diaper-changing or sexual practices) or indirectly by eating or drinking fecally contaminated food or water.

EPIDEMIOLOGY
A sample of returned travelers who sought health care from 2007 through 2011 at any of 53 international GeoSentinel-associated clinics showed that most people diagnosed with *E. histolytica* had traveled for tourism to India, Indonesia, Mexico, or Thailand, as opposed to visiting with friends and relatives or traveling for business. Nevertheless, cases of amebiasis are not restricted to these countries and are distributed worldwide, particularly in the tropics, most commonly in areas of poor sanitation. Long-term travelers (duration >6 months) are significantly more likely than short-term travelers (duration <1 month) to develop *E. histolytica* infection. Immigrants and refugees from these areas are also at risk. People at higher risk for severe disease are those who are pregnant,

immunocompromised, or receiving corticosteroids; associations with diabetes and alcohol use have also been reported.

CLINICAL PRESENTATION
Most patients have a gradual illness onset days or weeks after infection. Symptoms include cramps, watery or bloody diarrhea, and weight loss and may last several weeks. Occasionally, the parasite may spread to other organs (extraintestinal amebiasis), most commonly the liver. Amebic liver abscesses may be asymptomatic, but most patients present with fever and right upper quadrant abdominal pain, usually in the absence of diarrhea.

DIAGNOSIS
Microscopy does not distinguish between *E. histolytica* (known to be pathogenic), *E. bangladeshi*, *E. dispar*, and *E. moshkovskii*. *E. dispar* and *E. moshkovskii* have historically been considered nonpathogenic, but new evidence suggests they might cause illness; *E. bangladeshi* has only recently been identified, so its pathogenic potential is not well understood. More specific tests such as EIA or PCR are needed to confirm the diagnosis of *E. histolytica*. Additionally, serologic tests can help diagnose extraintestinal amebiasis.

TREATMENT

For symptomatic intestinal infection and extraintestinal disease, treatment with metronidazole or tinidazole should be followed by treatment with iodoquinol or paromomycin. Asymptomatic patients infected with *E. histolytica* should also be treated with iodoquinol or paromomycin, because they can infect others and because 4%–10% develop disease within a year if left untreated.

PREVENTION

Food and water precautions (see Chapter 2, Food & Water Precautions) and hand hygiene. Avoid fecal exposure during sexual activity.

CDC website: www.cdc.gov/parasites/amebiasis

BIBLIOGRAPHY

1. Bercu TE, Petri WA, Behm JW. Amebic colitis: new insights into pathogenesis and treatment. Curr Gastroenterol Rep. 2007 Oct;9(5):429–33.
2. Chen LH, Wilson ME, Davis X, Loutan L, Schwartz E, Keystone J, et al. Illness in long-term travelers visiting GeoSentinel clinics. Emerg Infect Dis. 2009 Nov;15(11):1773–82.
3. Choudhuri G, Rangan M. Amebic infection in humans. Indian J Gastroenterol. 2012 Jul;31(4):153–62.
4. Heredia RD, Fonseca JA, Lopez MC. *Entamoeba moshkovskii* perspectives of a new agent to be considered in the diagnosis of amebiasis. Acta Trop. 2012 Sep;123(3):139–45.
5. Leder K, Torresi J, Libman MD, Cramer JP, Castelli F, Schlagenhauf P, et al. GeoSentinel surveillance of illness in returned travelers, 2007–2011. Ann Intern Med. 2013 Mar 19;158(6):456–68.
6. Petri WA Jr, Singh U. Diagnosis and management of amebiasis. Clin Infect Dis. 1999 Nov;29(5):1117–25.
7. Stanley SL Jr. Amoebiasis. Lancet. 2003 Mar 22;361(9362):1025–34.
8. Ximenez C, Moran P, Rojas L, Valadez A, Gomez A, Ramiro M, et al. Novelties on amoebiasis: a neglected tropical disease. J Glob Infect Dis. 2011 Apr;3(2):166–74.

ANGIOSTRONGYLIASIS, NEUROLOGIC

Barbara L. Herwaldt, LeAnne M. Fox

INFECTIOUS AGENT

Angiostrongylus cantonensis, rat lungworm, a nematode parasite.

TRANSMISSION

Various species of rats are the definitive hosts of the parasite, known as the rat lungworm. Rats can infect only snails and slugs, which are the intermediate hosts. Transmission to humans occurs by consuming infected snails or slugs or contaminated raw produce or vegetable juices. Infective larvae have also been found in freshwater shrimp, crabs, and frogs.

EPIDEMIOLOGY

Most described cases have occurred in Asia and the Pacific Basin (such as in parts of Thailand, Taiwan, mainland China, the Hawaiian Islands, and other Pacific Islands); however, cases have been reported in many areas of the world, including the Caribbean.

CLINICAL PRESENTATION

Incubation period is typically 1–3 weeks but ranges from 1 day to >6 weeks. *A. cantonensis* is considered the most common infectious cause of eosinophilic meningitis in humans. Common manifestations include headache, photophobia, stiff neck, nausea, vomiting, fatigue, and body aches. Abnormal skin sensations (such as tingling or painful feelings) are more common than in other types of meningitis. A low-grade fever might be noted. Symptoms are usually self-limited but may persist for weeks or months. Severe cases can be associated with paralysis, blindness, or death.

DIAGNOSIS

Typically presumptive, on the basis of clinical and epidemiologic criteria in people with otherwise unexplained eosinophilic meningitis. Serum antibody testing may be available in reference laboratories. PCR testing of cerebrospinal fluid is available from CDC (www.dpd.cdc.gov/dpdx; 404-718-4745; parasites@cdc.gov).

TREATMENT

The larvae die spontaneously, and supportive care usually suffices. Clinicians may consult with CDC about evaluation and treatment of patients.

BIBLIOGRAPHY

1. Hochberg NS, Blackburn BG, Park SY, Sejvar JJ, Effler PV, Herwaldt BL. Eosinophilic meningitis attributable to *Angiostrongylus cantonensis* infection in Hawaii: clinical characteristics and potential exposures. Am J Trop Med Hyg. 2011 Oct;85(4):685–90.

2. Wang QP, Lai DH, Zhu XQ, Chen XG, Lun ZR. Human angiostrongyliasis. Lancet Infect Dis. 2008 Oct;8(10):621–30.

PREVENTION

Food and water precautions, particularly:

- Avoid eating raw or undercooked snails, slugs, and other possible hosts.
- Eat raw produce, such as lettuce, only if it has been thoroughly washed or treated with bleach. Such measures might provide some protection but may not eliminate the risk.
- Wear gloves (and wash hands) if snails or slugs are handled.

CDC website: www.cdc.gov/parasites/angiostrongylus

ANTHRAX

Sean V. Shadomy, Rita M. Traxler, Chung K. Marston

INFECTIOUS AGENT

Aerobic, gram-positive, encapsulated, spore-forming, nonmotile, nonhemolytic, rod-shaped bacterium *Bacillus anthracis*.

TRANSMISSION

B. anthracis is primarily transmitted by direct contact with *B. anthracis*–infected animals, their carcasses, or with contaminated products from infected animals. Such products include meat, hides, wool, or items made with those products, such as drums or wool clothing.

Anthrax normally presents in 3 forms: cutaneous, gastrointestinal, and inhalation. Introduction of the spores through the skin can result in cutaneous anthrax; abrasion of the skin increases susceptibility. Eating meat from infected animals can result in gastrointestinal anthrax. Inhalation anthrax typically occurs when a person inhales spores aerosolized from work with contaminated materials, such as hides or wool, in a way that can aerosolize dust and spores. Inhalation exposure was historically associated with industrial processing of hides or wool, but it has also resulted from bioterrorism. Rare inhalation anthrax cases have occurred in the United States and elsewhere where no source of exposure was identified. Since 2000, a new form of anthrax has been reported occurring among injecting heroin users; however, smoking and snorting heroin have also been identified as possible exposure routes. Anthrax in humans is not generally considered to be contagious; person-to-person transmission of cutaneous anthrax has rarely been reported.

EPIDEMIOLOGY

Anthrax is a zoonotic disease that primarily affects herbivores such as cattle, sheep, goats, antelope, and deer, which become infected by ingesting contaminated vegetation, water, or soil; humans are generally incidental hosts.

Anthrax is most common in agricultural regions in Central and South America, sub-Saharan Africa, Central and Southwestern Asia, and southern and Eastern Europe. Anthrax is now rare in the United States and Canada; however, sporadic outbreaks occur every year in livestock and wild herbivores in these countries. The most commonly reported form (95%–99%) of anthrax in humans worldwide is cutaneous anthrax. Outbreaks of cutaneous and gastrointestinal anthrax have been associated with handling infected animals, and butchering and consuming meat from those animals. Such outbreaks are primarily reported from endemic areas in Asia and Africa. Travelers to endemic areas have acquired cutaneous anthrax through either direct or indirect contact with carcasses of animals that died from anthrax. Cases of cutaneous, gastrointestinal, and inhalation anthrax have been reported among people who have handled or played drums made with contaminated goat hides from countries endemic for anthrax or who have been present at events where those drums have been played. Anthrax cases have also been reported among people making drums from contaminated goat hides imported from countries endemic for anthrax, as well as members of their households exposed to environments contaminated by the drum-making process.

Severe soft tissue infections, including cases with sepsis and systemic infection, have been reported in drug users in northern Europe and are suspected to be due to recreational use of heroin contaminated with B. anthracis spores. No associated cases have been identified in people who had not deliberately taken heroin. To date no heroin has been found to be contaminated with B. anthracis spores.

CLINICAL PRESENTATION

Cutaneous anthrax usually develops 1–7 days after exposure. The case-fatality ratio is as high as 20% if untreated, but typically is <1% with antimicrobial therapy. Cutaneous anthrax is characterized by localized itching, followed by the development of a painless papule, which turns vesicular and enlarges, ulcerates, and develops into a depressed black eschar within 7–10 days of the initial lesion. The head, neck, forearms, and hands are the most commonly affected sites. Edema usually surrounds the lesion, sometimes with secondary vesicles, hyperemia, and regional lymphadenopathy. Patients may have associated fever, malaise, and headache.

Gastrointestinal anthrax usually develops 1–7 days after consumption of contaminated meat and can present in either intestinal or oropharyngeal forms. Shock and death may occur within 2–5 days of onset; estimates of the case-fatality ratio for gastrointestinal anthrax are >50% if untreated, and <40% with treatment.

Inhalation anthrax usually develops within a week after exposure, but the incubation period may be prolonged (up to 2 months). Estimates for the case-fatality ratio are >85%; even with aggressive treatment, this ratio can be as high as 45%. Initial symptoms are nonspecific and may mimic those of influenza, including myalgia, fever, nonproductive cough, malaise, nausea, and vomiting; upper respiratory tract symptoms are rare. The patient's condition dramatically worsens 2–3 days after symptom onset, with the development of severe respiratory distress, diaphoresis, cyanosis, and shock.

Cases of anthrax in injection drug users reportedly developed within 1–4 days of exposure in most cases for which a suspected exposure could be identified; the case-fatality ratio was >25% in confirmed cases. Cases presented with severe soft tissue infection with or without localized swelling or with symptoms of sepsis, disseminated infection, and toxemia.

Hemorrhagic meningitis may develop from hematogenous spread of any of the clinical forms of anthrax. Anthrax meningitis is nearly always fatal.

DIAGNOSIS

Laboratory diagnosis depends on bacterial culture and isolation of B. anthracis; detection of bacterial DNA, antigens, or toxins; or detection of a host immune response to B. anthracis. Anthrax lethal toxin can be detected in acute-phase serum, while serologic testing of host antibody responses requires acute- and convalescent-phase sera for diagnosis.

Confirmatory testing, including isolate identification, antigen detection in tissues, or quantitative serology, should be performed in the United States by the state health department or Laboratory Response Network laboratories, or internationally by the relevant national reference laboratory. Guidelines for collecting and submitting clinical specimens for testing and algorithms for laboratory diagnosis can be found at www.bt.cdc.gov/agent/anthrax/lab-testing. Specimens for culture should be collected before initiating antimicrobial therapy. Diagnostic procedures for inhalation anthrax include thoracic imaging studies to detect a widened mediastinum or pleural effusion.

TREATMENT

Naturally occurring localized or uncomplicated cutaneous anthrax can be treated with 7–10 days of a single oral antimicrobial agent. First-line agents include ciprofloxacin or an equivalent fluoroquinolone or doxycycline; clindamycin is an alternative, as are penicillins if the isolate is penicillin susceptible. Ciprofloxacin is recommended as the primary antimicrobial component of an initial multidrug regimen for treating all forms of systemic anthrax until antimicrobial susceptibility data are available; levofloxacin and moxifloxacin are equivalent alternatives to ciprofloxacin. Because of intrinsic resistance, neither cephalosporins nor trimethoprim-sulfamethoxazole should be used.

Treatment recommendations for severe systemic or life-threatening disease are available at wwwnc.cdc.gov/eid/article/20/2/13-0687_intro. Additional recommendations to prevent or treat anthrax in pregnant, postpartum, and lactating women are available at wwwnc.cdc.gov/eid/article/20/2/13-0611_intro.

PREVENTION

The CDC published updated recommendations in 2010 for preexposure use of anthrax vaccine and for postexposure management for previously unvaccinated people (www.cdc.gov/mmwr/preview/mmwrhtml/rr5906a1.htm). Vaccination against anthrax is not recommended for travelers and is not available for civilian travelers. Travelers should not have direct or indirect contact with carcasses of animals found in anthrax-endemic regions or eat meat from animals that were not inspected by health officials and found to be healthy at the time of slaughter.

The risk of acquiring anthrax from playing with or handling an animal hide drum is very low. Since 2006, 6 cases of anthrax (including all 3 forms: cutaneous, gastrointestinal, and inhalation) in the United States and United Kingdom have been associated with making animal-hide drums or participating in drumming workshops or events where animal-hide drums were played. Some of these cases were fatal. Travelers who wish to bring back animal hides from anthrax-endemic regions to make drums should strongly consider the health risks before importing the hides.

No tests are available to determine if animal products are free of contamination with B. anthracis spores. Animal-hide drum owners or players should report any unexplained fever or new skin lesions to their health care provider and describe their recent contact with animal-hide drums.

The importation of goat-hide souvenirs, such as goat-hide drums, from Haiti is prohibited by CDC (see Chapter 6, Taking Animals & Animal Products across International Borders). Importation of animal products, including processed or unprocessed cattle and goat hides, is regulated by the United States Department of Agriculture (USDA). Animal products, trophies, or souvenirs from anthrax-endemic regions must be accompanied by an international veterinary certificate stating that they were harvested from animals that were free of anthrax, or that they have been disinfected in accordance with international regulations, for them to be allowed to be imported into the United States. Cattle or goat hides that have been tanned, pickled in a solution of salt and mineral acid, or treated with lime are considered to pose less of a risk for infectious diseases and may be imported under certain conditions. For more information, consult the USDA website at www.aphis.usda.gov/import_export/animals/animal_import/animal_imports.shtml and the World Organisation for Animal Health (OIE) Terrestrial Animal Health Code at www.oie.int/en/international-standard-setting/terrestrial-code/access-online.

CDC website: www.cdc.gov/anthrax/

BIBLIOGRAPHY

1. Bales ME, Dannenberg AL, Brachman PS, Kaufmann AF, Klatsky PC, Ashford DA. Epidemiologic response to anthrax outbreaks: field investigations, 1950–2001. Emerg Infect Dis. 2002 Oct;8(10):1163–74.

2. CDC. Gastrointestinal anthrax after an animal-hide drumming event—New Hampshire and Massachusetts, 2009. MMWR Morb Mortal Wkly Rep. 2010 Jul 23; 59(28):872–7.

3. Eurosurveillance editorial team. Probable human anthrax death in Scotland. Euro Surveill. 2006;11(8):E060817.2.

4. Griffith J, Blaney D, Shadomy S, Lehman M, Pesik N, Tostenson S, et al. Investigation of inhalation anthrax case, United States. Emerg Infect Dis. 2014 Feb;20(2): 280–3.

5. Hanczaruk M, Reischl U, Holzmann T, Frangoulidis D, Wagner DM, Keim PS, et al. Injectional anthrax in heroin users, Europe, 2000–2012. Emerg Infect Dis. 2014 Feb;20(2):322–3.

6. Hendricks KA, Wright ME, Shadomy SV, Bradley JS, Morrow MG, Pavia AT, et al. Centers for disease control and prevention expert panel meetings on prevention and treatment of anthrax in adults. Emerg Infect Dis. 2014 Feb;20(2).

7. Meaney-Delman D, Zotti ME, Creanga AA, Misegades LK, Wako E, Treadwell TA, et al. Special considerations for prophylaxis for and treatment of anthrax in pregnant and postpartum women. Emerg Infect Dis. 2014 Feb;20(2).

8. Van den Enden E, Van Gompel A, Van Esbroeck M. Cutaneous anthrax, Belgian traveler. Emerg Infect Dis. 2006 Mar;12(3):523–5.

B VIRUS

D. Scott Schmid

INFECTIOUS AGENT

Macacine herpesvirus or B virus, an enveloped, double-stranded DNA virus in the family Herpesviridae. B virus is also commonly referred to as herpes B, monkey B virus, herpesvirus simiae, and herpesvirus B. B virus is commonly found among macaques, a genus of Old World monkeys.

TRANSMISSION

Transmission is typically caused by bites or scratches from an infected macaque but may also be caused by contact with body fluids or tissues of an infected macaque. A single case of human-to-human spread has been documented, in which a woman became infected through direct contact with the lesions of her infected spouse.

EPIDEMIOLOGY

Macaque monkeys are the natural reservoir for B virus infection. No other primates are known to carry any risk of B virus infection unless they have become infected by contact with infected macaques. Although B virus infections in macaques are usually asymptomatic or cause only mild disease, approximately 70% of untreated infections in humans are fatal. People most at risk for B virus infection are veterinarians, laboratory workers, and others who have close contact with Old World macaques or monkey cell cultures, but infections in humans are rare. Since B virus was identified in 1932, there have been only 31 documented human infections.

CLINICAL PRESENTATION

Disease onset typically occurs within 1 month of exposure, although the incubation period can be as short as 3–7 days. The first signs of disease typically include influenzalike symptoms (fever, headache, myalgias) and sometimes vesicular lesions near the exposure site. Localized neurologic symptoms, such as pain, numbness, or itching, may occur near the wound site. Lymphadenitis, lymphangitis, nausea, vomiting, and abdominal pain may also occur. Spread of the infection to the central nervous system (CNS) causes acute ascending encephalomyelitis. Most patients with CNS involvement die despite antiviral therapy and supportive care, and those who survive usually suffer serious neurologic sequelae. Respiratory failure associated with ascending paralysis is the most common cause of death.

DIAGNOSIS

In the United States, diagnostic testing of human specimens for B virus infection is performed only at the National B Virus Resource Center at Georgia State University. Direct culture of B virus from clinical specimens has been the standard for diagnosis of infection, although this testing requires a biosafety level 4 containment facility. For more information, see www2.gsu.edu/~wwwvir/index.html.

TREATMENT

For any suspected exposure, immediate first aid is crucial. The wound should be immediately cleansed by thoroughly washing and scrubbing the area with soap, concentrated detergent solution, povidone-iodine, or chlorhexidine and water. The wound should then be irrigated with running water for 15–20 minutes. For urine splashes to the eyes, the eyes should be repeatedly flushed for 15 minutes with sterile saline solution or water. **Specimens for diagnostic testing should not be obtained from wound sites before washing because of the risk of forcing virus more deeply into the wound.**

Antiviral therapy is recommended as postexposure prophylaxis in high-risk exposures (see www.cdc.gov/herpesbvirus/firstaid-treatment.html). When recommended, the first choice of drug for postexposure prophylaxis is valacyclovir, and an alternative is acyclovir. If B virus infection is diagnosed, treatment consists of intravenous acyclovir or ganciclovir, depending on whether CNS symptoms are present.

PREVENTION

Adhering to laboratory and animal facility protocols will reduce the risk of B virus transmission among laboratory workers. Visitors to parks and other tourist destinations (such as certain religious temples) with free-roaming macaques should avoid contact with the animals (including feeding or petting them).

CDC website: www.cdc.gov/herpesbvirus/index.html

BIBLIOGRAPHY

1. Chosewood LC, Wilson DE, editors. Biosafety in Microbiological and Biomedical Laboratories. 5th ed. Washingon, DC: US Department of Health and Human Services; 2007. Section VIII—Agent summary statements; [cited 2014 Sep 22]; p. 205–8. Available from: http://www.cdc.gov/biosafety/publications/bmbl5/index.htm.

2. CDC. Notice to readers: Occupational safety and health in the care and use of nonhuman primates. MMWR. 2003;52(38):920.

3. Cohen JI, Davenport DS, Stewart JA, Deitchman S, Hilliard JK, Chapman LE, et al. Recommendations for prevention of and therapy for exposure to B virus (*Cercopithecine herpesvirus* 1). Clin Infect Dis. 2002 Nov 15;35(10):1191–203.

4. National Association of State Public Health Veterinarians. Compendium of measure to prevent disease associated with animals in public settings, 2009. MMWR Recomm Rep. 2009;58(RR-05):1–15.

5. National Institute for Occupational Safety and Health. Hazard ID 5: *Cercopithicine herpesvirus* 1 (B virus) infection resulting from ocular exposure. Atlanta: CDC; 1999 [cited 2014 Sep 19]. Available from: http://www.cdc.gov/niosh/docs/99-100/.

BARTONELLA INFECTIONS
Christina A. Nelson

INFECTIOUS AGENT

Gram-negative bacteria in the genus *Bartonella*. Human illness is primarily caused by *Bartonella henselae* (cat-scratch disease [CSD]), *B. quintana* (trench fever), and *B. bacilliformis* (Carrión disease). A variety of *Bartonella* spp. can cause culture-negative endocarditis; other clinical syndromes due to *Bartonella* spp. have also been reported. For example, in 2007, a newly recognized species of *Bartonella* (*B. rochalimae*) was identified in an ill traveler returning from Peru.

TRANSMISSION

CSD is contracted through scratches from domestic or feral cats, particularly kittens. Direct transmission to humans by the bite of infected cat fleas is likely but has not yet been proven. Trench fever is transmitted by the human body louse. Carrión disease is transmitted by sand flies (genus *Lutzomyia*) that are infected with B. *bacilliformis*.

EPIDEMIOLOGY

CSD and trench fever are distributed worldwide. In the United States, CSD is more common in children, and the incidence peaks from September through January. Trench fever typically occurs in populations that do not have access to proper hygiene, such as refugees and the homeless. Carrión disease has limited geographic distribution; transmission occurs in the Andes Mountains at 1–3 km (0.6–1.9 miles) elevation in Peru, Colombia, and Ecuador; sporadic cases have been reported in Bolivia, Chile, and possibly Guatemala. Most cases are reported in Peru. Short-term travelers to endemic areas are likely at low risk.

CLINICAL PRESENTATION

CSD symptoms include fever, a papule or pustule at the inoculation site, and enlarged, tender lymph nodes that develop ipsilateral to the inoculation site 1–3 weeks after exposure. B. *henselae* infection may also cause prolonged fever, follicular conjunctivitis, neuroretinitis, or encephalitis. Trench fever symptoms include fever, headache, transient rash, and bone pain (mainly in the shins, neck, and back).

Some *Bartonella* spp. can cause signs and symptoms of subacute endocarditis, which is often culture-negative. Bacillary angiomatosis (caused by B. *henselae* or B. *quintana*) and peliosis hepatis (caused by B. *henselae*) occur primarily in people infected with HIV. Bacillary angiomatosis may present as skin, subcutaneous, or bone lesions.

Carrión disease has 2 distinct phases: an acute phase (Oroya fever) characterized by fever, myalgia, headache, and anemia and an eruptive phase (verruga peruana) characterized by red-to-purple nodular skin lesions.

DIAGNOSIS

CSD can be diagnosed clinically in patients with typical presentation and a compatible exposure history. Serology can confirm the diagnosis, although cross-reactivity may limit interpretation in some circumstances. B. *henselae* DNA may also be detected by PCR or culture of pus or lymph node aspirates by using special techniques.

Trench fever can be diagnosed by isolating B. *quintana* from blood or by serology. PCR may also aid the diagnosis of disseminated *Bartonella* infections when performed by clinical laboratories using validated methods. Endocarditis caused by *Bartonella* spp. can be diagnosed by elevated serology of the patient and by PCR or culture of excised heart valve tissue.

Oroya fever is typically diagnosed via blood culture or direct observation of the bacilli in peripheral blood smears, though sensitivity of these methods is low. PCR and serologic testing may also aid diagnosis.

TREATMENT

Most cases of CSD eventually resolve without treatment, but a small percentage of people will develop disseminated disease with severe complications. The use of antibiotics to shorten the course of disease is debated, although azithromycin speeds the decrease in lymph node volume.

Various antibiotics are effective against *Bartonella* infections, including penicillins, tetracyclines, cephalosporins, and aminoglycosides. Recommended antibiotic regimens and duration of treatment vary by clinical disease.

PREVENTION

Avoid rough playing with cats, particularly strays and kittens, to prevent scratches. This is especially important for immunocompromised people. Wash hands promptly after handling cats. Protect against bites of sand flies and body lice (see Chapter 2, Protection against Mosquitoes, Ticks, & Other Arthropods).

CDC website: www.cdc.gov/bartonella

BIBLIOGRAPHY

1. Bass JW, Freitas BC, Freitas AD, Sisler CL, Chan DS, Vincent JM, et al. Prospective randomized double blind placebo-controlled evaluation of azithromycin for treatment of cat-scratch disease. Pediatr Infect Dis J. 1998 Jun;17(6):447–52.

2. Eremeeva ME, Gerns HL, Lydy SL, Goo JS, Ryan ET, Mathew SS, et al. Bacteremia, fever, and splenomegaly caused by a newly recognized *Bartonella* species. N Engl J Med. 2007 Jun 7;356(23):2381–7.

3. Florin TA, Zaoutis TE, Zaoutis LB. Beyond cat scratch disease: widening spectrum of *Bartonella henselae* infection. Pediatrics. 2008 May;121(5):e1413–25.

4. Fournier PE, Thuny F, Richet H, Lepidi H, Casalta JP, Arzouni JP, et al. Comprehensive diagnostic strategy for blood culture-negative endocarditis: a prospective study of 819 new cases. Clin Infect Dis. 2010 Jul 15;51(2):131–40.

5. Maguina C, Gotuzzo E. Bartonellosis. New and old. Infect Dis Clin North Am. 2000 Mar;14(1): 1–22, vii.

6. Rolain JM, Brouqui P, Koehler JE, Maguina C, Dolan MJ, Raoult D. Recommendations for treatment of human infections caused by *Bartonella* species. Antimicrob Agents Chemother. 2004 Jun;48(6):1921–33.

BRUCELLOSIS

Marta A. Guerra, Rebekah Tiller, Grishma A. Kharod

INFECTIOUS AGENT

Facultative, intracellular, gram-negative coccobacilli; known human pathogens include *Brucella abortus*, *B. melitensis*, *B. suis*, and *B. canis*.

TRANSMISSION

Most commonly through consumption of unpasteurized dairy products or undercooked meat from infected animals and direct contact with infected animals, especially those that have recently given birth. Since wildlife can be reservoirs for *Brucella* spp., hunting can be a risk for exposure as well. *Brucella* can enter the body via skin wounds, mucous membranes, or inhalation. Person-to-person transmission is rare.

EPIDEMIOLOGY

High-risk regions include the Mediterranean Basin, South and Central America, Eastern Europe, Asia, Africa, and the Middle East. In these areas, brucellosis is primarily enzootic in cattle, sheep, and goat populations, as well as feral swine.

CLINICAL PRESENTATION

Incubation period is 2–4 weeks (range, 5 days to 5 months). Initial presentation is nonspecific, including fever, muscle aches, fatigue, headache, and night sweats. Focal infections are common and can affect most organs in the body.

DIAGNOSIS

Blood culture is the diagnostic gold standard, but is not always positive. If culture of blood, bone marrow, or other clinical specimen is performed, the laboratory must be informed that *Brucella* is suspected, as the culture takes longer to grow and laboratory personnel require additional personnel protective equipment when handling cultures. A serum agglutination test is the most common serologic approach, but other serology, including ELISA, and PCR have been used to make a diagnosis.

TREATMENT

Doxycycline, rifampin, and trimethoprim-sulfamethoxazole have been used in various combinations for treatment for a minimum of 6–8 weeks. If bacteria localize in organs and tissues and cause focal infection, surgery could be indicated. Late diagnosis and inappropriate therapy can result in chronic disease or relapse.

PREVENTION

Avoid unpasteurized dairy products and undercooked meat. Wear protective equipment when dressing or butchering wild animals potentially infected with *Brucella* spp. In clinical microbiology laboratories, if *Brucella* spp. is suspected, culture isolates should be handled under BSL-3 conditions.

CDC website: www.cdc.gov/brucellosis

BIBLIOGRAPHY

1. Al Dahouk S, Nöckler K. Implications of laboratory diagnosis on brucellosis therapy. Expert Rev Anti Infect Ther. 2011 Jul;9(7):833–45.
2. Ariza J, Bosilkovski M, Cascio A, Colmenero JD, Corbel MJ, Falagas ME, et al. Perspectives for the treatment of brucellosis in the 21st century: the Ioannina recommendations. PLoS Med. 2007 Dec;4(12):e317.
3. Arnow PM, Smaron M, Ormiste V. Brucellosis in a group of travelers to Spain. JAMA. 1984 Jan 27;251(4):505–7.
4. Memish ZA, Balkhy HH. Brucellosis and international travel. J Travel Med. 2004 Jan–Feb;11(1):49–55.
5. Pappas G, Papadimitriou P, Akritidis N, Christou L, Tsianos EV. The new global map of human brucellosis. Lancet Infect Dis. 2006 Feb;6(2):91–9.
6. World Health Organization. Brucellosis. Geneva: World Health Organization; 2012 [cited 2014 Jun 23]. Available from: http://www.who.int/zoonoses/diseases/brucellosis/en.

CAMPYLOBACTERIOSIS
Aimee L. Geissler, Barbara E. Mahon

INFECTIOUS AGENT
Infection is caused by gram-negative, spiral-shaped microaerophilic bacteria of the family Campylobacteriaceae. Most infections are caused by *Campylobacter jejuni*; other species, including *C. coli*, also cause infection. *C. jejuni* and *C. coli* are carried normally in the intestinal tracts of many domestic and wild animals.

TRANSMISSION
The major modes of transmission include eating contaminated foods (especially undercooked chicken and foods contaminated by raw chicken), drinking contaminated water or milk (unpasteurized milk, most commonly), and having contact with animals, particularly farm animals such as cows and chickens, as well as domestic cats and dogs. *Campylobacter* can also be transmitted from person to person by the fecal-oral route.

EPIDEMIOLOGY
Campylobacter is a leading cause of bacterial diarrheal disease worldwide; in the United States, it is estimated to cause 1.3 million human illnesses every year. *Campylobacter* is the most common laboratory-confirmed enteric pathogen reported in travelers returning to the United States from every region of the world. The risk of infection is highest in travelers to Africa and South America, especially in areas with poor restaurant hygiene and inadequate sanitation. The infectious dose is thought to be small; <500 organisms can cause disease.

CLINICAL PRESENTATION
Incubation period is typically 2–4 days. Campylobacteriosis is characterized by diarrhea (frequently bloody), abdominal pain, fever, and occasionally nausea and vomiting. More severe illness can occur, including dehydration, bloodstream infection, and symptoms mimicking acute appendicitis or ulcerative colitis. *Campylobacter* is the most frequently observed antecedent infection in cases of Guillain-Barré syndrome (GBS). Symptoms of GBS usually begin 1–3 weeks after the onset of *Campylobacter* enteritis.

DIAGNOSIS
Diagnosis is traditionally based on isolation of the organism from stools by using selective media incubated under reduced oxygen tension at 42°C (107.6°F) for 72 hours.

Visualization of motile and curved, spiral, or S-shaped rods by stool phase-contrast or dark-field microscopy can provide rapid presumptive evidence for *Campylobacter* enteritis. Rapid culture-independent tests, including both antigen tests and nucleic acid–based tests, are becoming more widely available and commonly used. The sensitivity and specificity of stool antigen tests are variable, and in settings of low prevalence, the positive predictive value is likely to be low. Therefore, laboratories should confirm positive results of stool antigen tests by culture. Nucleic acid–based tests have recently been approved and appear to have higher sensitivity and specificity than the antigen tests.

TREATMENT

The disease is generally self-limited, lasting a week or less. Antibiotic therapy decreases the duration of symptoms if administered early in the course of disease. Because campylobacteriosis generally cannot be distinguished from other causes of travelers' diarrhea without a diagnostic test, the use of empiric antibiotics in travelers should follow the guidelines for travelers' diarrhea.

Rates of antibiotic resistance, especially fluoroquinolone resistance, have risen sharply in the past 20 years, and high rates of resistance are now seen in many regions of the world. Travel abroad is a risk factor for infection with resistant *Campylobacter*. Clinicians should suspect resistant infection in returning travelers with campylobacteriosis in whom empiric fluoroquinolone treatment has failed. When fluoroquinolone resistance is proven or suspected, azithromycin is usually the next choice of treatment, although resistance to macrolides has also been reported.

PREVENTION

No vaccine is available; food and water precautions are recommended (see Chapter 2, Food & Water Precautions). Antibiotic prophylaxis is not recommended.

CDC website: www.cdc.gov/nczved/divisions/dfbmd/diseases/campylobacter

BIBLIOGRAPHY

1. Coker AO, Isokpehi RD, Thomas BN, Amisu KO, Obi CL. Human campylobacteriosis in developing countries. Emerg Infect Dis. 2002 Mar;8(3):237–44.
2. Friedman CR, Hoekstra RM, Samuel M, Marcus R, Bender J, Shiferaw B, et al. Risk factors for sporadic *Campylobacter* infection in the United States: a case-control study in FoodNet sites. Clin Infect Dis. 2004 Apr 15;38 Suppl 3:S285–96.
3. Humphrey T, O'Brien S, Madsen M. Campylobacters as zoonotic pathogens: a food production perspective. Int J Food Microbiol. 2007 Jul 15;117(3):237–57.
4. Kassenborg HD, Smith KE, Vugia DJ, Rabatsky-Ehr T, Bates MR, Carter MA, et al. Fluoroquinolone-resistant *Campylobacter* infections: eating poultry outside of the home and foreign travel are risk factors. Clin Infect Dis. 2004 Apr 15;38 Suppl 3:S279–84.
5. Kendall ME, Crim S, Fullerton K, Han PV, Cronquist AB, Shiferaw B, et al. Travel-associated enteric infections diagnosed after return to the United States, Foodborne Diseases Active Surveillance Network (FoodNet), 2004–2009. Clin Infect Dis. 2012 Jun;54 Suppl 5:S480–7.
6. Moore JE, Barton MD, Blair IS, Corcoran D, Dooley JS, Fanning S, et al. The epidemiology of antibiotic resistance in *Campylobacter*. Microbes Infect. 2006 Jun;8(7):1955–66.
7. World Health Organization. The global view of campylobacteriosis: report of an expert consultation. Geneva: World Health Organization; 2012 [cited 2014 Sep 17]. Available from: http://apps.who.int/iris/bitstream/10665/80751/1/9789241564601_eng.pdf?ua=1.

CHIKUNGUNYA

J. Erin Staples, Susan L. Hills, Ann M. Powers

INFECTIOUS AGENT

Chikungunya virus (CHIKV) is a single-stranded RNA virus that belongs to the family Togaviridae, genus *Alphavirus*.

TRANSMISSION

CHIKV is transmitted to humans via the bite of an infected mosquito of the *Aedes* spp., predominantly *Aedes aegypti* and *Ae. albopictus*. Nonhuman and human primates are likely the main reservoirs of the virus, and anthroponotic (human-to-vector-to-human) transmission occurs during outbreaks of the disease. Bloodborne transmission is possible; 1 case was documented in a health care worker who was stuck with a needle after drawing blood from an infected patient. Cases have also been documented among laboratory personnel handling infected blood and through aerosol exposure in the laboratory.

The risk of a person transmitting the virus to a biting mosquito or through blood is highest when the patient is viremic, usually during the first 2–6 days of illness. Maternal–fetal transmission has been documented during pregnancy; the highest risk occurs when a woman is viremic at the time of delivery. Studies have not found CHIKV in breast milk.

EPIDEMIOLOGY

CHIKV often causes large outbreaks with high attack rates, affecting one-third to three-quarters of the population in areas where the virus is circulating. Outbreaks of CHIKV disease have occurred in Africa, Asia, Europe, and islands in the Indian and Pacific Oceans. In late 2013, the first locally acquired cases of chikungunya were reported in the Americas on islands in the Caribbean. Since that time, CHIKV has continued to spread in the Americas, with cases reported throughout the Caribbean and in several North, Central, and South American countries. Given the high level of viremia in humans and the worldwide distribution of *Ae. aegypti*

and *Ae. albopictus*, there is a risk of importation of CHIKV into new areas by infected travelers.

Risk to travelers is highest in areas experiencing ongoing epidemics of the disease (for the most updated information see the Travel Health Notices section on the CDC Travelers' Health website at wwwnc.cdc.gov/travel/notices). Most epidemics occur during the tropical rainy season and abate during the dry season. However, outbreaks in Africa have occurred after periods of drought, where open water containers served as vector-breeding sites. Risk of CHIKV infection exists throughout the day, as the primary vector, *Ae. aegypti*, aggressively bites during the daytime. *Ae. aegypti* mosquitoes bite indoors or outdoors near a dwelling. They typically breed in domestic containers that hold water, including buckets and flower pots.

Both adults and children can become infected and symptomatic with the disease. From 2010 through 2013, 110 cases of chikungunya fever were identified or reported among US travelers who predominantly traveled to areas with known ongoing outbreaks. Following the outbreaks in the Americas, however, >700 chikungunya cases have been reported from US states through the end of August 2014. Although most were in travelers, a few cases were acquired locally in the continental United States. In addition, several US territories (Puerto Rico, US Virgin Islands, and American Samoa) have reported locally acquired cases in 2014.

CLINICAL PRESENTATION

Approximately 3%–28% of people infected with CHIKV will remain asymptomatic. For people who develop symptomatic illness, the incubation period is typically 3–7 days (range, 1–12 days). Disease is most often characterized by sudden onset of high fever (temperature typically >102°F [39°C]) and joint pains. Other symptoms may include headache, myalgia, arthritis, conjunctivitis, nausea, vomiting, or a maculopapular rash. Fevers typically last from several days up to 1 week; the fever can be biphasic. Joint symptoms are often severe and can be debilitating. They usually involve multiple joints, typically bilateral and symmetric. They occur most commonly in hands and feet, but they can affect more proximal joints. Rash usually occurs after onset of fever. It typically involves the trunk and extremities but can also include palms, soles, and face.

Abnormal laboratory findings can include thrombocytopenia, lymphopenia, and elevated creatinine and liver function tests. Rare but serious complications of the disease can occur, including myocarditis, ocular disease (uveitis, retinitis), hepatitis, acute renal disease, severe bulbous lesions, and neurologic disease, such as meningoencephalitis, Guillain-Barré syndrome, myelitis, or cranial nerve palsies. Groups identified as having increased risk for more severe disease include neonates exposed intrapartum, adults >65 years of age, and people with underlying medical conditions, such as hypertension, diabetes, or heart disease.

Acute symptoms of chikungunya typically resolve in 7–10 days. Fatalities associated with CHIKV infection are rare and mostly occur in older adults. Some patients will have a relapse of rheumatologic symptoms such as polyarthralgia, polyarthritis, tenosynovitis, or Raynaud syndrome in the months after acute illness. Studies have reported variable proportions, ranging from 5% to 60%, of patients with persistent joint pains for months or years after their illness.

Pregnant women have symptoms and outcomes similar to those of other people, and most CHIKV infections that occur during pregnancy will not result in the virus being transmitted to the fetus. However, when intrapartum transmission occurs, it can result in complications for the baby, including neurologic disease, hemorrhagic symptoms, and myocardial disease. There are also rare reports of spontaneous abortions after maternal CHIKV infection.

DIAGNOSIS

The differential diagnosis of CHIKV infection depends on the clinical signs and symptoms as well as where the person was suspected of being infected. Diseases that should be considered in the differential diagnosis include dengue, malaria, leptospirosis, parvovirus, enterovirus, group A *Streptococcus*, rubella, measles, adenovirus, postinfectious arthritis, rheumatologic conditions, or alphavirus infections (including Mayaro, Ross River, Barmah Forest, O'nyong-nyong, and Sindbis viruses).

Preliminary diagnosis is based on the patient's clinical features, places and dates of travel, and activities. Laboratory diagnosis is generally accomplished by testing serum to detect virus, viral nucleic acid, or virus-specific IgM and neutralizing antibodies. During the first week after onset of symptoms, CHIKV infection can often be diagnosed by performing viral culture or nucleic acid amplification on serum. CHIKV-specific IgM and neutralizing antibodies normally develop toward the end of the first week of illness. Therefore, to definitively rule out the diagnosis, convalescent-phase samples should be obtained from patients whose acute-phase samples test negative.

Testing for CHIKV is performed at CDC, several state health department laboratories, and 1 commercial laboratory. Health care providers should report suspected chikungunya cases to their state or local health departments to facilitate diagnosis and mitigate the risk of local transmission. State health departments are encouraged to report laboratory-confirmed cases to CDC through ArboNET, the national surveillance system for arboviral diseases.

TREATMENT

No specific antiviral treatment is available for chikungunya. Treatment is for symptoms and can include rest, fluids, and use of analgesics and antipyretics. Nonsteroidal anti-inflammatory drugs can be used to help with acute fever and pain. In dengue-endemic areas, however, acetaminophen is the preferred first-line treatment for fever and joint pain until dengue can be ruled out, to reduce the risk of hemorrhage. For patients with persistent joint pain, use of nonsteroidal anti-inflammatory drugs, corticosteroids including topical preparations, and physiotherapy may help lessen the symptoms.

PREVENTION

No vaccine or preventive drug is available. The best way to prevent CHIKV infection is to avoid mosquito bites (see Chapter 2, Protection against Mosquitoes, Ticks, & Other Arthropods). Travelers at increased risk for more severe disease, including travelers with underlying medical conditions and women who are late in their pregnancy (as their unborn infants are at increased risk), may consider avoiding travel to areas with ongoing outbreaks. If travel is unavoidable, emphasize the need for protective measures against mosquito bites.

CDC website: www.cdc.gov/chikungunya

BIBLIOGRAPHY

1. CDC. Geographic distribution of chikungunya virus. Atlanta: CDC; 2014 [updated March 2014; cited 2014 Mar 31]. Available from: http://www.cdc.gov/chikungunya/geo/index.html.
2. Kularatne SA, Gihan MC, Weerasinghe SC, Gunasena S. Concurrent outbreaks of chikungunya and dengue fever in Kandy, Sri Lanka, 2006–07: a comparative analysis of clinical and laboratory features. Postgrad Med J. 2009 Jul;85(1005):342–6.
3. Lee VJ, Chow A, Zheng X, Carrasco LR, Cook AR, Lye DC, et al. Simple clinical and laboratory predictors of chikungunya versus dengue infections in adults. PLoS Negl Trop Dis. 2012;6(9):e1786.
4. Leparc-Goffart I, Nougairede A, Cassadou S, Prat C, de Lamballerie X. Chikungunya in the Americas. Lancet. 2014 Feb 8;383(9916):514.
5. Lindsey NP PH, Kosoy O, Laven J, Messenger S, Staples JE, Fischer M. Chikungunya virus disease in travelers—United States, 2010–2013. Poster session presented at: Council of State and Territorial Epidemiologist Annual Meeting; 2014 Jun 22–26; Nashville, TN.
6. Pan American Health Organization and CDC. Preparedness and response for chikungunya virus introduction in the Americas. Washington, DC: Pan American Health Organization; 2011 [cited 2014 Sep 17]. Available from: http://new.paho.org/hq/index.php?option=com_content&view=article&id=3545&Itemid=2545&lang=en.
7. Rajapakse S, Rodrigo C, Rajapakse A. Atypical manifestations of chikungunya infection. Trans R Soc Trop Med Hyg. 2010 Feb;104(2):89–96.
8. Rezza G, Nicoletti L, Angelini R, Romi R, Finarelli AC, Panning M, et al. Infection with chikungunya virus in Italy: an outbreak in a temperate region. Lancet. 2007 Dec 1;370(9602):1840–6.
9. Thiberville SD, Moyen N, Dupuis-Maguiraga L, Nougairede A, Gould EA, Roques P, et al. Chikungunya fever: epidemiology, clinical syndrome, pathogenesis and therapy. Antiviral Res. 2013 Sep;99(3):345–70.

CHOLERA

Janell A. Routh, Anna E. Newton, Eric Mintz

INFECTIOUS AGENT

Cholera is an acute bacterial, intestinal infection caused by toxigenic *Vibrio cholerae* O-group 1 or O-group 139. Many other serogroups of *V. cholerae*, with or without the cholera toxin gene (including the nontoxigenic strains of the O1 and O139 serogroups), can cause a choleralike illness. Only toxigenic strains of serogroups O1 and O139 have caused widespread epidemics and are reportable to the World Health Organization (WHO) as "cholera."

V. cholerae O1 has 2 biotypes, classical and El Tor, and each biotype has 2 distinct serotypes, Inaba and Ogawa. The symptoms of infection are indistinguishable, although more people infected with the El Tor biotype remain asymptomatic or have only a mild illness. Globally, most cases of cholera are caused by O1 El Tor organisms. In recent years, an El Tor variant that has characteristics of both classical and El Tor biotypes and may be more virulent than older El Tor strains has emerged in Asia and spread to Africa and the Caribbean. This strain is responsible for the epidemic on Hispaniola and may cause more severe episodes of cholera and higher death rates.

TRANSMISSION

Toxigenic *V. cholerae* O1 and O139 are free-living bacterial organisms found in fresh and brackish water, often in association with copepods or other zooplankton, shellfish, and aquatic plants. Cholera infections are most commonly acquired from drinking water in which *V. cholerae* is found naturally or into which it has been introduced from the feces of an infected person. Other common vehicles include contaminated fish and shellfish. Other foods, including produce, are less commonly implicated. Direct transmission from person to person, even to health care workers during epidemics, has been reported but is not frequent.

EPIDEMIOLOGY

Cholera is endemic in approximately 50 countries and has the potential to emerge in dramatic epidemics; unfortunately, most cases go unreported. *V. cholerae* O1 is endemic in much of Africa and South and Southeast Asia. *V. cholerae* O139 spread rapidly through Asia in the early 1990s but has since remained localized to a few areas in Asia. In October 2010, a large cholera epidemic began in Haiti, just 10 months after a devastating earthquake destroyed the Haitian capital of Port-au-Prince and surrounding areas. Cholera is likely to persist in Haiti at endemic levels with the potential for localized outbreaks and elevated case counts, especially during the rainy season, for the foreseeable future. After it emerged in Haiti, cholera spread to a number of other countries, including the Dominican Republic and Cuba. Sporadic cases associated with travel to or from the Caribbean may continue to occur.

From 2001 through 2013, 123 confirmed cases of cholera in the United States were acquired abroad; of these, 63 were associated with the epidemic in Hispaniola. Risk of infection is highest for travelers who are traveling to countries where cholera is endemic or there is an active epidemic. Haiti continues to be the primary source of travel-associated cholera cases, even though cases among US travelers in 2013 declined to 2010 levels. Travelers who follow the usual tourist itineraries and who observe safe food and water recommendations and hygiene precautions while in countries reporting cholera have virtually no risk of acquiring cholera. The risk is increased for those who drink untreated water, do not follow proper hygiene recommendations, or eat raw or poorly cooked food, especially seafood, in endemic or outbreak settings. Although rare, several cases of cholera have been reported among US health care workers caring for cholera patients in Haiti and in the United States.

CLINICAL PRESENTATION

Cholera most commonly manifests as watery diarrhea in an afebrile person. Severe cholera is characterized by acute, profuse watery diarrhea, described as "rice-water stools," and often nausea and vomiting and can rapidly lead to severe volume depletion. Signs and symptoms include tachycardia, loss of skin turgor, dry mucous membranes, hypotension, and thirst. Additional symptoms, including muscle cramps, are secondary to the resulting electrolyte imbalances. If untreated, rapid loss of body fluids can lead to severe dehydration, hypovolemic shock, and death within hours. With adequate and timely rehydration, case-fatality rates (CFRs) are <1%.

DIAGNOSIS

Cholera is confirmed through culture of a stool specimen or rectal swab. Cary-Blair medium can be used for transport, and selective media such as taurocholate-tellurite-gelatin agar and thiosulfate-citrate-bile salts agar may be used for isolation and identification. Reagents for serogrouping *V. cholerae* isolates are available in state health department laboratories. Commercially available rapid test kits do not yield an isolate for antimicrobial susceptibility testing and subtyping and should not be used for routine diagnosis. All isolates obtained in the United States should be sent to CDC via state health department laboratories for cholera toxin testing and subtyping. Cholera is a nationally reportable disease.

TREATMENT

Rehydration is the cornerstone of cholera treatment. Oral rehydration solution and, when necessary, intravenous fluids and electrolytes, if administered in a timely manner and in adequate volumes, will reduce CFRs to <1%. Antibiotics reduce fluid requirements and duration of illness and are indicated for moderate and severe cases. Whenever possible, antimicrobial susceptibility testing should inform treatment choices, which may include doxycycline, tetracycline, erythromycin, azithromycin, or ciprofloxacin. Multidrug-resistant isolates are emerging, particularly in South Asia, with resistance to quinolones, trimethoprim-sulfamethoxazole, and tetracycline. The strain from Hispaniola is also multidrug resistant; however, it is still sensitive to doxycycline and tetracycline. Zinc supplementation reduces the severity and duration of cholera and other diarrheal diseases in children in resource-limited areas.

PREVENTION

Safe food and water precautions and frequent handwashing are critical in preventing cholera (see Chapter 2, Food & Water Precautions). Chemoprophylaxis is not indicated.

No cholera vaccine is currently licensed in the United States. Two oral vaccines are prequalified by WHO and are available in many countries outside the United States: Dukoral (Crucell, the Netherlands) and Shanchol (ShanthaBiotechnics, India). No country or territory requires vaccination against cholera as a condition for entry.

Further information on Dukoral can be obtained from Crucell (www.crucell.com). Information on Shanchol can be obtained from ShanthaBiotechnics (www.shanthabiotech. com).

CDC website: www.cdc.gov/cholera

BIBLIOGRAPHY

1. Gaffga NH, Tauxe RV, Mintz ED. Cholera: a new homeland in Africa? Am J Trop Med Hyg. 2007 Oct;77(4):705–13.
2. Haitian Ministry of Public Health and Population (MSPP). Ministere de la SantePubliqueet de la Population. Port-au-Prince, Haiti: Haitian Ministry of Public Health and Population; 2013 [cited 2014 Jun 19]. Available from: http://mspp.gouv.ht.
3. Harris JB, Larocque RC, Charles RC, Mazumder RN, Khan AI, Bardhan PK. Cholera's western front. Lancet. 2010 Dec 11;376(9757):1961–5.
4. Harris JB, LaRocque RC, Qadri F, Ryan ET, Calderwood SB. Cholera. Lancet. 2012 Jun 30;379(9835):2466–76.
5. Loharikar A, Newton AE, Stroika S, Freeman M, Greene KD, Parsons MB, et al. Cholera in the United States, 2001–2011: a reflection of patterns of global epidemiology and travel. Epidemiol Infect. 2014 May 27:1–9.
6. Lucas ME, Deen JL, von Seidlein L, Wang XY, Ampuero J, Puri M, et al. Effectiveness of mass oral cholera vaccination in Beira, Mozambique. N Engl J Med. 2005 Feb 24;352(8):757–67.
7. Schilling KA, Cartwright EJ, Stamper J, Locke M, Esposito DH, Balaban V, et al. Diarrheal illness among US residents providing medical services in Haiti during the cholera epidemic, 2010–2011. J Travel Med. 2014 Jan-Feb;21(1):55–7.
8. Sur D, Lopez AL, Kanungo S, Paisley A, Manna B, Ali M, et al. Efficacy and safety of a modified killed-whole-cell oral cholera vaccine in India: an interim analysis of a cluster-randomised, double-blind, placebo-controlled trial. Lancet. 2009 Nov 14;374(9702):1694–702.
9. World Health Organization. Cholera, 2012. Wkly Epidemiol Rec. 2013 Aug 2;88(31):321–34.

COCCIDIOIDOMYCOSIS

Tom M. Chiller

INFECTIOUS AGENT

The fungi *Coccidioides immitis* and *C. posadasii*.

TRANSMISSION

Inhalation of fungal conidia from dust in ambient air or generated by soil-disrupting human activities or natural disasters. Not transmitted from person to person.

EPIDEMIOLOGY

Endemic in arid regions, including those in the southwestern United States. Outside the United States, coccidioidomycosis is endemic in parts of Central and South America. Travelers are at increased risk if they participate in activities that expose them to dust, such as construction, landscaping, mining, agriculture, archaeological excavation, military maneuvers, and recreational pursuits such as dirt biking.

CLINICAL PRESENTATION

The incubation period is 7–21 days. Most infections (60%) are asymptomatic. Symptomatic infection ranges from a self-limited influenzalike illness, characterized by fever, rash, muscle aches, dry cough, weight loss, and malaise, to primary pulmonary coccidioidomycosis, characterized by pneumonia with changes on chest radiography.

In rare instances, severe lung disease (such as cavitary pneumonia) or dissemination to the central nervous system, joints, bones, or skin may develop. People at increased risk for severe pulmonary disease are the elderly, those with diabetes or recent smoking history, and people of low socioeconomic status. People at increased risk for disseminated disease include African Americans and Filipinos, those with immunocompromising conditions (such as HIV), and pregnant women, particularly in the third trimester of pregnancy.

DIAGNOSIS

Best diagnosed by using serologic, histopathologic, and culture methods. Serologic tests are useful to confirm diagnoses and provide prognostic information.

TREATMENT

Some experts recommend that people without risk factors for severe or disseminated disease do not require treatment, because the illness is self-limited; others propose treatment to reduce the intensity or duration of symptoms. People at high risk for dissemination should receive antifungal therapy when diagnosed with acute coccidioidomycosis. Additionally, people with severe acute pulmonary disease, chronic pulmonary infection, or disseminated disease should receive antifungal therapy. Depending on the clinical situation, azole antifungal agents (such as fluconazole or itraconazole) or amphotericin B may be used.

PREVENTION

Limit exposure to outdoor dust in endemic areas.

CDC website: www.cdc.gov/fungal/diseases/ coccidioidomycosis

BIBLIOGRAPHY

1. Ampel NM. Coccidioidomycosis: a review of recent advances. Clin Chest Med. 2009 Jun;30(2):241–51.
2. CDC. Coccidioidomycosis in travelers returning from Mexico—Pennsylvania, 2000. MMWR. 2000;49(44):1004–6.
3. Chiller TM, Galgiani JN, Stevens DA. Coccidioidomycosis. Infect Dis Clin North Am. 2003 Mar;17(1):41–57, viii.
4. Crum NF, Lederman ER, Stafford CM, Parrish JS, Wallace MR. Coccidioidomycosis: a descriptive survey of a reemerging disease. Clinical characteristics and current controversies. Medicine (Baltimore). 2004 May;83(3):149–75.
5. Galgiani JN, Ampel NM, Blair JE, Catanzaro A, Johnson RH, Stevens DA, et al. Coccidioidomycosis. Clin Infect Dis. 2005 Nov 1;41(9):1217–23.
6. Rosenstein NE, Emery KW, Werner SB, Kao A, Johnson R, Rogers D, et al. Risk factors for severe pulmonary and disseminated coccidioidomycosis: Kern County, California, 1995–1996. Clin Infect Dis. 2001 Mar 1;32(5):708–15.

CRYPTOSPORIDIOSIS

Michele C. Hlavsa, Lihua Xiao

INFECTIOUS AGENT

Among the many protozoan parasites in the genus *Cryptosporidium, Cryptosporidium hominis* and *C. parvum* most frequently cause human infections.

TRANSMISSION

Cryptosporidium is transmitted via the fecal-oral route. Its low infectious dose, prolonged survival in moist environments, protracted communicability, and extreme chlorine tolerance make *Cryptosporidium* ideally suited for transmission through contaminated drinking or recreational water, such as swimming pools. Transmission can also occur through contaminated food, or contact with infected people, or contaminated surfaces.

EPIDEMIOLOGY

Cryptosporidiosis is endemic worldwide. Of 22 US Peace Corps volunteers, 9 developed anti-*Cryptosporidium* IgG while serving in Africa. International travel is a risk factor for sporadic cryptosporidiosis in the United States and other industrialized nations; however, few studies have assessed the prevalence of cryptosporidiosis in travelers. One study found 2.9% prevalence of *Cryptosporidium* infection among those with travel-associated diarrhea; cryptosporidiosis was significantly associated with travel to Asia, particularly India, and Latin America. Another study found a 6.4% prevalence of *Cryptosporidium* infection among North Americans with diarrhea associated with travel to 2 Mexican cities. This study suggests an association between cryptosporidiosis and length of travel.

CLINICAL PRESENTATION

Symptoms begin within 2 weeks (typically 5–7 days) after infection and are generally self-limited. The most common symptom is watery diarrhea. Other symptoms can include urgency, tenesmus, abdominal cramps, flatulence, nausea, vomiting, weight loss, fever, decreased appetite, fatigue, joint pain, and headache. In immunocompetent people, symptoms typically resolve within 2–3 weeks; patients might experience a recurrence of symptoms after a brief period of recovery before complete symptom resolution. Clinical presentation of cryptosporidiosis in HIV-infected patients varies with level of immunosuppression, ranging from no symptoms or transient disease to relapsing or chronic diarrhea or even choleralike diarrhea, which can lead to life-threatening wasting and malabsorption. Extraintestinal cryptosporidiosis (in the biliary or respiratory tract or rarely the pancreas) has been documented in children and immunocompromised people.

DIAGNOSIS

Tests for *Cryptosporidium* are typically not included in routine ova and parasite testing. Therefore, clinicians should specifically request testing for this parasite, when suspected. Because *Cryptosporidium* can be excreted intermittently, multiple stool collections (3 stool specimens collected on separate days) increase test sensitivity. Diagnostic techniques include direct fluorescent antibody (considered the gold standard), EIA testing, rapid immunochromatographic cartridge assays, and microscopy with modified acid-fast staining. False-positive results might occur when using rapid immunochromatographic cartridge assays if they are not used according to the manufacturer's directions. Confirmation by microscopy might be considered.

TREATMENT

Most immunocompetent people will recover without treatment. Nitazoxanide is approved to treat cryptosporidiosis in immunocompetent people aged ≥1 year. Nitazoxanide has not been shown to be an effective treatment of cryptosporidiosis in HIV-infected patients. However, dramatic clinical and parasitologic responses have been reported in these patients after the immune system has been reconstituted with active combination antiretroviral therapy. Protease inhibitors might have direct anti-*Cryptosporidium* activity.

PREVENTION

Food and water precautions (see Chapter 2, Food & Water Precautions) and handwashing(www.cdc.gov/handwashing). *Cryptosporidium* is extremely tolerant to halogens (such as chlorine or iodine). Water can be treated effectively by heating it to a rolling boil for 1 minute or filtering with an absolute 1-µm filter. Alcohol-based hand sanitizers are not effective against the parasite. Prevention recommendations can be found at www.cdc.gov/parasites/crypto/gen_info/prevent.html.

CDC website: www.cdc.gov/parasites/crypto

BIBLIOGRAPHY

1. Alinia (nitazoxanide) prescribing information. Tampa, FL: Romark Pharmaceuticals; 2005 [cited 2014 Jun 14]. Available from: http://www.accessdata.fda.gov/drugsatfda_docs/label/2005/021818lbl.pdf.
2. Cartwright RY. Food and waterborne infections associated with package holidays. J Appl Microbiol. 2003;94 Suppl:12S–24S.
3. Kotloff KL, Nataro JP, Blackwelder WC, Nasrin D, Farag TH, Panchalingam S, et al. Burden and aetiology of diarrhoeal disease in infants and young children in developing countries (the Global Enteric Multicenter Study, GEMS): a prospective, case-control study. Lancet. 2013 Jul 20;382(9888):209–22.
4. Nair P, Mohamed JA, DuPont HL, Figueroa JF, Carlin LG, Jiang ZD, et al. Epidemiology of cryptosporidiosis in North American travelers to Mexico. Am J Trop Med Hyg. 2008 Aug;79(2):210–4.
5. Pantenburg B, Cabada MM, White AC, Jr. Treatment of cryptosporidiosis. Expert Rev Anti Infect Ther. 2009 May;7(4):385–91.
6. Roy SL, DeLong SM, Stenzel SA, Shiferaw B, Roberts JM, Khalakdina A, et al. Risk factors for sporadic cryptosporidiosis among immunocompetent persons in the United States from 1999–2001. J Clin Microbiol. 2004 Jul;42(7):2944–51.
7. Ungar BL, Mulligan M, Nutman TB. Serologic evidence of *Cryptosporidium* infection in US volunteers before and during Peace Corps service in Africa. Arch Intern Med. 1989 Apr;149(4):894–7.
8. Weitzel T, Wichmann O, Muhlberger N, Reuter B, Hoof HD, Jelinek T. Epidemiological and clinical features of travel-associated cryptosporidiosis. Clin Microbiol Infect. 2006 Sep;12(9):921–4.

CUTANEOUS LARVA MIGRANS

Susan Montgomery

INFECTIOUS AGENT

Larval stages of dog and cat hookworms (usually *Ancylostoma* spp.).

TRANSMISSION

Skin contact with contaminated soil or sand.

EPIDEMIOLOGY

Most cases are reported in travelers to the Caribbean, Africa, Asia, and South America. Beaches where domestic animals may roam are a common source of infection. Infection occurs in short- as well as long-term travelers.

CLINICAL PRESENTATION

Creeping eruption usually appears 1–5 days after skin penetration, but the incubation period may be ≥1 month. Typically, a serpiginous, erythematous track appears in the skin and is associated with intense itchiness and mild swelling. Usual locations are the foot and buttocks, although any skin surface coming in contact with contaminated soil can be affected.

DIAGNOSIS

Diagnosed on the basis of characteristic skin lesions. Biopsy is not recommended.

TREATMENT

Cutaneous larva migrans is self-limiting; migrating larvae usually die after 5–6 weeks. Albendazole is the treatment of choice. Ivermectin is effective but not approved for this indication.

PREVENTION

Reduce contact with contaminated soil by wearing shoes and protective clothing and using barriers such as towels when seated on the ground.

BIBLIOGRAPHY

1. Caumes E. Treatment of cutaneous larva migrans. Clin Infect Dis. 2000 May;30(5):811–4.
2. Gillespie SH. Cutaneous larva migrans. Curr Infect Dis Rep. 2004 Feb;6(1):50–3.
3. Heukelbach J, Feldmeier H. Epidemiological and clinical characteristics of hookworm-related cutaneous larva migrans. Lancet Infect Dis. 2008 May;8(5):302–9.
4. Hochedez P, Caumes E. Hookworm-related cutaneous larva migrans. J Travel Med. 2007 Sep–Oct;14(5):326–33.
5. Lederman ER, Weld LH, Elyazar IR, von Sonnenburg F, Loutan L, Schwartz E, et al. Dermatologic conditions of the ill returned traveler: an analysis from the GeoSentinel Surveillance Network. Int J Infect Dis. 2008 Nov;12(6):593–602.

CDC website: www.cdc.gov/parasites/zoonotichookworm

CYCLOSPORIASIS

Barbara L. Herwaldt

INFECTIOUS AGENT

Cyclospora cayetanensis, a coccidian protozoan parasite.

TRANSMISSION

Ingestion of infective *Cyclospora* oocysts, such as in contaminated food or water.

EPIDEMIOLOGY

Most common in tropical and subtropical regions, where outbreaks are frequently seasonal (such as during summers and rainy season in Nepal); even short-term travelers can become infected. Outbreaks in the United States and Canada have been linked to imported fresh produce.

CLINICAL PRESENTATION

Incubation period averages 1 week (range, 2 days to >2 weeks). Onset of symptoms is often abrupt but can be gradual; some people have an influenzalike prodrome. The most common symptom is watery diarrhea, which can be profuse. Other symptoms can include anorexia, weight loss, abdominal cramps, bloating, nausea, body aches, vomiting, and low-grade fever. If untreated, the illness can last for several weeks or months, with a remitting-relapsing course.

DIAGNOSIS

Diagnosed by detecting *Cyclospora* oocysts in stool specimens. Stool examinations for ova and parasites usually do not include methods for detecting *Cyclospora* unless testing for this parasite is specifically requested. Diagnostic assistance is also available from CDC (www.dpd.cdc.gov/dpdx; 404-718-4745; parasites@cdc.gov).

TREATMENT

Trimethoprim-sulfamethoxazole; no highly effective alternatives have been identified.

PREVENTION

Food and water precautions (see Chapter 2, Food & Water Precautions); disinfection with chlorine or iodine is unlikely to be effective.

CDC website: www.cdc.gov/parasites/cyclosporiasis

BIBLIOGRAPHY

1. Hall RL, Jones JL, Herwaldt BL. Surveillance for laboratory-confirmed sporadic cases of cyclosporiasis—United States, 1997–2008. MMWR Surveill Summ. 2011 Apr 8;60(2):1–11.
2. Herwaldt BL. *Cyclospora cayetanensis*: a review, focusing on the outbreaks of cyclosporiasis in the 1990s. Clin Infect Dis. 2000 Oct;31(4):1040–57.

3. Herwaldt BL. The ongoing sage of US outbreaks of cyclosporiasis associated with imported fresh produce: what *Cyclospora cayetanensis* has taught us and what we have yet to learn. In: Institute of Medicine, editor. Addressing Foodborne Threats to Health: Policies, Practices, and Global Coordination, Workshop Summary. Washington, DC: National Academies Press; 2006. p. 85–115, 133–40.

4. Ortega YR, Sanchez R. Update on *Cyclospora cayetanensis*, a food-borne and waterborne parasite. Clin Microbiol Rev. 2010 Jan;23(1):218–34.

5. Shlim DR. *Cyclospora cayetanensis*. Clin Lab Med. 2002 Dec;22(4):927–36.

CYSTICERCOSIS
Paul T. Cantey

INFECTIOUS AGENT
Taenia solium, a cestode parasite.

TRANSMISSION
Ingestion of eggs, excreted by a human carrier of the adult *T. solium* tapeworm, on fecally contaminated food or through close contact with the carrier. Autoinfection is also possible. Eating undercooked pork with cysticerci results in tapeworm infection (taeniasis), not human cysticercosis.

EPIDEMIOLOGY
Common where sanitary conditions are poor and where pigs have access to human feces. Endemic areas include Mexico, Latin America, sub-Saharan Africa, India, and East Asia. Uncommon in travelers. Seen in immigrants from endemic regions.

CLINICAL PRESENTATION
Median latent period of 5 years (range, 1–30 years). Symptoms depend on the number, location, and stage of cysts. The most common location is brain parenchyma, with late-onset seizures. Other presentations include increased intracranial pressure, encephalitis, symptoms of space-occupying lesion, and hydrocephalus. Cysticercosis should be excluded in any adult with new-onset seizures who comes from an endemic area or has potential exposure to a tapeworm carrier.

DIAGNOSIS
Neuroimaging studies (CT or MRI) and confirmatory serologic testing. The most specific serologic test is the enzyme-linked immunotransfer blot, but this test may be negative in up to 30% of patients with a single parenchymal lesion.

TREATMENT
Control of symptoms is the cornerstone of therapy. Anticonvulsants, corticosteroids, or both may be indicated. For some lesions, surgical intervention may be the treatment of choice. Antiparasitic treatment (albendazole, praziquantel) should *not* be initiated in patients with heavy infections, cysticercotic encephalitis, or increased intracranial pressure, as dying cysts can cause or worsen some symptoms. In these cases, the priority is neurologic management (steroids, mannitol), neurosurgical management, or both. Clinicians can consult CDC to obtain more information about diagnosis and treatment (CDC Parasitic Diseases Inquiries: 404-718-4745 or parasites@cdc.gov).

PREVENTION
Food and water precautions (see Chapter 2, Food & Water Precautions).

CDC website: www.cdc.gov/parasites/cysticercosis

BIBLIOGRAPHY
1. Garcia HH, Del Brutto OH. Neurocysticercosis: updated concepts about an old disease. Lancet Neurol. 2005 Oct;4(10):653–61.

2. Garcia HH, Del Brutto OH, Nash TE, White AC, Jr., Tsang VC, Gilman RH. New concepts in the diagnosis and management of neurocysticercosis

(*Taenia solium*). Am J Trop Med Hyg. 2005
Jan;72(1):3–9.

3. Garcia HH, Gonzalez AE, Evans CA, Gilman
RH, Cysticercosis Working Group in Peru.

Taenia solium cysticercosis. Lancet. 2003 Aug
16;362(9383):547–56.

4. Sorvillo FJ, DeGiorgio C, Waterman SH. Deaths from
cysticercosis, United States. EID 2007 Feb;13(2):230–5.

DENGUE

Kay M. Tomashek, Tyler M. Sharp, Harold S. Margolis

INFECTIOUS AGENT

Dengue, an acute febrile illness, is caused by infection with any of 4 related positive-sense, single-stranded RNA viruses of the genus *Flavivirus*, dengue viruses (DENV) 1, 2, 3, or 4.

TRANSMISSION

Transmission occurs through the bite of infected *Aedes* mosquitoes, primarily *Aedes aegypti* and *Ae. albopictus*. Because of the approximately 7-day viremia in humans, bloodborne transmission is possible through exposure to infected blood, organs, or other tissues (such as bone marrow). In addition, perinatal DENV transmission occurs, and the highest risk appears to be among infants whose mothers are acutely ill around the time of delivery. DENV may also be transmitted through breast milk.

EPIDEMIOLOGY

Dengue is endemic throughout the tropics and subtropics and is a leading cause of febrile illness among travelers returning from Latin America, the Caribbean, and Southeast Asia, according to an analysis of data collected by the GeoSentinel Surveillance Network. Dengue occurs in >100 countries worldwide (Maps 3-1 through 3-3,), including Puerto Rico, the US Virgin Islands, and US-affiliated Pacific Islands. Sporadic outbreaks with local transmission have occurred in Florida, Hawaii, and along the Texas–Mexico border. Although the geographic distribution of dengue is similar to that of malaria, dengue is more of a risk in urban and residential areas than is malaria. DengueMap (www.healthmap.org/dengue/index.php) shows up-to-date information on areas of ongoing transmission.

CLINICAL PRESENTATION

About 75% of all DENV infections are asymptomatic. Symptomatic infection (dengue) most commonly presents as a mild to moderate, nonspecific, acute, febrile illness. However, as many as 5% of all dengue patients develop severe, life-threatening disease. Early clinical findings are nonspecific but require a high index of suspicion, because recognizing early signs of shock and promptly initiating intensive supportive therapy can reduce risk of death among patients with severe dengue from 10% to <1%. See Box 3-1 for information regarding the World Health Organization guidelines for classifying dengue.

Dengue begins abruptly after an incubation period of 5–7 days (range, 3–10 days), and the course follows 3 phases: febrile, critical, and convalescent. Fever typically lasts 2–7 days and can be biphasic. Other signs and symptoms may include severe headache; retroorbital pain; muscle, joint, and bone pain; macular or maculopapular rash; and minor hemorrhagic manifestations, including petechiae, ecchymosis, purpura, epistaxis, bleeding gums, hematuria, or a positive tourniquet test result. Some patients have injected oropharynx and facial erythema in the first 24–48 hours after onset. Warning signs of progression to severe dengue occur in the late febrile phase around the time of defervescence and include persistent vomiting, severe abdominal pain, mucosal bleeding, difficulty breathing, signs of hypovolemic shock, and rapid decline in platelet count with an increase in hematocrit (hemoconcentration).

The critical phase of dengue begins at defervescence and typically lasts 24–48

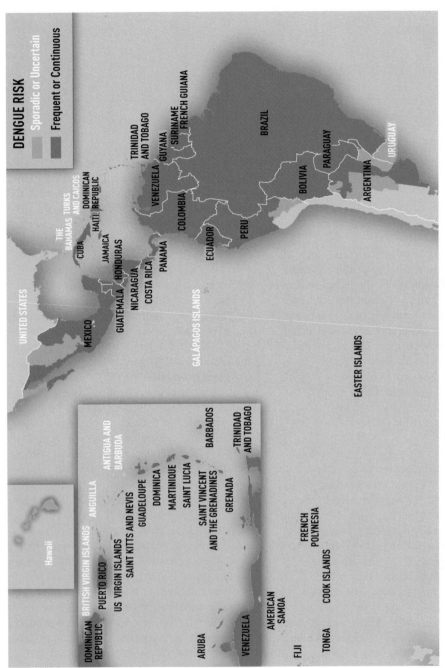

MAP 3-1. DISTRIBUTION OF DENGUE IN THE AMERICAS AND THE CARIBBEAN.[1,2]

[1] Risk areas are shown on a national level except for where evidence exists of different risk levels at sub-national regions. Areas that are too small to be seen on the regional maps are labeled in white or gray depending on their risk categorization.

[2] Based on surveillance data, official reports, published research, and expert opinion, including data from Brady et al. Refining the Global Spatial Limits of Dengue Virus Transmission by Evidence-Based Consensus. PLoS Negl Trop Dis. 2012 Aug 7; 6(8): e1760. Compiled by CDC Dengue Branch in collaboration with University of Oxford.

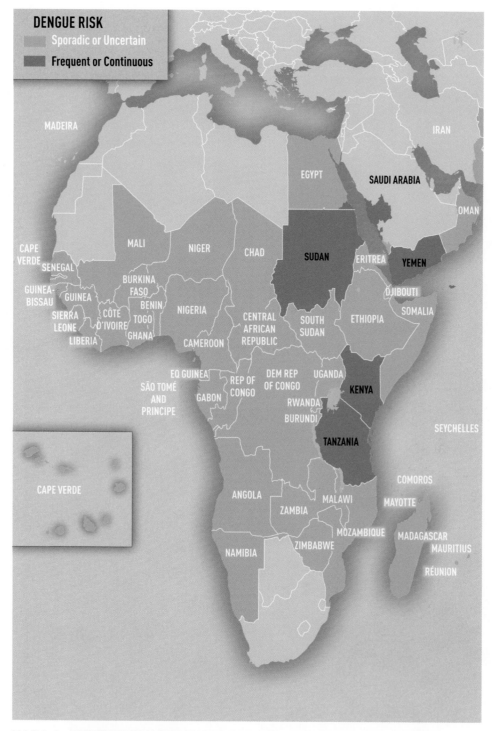

DENGUE RISK

- Sporadic or Uncertain
- Frequent or Continuous

MAP 3-2. DISTRIBUTION OF DENGUE IN AFRICA AND THE MIDDLE EAST.[1,2]

[1] Risk areas are shown on a national level except for where evidence exists of different risk levels at sub-national regions. Areas that are too small to be seen on the regional maps are labeled in white or gray depending on their risk categorization.

[2] Based on surveillance data, official reports, published research, and expert opinion, including data from Brady et al. Refining the Global Spatial Limits of Dengue Virus Transmission by Evidence-Based Consensus. PLoS Negl Trop Dis. 2012 Aug 7; 6(8): e1760. Compiled by CDC Dengue Branch in collaboration with University of Oxford.

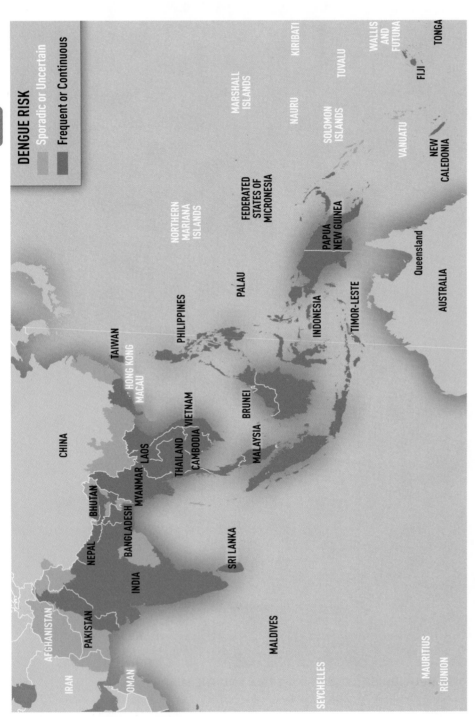

MAP 3-3. DISTRIBUTION OF DENGUE IN ASIA AND OCEANIA.[1,2]

[1] Risk areas are shown on a national level except for where evidence exists of different risk levels at sub-national regions. Areas that are too small to be seen on the regional maps are labeled in white or gray depending on their risk categorization.

[2] Based on surveillance data, official reports, published research, and expert opinion, including data from Brady et al. Refining the Global Spatial Limits of Dengue Virus Transmission by Evidence-Based Consensus. PLoS Negl Trop Dis. 2012 Aug 7; 6(8): e1760. Compiled by CDC Dengue Branch in collaboration with University of Oxford.

BOX 3-1. GUIDELINES FOR CLASSIFYING DENGUE

In November 2009, World Health Organization (WHO) issued a new guideline that classifies symptomatic cases as dengue or severe dengue.

Dengue is defined by a combination of ≥2 clinical findings in a febrile person who traveled to or lives in a dengue-endemic area. Clinical findings include nausea, vomiting, rash, aches and pains, a positive tourniquet test, leukopenia, and the following warning signs: abdominal pain or tenderness, persistent vomiting, clinical fluid accumulation, mucosal bleeding, lethargy, restlessness, and liver enlargement. The presence of a warning sign may predict severe dengue in a patient.

Severe dengue is classified as dengue with any of the following symptoms: severe plasma leakage leading to shock or fluid accumulation with respiratory distress; severe bleeding; or severe organ impairment such as elevated transaminases ≥1,000 IU/L, impaired consciousness, or heart impairment.

From 1975 through 2009, symptomatic dengue virus infections were classified according to the WHO guidelines as dengue fever, dengue hemorrhagic fever (DHF), and dengue shock syndrome (the most severe form of DHF). The case definition was changed to the 2009 clinical classification after reports that the case definition of DHF was both too difficult to apply in resource-limited settings and too specific, as it failed to identify a substantial proportion of severe dengue cases, including cases of hepatic failure and encephalitis. Many dengue experts felt that the original case definitions, which were developed based on data from pediatric cases in Southeast Asia, were not applicable to other regions and populations. The 2009 clinical classification has been criticized because it is felt to be overly inclusive, as it allows several different ways to qualify for severe dengue, and nonspecific warning signs are used as diagnostic criteria for dengue. Last, the new guidelines have been criticized because they do not define the clinical criteria for establishing severe dengue (with the exception of providing laboratory cutoff values for transaminase levels), thereby leaving severity determination up to individual clinical judgment.

hours. Most patients clinically improve during this phase, but those with substantial plasma leakage develop severe dengue as a result of a marked increase in vascular permeability. Initially, physiologic compensatory mechanisms maintain adequate circulation, which narrows pulse pressure as diastolic blood pressure increases. Patients with severe plasma leakage have pleural effusions or ascites, hypoproteinemia, and hemoconcentration. Patients may appear to be well despite early signs of shock. However, once hypotension develops, systolic blood pressure rapidly declines, and irreversible shock and death may ensue despite resuscitation. Patients can also develop severe hemorrhagic manifestations, including hematemesis, bloody stool, melena, or menorrhagia, especially if they have prolonged shock. Atypical manifestations include hepatitis, myocarditis, pancreatitis, and encephalitis.

As plasma leakage subsides, the patient enters the convalescent phase and begins to reabsorb extravasated intravenous fluids and pleural and abdominal effusions. As a patient's well-being improves, hemodynamic status stabilizes (although he or she may manifest bradycardia), and diuresis ensues. The patient's hematocrit stabilizes or may fall because of the dilutional effect of the reabsorbed fluid, and the white cell count usually starts to rise, followed by a recovery of platelet count. The convalescent-phase rash may desquamate and be pruritic.

Laboratory findings commonly include leucopenia, thrombocytopenia, hyponatremia, elevated aspartate aminotransferase and alanine aminotransferase, and a normal erythrocyte sedimentation rate.

Data are limited on health outcomes of dengue in pregnancy and effects of maternal DENV infection on the developing fetus. Perinatal DENV transmission can occur, and peripartum maternal infection may increase the likelihood of symptomatic infection in the newborn. Of the 34 perinatal transmission cases described in the literature, all developed thrombocytopenia and all but 1 had fever in the first 2 weeks after birth. Nearly 40% had a hemorrhagic manifestation, and one-fourth had hypotension. Placental transfer of maternal IgG anti-DENV (from a previous maternal infection) may increase risk for severe dengue among infants infected at 6–12 months of age, when the protective effect of these antibodies wanes.

DIAGNOSIS

Clinicians should consider dengue in a patient who was in an endemic area within 2 weeks before symptom onset. All suspected cases should be reported to the local health department, because dengue is a nationally reportable disease. Laboratory confirmation can be made from a single acute-phase serum specimen obtained early (≤5 days after fever onset) in the illness by detecting DENV genomic sequences with RT-PCR or DENV nonstructural protein 1 (NS1) antigen by immunoassay. Later in the illness (≥4 days after fever onset), IgM anti-DENV can be detected with ELISA. For patients presenting during the first week after fever onset, diagnostic testing should include a test for DENV (PCR or NS1) and IgM anti-DENV. For patients presenting

>1 week after fever onset, IgM anti-DENV is most useful, although NS1 has been reported positive up to 12 days after fever onset (Figure 3-1). In the United States, both IgM anti-DENV ELISA and DENV real-time RT-PCR are approved as in vitro diagnostic tests.

Presence of DENV by PCR or NS1 antigen in a single diagnostic specimen is considered laboratory confirmation of dengue in patients with a compatible clinical and travel history. IgM anti-DENV in a single serum sample suggests a probable, recent DENV infection and should be considered diagnostic for dengue if the infection most likely occurred in a place (such as Puerto Rico and much of the Caribbean) where other potentially cross-reactive flaviviruses (such as West Nile, yellow fever, and Japanese encephalitis viruses) are not a risk. IgM anti-DENV seroconversion in acute- and convalescent-phase serum specimens is considered laboratory confirmation of dengue.

IgG anti-DENV by ELISA in a single serum sample is not useful for diagnostic testing because it remains detectable for life after a DENV infection. In addition, people infected with or vaccinated against other flaviviruses may produce

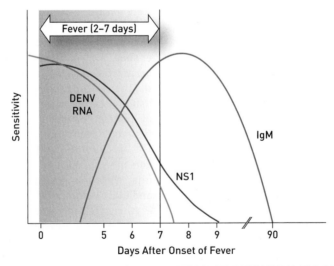

FIGURE 3-1. RELATIVE SENSITIVITY OF DETECTION OF DENV NUCLEIC ACID, ANTIGEN, AND IGM[1]

Abbreviations: DENV, dengue virus; NS1, nonstructural protein 1.
[1] DENV RNA and NS1 are detectable during the first week of illness. Anti-DENV IgM is detectable starting approximately 5 days after illness onset. Although most cases only have detectable IgM anti-DENV for 14–20 days after illness onset, in some cases it may be detectable for up to 90 days. Detection of anti-DENV IgG is neither sensitive nor specific in identifying patients with dengue.

cross-reactive flavivirus antibodies, yielding false-positive serologic dengue diagnostic test results.

Dengue diagnostic testing (molecular and immunoassay) is available from several commercial reference diagnostic laboratories, state public health laboratories, and CDC (www.cdc.gov/Dengue/clinicalLab/index.html). Consultation on dengue diagnostic testing can be obtained from CDC at 787-706-2399.

TREATMENT

No specific antiviral agents exist for dengue. Patients should be advised to stay well hydrated and to avoid aspirin (acetylsalicylic acid), aspirin-containing drugs, and other nonsteroidal anti-inflammatory drugs (such as ibuprofen) because of their anticoagulant properties. Fever should be controlled with acetaminophen and tepid sponge baths. Febrile patients should avoid mosquito bites to reduce risk of further transmission. For those who develop severe dengue, close observation and frequent monitoring in an intensive care unit setting may be required. Prophylactic platelet transfusions in dengue patients are not beneficial and may contribute to fluid overload.

PREVENTION

No vaccine is available, although several are in clinical trials; no chemoprophylaxis

is available to prevent dengue. Travelers to dengue-endemic areas are at risk of getting dengue; risk increases with longer duration of travel and disease incidence in the travel destination (such as during the rainy season and during epidemics). Travelers going to the tropics for any length of time should be advised to avoid mosquito bites by taking the following preventive measures:

- Select accommodations with well-screened windows and doors or air conditioning when possible. *Aedes* mosquitoes typically live indoors and are often found in dark, cool places, such as in closets, under beds, behind curtains, in bathrooms, and on porches. Travelers should be advised to use insecticides to get rid of mosquitoes in these areas.
- Wear clothing that adequately covers the arms and legs, especially during the early morning and late afternoon, when risk of being bitten is the highest.
- Use insect repellent (see Chapter 2, Protection against Mosquitoes, Ticks, & Other Arthropods).
- For longer-term travelers, empty and clean or cover any standing water that can be mosquito-breeding sites in the local residence (such as water storage tanks or flowerpot trays).

CDC website: www.cdc.gov/dengue

BIBLIOGRAPHY

1. Barthel A, Gourinat AC, Cazorla C, Joubert C, Dupont-Rouzeyrol M, Descloux E. Breast milk as a possible route of vertical transmission of dengue virus? Clin Infect Dis. 2013 Aug;57(3):415–7.
2. Bhatt S, Gething PW, Brady OJ, Messina JP, Farlow AW, Moyes CL, et al. The global distribution and burden of dengue. Nature. 2013 Apr 25;496(7446):504–7.
3. Guzman MG, Halstead SB, Artsob H, Buchy P, Farrar J, Gubler DJ, et al. Dengue: a continuing global threat. Nat Rev Microbiol. 2010 Dec;8(12 Suppl):S7–16.
4. Leder K, Torresi J, Libman MD, Cramer JP, Castelli F, Schlagenhauf P, et al. GeoSentinel surveillance of illness in returned travelers, 2007–2011. Ann Intern Med. 2013 Mar 19;158(6):456–68.
5. Schwartz E, Weld LH, Wilder-Smith A, von Sonnenburg F, Keystone JS, Kain KC, et al. Seasonality, annual trends, and characteristics of dengue among ill returned travelers, 1997–2006. Emerg Infect Dis. 2008 Jul;14(7):1081–8.
6. Simmons CP, Farrar JJ, van Vinh Chau N, Wills B. Dengue. N Engl J Med. 2012 Apr 12;366(15): 1423–32.
7. Srikiatkhachorn A, Rothman AL, Gibbons RV, Sittisombut N, Malasit P, Ennis FA, et al. Dengue—how best to classify it. Clin Infect Dis. 2011 Sep;53(6):563–7.
8. Streit JA, Yang M, Cavanaugh JE, Polgreen PM. Upward trend in dengue incidence among hospitalized patients, United States. Emerg Infect Dis. 2011 May;17(5):914–6.
9. Tomashek KM, Margolis HS. Dengue: a potential transfusion-transmitted disease. Transfusion. 2011 Aug;51(8):1654–60.
10. World Health Organization. Dengue: guidelines for diagnosis, treatment, prevention and control. Geneva: World Health Organization; 2009.

DIPHTHERIA

Tejpratap S. P. Tiwari

INFECTIOUS AGENT

Toxigenic strains of *Corynebacterium diphtheriae* biotype *mitis*, *gravis*, *intermedius*, or *belfanti*.

TRANSMISSION

Person-to-person through oral or respiratory droplets, close physical contact, and rarely, by fomites. Cutaneous diphtheria is common in tropical countries, and contact with discharge from skin lesions may transmit infection in these environments.

EPIDEMIOLOGY

Endemic in many countries in Asia, the South Pacific, the Middle East, and Eastern Europe and in Haiti and the Dominican Republic; large outbreaks in Indonesia, Thailand, and Laos have occurred since 2011.

CLINICAL PRESENTATION

The incubation period is 2–5 days (range, 1–10 days). Affected anatomic sites include the mucous membrane of the upper respiratory tract (nose, pharynx, tonsils, larynx, and trachea [respiratory diphtheria]), skin (cutaneous diphtheria), or rarely, mucous membranes at other sites (eye, ear, vulva). Nasal diphtheria can be asymptomatic or mild, with a blood-tinged discharge.

Respiratory diphtheria has a gradual onset and is characterized by a mild fever (rarely >101°F [38.3°C]), sore throat, difficulty swallowing, malaise, loss of appetite, and if the larynx is involved, hoarseness. The hallmark of respiratory diphtheria is a pseudomembrane that appears within 2–3 days of illness over the mucous lining of the tonsils, pharynx, larynx, or nares and that can extend into the trachea. The pseudomembrane is firm, fleshy, grey, and adherent; it will bleed after attempts to remove or dislodge it. Fatal airway obstruction can result if the pseudomembrane extends into the larynx or trachea, or if a piece of it becomes dislodged.

DIAGNOSIS

A presumptive diagnosis is usually based on clinical features. Diagnosis is confirmed by isolating *C. diphtheriae* from culture of nasal or throat swabs or membrane tissue.

TREATMENT

Patients with respiratory diphtheria require hospitalization to monitor response to treatment and manage complications. Equine diphtheria antitoxin (DAT) is the mainstay of treatment and is administered after specimen testing, without waiting for laboratory confirmation. In the United States, DAT is available to physicians under an investigational new drug protocol by contacting CDC at 770-488-7100.

An antibiotic (erythromycin or penicillin) should be used to eliminate the causative organisms, stop exotoxin production, and reduce communicability. Supportive care (airway, cardiac monitoring) is required. Antimicrobial prophylaxis (erythromycin or penicillin) is recommended for close contacts of patients.

PREVENTION

All travelers should be up-to-date with diphtheria toxoid vaccine before departure. After a childhood primary series and a booster dose during adolescence, routine booster doses with Td (tetanus-diphtheria) should be given to all adults every 10 years. This booster is particularly important for travelers who will live or work with local populations in countries where diphtheria is endemic.

CDC website: http://www.cdc.gov/diphtheria/index.html

BIBLIOGRAPHY

1. CDC. Fatal respiratory diphtheria in a US traveler to Haiti—Pennsylvania, 2003. MMWR Morb Mortal Wkly Rep. 2004 Jan 9;52(53):1285–6.

2. CDC. Updated recommendations for use of tetanus toxoid, reduced diphtheria toxoid and acellular pertussis (Tdap) vaccine from the Advisory

Committee on Immunization Practices, 2010. MMWR Morb Mortal Wkly Rep. 2011 Jan 14;60(1):13–5.

3. Galazka A. The changing epidemiology of diphtheria in the vaccine era. J Infect Dis. 2000 Feb;181 Suppl 1:S2–9.

4. World Health Organization. Diphtheria vaccine. Wkly Epidemiol Rec. 2006 Jan 20;81(3): 24–32.

ECHINOCOCCOSIS

Pedro L. Moro

INFECTIOUS AGENT

Larval stages of taeniid cestodes of the genus *Echinococcus*.

TRANSMISSION

Oral contact with contaminated dog feces, particularly in the course of playful and close contact between children and dogs, or through contaminated food or water.

EPIDEMIOLOGY

Echinococcus granulosus is prevalent in broad regions of Eurasia, several South American countries, North and Central America, and Africa. Foci of transmission are found in many other countries. *E. multilocularis* is endemic in the central part of Europe, parts of the Near East, Russia, the Central Asian Republics, China, northern Japan, northwestern Canada, and Alaska. In nonendemic countries, *E. granulosus* is typically seen among immigrants or refugees coming from endemic countries. *E. vogeli* is indigenous to the humid tropical forests in central and northern South America. A small number of polycystic echinococcosis cases in these areas are caused by *E. oligarthrus*.

CLINICAL PRESENTATION
Cystic Echinococcosis or Cystic Hydatid Disease

In humans, hydatid cysts of *E. granulosus* are slowly enlarging masses comparable to benign neoplasms; most human infections remain asymptomatic. Clinical manifestations are determined by the site, size, and condition of the cysts. Hydatid cysts in the liver and the lungs together account for 90% of affected localizations.

Alveolar Echinococcosis or Alveolar Hydatid Disease

The embryo of *E. multilocularis* seems to localize invariably in the liver of the intermediate host (such as wild rodents) and humans. Patients eventually die from hepatic failure, invasion of contiguous structures, or less frequently, metastases to the brain.

Polycystic Echinococcosis or Polycystic Hydatid Disease

Polycystic echinococcosis is usually caused by *E. vogeli* or *E. oligarthrus*. Relatively large cysts develop over years and are primarily found in the liver and occasionally in the thorax or abdominal cavity. Those who are symptomatic may present with a painful right hypochondrial mass, progressive jaundice, or, as in the other forms of disease, liver abscess(es).

DIAGNOSIS

A presumptive diagnosis can be made on the basis of a combination of the individual's history and imaging studies, such as an ultrasound or CT scan. Lesions may be found incidentally in an asymptomatic person. Serologic assays may also be performed, and newer ones are under development. Additional information and diagnostic assistance are available through CDC (www.dpd.cdc.gov/dpdx; 404-718-4745; parasites@cdc.gov).

TREATMENT

For cystic echinococcosis, treatment depends on cyst characteristics and cyst type. Some uncomplicated cysts do not require any treatment. Surgical removal is preferred when cysts are large (>10 cm), secondarily infected, or located in certain organs (brain, lung, or kidney). PAIR (puncture, aspiration, injection, reaspiration) is a minimally invasive technique used to treat cysts in the liver and other abdominal locations. It is less risky and less expensive than surgery. Benzimidazoles (albendazole, mebendazole) should be given to prevent recurrence after surgery or PAIR. Benzimidazoles may be used to treat small cysts (<5 cm). Albendazole should be given continuously, with no monthly treatment interruptions and in 2 divided doses, with a fat-rich meal to increase its bioavailability. Approximately 30% of patients treated with albendazole are cured after 3–6 months, and even higher proportions (30%–50%) demonstrate regression of cyst size and alleviation of symptoms.

Alveolar hydatid disease may require surgery and long-term albendazole but has a high case-fatality ratio. Praziquantel is used in some circumstances. Management of complex cases may require consultation with a tropical medicine specialist.

PREVENTION

Advise travelers to avoid contact with dogs or wild canids in endemic areas. Also advise them not to drink untreated water from streams, canals, lakes, or rivers and to observe food and water precautions (see Chapter 2, Food & Water Precautions).

CDC website: www.cdc.gov/parasites/echinococcosis

BIBLIOGRAPHY

1. Brunetti E, Kern P, Vuitton DA. Expert consensus for the diagnosis and treatment of cystic and alveolar echinococcosis in humans. Acta Trop. 2010 Apr;114(1):1–16.
2. Eckert J, Gottstein B, Heath D, Liu FJ. Prevention of echinococcosis in humans and safety precautions. In: Eckert J, Gemmell MA, Meslin FX, Pawlowski ZS, editors. WHO/OIE Manual on Echinococcosis in Humans and Animals: A Public Health Problem of Global Concern. Paris: World Organization for Animal Health; 2001. p. 238–45.
3. McManus DP, Zhang W, Li J, Bartley PB. Echinococcosis. Lancet. 2003 Oct 18;362(9392):1295–304.
4. Moro PL, Schantz PM. Echinococcosis: historical landmarks and progress in research and control. Ann Trop Med Parasitol. 2006 Dec;100(8):703–14.

ESCHERICHIA COLI

Rajal Mody, Ciara E. O'Reilly

INFECTIOUS AGENT

Most *Escherichia coli* strains do not cause illness. Pathogenic *E. coli* strains are categorized into pathotypes on the basis of their virulence genes. Six pathotypes are associated with diarrhea (diarrheagenic): enterotoxigenic *E. coli* (ETEC), Shiga toxin–producing *E. coli* (STEC), enteropathogenic *E. coli* (EPEC), enteroaggregative *E. coli* (EAEC), enteroinvasive *E. coli* (EIEC), and possibly diffusely adherent *E. coli* (DAEC). Other pathotypes that are common causes of urinary tract infections, bloodstream infections, and meningitis are not covered here. Serotypes of *E. coli* are determined by surface antigens (H and O), and specific serotypes tend to cluster within specific pathotypes.

STEC are also called verotoxigenic *E. coli* (VTEC), and the term enterohemorrhagic *E. coli* (EHEC) is commonly used to specify STEC strains capable of causing human illness, especially bloody diarrhea and hemolytic uremic syndrome (HUS).

TRANSMISSION

Diarrheagenic pathotypes can be passed in the feces of humans and other animals. Transmission of *E. coli* occurs through the fecal-oral route, primarily via contaminated food or water. Transmission also occurs through person-to-person contact, as well as contact with animals or their environment. Although some animals may carry non-STEC diarrheagenic E. coli, people constitute the main reservoir for strains causing diarrhea in humans. The intestinal tracts of animals, especially cattle and other ruminants, are the primary reservoirs of STEC.

EPIDEMIOLOGY

Travel to less-developed countries is associated with higher risk for travelers' diarrhea, including E. coli infection. ETEC is the most common pathotype that causes diarrhea among travelers returning from most regions, but other pathotypes can also cause travelers' diarrhea. Travel-associated infections caused by non-STEC diarrheagenic E. coli are likely underrecognized because most clinical laboratories do not use methods that can detect them. Risk of non-STEC diarrheagenic E. coli infections (primarily ETEC) can be divided into 3 grades, according to the destination country:

- Low-risk countries include the United States, Canada, Australia, New Zealand, Japan, and countries in Northern and Western Europe.
- Intermediate-risk countries include those in Eastern Europe, South Africa, and some of the Caribbean islands.
- High-risk areas include most of Asia, the Middle East, Africa, Mexico, and Central and South America.

Additional information about travelers' diarrhea is available in Chapter 2, Travelers' Diarrhea.

CLINICAL PRESENTATION

Where information is available, non-STEC diarrheagenic E. coli infections have an incubation period ranging from 9 hours to 3 days. The median incubation period of STEC infections is 3–4 days, with a range of 1–10 days. The clinical manifestations of diarrheagenic E. coli vary by pathotype (Table 3-1).

DIAGNOSIS

Many patients with travel-associated E. coli infections, especially those with nonbloody diarrhea, as commonly occurs with ETEC infection, are likely to be managed symptomatically and are unlikely to have the diagnosis

confirmed by a laboratory. Most US clinical laboratories do not use tests that can detect diarrheagenic E. coli other than STEC, although recently approved nucleic acid amplification tests that can detect ETEC are now available in some clinical laboratories. Testing for non-STEC pathotypes is typically done at public health laboratories and only when an outbreak of diarrheal illness of unknown origin is being investigated. In this situation, isolates may be submitted for testing to CDC via state health departments. These tests typically involve PCR testing or whole genome sequence analysis for the specific virulence genes of ETEC, EPEC, EAEC, EIEC, and DAEC.

When a decision is made to identify a cause of an acute diarrheal illness, in addition to routine culture for Salmonella, Shigella, and Campylobacter, the stool sample should be cultured for E. coli O157:H7 and simultaneously assayed for non-O157 STEC with a test that detects Shiga toxins (or the genes that encode them). For more information, see www.cdc.gov/mmwr/preview/mmwrhtml/rr5812a1.htm. All presumptive E. coli O157 isolates and Shiga toxin–positive specimens should be sent to a public health laboratory for further characterization. Rapid, accurate diagnosis of STEC infection is important, because early clinical management decisions can affect patient outcomes, and early detection can help prevent secondary spread.

TREATMENT

Patients with profuse diarrhea or vomiting should be rehydrated. Evidence from pediatric studies indicates that early use of intravenous fluids (within the first 4 days of diarrhea onset) may decrease the risk of oligoanuric renal failure in patients with STEC O157 infections. Where indicated for non-STEC diarrheagenic E. coli, antibiotics for treatment include those of the fluoroquinolone class (such as ciprofloxacin), macrolides such as azithromycin, or rifaximin. Clinicians treating a patient whose clinical syndrome suggests STEC infection (Table 3-1) should be aware that administering antimicrobial agents may increase the risk of HUS. Because resistance to antibiotics is increasing worldwide, the decision to use an antibiotic should be carefully weighed against the severity of illness and the risk of adverse reactions, such as rash,

Table 3-1. Mechanism of pathogenesis and typical clinical syndrome of *Escherichia coli* pathotypes

PATHOTYPE	MECHANISM OF PATHOGENESIS	TYPICAL CLINICAL SYNDROME
ETEC	Heat stable/heat labile enterotoxin production	Acute watery diarrhea, afebrile, occasionally severe
EAEC	Small and large bowel adherence; enterotoxin and cytotoxin production	Watery diarrhea, bloody diarrhea; can cause prolonged or persistent diarrhea in children
EPEC	Small bowel adherence and epithelial cell effacement mediated by intimin	Severe acute watery diarrhea, bloody diarrhea; may be persistent; common cause of infant diarrhea in developing countries
EIEC	Adherence, mucosal invasion and inflammation of large bowel	Watery diarrhea, dysenterylike diarrhea, fever
DAEC	Diffuse adherence to epithelial cells	Watery diarrhea, but pathogenicity not conclusively demonstrated
STEC	Large bowel adherence (frequently mediated via intimin); Shiga toxin 1, Shiga toxin 2 production	Watery diarrhea that often progresses to bloody diarrhea in 1–3 days; pain with defecation; abdominal tenderness; patients may report a history of fever but are often afebrile on presentation; often >5 stools in 24 hours

Abbreviations: ETEC, enterotoxigenic *E. coli*; EAEC, enteroaggregative *E. coli*; EPEC, enteropathogenic *E. coli*; EIEC, enteroinvasive *E. coli*; DAEC, diffusely adherent *E. coli*; STEC, Shiga toxin–producing *E. coli*.

antibiotic-associated colitis, and vaginal yeast infection. Additionally, antimotility agents should be avoided in patients with bloody diarrhea or patients with confirmed STEC infections, because some studies have found that these agents may increase the risk of complications, including HUS, neurologic complications, and toxic megacolon. (See Chapter 2, Travelers' Diarrhea and Chapter 7, Traveling Safely with Infants & Children for information about managing travelers' diarrhea in children.)

PREVENTION

There is no vaccine for *E. coli* infection, nor are any medications recommended for prevention. Food and water are primary sources of *E. coli* infection, so travelers should be reminded of the importance of adhering to food and water precautions (see Chapter 2, Food & Water Precautions). People who may be exposed to livestock, especially ruminants, should be instructed about the importance of handwashing in preventing infection. Since soap and water may not be readily available in at-risk areas, travelers should consider taking hand sanitizer that contains ≥60% alcohol. During *E. coli* outbreaks, clinicians should alert people traveling to affected areas and be cognizant of possible infections among returning travelers.

CDC website: www.cdc.gov/ecoli

BIBLIOGRAPHY

1. CDC. Outbreak of *Escherichia coli* O104:H4 infections associated with sprout consumption—Europe and North America, May–July 2011. MMWR Morb Mortal Wkly Rep. 2013 Dec. 20, 2013;62(50):1029–31.

2. DuPont HL. Systematic review: the epidemiology and clinical features of travellers' diarrhoea. Aliment Pharmacol Ther. 2009 Aug;30(3):187–96.

3. Hedican EB, Medus C, Besser JM, Juni BA, Koziol B, Taylor C, et al. Characteristics of O157 versus non-O157 Shiga toxin-producing *Escherichia coli* infections in Minnesota, 2000–2006. Clin Infect Dis. 2009 Aug 1;49(3):358–64.

4. Hickey CA, Beattie TJ, Cowieson J, Miyashita Y, Strife CF, Frem JC, et al. Early volume expansion during diarrhea and relative nephroprotection during subsequent hemolytic uremic syndrome. Arch Pediatr Adolesc Med. 2011 Oct;165(10):884–9.

5. Kaper JB, Nataro JP, Mobley HL. Pathogenic *Escherichia coli*. Nat Rev Microbiol. 2004 Feb;2(2):123–40.

6. Kendall ME, Crim S, Fullerton K, Han PV, Cronquist AB, Shiferaw B, et al. Travel-associated enteric infections diagnosed after return to the United States, Foodborne Diseases Active Surveillance Network (FoodNet), 2004–2009. Clin Infect Dis. 2012 Jun;54 Suppl 5:S480–7.

7. Mintz ED. Enterotoxigenic *Escherichia coli*: outbreak surveillance and molecular testing. Clin Infect Dis. 2006 Jun 1;42(11):1518–20.

8. Ouyang-Latimer J, Jafri S, VanTassel A, Jiang ZD, Gurleen K, Rodriguez S, et al. In vitro antimicrobial susceptibility of bacterial enteropathogens isolated from international travelers to Mexico, Guatemala, and India from 2006–2008. Antimicrob Agents Chemother. 2011 Feb;55(2):874–8.

9. Shah N, DuPont HL, Ramsey DJ. Global etiology of travelers' diarrhea: systematic review from 1973 to the present. Am J Trop Med Hyg. 2009 Apr;80(4):609–14.

10. Wong CS, Mooney JC, Brandt JR, Staples AO, Jelacic S, Boster DR, et al. Risk factors for the hemolytic uremic syndrome in children infected with *Escherichia coli* O157:H7: a multivariable analysis. Clin Infect Dis. 2012 Jul;55(1):33–41.

FASCIOLIASIS

LeAnne M. Fox

INFECTIOUS AGENT

Trematode flatworms *Fasciola hepatica* and *F. gigantica*.

TRANSMISSION

Consumption of watercress or other aquatic plants contaminated with infective metacercariae or contaminated freshwater.

EPIDEMIOLOGY

Broadly distributed. The highest rates of *F. hepatica* infection have been reported from Bolivia, Peru, Egypt, Iran, Portugal, and France. *F. gigantica* has a more limited distribution (parts of Africa, the Middle East, and South and East Asia).

CLINICAL PRESENTATION

The acute phase begins 6–12 weeks after exposure and can last up to 4 months. Most infected people are asymptomatic, but symptoms might include marked eosinophilia, abdominal pain, intermittent high fever, weight loss, or urticaria. Within weeks to months, symptoms of the acute phase subside as worms enter the bile ducts, beginning the chronic phase. Chronically infected people in this phase may also be asymptomatic or may present with biliary colic, epigastric pain, nausea, jaundice, or pruritus. The long-term prognosis depends on the extent of the liver and biliary damage.

DIAGNOSIS

Detection of eggs in stool or duodenal or biliary aspirates. Serologic tests may be useful during the acute phase, since egg production does not start until 3–4 months after exposure. Radiologic examinations, including ultrasonogram and CT of the liver, can be helpful, especially during the hepatic or migratory acute phase.

TREATMENT

First-line treatment is with triclabendazole, which is not commercially available for human use in the United States, although it is available through CDC under an investigational protocol (404-718-4745; parasites@cdc.gov). An alternative drug is nitazoxanide. Surgical resection or endoscopic retrograde cholangiopancreatographic removal of adult flukes can be done in cases with biliary tract obstruction.

BIBLIOGRAPHY

1. Garcia HH, Moro PL, Schantz PM. Zoonotic helminth infections of humans: echinococcosis, cysticercosis and fascioliasis. Curr Opin Infect Dis. 2007 Oct;20(5):489–94.
2. Mas-Coma S, Bargues MD, Valero MA. Fascioliasis and other plant-borne trematode zoonoses. Int J Parasitol. 2005 Oct;35(11–12):1255–78.
3. Rowan SE, Levi ME, Youngwerth JM, Brauer B, Everson GT, Johnson SC. The variable presentations and broadening geographic distribution of hepatic fascioliasis. Clin Gastroenterol Hepatol. 2012 Jun;10(6):598–602.

PREVENTION
Avoid eating uncooked aquatic plants, including watercress, especially from endemic grazing areas; avoid drinking untreated freshwater.

CDC website: www.cdc.gov/parasites/fasciola

FILARIASIS, LYMPHATIC
LeAnne M. Fox

INFECTIOUS AGENT
Filarial nematodes *Wuchereria bancrofti*, *Brugia malayi*, and *B. timori*.

TRANSMISSION
Through the bite of infected *Aedes*, *Culex*, *Anopheles*, and *Mansonia* mosquitoes.

EPIDEMIOLOGY
Found in sub-Saharan Africa, Egypt, southern Asia, the western Pacific Islands, the northeastern coast of Brazil, Guyana, Haiti, and the Dominican Republic. Travelers are at low risk, although infection has been documented in long-term travelers. Most infections are seen in immigrants and refugees.

CLINICAL PRESENTATION
Most infections are asymptomatic, but lymphatic dysfunction may lead to lymphedema of the leg, scrotum, penis, arm, or breast years after infection. Acute episodes in people with lymphatic dysfunction are associated with painful swelling of an affected limb, fever, or chills due to bacterial superinfection. Tropical pulmonary eosinophilia is a potentially serious progressive lung disease that presents with nocturnal cough, wheezing, and fever, resulting from immune hyperresponsiveness to microfilariae in the pulmonary capillaries.

DIAGNOSIS
Microscopic detection of microfilariae on an appropriately timed thick blood film. Determination of serum antifilarial IgG is also a diagnostically useful test. This assay is available through the Parasitic Diseases Laboratory at the National Institutes of Health (301-496-5398) or through CDC (www.dpd.cdc.gov/dpdx; 404-718-4745; parasites@cdc.gov). Microfilariae are usually not detected in patients with tropical pulmonary eosinophilia. Diagnosis requires epidemiologic risk and filarial antibody testing.

TREATMENT
The drug of choice, diethylcarbamazine, can be obtained from CDC under an investigational new drug protocol. Patients with lymphedema and hydrocele can benefit from lymphedema management and, in the case of hydrocele, surgical repair.

PREVENTION

Mosquito precautions (see Chapter 2, Protection against Mosquitoes, Ticks, & Other Arthropods).

BIBLIOGRAPHY

1. Eberhard ML, Lammie PJ. Laboratory diagnosis of filariasis. Clin Lab Med. 1991 Dec;11(4):977–1010.
2. Lipner EM, Law MA, Barnett E, Keystone JS, von Sonnenburg F, Loutan L, et al. Filariasis in travelers presenting to the GeoSentinel Surveillance Network. PLoS Negl Trop Dis. 2007;1(3):e88.
3. Nutman TB, editor. Lymphatic Filariasis. London: Imperial College Press; 2000.

CDC website: www.cdc.gov/parasites/lymphaticfilariasis

GIARDIASIS

Julia Warner Gargano, Jonathan S. Yoder

INFECTIOUS AGENT

The anaerobic protozoan parasite *Giardia intestinalis* (formerly known as *G. lamblia* or *G. duodenalis*).

TRANSMISSION

By ingesting *Giardia* cysts in contaminated food or water, including water swallowed while swimming. Its low infectious dose, protracted communicability, and moderate chlorine tolerance make *Giardia* ideally suited for transmission through drinking and recreational water. Transmission also occurs through person-to-person contact, such as caring for an infected person, through sexual contact, through ingestion of food contaminated by ill food handlers or irrigated or washed with contaminated water, and by contact with fecally contaminated surfaces.

EPIDEMIOLOGY

Giardia is endemic worldwide. *Giardia* was the most commonly diagnosed pathogen in travelers seeking medical attention for a gastrointestinal infection at GeoSentinel surveillance clinics worldwide after returning from the Caribbean, Central and South America, Western Europe, North Africa, sub-Saharan Africa, the Middle East, South Asia, and East Asia and was the second most commonly diagnosed pathogen in travelers returning from Southeast Asia and Australasia. The risk of infection increases with duration of travel; backpackers or campers who drink untreated water from lakes or rivers are also more likely to be infected. *Giardia* infections are commonly identified in internationally adopted children, although many are asymptomatic.

CLINICAL PRESENTATION

Symptoms typically develop 1–2 weeks after infection and generally resolve within 2–4 weeks. Signs and symptoms include diarrhea (often with foul-smelling, greasy stools), abdominal cramps, bloating, flatulence, fatigue, anorexia, and nausea. Typically, a patient presents with the gradual onset of 2–5 loose stools per day and gradually increasing fatigue. Sometimes upper gastrointestinal symptoms are more prominent. Weight loss may occur over time. Fever and vomiting are uncommon. Reactive arthritis, irritable bowel, and other chronic symptoms sometimes occur after infection with *Giardia* (see Chapter 5, Persistent Travelers' Diarrhea).

DIAGNOSIS

Giardia cysts or trophozoites are not consistently seen in the stools of infected patients. Diagnostic yield can be increased by examining up to 3 stool samples over several days. Direct fluorescent antibody testing is extremely sensitive and specific. Other immunodiagnostic kits that do not require microscopy also detect *Giardia* antigens but do not take the place of ova and parasite examinations. Retesting is only recommended if symptoms persist after treatment.

TREATMENT

Tinidazole, metronidazole, and nitazoxanide are the drugs of choice; paromomycin is an alternative drug available in the United States. Because making a definitive diagnosis is difficult, empiric treatment can be used in patients with the appropriate history and typical symptoms.

PREVENTION

Food and water precautions (see Chapter 2, Food & Water Precautions and Water Disinfection for Travelers) and hand hygiene.

CDC website: www.cdc.gov/parasites/giardia

BIBLIOGRAPHY

1. Abramowicz M, editor. Drugs for Parasitic Infections. New Rochelle, NY: The Medical Letter, Inc.; 2013.
2. Cantey PT, Roy S, Lee B, Cronquist A, Smith K, Liang J, et al. Study of nonoutbreak giardiasis: novel findings and implications for research. Am J Med. 2011 Dec;124(12):1175 e1–8.
3. Greenwood Z, Black J, Weld L, O'Brien D, Leder K, Von Sonnenburg F, et al. Gastrointestinal infection among international travelers globally. J Travel Med. 2008 Jul–Aug;15(4):221–8.
4. Harvey K, Esposito DH, Han P, Kozarsky P, Freedman DO, Plier DA, et al. Surveillance for travel-related disease—GeoSentinel Surveillance System, United States, 1997–2011. MMWR Surveill Summ. 2013 Jul 19;62:1–23.
5. Okhuysen PC. Traveler's diarrhea due to intestinal protozoa. Clin Infect Dis. 2001 Jul 1;33(1):110–4.
6. Ross AG, Cripps AW. Enteropathogens and chronic illness in returning travelers. N Engl J Med. 2013 Aug 22;369(8):784.
7. Saiman L, Aronson J, Zhou J, Gomez-Duarte C, Gabriel PS, Alonso M, et al. Prevalence of infectious diseases among internationally adopted children. Pediatrics. 2001 Sep 3;108(3):608–12.
8. Staat MA, Rice M, Donauer S, Mukkada S, Holloway M, Cassedy A, et al. Intestinal parasite screening in internationally adopted children: importance of multiple stool specimens. Pediatrics. 2011 Sep;128(3):e613–22.
9. Swaminathan A, Torresi J, Schlagenhauf P, Thursky K, Wilder-Smith A, Connor BA, et al. A global study of pathogens and host risk factors associated with infectious gastrointestinal disease in returned international travellers. J Infect. 2009 Jul;59(1):19–27.
10. Wensaas KA, Langeland N, Hanevik K, Morch K, Eide GE, Rortveit G. Irritable bowel syndrome and chronic fatigue 3 years after acute giardiasis: historic cohort study. Gut. 2012 Feb;61(2):214–9.

HAND, FOOT, & MOUTH DISEASE

Ronnie Henry, John T. Watson

INFECTIOUS AGENT

In the United States, coxsackievirus A16 is most commonly detected, but other enteroviruses (such as coxsackievirus A10) can cause hand, foot, and mouth disease. Recently, coxsackievirus A6 has been detected in outbreaks. Internationally, enterovirus 71 is a common etiologic agent.

TRANSMISSION

Person-to-person, through contact with saliva, sputum, fluid in blisters, or stool of an infected person.

EPIDEMIOLOGY

A common illness in young children, with worldwide distribution. Recent large outbreaks have been reported in Cambodia, China, Japan, Korea, Malaysia, Singapore, Thailand, Taiwan, and Vietnam.

CLINICAL PRESENTATION

Incubation period is 4–6 days. Patients usually present with fever and malaise, followed by sore throat and the development of vesicles in the mouth and a rash, often vesicular, on the hands (palms) and feet (soles).

In some cases, the rash may be more wide-spread. Lesions usually resolve in 1 week, but rare complications can include aseptic meningitis and encephalitis.

DIAGNOSIS
Diagnosis is most often made clinically. Laboratory testing (such as PCR) is available and is usually performed on atypical or severe cases.

BIBLIOGRAPHY
1. Ooi MH, Wong SC, Lewthwaite P, Cardosa MJ, Solomon T. Clinical features, diagnosis, and management of enterovirus 71. Lancet Neurol. 2010 Nov;9(11):1097–105.
2. World Health Organization. A guide to clinical management and public health response for hand, foot and mouth disease (HFMD). Geneva: World Health Organization; 2011 [cited 2014 Sep 17]. Available from: http://www.wpro.who.int/publications/docs/GuidancefortheclinicalmanagementofHFMD.pdf.

TREATMENT
Supportive care.

PREVENTION
Avoiding close contact with infected people, maintaining good hand hygiene, and disinfecting potentially contaminated surfaces, including toys.

CDC website: www.cdc.gov/hand-foot-mouth

HELICOBACTER PYLORI
Ronnie Henry

INFECTIOUS AGENT
Helicobacter pylori is a small, curved, microaerophilic, gram-negative, rod-shaped bacterium.

TRANSMISSION
Believed to be fecal-oral or possibly oral-oral.

EPIDEMIOLOGY
Common worldwide. Estimated prevalence is 70% in developing countries and 30%–40% in the United States and other industrialized countries.

CLINICAL PRESENTATION
Usually asymptomatic, but *H. pylori* is the major cause of peptic ulcer disease and gastritis, which presents as gnawing or burning epigastric pain. Less commonly, symptoms include nausea, vomiting, loss of appetite, or bleeding.

DIAGNOSIS
Fecal antigen assay, urea breath test, rapid urease test, or histology of biopsy specimen. A positive serology indicates present or past infection.

TREATMENT
Treatment should be determined on an individual basis. Clarithromycin triple therapy (proton pump inhibitor [PPI] + clarithromycin + amoxicillin or metronidazole) or bismuth quadruple therapy (PPI or H_2-blocker + bismuth + metronidazole + tetracycline). See www.acg.gi.org/physicians/guidelines/ManagementofHpylori.pdf.

PREVENTION
No specific recommendations.

BIBLIOGRAPHY
1. Chey WD, Wong BC. American College of Gastroenterology guideline on the management of *Helicobacter pylori* infection. Am J Gastroenterol. 2007 Aug;102(8):1808–25.
2. Lindkvist P, Wadstrom T, Giesecke J. *Helicobacter pylori* infection and foreign travel. J Infect Dis. 1995 Oct;172(4):1135–6.

3. Peterson WL, Fendrick AM, Cave DR, Peura DA, Garabedian-Ruffalo SM, Laine L. *Helicobacter pylori*-related disease: guidelines for testing and treatment. Arch Intern Med. 2000 May 8;160(9):1285–91.

HELMINTHS, SOIL-TRANSMITTED

Christine Dubray

INFECTIOUS AGENTS

Ascaris lumbricoides (roundworm), *Ancylostoma duodenale* (hookworm), *Necator americanus* (hookworm), and *Trichuris trichiura* (whipworm) are helminths (parasitic worms) that infect the intestine and are transmitted via contaminated soil.

TRANSMISSION

Eggs are passed in feces from an infected person. Infection with roundworm and whipworm occurs when eggs in soil have become infective and are ingested. Hookworm infection (see the Cutaneous Larva Migrans section earlier in this chapter) usually occurs when larvae penetrate the skin of people walking barefoot on contaminated soil. One kind of hookworm (*Ancylostoma duodenale*) can also be transmitted when larvae are ingested.

EPIDEMIOLOGY

A large part of the world's population is infected with 1 or more of these helminths, but the prevalence is highest in tropical and subtropical countries where water supplies and sanitation are poor. Travelers to these countries should be at low risk of infection if prevention measures are taken. Since these worms do not multiply in hosts, reinfection occurs only as a result of multiple contacts with the infective stages.

CLINICAL PRESENTATION

Most infections are asymptomatic, especially when few worms are present. Pulmonary symptoms occur in a small percentage of patients when roundworm larvae pass through the lungs. Roundworm can also cause intestinal discomfort, obstruction, and impaired nutritional status. Hookworm infection can lead to anemia due to blood loss and chronic protein deficiency. Whipworm infection can cause chronic abdominal pain, diarrhea, blood loss, dysentery, and rectal prolapse. However, travelers are rarely at risk because these more severe manifestations are generally associated with high worm burdens seen in indigenous populations.

DIAGNOSIS

The standard method for diagnosing soil-transmitted helminths is by identifying eggs in a stool specimen using a microscope.

TREATMENT

The drugs most commonly used are albendazole and mebendazole.

PREVENTION

Food and water precautions (see Chapter 2, Food & Water Precautions). To avoid hookworm infection, travelers should not walk barefoot in areas where hookworm is common and where there may be human fecal contamination of the soil. In general, avoid ingesting soil that may be contaminated with human feces, including where human fecal matter or wastewater is used to fertilize crops.

CDC website: www.cdc.gov/parasites/sth

BIBLIOGRAPHY

1. Bethony J, Brooker S, Albonico M, Geiger SM, Loukas A, Diemert D, et al. Soil-transmitted helminth infections: ascariasis, trichuriasis, and hookworm. Lancet. 2006 May 6;367(9521):1521–32.

2. Brooker S, Bundy DAP. Soil-transmitted helminths (geohelminths). In: Cook GC, Zumla A, editors. Manson's Tropical Diseases. 22nd ed. London: Saunders; 2009. p 1515–48.

3. Brooker S, Clements AC, Bundy DA. Global epidemiology, ecology and control of soil-transmitted helminth infections. Adv Parasitol. 2006;62:221–61.

HEPATITIS A

Noele P. Nelson, Trudy V. Murphy

INFECTIOUS AGENT

Hepatitis A virus (HAV) is a nonenveloped RNA virus classified as a picornavirus. HAV can survive in the environment for prolonged periods at low pH and in freezing to moderate temperatures.

TRANSMISSION

Through direct person-to-person contact (fecal-oral transmission); contaminated water, ice, or shellfish harvested from sewage-contaminated water; or from contaminated raw, inadequately cooked, or frozen fruits, vegetables, or other foods. HAV is shed in the feces of infected people. People are most infectious 1–2 weeks before the onset of clinical signs and symptoms (jaundice or elevation of liver enzymes), when the concentration of virus is highest in the stool and serum. Viral excretion and the risk of transmission diminish rapidly after liver dysfunction or symptoms appear, which is concurrent with the appearance of circulating antibodies to HAV. Infants and children can shed virus for up to 6 months after infection.

EPIDEMIOLOGY

HAV is common in areas with inadequate sanitation and limited access to clean water. In highly endemic areas (such as parts of Africa and Asia), a large proportion of adults in the population are immune to HAV, and epidemics of hepatitis A are uncommon. In intermediately endemic areas (such as Central and South America, Eastern Europe, and parts of Asia), childhood transmission is less frequent, more adolescents and adults are susceptible to infection, and outbreaks are common. In less endemic areas (such as the United States and Western Europe), infection is less common, but disease occurs among people in high-risk groups and as communitywide outbreaks.

Hepatitis A is among the most common vaccine-preventable infections acquired during travel. In the United States the most frequently identified risk factor for hepatitis A is international travel. Cases of travel-related hepatitis A can occur in travelers to developing countries with "standard" tourist itineraries, accommodations, and eating behaviors. Risk is highest for those who live in or visit rural areas, trek in backcountry areas, or frequently eat or drink in settings of poor sanitation.

CLINICAL PRESENTATION

The incubation period averages 28 days (range, 15–50 days). Infection can be asymptomatic or range in severity from a mild illness lasting 1–2 weeks to a severely disabling disease lasting several months. Clinical manifestations include the abrupt onset of fever, malaise, anorexia, nausea, and abdominal discomfort, followed within a few days by jaundice. The likelihood of having symptoms with HAV infection is related to the age of the infected person. In children aged <6 years, most (70%) infections are asymptomatic; jaundice is uncommon in symptomatic young children. Among older children and adults, the illness usually lasts <2 months, although approximately 10%–15% of infected people have prolonged or relapsing symptoms over a 6- to 9-month period. Severe hepatic and extrahepatic complications, including fulminant hepatitis and liver failure, are rare but more common in older adults and people with underlying liver disease. Chronic infection does not occur. The overall case-fatality ratio is 0.3%; however, the ratio is 1.8% among adults aged >50 years.

DIAGNOSIS

HAV cannot be differentiated from other types of viral hepatitis on the basis of clinical or epidemiologic features. Diagnosis requires a positive test for antibody to HAV (anti-HAV) IgM in serum, detectable from 2 weeks before the onset of symptoms to approximately 6 months afterward.

Serologic tests for total anti-HAV (IgG and IgM) are available commercially. A positive total anti-HAV result and a negative IgM anti-HAV result indicate past infection or vaccination and immunity. The presence of serum IgM anti-HAV usually indicates current or recent infection and does not distinguish between immunity from infection and vaccination.

TREATMENT

Supportive care.

PREVENTION

Vaccination or immune globulin (IG), food and water precautions, maintaining standards of hygiene and sanitation.

Vaccine

Two monovalent hepatitis A vaccines, Vaqta (Merck & Co, Inc, Whitehouse Station, NJ) and Havrix (GlaxoSmithKline Beecham Biologicals, Rixensart, Belgium), are approved for people ≥12 months of age in a 2-dose series, and a combined hepatitis A and hepatitis B (Twinrix, GlaxoSmithKline) vaccine is approved for people ≥18 years of age in the United States (Table 3-2). The immunogenicity of the combination vaccine is equivalent to that of the monovalent hepatitis A and hepatitis B vaccines when tested after completion of the recommended schedule.

Indications for Use

All susceptible people traveling for any purpose, frequency, or duration to countries with high or intermediate HAV endemicity should be vaccinated or receive IG before departure. Although the Advisory Committee for Immunization Practices recommends hepatitis A vaccination for

travelers, published maps may not be the best guide for determining endemicity in developing countries. Prevalence patterns of HAV infection vary among regions within a country, and missing or obsolete data present a challenge. Countries where the prevalence of HAV infection is decreasing have growing numbers of susceptible people and risk for large outbreaks of hepatitis A. In recent years, large outbreaks of hepatitis A were reported in developed countries among people who had been exposed to imported food contaminated with HAV. Recognized exposures to hepatitis A through infection in food handlers have also increased. Taking into account the complexity of interpreting hepatitis A risk maps and potential risk of foodborne hepatitis A in countries with low endemicity, some experts advise people traveling outside the United States to consider hepatitis A vaccination regardless of their destination.

Vaccination is recommended for unvaccinated household members and other people who anticipate close personal contact (such as household contacts or regular babysitters) with an international adoptee from a country of high or intermediate endemicity during the 60 days after arrival of the child in the United States. The first dose of the 2-dose hepatitis A vaccine series should be administered as soon as adoption is planned, ideally ≥2 weeks before the arrival of the child (see Chapter 7, International Adoption).

Vaccine Administration

One dose of a monovalent hepatitis A vaccine protects most healthy people aged 1–40 years and should be administered as soon as travel is considered. The monovalent vaccine series should be completed according to the licensed schedule for long-term protection. No data on single-dose hepatitis A vaccine efficacy are available for Twinrix. An alternate, accelerated 4-dose schedule is available for Twinrix; doses can be administered at 0, 7, and 21–30 days, followed by a dose at 12 months.

Hepatitis A vaccine at the age-appropriate dose is preferred to IG for children and adults aged 1–40 years. For optimal protection, adults aged >40 years, immunocompromised people, and people with chronic liver disease or other chronic

Table 3-2. Vaccines to prevent hepatitis A

VACCINE	TRADE NAME (MANUFACTURER)	AGE (Y)	DOSE	ROUTE	SCHEDULE	BOOSTER
Hepatitis A vaccine, inactivated	Havrix (GlaxoSmithKline)	1–18	0.5 mL (720 ELU)	IM	0, 6–12 mo	None
		≥19	1.0 mL (1,440 ELU)	IM	0, 6–12 mo	None
Hepatitis A vaccine, inactivated	Vaqta (Merck & Co., Inc.)	1–18	0.5 mL (25 U)	IM	0, 6–18 mo	None
		≥19	1.0 mL (50 U)	IM	0, 6–18 mo	None
Combined hepatitis A and B vaccine	Twinrix (GlaxoSmithKline)	≥18 (primary)	1.0 mL (720 ELU HAV + 20 μg HBsAg)	IM	0, 1, 6 mo	None
		≥18 (accelerated)	same as above	IM	0, 7, 21–30 d	12 mo

Abbreviations: ELU, ELISA units of inactivated HAV; IM, intramuscular; U, units HAV antigen; HAV, hepatitis A virus; HBsAg, hepatitis B surface antigen.

3

medical conditions planning to depart to an area in <2 weeks should receive the initial dose of vaccine along with IG (0.02 mL/kg) at a separate injection site.

Travelers who are aged <12 months, are allergic to a vaccine component, or who otherwise elect not to receive vaccine should receive a single dose of IG (0.02 mL/kg), which provides effective protection against HAV infection for up to 3 months. Those who do not receive vaccination and plan to travel for >3 months should receive an IG dose of 0.06 mL/kg, which must be repeated if the duration of travel is >5 months. IG can be repeated every 6 months thereafter if the traveler remains in a high-risk setting, though hepatitis A vaccination should be encouraged if not contraindicated.

Although vaccinating an immune traveler is not contraindicated and does not increase the risk for adverse effects, screening for total anti-HAV before travel can be useful in some circumstances to determine susceptibility and eliminate unnecessary vaccination. Postvaccination testing for serologic response is not indicated.

Other Vaccine Considerations

Using vaccine according to the licensed schedule is preferable. An interrupted series does not need to be restarted. More than 95% of vaccinated people develop levels of anti-HAV that correlate with protection 1 month after the first dose. Given their similar immunogenicity, a series that has been started with one brand of hepatitis A monovalent vaccine may be completed with the other brand of monovalent vaccine. For children and adults who complete the primary series, booster doses of vaccine are not recommended.

Vaccine Safety and Adverse Reactions

Among adults, the most frequently reported side effects after hepatitis A vaccination are tenderness or pain at the injection site (56%–67%) and headache (14%–16%). Among children (11–25 months of age), the most common reported side effects are pain or tenderness at the injection site (32%–37%) and redness (21%–29%). No serious adverse events in children or adults have been reported that could be attributed definitively to the vaccine; no increase in serious adverse events has been identified among vaccinated people compared with baseline rates.

Precautions and Contraindications

Hepatitis A–containing vaccines should not be administered to travelers with a history of hypersensitivity to any vaccine component, including neomycin. Twinrix should not be administered to people with a history of hypersensitivity to yeast. The tip caps of prefilled syringes of Havrix and Twinrix and the vial stopper, syringe plunger stopper, and tip caps of Vaqta may contain dry natural rubber, which may cause allergic reactions in latex-sensitive people. Because hepatitis A vaccine consists of inactivated virus and hepatitis B vaccine consists of a recombinant protein, no special precautions are needed for vaccination of immunocompromised travelers. Providers should check precautions and contraindications before administering IG.

Pregnancy

The safety of hepatitis A vaccine for pregnant women has not been determined. However, because hepatitis A vaccine is produced from inactivated HAV, the theoretical risk to either the pregnant woman or the developing fetus is thought to be low. The risk of vaccination should be weighed against the risk of hepatitis A among female travelers who might be at high risk for exposure to HAV.

Postexposure Prophylaxis

Travelers who are exposed to HAV and who have not received hepatitis A vaccine previously should be administered 1 dose of monovalent hepatitis A vaccine or IG (0.02 mL/kg) as soon as possible, ideally within 2 weeks of exposure. The efficacy of IG or vaccine when administered >2 weeks after exposure has not been established. The relative efficacy of vaccine is comparable to IG for postexposure prophylaxis among people aged 1–40 years.

For healthy people aged 1–40 years, a dose of monovalent hepatitis A vaccine is recommended. For people aged >40 years, IG is preferred, but vaccine can be used if IG is unavailable. IG is recommended for people aged <12 months, people who are immunocompromised, people who have chronic liver disease, and people for whom vaccine is contraindicated. Twinrix is not approved for postexposure prophylaxis. More detailed information can be found in the Advisory Committee on Immunization Practices recommendations at www.cdc. gov/mmwr/preview/mmwrhtml/ mm5641a3.htm.

CDC website: www.cdc.gov/hepatitis/HAV

BIBLIOGRAPHY

1. Bacaner N, Stauffer B, Boulware DR, Walker PF, Keystone JS. Travel medicine considerations for North American immigrants visiting friends and relatives. JAMA. 2004 Jun 16;291(23):2856–64.
2. CDC. Update: Prevention of hepatitis A after exposure to hepatitis A virus and in international travelers. Updated recommendations of the Advisory Committee on Immunization Practices (ACIP). MMWR Morb Mortal Wkly Rep. 2007 Oct 19;56(41):1080–4.
3. CDC. Updated recommendations from the Advisory Committee on Immunization Practices (ACIP) for use of hepatitis A vaccine in close contacts of newly arriving international adoptees. MMWR Morb Mortal Wkly Rep. 2009 Sep 18;58(36):1006–7.
4. CDC. Viral hepatitis surveillance: United States, 2011. Atlanta: CDC; 2011 [cited 2014 Sep 17]. Available from: http://www.cdc. gov/hepatitis/Statistics/2011Surveillance/ PDFs/2011HepSurveillanceRpt.pdf.
5. Fiore AE, Wasley A, Bell BP. Prevention of hepatitis A through active or passive immunization: recommendations of the Advisory Committee on Immunization Practices (ACIP). MMWR Recomm Rep. 2006 May 19;55(RR-7):1–23.
6. Klevens RM, Miller JT, Iqbal K, Thomas A, Rizzo EM, Hanson H, et al. The evolving epidemiology of hepatitis A in the United States: incidence and molecular epidemiology from population-based surveillance, 2005–2007. Arch Intern Med. 2010 Nov 8;170(20):1811–8.
7. Mohd Hanafiah K, Jacobsen KH, Wiersma ST. Challenges to mapping the health risk of hepatitis A virus infection. Int J Health Geogr. 2011;10:57.
8. Murphy TV, Feinstone SM, Bell BP. Hepatitis A vaccines. In: Plotkin SA, Orenstein WA, Offit PA, editors. Vaccines. 6th ed. Philadelphia: Saunders Elsevier; 2012. p. 183–204.
9. Mutsch M, Spicher VM, Gut C, Steffen R. Hepatitis A virus infections in travelers, 1988–2004. Clin Infect Dis. 2006 Feb 15;42(4):490–7.
10. Nelson NP, Murphy TV. Hepatitis A: the changing epidemiology of hepatitis A. Clin Liver Dis. 2013 Dec 20;2(6):227–30.

HEPATITIS B

Francisco Averhoff

INFECTIOUS AGENT

Hepatitis B is a disease caused by hepatitis B virus (HBV), a small, circular, partially double-stranded DNA virus in the Hepadnaviridae family.

TRANSMISSION

HBV is transmitted by contact with contaminated blood, blood products, and other body fluids (such as semen). Examples of exposures that travelers may encounter that are associated with transmission include poor infection control during medical or dental procedures, receipt of blood products, injection drug use, tattooing or acupuncture, and unprotected sex.

EPIDEMIOLOGY

An estimated 240 million people have chronic HBV infection globally. Map 3-4 shows the estimated prevalence of chronic HBV infection by country. No data are available to show the specific risk to travelers; however, published reports of travelers acquiring hepatitis B are rare, and the risk for travelers who do not have high-risk behaviors or exposures is low. The risk for HBV infection may be higher in countries where the prevalence of chronic HBV infection is high or intermediate; expatriates, missionaries, and long-term development workers may be at increased risk for HBV infection in such countries. All travelers should be aware of

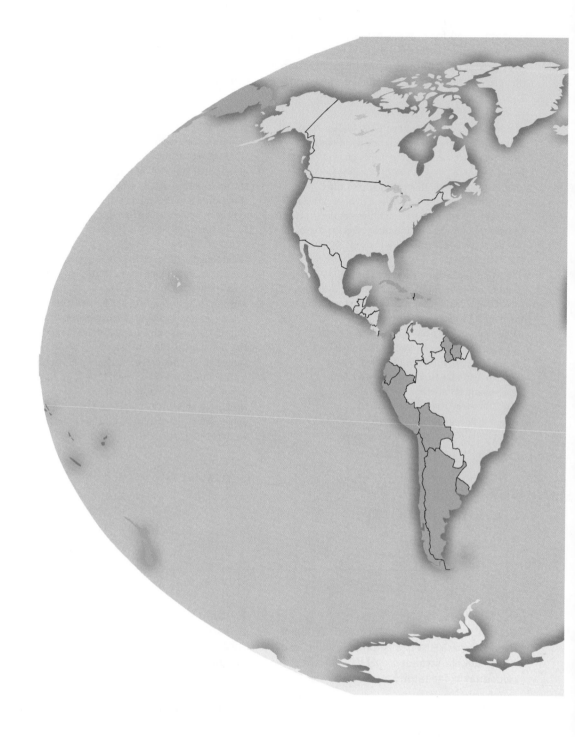

MAP 3-4. PREVALENCE OF CHRONIC HEPATITIS B VIRUS INFECTION AMONG ADULTS

Disease data source: Ott JJ, Stevens GA, Groeger J, Wiersma ST. Global epidemiology of hepatitis B virus infection: new estimates of age-specific HBsAg seroprevalence and endemicity. Vaccine. 2012; 30(12):2212–2219.

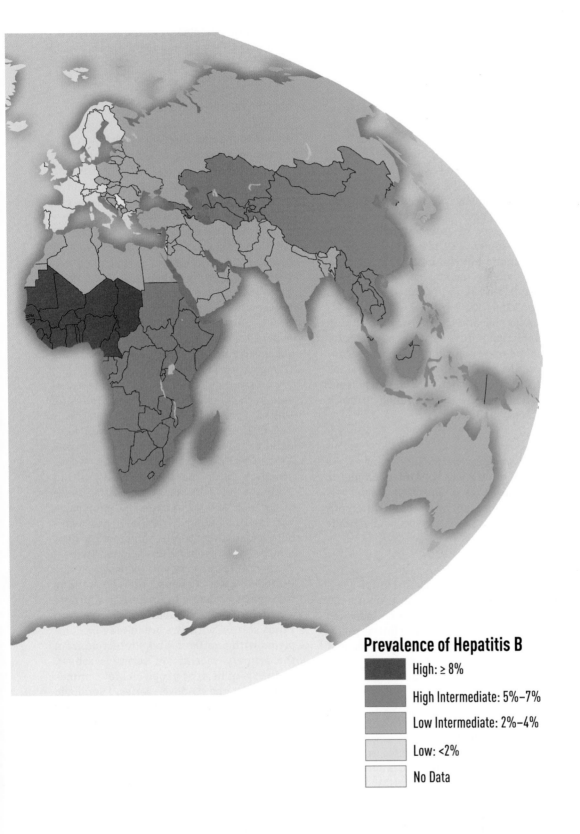

Prevalence of Hepatitis B

- High: ≥ 8%
- High Intermediate: 5%–7%
- Low Intermediate: 2%–4%
- Low: <2%
- No Data

how HBV is transmitted and take measures to minimize their exposures.

CLINICAL PRESENTATION
HBV infection primarily affects the liver. Typically, the incubation period for hepatitis B is 90 days (range, 60–150 days). The typical signs and symptoms include malaise, fatigue, anorexia, nausea, vomiting, abdominal pain, and jaundice. In some cases skin rashes, joint pain, and arthritis may occur. Among people aged ≥5 years, 30%–50% will develop signs and symptoms. In children aged <5 years and immunocompromised adults, HBV infection is typically asymptomatic but can be asymptomatic at any age among healthy people. The overall case-fatality ratio of acute hepatitis B is approximately 1%.

Acute hepatitis B progresses to chronic HBV infection in 30%–90% of people infected as infants or young children and in <5% of people infected during adolescence or adulthood. Chronic infection with HBV may result in chronic liver disease, including cirrhosis, liver cancer, and death.

DIAGNOSIS
Serologic markers specific for hepatitis B are necessary to diagnose HBV infection and to identify the stage of infection (Table 3-3). These markers can be used to differentiate between acute, resolving, and chronic infection.

TREATMENT
No specific treatment is available for acute hepatitis B; however, supportive treatment, including hospitalization, may be indicated for some people with severe clinical manifestations. Antiviral drugs are approved and available to treat chronic hepatitis B.

PREVENTION
Vaccine
Indications for Use
Hepatitis B vaccination should be administered to all unvaccinated people traveling to areas with intermediate to high prevalence of chronic hepatitis B (HBV surface antigen prevalence ≥2%). Complete vaccination information and recommendations for the United States are available at www.cdc.gov/vaccines/vpd-vac/hepb/

default.htm. Vaccination to prevent hepatitis B may be considered for all international travelers, regardless of destination, depending on the traveler's behavioral risk.

Vaccine Administration
Hepatitis B vaccine (see Table 3-4) is usually administered as a 3-dose series on a 0-, 1-, 6-month schedule to achieve immunity. The second dose should be given ≥1 month after the first dose; the third dose should be given ≥2 months after the second dose and ≥4 months after the first dose. The third dose should not be administered before age 24 weeks. Administration of 4 doses of hepatitis B vaccine is permitted when a combination vaccine containing hepatitis B is administered after the birth dose. Postexposure prophylaxis with hepatitis B immune globulin (HBIG) administered in conjunction with hepatitis B vaccine, as well as hepatitis B vaccine alone, are effective in preventing transmission after exposure to HBV.

Exceptions to this schedule are available with specific licensed products in the United States; Recombivax HB (Merck & Co.) is licensed for a 2-dose schedule for children aged 11–15 years, and Engerix-B (GlaxoSmithKline) is licensed for a 4-dose schedule, with the first 3 doses within 2 months and a booster at 12 months (doses at 0, 1, 2, and 12 months). Combination vaccines including hepatitis B are available for children, and a combination hepatitis A and hepatitis B vaccine, Twinrix (GlaxoSmithKline), is also licensed in the United States. Consult the prescribing information when administering alternate schedules and formulations. Vaccination series started with one brand may be completed with another brand. Protection from the primary vaccination series is robust, and >95% of healthy people achieve immunity with the 3-dose series. Serologic testing and booster vaccination are not recommended before travel for immunocompetent adults who have been previously vaccinated.

Special Situations
Ideally, hepatitis B vaccination should begin ≥6 months before travel so the full vaccine series can be completed before departure. Because some protection is provided by 1 or

Table 3-3. Interpretation of serologic test results for hepatitis B virus infection[1]

SEROLOGIC MARKER				INTERPRETATION
HBSAG[2]	TOTAL ANTI-HBC	IGM ANTI-HBC	ANTI-HBS	
–	–	–	–	Never infected
+	–	–	–	Early acute infection; transient (up to 18 days) after vaccination
+	+	+	–	Acute infection
–	+	+	+ or –	Acute resolving infection
–	+	–	+	Recovered from past infection and immune
+	+	–	–	Chronic infection
–	+	–	–	False-positive (susceptible); past infection; occult infection;[3] or passive transfer of anti-HBc to infant born to HBsAg-positive mother
–	–	–	+	Immune if concentration is ≥10 mIU/mL after vaccine series completion; passive transfer after hepatitis B immune globulin administration

Abbreviations: HBsAg, hepatitis B surface antigen; anti-HBc, antibody to hepatitis B core antigen; anti-HBs, antibody to hepatitis B surface antigen.

[1] From: CDC. A comprehensive immunization strategy to eliminate transmission of hepatitis B virus infection in the United States: recommendations of the Advisory Committee on Immunization Practices (ACIP). Part II: immunization of adults. MMWR Recomm Rep. 2006 Dec 8;55(RR-16):1–33.

[2] To ensure that an HBsAg-positive test result is not a false positive, samples with reactive HBsAg results should be tested with a licensed neutralizing confirmatory test, if recommended in the manufacturer's package insert.

[3] People positive only for anti-HBc are unlikely to be infectious except under unusual circumstances in which they are the source for direct percutaneous exposure of susceptible recipients to large quantities of virus (such as blood transfusion or organ transplant).

2 doses, the vaccine series should be initiated, if indicated, even if it cannot be completed before departure. Optimal protection, however, is not conferred until after the final vaccine dose is received, and travelers should be advised to complete the vaccine series. An approved accelerated vaccination schedule can be used for people traveling on short notice who face imminent exposure or for emergency responders to disaster areas. The accelerated vaccination schedule calls for vaccine doses administered at days 0, 7, and 21–30; a booster should be administered at 12 months to promote long-term immunity. A combined hepatitis A and hepatitis B vaccine can also be used on the same 3-dose

Table 3-4. Vaccines to prevent hepatitis B

VACCINE	TRADE NAME (MANUFACTURER)	AGE (Y)	DOSE	ROUTE	SCHEDULE	BOOSTER
Hepatitis B vaccine, recom-binant[1]	Engerix-B (GlaxoSmithKline)	0–19 (primary)	0.5 mL (10 µg HBsAg)	IM	0, 1, 6 mo	None
		0–10 (accelerated)	0.5 mL (10 µg HBsAg)	IM	0, 1, 2 mo	12 mo
		11–19 (accelerated)	1.0 mL (20 µg HBsAg)	IM	0, 1, 2 mo	12 mo
		≥20 (primary)	1.0 mL (20 µg HBsAg)	IM	0, 1, 6 mo	None
		≥20 (accelerated)	1.0 mL (20 µg HBsAg)	IM	0, 1, 2 mo	12 mo
Hepatitis B vaccine, recom-binant[1]	Recombivax HB (Merck & Co., Inc.)	0–19 (primary)	0.5 mL (5 µg HBsAg)	IM	0, 1, 6 mo	None
		11–15 (adolescent accelerated)	1.0 mL (10 µg HBsAg)	IM	0, 4–6 mo	None
		≥20 (primary)	1.0 mL (10 µg HBsAg)	IM	0, 1, 6 mo	None
Combined hepatitis A and B vaccine	Twinrix (GlaxoSmithKline)	≥18 (primary)	1.0 mL (720 ELU HAV + 20 µg HBsAg)	IM	0, 1, 6 mo	None
		≥18 (accelerated)	same as above	IM	0, 7, 21–30 d	12 mo

Abbreviations: HBsAg, hepatitis B surface antigen; IM, intramuscular; ELU, ELISA units of inactivated HAV; HAV, hepatitis A virus.
[1] Consult the package insert for differences in dosing for hemodialysis and other immunocompromised patients.

schedule (0, 7, and 21–30 days), with a booster at 12 months.

Vaccine Safety and Adverse Reactions
Hepatitis B vaccines are safe for people of all ages. Pain at the injection site (3%–29%) and fever (temperature >99.9°F [37.7°C]; 1%–6%) are the most frequently reported side effects among vaccine recipients. Hepatitis B vaccines should not be administered to people with a history of hypersensitivity to any vaccine component, including yeast. The vaccine contains a recombinant protein (hepatitis B surface antigen) that is noninfectious.

Limited data indicate no apparent risk of adverse events to the mother or the developing fetus when hepatitis B vaccine is administered to pregnant women. HBV infection affecting a pregnant woman can result in serious disease for the mother and chronic infection for the newborn. Neither pregnancy nor lactation should be considered a contraindication for vaccination.

Personal Protection Measures
As part of the pre-travel education process, all travelers should be counseled and given information about the risks for hepatitis B and other bloodborne pathogens from contaminated equipment or items used during medical, dental, or cosmetic procedures; blood products; injection drug use; any activities or procedures that involve piercing the skin or mucosa; or unprotected sexual activity, and should be informed about prevention measures. When seeking medical or dental care or cosmetic procedures (such as tattooing or piercing), travelers should be alert to the use of equipment that has not been adequately sterilized or disinfected, reuse

of contaminated equipment, and unsafe injecting practices (such as reuse of disposable needles and syringes). HBV and other bloodborne pathogens can be transmitted if tools are not sterile or if personnel do not follow proper infection control procedures. Travelers should consider the health risks when receiving medical or dental care overseas; information may be available from the US embassy. The health risks should be strongly considered when deciding to obtain a tattoo or body piercing in areas where adequate sterilization or disinfection procedures might not be available or practiced.

CDC website: www.cdc.gov/hepatitis/HBV

BIBLIOGRAPHY

1. CDC. A comprehensive immunization strategy to eliminate transmission of hepatitis B virus infection in the United States: recommendations of the Advisory Committee on Immunization Practices (ACIP) Part 1: immunization of infants, children, and adolescents. MMWR Recomm Rep. 2005 Dec 23;54(RR-16):1–31.

2. CDC. A comprehensive immunization strategy to eliminate transmission of hepatitis B virus infection in the United States: recommendations of the Advisory Committee on Immunization Practices (ACIP) Part II: immunization of adults. MMWR Recomm Rep. 2006 Dec 8;55(RR-16):1–33.

3. CDC. Updated US Public Health Service guidelines for the management of occupational exposures to HBV, HCV, and HIV and recommendations for postexposure prophylaxis. MMWR Recomm Rep. 2001 Jun 29;50(RR-11):1–42.

4. Lok AS, McMahon BJ. Chronic hepatitis B: update of recommendations. Hepatology. 2004 Mar;39(3):857–61.

5. Mariano A, Mele A, Tosti ME, Parlato A, Gallo G, Ragni P, et al. Role of beauty treatment in the spread of parenterally transmitted hepatitis viruses in Italy. J Med Virol. 2004 Oct;74(2):216–20.

6. Mast EE, Ward JW. Hepatitis B vaccine. In: Plotkin S, Orenstein W, Offit P, editors. Vaccines. 5th ed. Philadelphia: Elsevier; 2008. p. 205–42.

7. Ott JJ, Stevens GA, Groeger J, Wiersma ST. Global epidemiology of hepatitis B virus infection: new estimates of age-specific HBsAg seroprevalence and endemicity. Vaccine. 2012 Mar 9;30(12):2212–9.

8. Sagliocca L, Stroffolini T, Amoroso P, Manzillo G, Ferrigno L, Converti F, et al. Risk factors for acute hepatitis B: a case-control study. J Viral Hepat. 1997 Jan;4(1):63–6.

9. Simonsen L, Kane A, Lloyd J, Zaffran M, Kane M. Unsafe injections in the developing world and transmission of bloodborne pathogens: a review. Bull World Health Organ. 1999;77(10):789–800.

HEPATITIS C

Deborah Holtzman

INFECTIOUS AGENT

Hepatitis C virus (HCV), a spherical, enveloped, positive-strand RNA virus.

TRANSMISSION

Transmission of HCV is bloodborne and most often involves exposure to contaminated needles or syringes or receipt of blood or blood products that have not been screened for HCV. Although infrequent, HCV can be transmitted through other procedures that involve blood exposure, such as tattooing, during sexual contact, or perinatally from mother to child.

EPIDEMIOLOGY

Globally, an estimated 170 million people are living with HCV infection (chronically infected), and almost 500,000 were estimated to have died from HCV-related liver disease in 2010. Although the quality of epidemiologic data varies widely across countries and regions, the most recent global estimates indicate that the prevalence of HCV infection is <2% in many developed countries, including the United States (Map 3-5). The prevalence is higher (≥2%) in several countries in Latin America, Eastern Europe and the former Soviet Union, and certain countries in Africa,

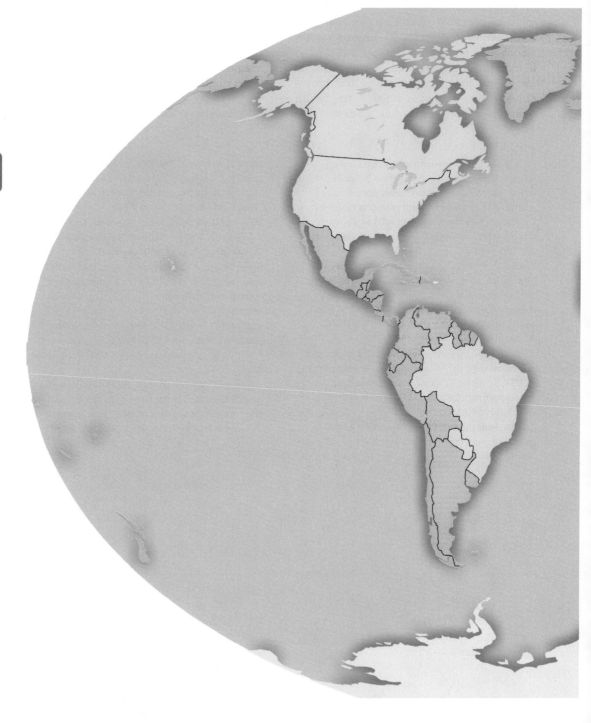

MAP 3-5. GLOBAL EPIDEMIOLOGY OF HEPATITIS C VIRUS INFECTION[1]

[1] Disease data source: Mohd Hanafiah K, Groeger J, Flaxman AD, Wiersma ST. Global Epidemiology of Hepatitis C Virus Infection; New Estimates of Age-Specific Antibody to HCV and Seroprevalence. Hepatology. 2013; 57:1333–1342.

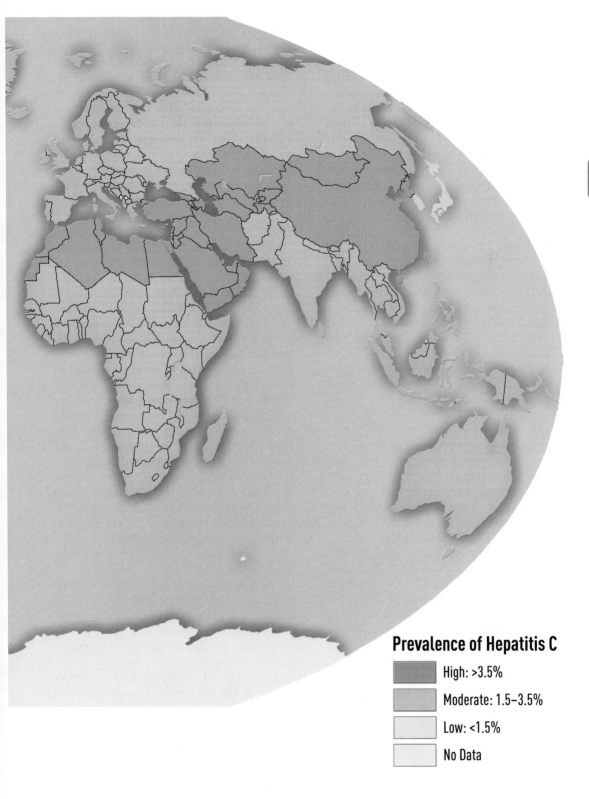

Prevalence of Hepatitis C

- High: >3.5%
- Moderate: 1.5–3.5%
- Low: <1.5%
- No Data

the Middle East, and South Asia; the prevalence is reported to be highest (approximately 10%) in Egypt. The most frequent mode of transmission in the United States and most developed countries is through sharing drug-injection equipment. In countries where HCV is more common (≥2% prevalence), the predominant mode of transmission is from unsafe injections and other health care exposures where infection control practices are poor. Travelers' risk for contracting HCV infection is generally low, but they should exercise caution, as the following activities can result in blood exposure:

- Receiving blood transfusions that have not been screened for HCV
- Having medical or dental procedures
- Activities such as acupuncture, tattooing, being shaved, or injection drug use in which equipment has not been adequately sterilized or disinfected or in which contaminated equipment is reused
- Working in health care fields (medical, dental, or laboratory) that entail direct exposure to human blood

CLINICAL PRESENTATION

Most people (80%) with acute HCV infection have no symptoms. If symptoms occur, they may include loss of appetite, abdominal pain, fatigue, nausea, dark urine, and jaundice. Of those who develop chronic HCV infection, the most common symptom is fatigue. Severe liver disease develops in approximately 10%–20% of chronically infected people, but progression to end-stage liver disease is slow and typically does not occur until ≥20 years after infection. This progression is often clinically silent until late in the course of disease, and in the absence of HCV testing, most people are unaware of their infection. Nonetheless, HCV is a major cause of cirrhosis and hepatocellular cancer and is the leading reason for liver transplantation in the United States.

DIAGNOSIS

Two major types of tests are available: IgG assays for HCV antibodies and nucleic acid amplification testing to detect HCV RNA in blood (viremia). Assays for IgM, to detect early or acute infection, are not available. Approximately 75%–85% of people who seroconvert to anti-HCV, indicative of acute infection, will progress to chronic infection and persistently detectable viremia. Because a positive HCV antibody test cannot discriminate between someone who was previously infected but resolved or cleared the infection and someone with current infection, it is essential that HCV RNA testing follow a positive HCV antibody test to assess current (chronic) HCV infection. False-negative antibody test results, while rare, may occur early in acute infection, usually in the first 15 weeks after exposure and infection.

TREATMENT

Treatment for hepatitis C has evolved dramatically since the approval of 2 protease inhibitors (boceprevir and telaprevir) in 2011 in the United States. Since then, a number of new direct-acting antiviral agents have been approved or will be approved in the next few years that will obviate the need for injectable interferon. The new treatments offer all-oral regimens, short duration of therapy (from 6–12 weeks to 24–48 weeks), few side effects, and high cure rates (>90%). Travelers who think they may have been exposed should see their health care provider upon return and get tested for HCV, and if found to have evidence of infection, be referred for care. No therapies for HCV postexposure prophylaxis are available; however, this may change as new treatments are approved. The most up-to-date treatment information can be found at www.hcvguidelines.org.

PREVENTION

No vaccine is available to prevent HCV infection, nor does immune globulin provide protection. Before traveling, people should check with their health care providers to understand the potential risk of infection and any precautions they should take. When seeking medical or dental care, travelers should be alert to the use of medical, surgical, or dental equipment that has not been adequately sterilized or disinfected; reuse of contaminated equipment; and unsafe injection practices (such as reuse of disposable needles and syringes). HCV and other bloodborne pathogens can be transmitted if instruments are not sterile or the clinician does not follow other proper infection-control procedures (washing hands, using latex gloves, and cleaning and disinfecting surfaces and instruments). In some parts of the world, such as parts of sub-Saharan Africa, blood donors may not be screened for HCV. Travelers should be advised to consider the health risks if they are thinking about getting a tattoo or body piercing or having a medical procedure in areas where adequate

sterilization or disinfection procedures might not be practiced. Travelers should be advised to seek testing for HCV upon return if they received blood transfusions or sustained other blood exposures for which they could not assess the risks.

CDC website: www.cdc.gov/hepatitis/HCV

BIBLIOGRAPHY

1. American Association for Study of Liver Diseases (AASLD), Infectious Diseases Society of America (IDSA). Recommendations for testing, managing, and treating hepatitis C. [updated 2014 Aug 11; cited 2014 Sep 17]. Available from: http://www.hcvguidelines.org/.
2. Averhoff FM, Glass N, Holtzman D. Global burden of hepatitis C: considerations for healthcare providers in the United States. Clin Infect Dis. 2012 Jul;55 Suppl 1:S10–5.
3. CDC. Testing for HCV infection: an update of guidance for clinicians and laboratorians. MMWR Morb Mortal Wkly Rep. 2013 May 10;62(18):362–5.
4. Dore GJ. The changing therapeutic landscape for hepatitis C. Med J Aust. 2012 Jun 4;196(10):629–32.
5. Lozano R, Naghavi M, Foreman K, Lim S, Shibuya K, Aboyans V, et al. Global and regional mortality from 235 causes of death for 20 age groups in 1990 and 2010: a systematic analysis for the Global Burden of Disease Study 2010. Lancet. 2012 Dec 15;380(9859):2095–128.
6. Mohd Hanafiah K, Groeger J, Flaxman AD, Wiersma ST. Global epidemiology of hepatitis C virus infection: new estimates of age-specific antibody to HCV seroprevalence. Hepatology. 2013 Apr;57(4):1333–42.
7. Prati D. Transmission of hepatitis C virus by blood transfusions and other medical procedures: a global review. J Hepatol. 2006 Oct;45(4):607–16.
8. Seeff LB. The history of the "natural history" of hepatitis C (1968–2009). Liver Int. 2009 Jan;29 Suppl 1:89–99.
9. Simonsen L, Kane A, Lloyd J, Zaffran M, Kane M. Unsafe injections in the developing world and transmission of bloodborne pathogens: a review. Bull World Health Organ. 1999;77(10):789–800.
10. World Health Organization. Global surveillance and control of hepatitis C. J Viral Hepat. 1999 Jan;6(1):35–47.

HEPATITIS E

Chong-Gee Teo

INFECTIOUS AGENT
Infection is caused by hepatitis E virus (HEV), a single-stranded, RNA virus belonging to the Hepeviridae family.

TRANSMISSION
HEV is transmitted primarily by the fecal-oral route. In regions with poor sanitation and limited access to safe drinking water, epidemics and interepidemic occurrences of hepatitis E are largely waterborne. Transmission to fetuses and neonates by women infected during pregnancy is common. In Japan and Europe, sporadic disease can be zoonotic and foodborne, associated with eating meat and offal (including liver) of

deer, boars, and pigs. In France, disease can be acquired from eating *figatellu*, a sausage delicacy prepared from raw pig liver. Sporadic disease also is observed in the United States and other temperate countries, but its cause is generally unknown. Shellfish can transmit HEV. Transmission from blood transfusion has been reported, although rare.

EPIDEMIOLOGY
Waterborne outbreaks (which can be large, involving hundreds to thousands of people) have occurred in South and Central Asia, tropical East Asia, Africa, and Central America (Map 3-6). Of note, Hong Kong SAR and Singapore have been identified

MAP 3-6. DISTRIBUTION OF HEPATITIS E VIRUS INFECTION[1]

[1] Disease data adapted from: World Health Organization. The Global Prevalence of Hepatitis E Virus Infection and Susceptibility: A Systematic Review. http://whqlibdoc.who.int/hq/2010/WHO_IVB_10.14_eng.pdf. Accessed November 13, 1024.
[2] Defined as waterborne outbreaks or confirmed Hepatitis E virus infection ⩾25% of sporadic non-A, non-B hepatitis
[3] Defined as confirmed Hepatits E virus infection in <25% of sporadic non-A, non-B hepatits

Hepatitis E Endemicity

- Highly Endemic[2]
- Endemic[3]
- Not Endemic or Endemicity Unknown

as endemic areas. Clinical attack rates are highest in young adults aged 15–49 years. In outbreak-prone areas, interepidemic disease is sporadically encountered. In these areas, pregnant women—whether infected sporadically or during an epidemic—are at risk of their HEV disease progressing to liver failure and death. Miscarriages and neonatal deaths are common complications of HEV infection.

Sporadic disease also occurs in regions that are not prone to outbreaks, such as the Middle East, temperate East Asia (including China), North and South America, and Europe. Symptomatic disease is observed most frequently in adults aged >50 years. Primary infection acquired by people who are immunosuppressed, particularly recipients of solid-organ allografts, may progress to chronic infection.

People living in the United States are at risk of HEV infection when they travel to areas where epidemics have occurred. When traveling in Japan and Europe, eating raw or inadequately cooked venison, boar meat, pig liver, pig meat, or food products derived from these is a risk factor for infection.

CLINICAL PRESENTATION

The incubation period of acute hepatitis E is 2–9 weeks (mean 6 weeks). Signs and symptoms of disease during acute infection include jaundice, fever, loss of appetite, abdominal pain, and lethargy. A wide range of neurologic manifestations have been associated with HEV. For most people, HEV infection and disease is self-limited. Pregnant women (especially those infected during the second or third trimester) may present with or progress to liver failure, and their fetuses are at risk of spontaneous abortion and premature delivery. People with preexisting liver disease may undergo further hepatic decompensation with HEV infection. Recipients of organ transplants tend to have no symptoms associated with acute and chronic HEV infection.

DIAGNOSIS

The diagnosis of acute hepatitis E is established by detecting anti-HEV IgM and IgG in serum. Detecting HEV RNA in serum or stools further confirms the serologic diagnosis but is seldom required. Longer-term, serial detection of HEV RNA in serum or stools, regardless of the HEV antibody serostatus, suggests chronic HEV infection. No diagnostic test for HEV has been approved by the Food and Drug Administration.

TREATMENT

Treatment is supportive. Oral ribavirin has been used to treat chronic hepatitis E in solid-organ transplant recipients.

PREVENTION

No vaccine is available, nor are drugs for preventing infection. Travelers should avoid drinking unboiled or unchlorinated water and beverages that contain unboiled water or ice. Travelers should eat only thoroughly cooked food, including seafood, meat, offal, and products derived from these (see Chapter 2, Food & Water Precautions).

CDC website: www.cdc.gov/hepatitis/HEV

BIBLIOGRAPHY

1. Kamar N, Izopet J, Tripon S, Bismuth M, Hillaire S, Dumortier J, et al. Ribavirin for chronic hepatitis E virus infection in transplant recipients. N Engl J Med. 2014 Mar 20;370(12):1111–20.
2. Krawczynski K. Hepatitis E virus. Semin Liver Dis. 2013 Feb;33(1):1–93.
3. Riveiro-Barciela M, Minguez B, Girones R, Rodriguez-Frias F, Quer J, Buti M. Phylogenetic demonstration of hepatitis E infection transmitted by pork meat ingestion. J Clin Gastroenterol. Forthcoming 2014.

HISTOPLASMOSIS

Tom M. Chiller

INFECTIOUS AGENT

Histoplasma capsulatum, a dimorphic fungus that grows as a mold in soil and as a yeast in animal and human hosts.

TRANSMISSION

Through inhalation of spores (conidia) from soil (often soil contaminated with bat guano or bird droppings); not transmitted from person to person.

EPIDEMIOLOGY

Distributed worldwide, except in Antarctica, but most often associated with river valleys. Activities such as spelunking, mining, construction, excavation, demolition, roofing, chimney cleaning, farming, gardening, and installing heating and air-conditioning systems are associated with histoplasmosis. Activities that expose people to areas where bats live and birds roost also increase risk. Outbreaks have been reported associated with travel to many countries in Central and South America, most often associated with visiting caves.

CLINICAL PRESENTATION

Incubation period is typically 3–17 days for acute disease. Ninety percent of infections are asymptomatic or result in a mild influenza-like illness. Some infections may cause acute pulmonary histoplasmosis, manifested by high fever, headache, nonproductive cough, chills, weakness, pleuritic chest pain, and fatigue. Most people spontaneously recover 2–3 weeks after onset of symptoms, although fatigue may persist longer. Dissemination, especially to the gastrointestinal tract and central nervous system, can occur in people who are immunocompromised.

DIAGNOSIS

Culture of *H. capsulatum* from bone marrow, blood, sputum, and tissue specimens is the definitive method. Demonstration of the typical intracellular yeast forms by microscopic examination strongly supports the diagnosis of histoplasmosis when clinical, epidemiologic, and other laboratory studies are compatible. EIA on urine, serum, plasma, bronchoalveolar lavage, or cerebrospinal fluid is a rapid diagnostic test commercially available in the United States.

TREATMENT

Treatment is not usually indicated for immunocompetent people with acute, localized pulmonary infection. People with more extensive disease or persistent symptoms beyond 1 month are generally treated with an azole drug, such as itraconazole, for mild to moderate illness or amphotericin B for severe infection.

PREVENTION

People at increased risk for severe disease should avoid high-risk areas, such as bat-inhabited caves.

CDC website: www.cdc.gov/fungal/diseases/histoplasmosis

BIBLIOGRAPHY

1. CDC. Outbreak of histoplasmosis among travelers returning from El Salvador—Pennsylvania and Virginia, 2008. MMWR Morb Mortal Wkly Rep. 2008 Dec 19;57(50):1349–53.
2. Kauffman CA. Histoplasmosis. Clin Chest Med. 2009 Jun;30(2):217–25.
3. Kauffman CA. Histoplasmosis: a clinical and laboratory update. Clin Microbiol Rev. 2007 Jan;20(1):115–32.
4. Morgan J, Cano MV, Feikin DR, et al. A large outbreak of histoplasmosis among American travelers associated with a hotel in Acapulco, Mexico, spring 2001. Am J Trop Med Hyg. 2003;69:663–9.
5. Weinberg M, Weeks J, Lance-Parker S, Traeger M, Wiersma S, Phan QN, et al. Severe histoplasmosis in travelers to Nicaragua. Emerg Infect Dis. 2003 Oct;9(10):1322–5.
6. Wheat LJ. Histoplasmosis: a review for clinicians from non-endemic areas. Mycoses. 2006 Jul;49(4):274–82.

HIV INFECTION

John T. Brooks

INFECTIOUS AGENT

HIV, a single-stranded, positive-sense, enveloped RNA virus in the genus *Lentivirus*.

TRANSMISSION

HIV can be transmitted through sexual contact, needle- or syringe-sharing, medical use of blood or blood components, organ or tissue transplantation, and artificial insemination. It can also be transmitted from mother to child during pregnancy, at birth, and postpartum through breastfeeding. HIV may be transmitted occupationally to health care workers who are exposed to blood and other potentially infectious bodily fluids via percutaneous injury or splash exposures to mucous membranes or non-intact skin (see Chapter 8, Health Care Workers). HIV is not transmitted through casual person-to-person contact; air, food, or water; contact with inanimate objects; or by mosquitoes or other arthropod vectors. The use of any public conveyance (such as airplanes, automobiles, boats, buses, or trains) by people with HIV infection does not pose a risk of HIV infection for the crew members or other travelers.

EPIDEMIOLOGY

HIV infection occurs worldwide. As of the end of 2012, an estimated 35 million people were living with HIV infection. Although sub-Saharan Africa has experienced a substantial decline in the number of new infections annually, from 2,600,000 in 2001 to 1,600,000 in 2012, and a decline in prevalence during the same period, from an estimated 5.8 to 4.7 infections per 100,000 people, it remains the most affected part of the world (25 million cases or 71% of all people living with HIV infection). Notable increases in HIV infection have occurred in Eastern Europe and Central Asia, where the number of people living with HIV infection from 2001 to 2012 rose from an estimated 860,000 to 1,300,000. Most new infections come from low- and middle-income countries. Many countries lack comprehensive surveillance systems and, despite improvements, the true number of cases may be higher than officially reported, particularly in developing countries.

The risk of HIV infection for international travelers is generally low, although the risk is determined less by geographic destination and more by behaviors such as drug use and unprotected sex. Travelers who might undergo medical procedures, whether scheduled or in an emergency, should be aware that in developing countries the blood supply (and organs and tissues used for transplantation) might not be adequately screened, increasing the risk of HIV transmission.

DIAGNOSIS

Any person who suspects that she or he may have been exposed to HIV should be tested. Most people develop detectable antibodies within 2–8 weeks (mean, 25 days). Ninety-seven percent of people develop antibodies in the first 3 months after infection. In rare cases, it can take up to 6 months to develop antibodies to HIV. After being infected, a person remains antibody positive for life, except when people lose the capacity to mount detectable antibodies in the latest stages of the disease. The earliest time after exposure that HIV infection can be diagnosed is approximately 9 days, when HIV RNA becomes detectable in blood; however, tests needed to measure HIV RNA are costly and may not be available. Any person not known to be HIV-infected who is diagnosed with an AIDS-compatible illness, such as *Pneumocystis* pneumonia, should be tested for HIV. For further information on HIV testing, travelers should talk to their health care provider, or identify an HIV testing site near them by visiting the National HIV Testing Resources website at www.hivtest.org or call CDC-INFO toll-free at 800-CDC-INFO (800-232-4636) or 888-232-6348 (TTY). Both these resources are confidential.

3

TREATMENT

Prompt medical care and effective treatment with antiretrovirals can inhibit HIV from damaging the immune system and delay progression of disease. Effective treatment also substantially reduces the risk of HIV transmission to others. US guidelines recommend all people with HIV infection be treated for their own health and to prevent transmission to others. Detailed information on specific treatments is available from the Department of Health and Human Services AIDSinfo (www.aidsinfo.nih.gov). Information on enrolling in clinical trials is also available at AIDSinfo. Travelers may contact AIDSinfo toll-free at 800-448-0440 (English or Spanish) or 888-480-3739 (TTY).

PREVENTION

No vaccine is available to prevent infection with HIV. Travelers should be advised that they are at risk if they

- Have sexual contact (heterosexual or homosexual) with an infected person or a person whose HIV infection status is unknown.
- Use or allow the use of contaminated, unsterilized syringes or needles for any injections or other procedures that pierce the skin, including acupuncture, use of illicit drugs, steroid or vitamin injections, medical or dental procedures, ear or body piercing, or tattooing.
- Receive infected blood, blood components, or clotting factor concentrates. HIV infection by this route is rare in countries or cities where donated blood and plasma are screened for antibodies to HIV.
- Work in a health care setting. Typically, exposures occur as a result of percutaneous exposure to contaminated sharps, including needles, lancets, scalpels, and broken glass (from capillary or test tubes). See Chapter 8, Health Care Workers.

To reduce their risk of acquiring HIV, travelers should

- Avoid sexual encounters with people who are infected with HIV, whose HIV infection status is unknown, or who are at high risk for HIV infection, such as intravenous drug users, commercial sex workers (both male and female), and other people with multiple sexual partners
- Use condoms consistently and correctly, especially if engaging in vaginal, anal, or oral sex with a person who is HIV infected or whose HIV status is unknown
- Avoid injecting drugs
- Avoid sharing needles or other devices that can puncture skin
- Avoid, if at all possible, blood transfusions or use of clotting factor concentrates
- Ensure that if traveling for purposes of medical treatment (see Chapter 2, Medical Tourism), the blood and blood products used in the facility where the traveler will be treated are screened for HIV, and that such facilities exercise proper infection control practices
- Consider discussing using preexposure prophylaxis (www.cdc.gov/hiv/prep) with a health care provider, especially if the traveler is sexually active with >1 partner and does not use condoms consistently during sex

Condoms

People who are sensitive to latex should use condoms made of polyurethane or other synthetic materials (not lambskin) and should carry their own supply of male or female condoms. If no condom is available, travelers should abstain from sex with people who are HIV-infected or whose HIV status is unknown. Barrier methods other than condoms do not prevent HIV transmission. Spermicides alone are also not effective. The widely used spermicide nonoxynol-9 can increase the risk of HIV transmission and should not be used.

Needles

Needles used to draw blood or administer injections should be sterile, single use, disposable, and prepackaged in a sealed container. If at all possible, travelers should avoid receiving medications from multidose vials, which may have become contaminated by used needles. Travelers with type 1 diabetes, hemophilia, or other conditions that necessitate routine or frequent injections should be advised to carry a supply of medication, syringes, needles, and disinfectant swabs sufficient to last their entire stay abroad. These travelers should request documentation of the medical necessity for traveling with these items (a letter from a licensed health care provider) to avoid having them confiscated, such as by inspection personnel at ports of entry (see Chapter 2, Travel Health Kits for more information about traveling with medications).

Transfusions

In many developed countries, the risk of HIV infection through transfusion of blood or blood products has been virtually eliminated through required testing of all donated blood. Developing countries may have no formal program, or may have inadequate technology for testing blood or biological products for contamination with HIV. If transfusion is necessary, the blood should be tested for HIV antibodies by trained laboratory technicians using a reliable test.

Postexposure Prophylaxis

Travelers who will be working in a medical setting (such as a nurse volunteer drawing blood or medical missionary performing surgeries) may have contact with HIV-infected or potentially infected biological materials. Detailed advice regarding management of postexposure prophylaxis in the occupational setting is found in Chapter 8, Health Care Workers. General recommendations on postexposure prophylaxis include the following:

- People who have been exposed to HIV in a nonoccupational setting (through sex or needle sharing) should seek immediate medical consultation to consider postexposure prophylaxis.
- Postexposure prophylaxis for potential exposure to HIV as a result of mass-casualty events is generally not warranted, except in special circumstances (for example, a blast injury in a facility that contained a large archive of HIV-infected blood specimens).
- Clinicians seeking advice on postexposure prophylaxis can call the US National HIV/AIDS Clinicians' Consultation Center PEPline toll-free at 888-448-4911 (www.nccc.ucsf.edu).

HIV TESTING REQUIREMENTS FOR US TRAVELERS ENTERING FOREIGN COUNTRIES

International travelers should be advised that some countries screen incoming travelers for HIV infection and may deny entry to people with AIDS or evidence of HIV infection. These countries usually screen only people planning extended visits, such as for work or study. People intending to visit a country for an extended stay should review that country's policies and requirements. This information is usually available from the consular officials of the individual nations. Information about entry and exit requirements compiled by the Department of State can be found at http://travel.state.gov/travel/tips/tips_1232.html#requirement.

CDC website: www.cdc.gov/hiv

BIBLIOGRAPHY

1. CDC. Preexposure prophylaxis for the prevention of HIV in the United States: a clinical practice guideline. Atlanta: US Public Health Service; 2014 [cited 2014 Sep 17]. Available from: http://www.cdc.gov/hiv/pdf/PrEPguidelines2014.pdf.

2. CDC. Preexposure prophylaxis for the prevention of HIV in the United States: clinical providers' supplement. Atlanta: US Public Health Service; 2014 [cited 2014 Sep 17]. Available from: http://www.cdc.gov/hiv/pdf/PrEPProviderSupplement2014.pdf.

3. Chapman LE, Sullivent EE, Grohskopf LA, Beltrami EM, Perz JF, Kretsinger K, et al. Recommendations for postexposure interventions to prevent infection with hepatitis B virus, hepatitis C virus, or human immunodeficiency virus, and tetanus in persons wounded during bombings and other mass-casualty events—United States, 2008: recommendations of the Centers for Disease Control and Prevention (CDC). MMWR Recomm Rep. 2008 Aug 1;57(RR-6):1–21.

4. Joint United Nations Programme on HIV/AIDS (UNAIDS). UNAIDS World AIDS Day report, 2012. Geneva: Joint United Nations Programme on HIV/AIDS (UNAIDS); 2012 [cited 2012 Dec 20]. Available from: http://www.unaids.org/en/resources/campaigns/20121120_globalreport2012/.

5. Kuhar DT, Henderson DK, Struble KA, Heneine W, Thomas V, Cheever LW, et al. Updated US Public Health Service guidelines for the management of occupational exposures to human immunodeficiency virus and recommendations for postexposure prophylaxis. Infect Control Hosp Epidemiol. 2013 Sep;34(9):875–92.

6. Rice B, Gilbart VL, Lawrence J, Smith R, Kall M, Delpech V. Safe travels? HIV transmission among Britons travelling abroad. HIV Med. 2012 May;13(5):315–7.

7. Smith DK, Grohskopf LA, Black RJ, Auerbach JD, Veronese F, Struble KA, et al. Antiretroviral postexposure prophylaxis after sexual, injection-drug use, or other nonoccupational exposure to HIV in the United States: recommendations from the US Department of Health and Human Services. MMWR Recomm Rep. 2005 Jan 21;54(RR-2):1–20.

INFLUENZA

Scott Epperson, Joseph Bresee

INFECTIOUS AGENT

Influenza is caused by infection of the respiratory tract with influenza viruses, which are classified into 3 types: A, B, and C. Only virus types A and B commonly cause illness in humans. Influenza A viruses are further classified into subtypes based on 2 surface proteins, hemagglutinin (H) and neuraminidase (N). Although 3 types and subtypes of influenza virus cocirculate in humans worldwide (influenza A(H1N1)pdm09, A (H3N2), and influenza B viruses, the distribution of these viruses can vary from year to year and between geographic areas and time of year. Information on circulating virus strains in various regions can be found via CDC (www.cdc.gov/flu/weekly/) or the World Health Organization (www.who.int/topics/influenza/en/). Avian and swine influenza viruses can occasionally infect and cause disease in humans, usually associated with close exposure to infected animal populations. Notably, avian influenza A (H5N1) and A (H7N9) have led to sporadic human cases in recent years, and swine-origin A(H3N2) variant viruses have been associated with disease in the United States.

TRANSMISSION

Influenza viruses spread from person to person, primarily through respiratory droplet transmission (such as when an infected person coughs or sneezes near a susceptible person). Transmission via large-particle droplets requires close contact between the source and the recipient, because droplets generally travel only short distances (approximately 6 feet or less) through the air, before settling onto surfaces. Airborne transmission via small-particle aerosols in the vicinity of the infectious person may also occur. Indirect transmission can also occur when a person touches a virus-contaminated surface and then touches his or her face. However, the relative contribution of the different modes of transmission to the spread of influenza viruses is unclear.

Most adults who are ill with influenza shed the virus in the upper respiratory tract and are infectious from the day before symptom onset to approximately 5–7 days after symptom onset. Ninety-five percent of virus transmission occurs within 3 days after illness onset. Children and those who are immunocompromised or severely ill, including those who are hospitalized, may shed influenza virus for 10 days or more after the onset of symptoms. Seasonal influenza viruses have rarely been detected from non-respiratory sources such as stool or blood.

EPIDEMIOLOGY
Seasonal Influenza

Influenza circulation varies geographically. The risk for exposure to influenza during travel depends on the time of year and destination. In temperate regions, influenza typically circulates at higher levels during colder winter months: October to May in the Northern Hemisphere and April to September in the Southern Hemisphere. In tropical or subtropical regions, although influenza activity may peak during rainy or dry seasons, or even have 2 annual peaks, year-round circulation is commonly observed.

Influenza virus can cause disease in all age groups. Infection rates are typically highest in children, especially in school-aged children. Rates of severe illness and death are typically highest among people aged ≥65, children <2 years, and people of any age who have underlying medical conditions that place them at increased risk for complications of influenza. Children aged <2 years have rates of influenza-associated hospitalizations that are as high as those in the elderly, although with much lower death rates. CDC estimates that from 1976 through 2006, annual influenza-associated deaths in the United States ranged from a low of approximately 3,000 people to a high of approximately 49,000 people; approximately 90% of these deaths occurred among people aged ≥65 years.

Zoonotic Influenza

Although influenza B viruses circulate only among humans, influenza A viruses circulate among many animal populations. The primary reservoir for influenza A viruses is wild waterfowl. Influenza A viruses can also be found in other animal species, such as poultry, cats, dogs, horses, sea lions, and bats.

Human infections with animal-origin influenza A viruses are uncommon, but they do occur. In the United States, human influenza illnesses caused by swine-origin influenza A viruses (called "variant" influenza virus infections) have been sporadically identified. In 2012, a large number of human illnesses caused by an influenza A(H3N2) variant virus were identified, and >300 confirmed cases were reported in the United States from July through September. A smaller outbreak of this virus was seen in the summer months of 2013 with 18 cases identified in 4 states. Most illnesses caused by the H3N2 variant have occurred after direct or indirect contact with an infected pig, often among exhibitors or visitors to agricultural fairs. Limited person-to-person transmission has occurred with this virus and the severity of illness has been similar to that seen with seasonal influenza.

Although avian influenza viruses do not commonly infect humans, disease resulting from these viruses has been reported. From 2003 through March 2014, 650 human illnesses caused by avian influenza A(H5N1) were reported globally, approximately 60% of which were fatal. Most disease from H5N1 has occurred after direct or close contact with sick or dead infected poultry. H5N1 is widespread among poultry in some countries in Asia and the Middle East and is considered to be endemic among poultry in 6 countries: Bangladesh, China, Egypt, India (West Bengal), Indonesia, and Vietnam (Map 3-7). Distribution of H5N1 avian influenza. From January 2013 through March 2014, 65% of human H5N1 cases have been from Cambodia, where it is not considered endemic among poultry. Instances of limited, nonsustained human-to-human transmission of H5N1 virus have been reported.

Avian influenza A(H7N9) virus emerged in China in 2013, and as of March 2014, has caused nearly 400 confirmed human illnesses. Most cases have been identified in mainland China, but several cases associated with exposure in mainland China and subsequent travel have been identified in Malaysia, Taiwan, and Hong Kong. Most of the people with illness due to H7N9 had exposure to infected poultry or contaminated environments, as the virus has been found in poultry and environmental samples collected in China. While a small proportion of human H7N9 illnesses has been mild, most patients have developed severe respiratory illness, and 32% have died.

Human infections with other avian influenza A viruses, including H7N7, H9N2, and H10N8 viruses, although rare, have been reported in recent years.

CLINICAL PRESENTATION

Uncomplicated influenza illness is characterized by the abrupt onset of signs and symptoms that include fever, muscle aches, headache, malaise, nonproductive cough, sore throat, vomiting, and rhinitis. Illness without fever can occur, especially in the elderly. Children are more likely than adults to also experience nausea, vomiting, or diarrhea when ill with influenza. Physical findings are predominantly localized to the respiratory tract and include nasal discharge, pharyngeal inflammation without exudates, and occasionally rales on chest auscultation. The incubation period is usually 1–4 days after exposure. Influenza illness typically resolves within 1 week for most previously healthy children and adults who do not receive antiviral medication, although cough and malaise can persist for >2 weeks, especially in the elderly. Complications of influenza virus infection include primary influenza viral pneumonia, secondary bacterial pneumonia, exacerbation of underlying medical conditions (such as pulmonary and cardiac disease), encephalopathy, myocarditis, myositis, and coinfections with other viral or bacterial pathogens.

DIAGNOSIS

Influenza can be difficult to distinguish from respiratory illnesses caused by other pathogens on the basis of signs and symptoms alone. The positive predictive value of clinical signs and symptoms for influenzalike illness (fever with either cough or sore throat) for laboratory-confirmed influenza virus infection is 30%–88%, depending on the level of influenza activity.

Diagnostic tests available for influenza include viral culture, rapid influenza diagnostic tests (RIDTs), immunofluorescence assays, and RT-PCR. Most patients with clinical illness consistent with uncomplicated influenza in an area where influenza viruses are circulating do not require diagnostic testing for clinical management. Patients who should be considered for influenza diagnostic testing include the following:

- Hospitalized patients with suspected influenza
- Patients for whom a diagnosis of influenza will inform decisions regarding clinical care, especially those with medical conditions that place them at high risk of complications
- Patients for whom results of influenza testing would affect infection control or management of close contacts, including other patients, such as in institutional outbreaks or other settings (cruise ships or tour groups, for example)

The sensitivity of RIDTs varies but is substantially lower than for RT-PCR or viral culture. The sensitivity of RIDTs to detect animal-origin influenza viruses, including avian influenza viruses, can vary by test type and virus subtype. Therefore, a negative RIDT result does not rule out influenza virus infection, and health care providers should not rely on a negative RIDT result to make decisions about treatment.

TREATMENT

Early antiviral treatment can shorten the duration of fever and other symptoms and reduce the risk of complications from influenza. Antiviral treatment is recommended as early as possible for any patient with confirmed or suspected influenza who is hospitalized; has severe, complicated, or progressive illness; or is at a higher risk for influenza-associated complications (www.cdc.gov/flu/professionals/antivirals/summary-clinicians.htm). Antiviral treatment can also be considered for any previously healthy patient with confirmed or suspected influenza not at high risk of complications, if treatment can be initiated within 48 hours of illness onset.

Although antiviral therapy is ideally initiated within the first 48 hours of illness, for hospitalized patients, those with severe illness, or those at higher risk of complications, antiviral therapy may still be beneficial if started >48 hours after illness onset. Two influenza antiviral medications are available for the treatment and prophylaxis of influenza: oral oseltamivir (Tamiflu) and inhaled zanamivir (Relenza). Both are active against influenza A and B viruses. Oseltamivir is approved for treatment in children aged ≥14 days and for chemoprophylaxis of patients aged ≥1 year. Zanamivir is approved for treatment in those aged ≥7 years and for chemoprophylaxis in those aged ≥5 years (Table 3-5). Two other medications, amantadine and rimantadine, are not recommended for treatment or chemoprophylaxis of influenza because of widespread viral resistance among circulating influenza A viruses. Amantadine and rimantadine are not active against influenza B viruses.

People at increased risk for complications of influenza should discuss antiviral treatment and chemoprophylaxis with their health care provider before travel if traveling to areas where influenza activity is occurring. CDC recommends treatment with oseltamivir or zanamivir for human infection with avian or swine influenza viruses.

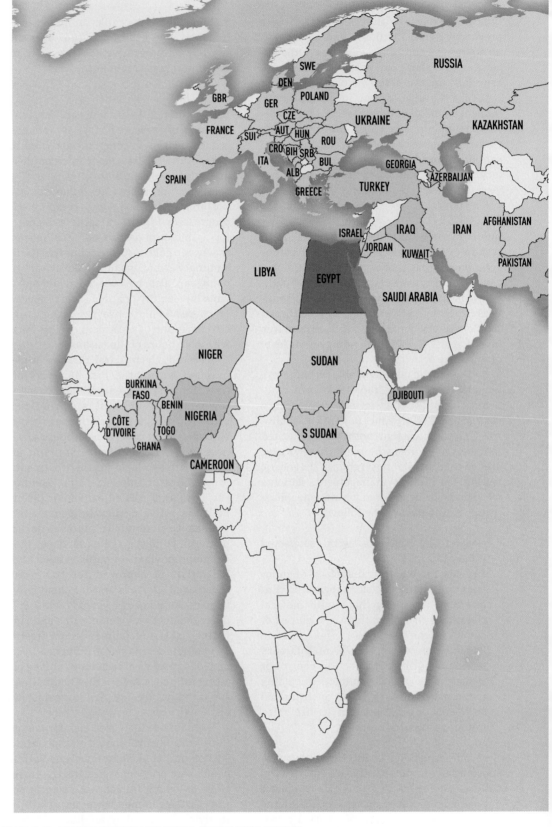

MAP 3-7. DISTRIBUTION OF H5N1 AVIAN INFLUENZA

INFECTIOUS DISEASES RELATED TO TRAVEL

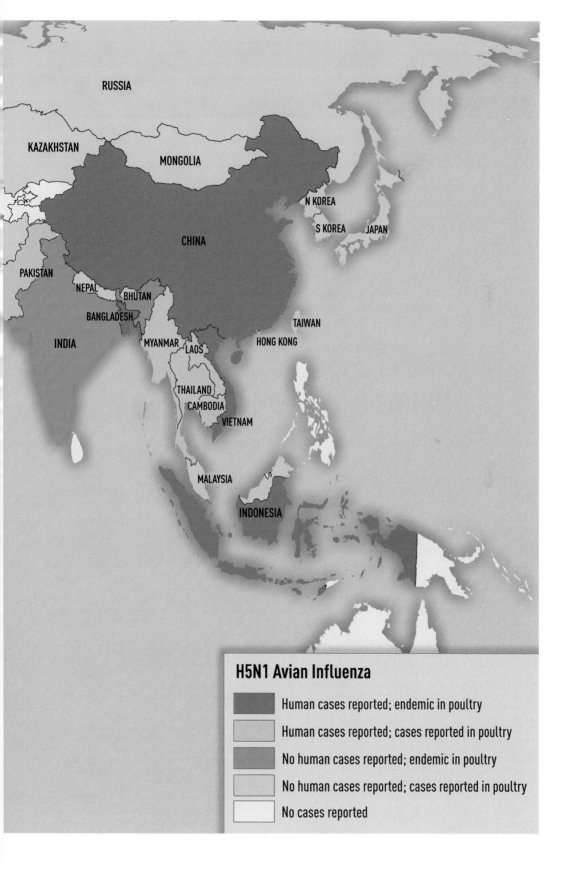

H5N1 Avian Influenza

Human cases reported; endemic in poultry

Human cases reported; cases reported in poultry

No human cases reported; endemic in poultry

No human cases reported; cases reported in poultry

No cases reported

Table 3-5. Recommended dosage and duration of influenza antiviral medications for treatment and prophylaxis

ANTIVIRAL AGENT	USE	CHILDREN	ADULTS
Oseltamivir (Tamiflu)	Treatment (5 days)	**If child is <1 year old[1]:** 3 mg/kg/dose twice daily[2,3] **If ≥1 year old, dose varies by child's weight:** ≤15 kg, the dose is 30 mg twice a day. >15–23 kg, the dose is 45 mg twice a day. >23–40 kg, the dose is 60 mg twice a day. >40 kg, the dose is 75 mg twice a day.	75 mg twice daily
	Chemo-prophylaxis (7 days)	**If child is <3 months old:** use of oseltamivir for chemoprophylaxis is not recommended unless situation is judged critical because data in this age group are limited. **If child is ≥3 months and <1 year old[1]:** 3 mg/kg/dose once daily.[2] **If ≥1 year old, dose varies by child's weight:** ≤15 kg, the dose is 30 mg once a day. >15–23 kg, the dose is 45 mg once a day. >23–40 kg, the dose is 60 mg once a day. >40 kg, the dose is 75 mg once a day.	75 mg once daily
Zanamivir	Treatment (5 days)	10 mg (2 5-mg inhalations) twice daily (**FDA approved and recommended for use in children ≥7 years**)	10 mg (2 5-mg inhalations) twice daily
	Chemo-prophylaxis (7 days)	10 mg (2 5-mg inhalations) once daily (**FDA approved for and recommended for use in children ≥5 years**)	10 mg (2 5-mg inhalations) once daily

[1] Oral oseltamivir is approved by the FDA for treatment of acute uncomplicated influenza with twice-daily dosing in people aged ≥14 days and for chemoprophylaxis with once-daily dosing in people aged ≥1 year. Although not part of the FDA-approved indications, use of oral oseltamivir for treatment of influenza in infants <14 days old, and for chemoprophylaxis in infants 3 months to 1 year of age, is recommended by CDC and the American Academy of Pediatrics.

[2] This is the FDA-approved oral oseltamivir treatment dose for infants aged ≥14 days and <1 year old and provides oseltamivir exposure in children similar to that achieved by the approved dose of 75 mg orally twice daily for adults, as shown in 2 studies of oseltamivir pharmacokinetics in children. The American Academy of Pediatrics has recommended an oseltamivir treatment dose of 3.5 mg/kg orally twice daily for infants aged 9–11 months for the 2013–2014 season. It is unknown whether this higher dose will improve efficacy or prevent the development of antiviral resistance. However, there is no evidence that the 3.5-mg/kg dose is harmful or causes more adverse events to infants in this age group.

[3] Current weight-based dosing recommendations are not appropriate for premature infants. Premature infants might have slower clearance of oral oseltamivir because of immature renal function, and doses recommended for full-term infants might lead to very high drug concentrations in this age group. CDC recommends dosing as also recommended by the American Academy of Pediatrics: 1.0 mg/kg/dose, orally, twice daily, for those <38 weeks postmenstrual age; 1.5 mg/kg/dose, orally, twice daily, for those 38–40 weeks postmenstrual age; 3.0 mg/kg/dose, orally, twice daily, for those >40 weeks postmenstrual age.

[4] Inhaled zanamivir is approved to treat acute uncomplicated influenza with twice-daily dosing in people aged ≥7 years and for chemoprophylaxis with once-daily dosing in people aged ≥5 years.

PREVENTION
Vaccine
Indications for Use

Annual seasonal influenza vaccination is recommended for those aged ≥6 months and is the most effective way to prevent influenza and its complications. In the United States, annual influenza vaccination is recommended by the Advisory Committee on Immunization Practices for all US residents aged ≥6 months who do not have contraindications.

Many influenza vaccine products are available for use in the United States (www.cdc.gov/flu/protect/vaccine/vaccines.htm) and can be grouped into categories: inactivated influenza vaccine (IIV), live attenuated influenza vaccine (LAIV), and recombinant influenza vaccine (RIV). IIV can be administered by intramuscular or intradermal injection and is available for people ≥6 months of age. Specific age indications vary by manufacturer and product; label instructions should be followed. LAIV, administered by nasal spray, is approved for use only in healthy people aged 2–49 years who are not pregnant. RIV is indicated for people aged 18–49 years. Within indicated groups, there is no preference for any particular vaccine.

Any traveler, including people at high risk for complications of influenza, who did not receive influenza vaccine during the preceding fall or winter and wants to reduce the risk for influenza infection should consider influenza vaccination ≥2 weeks before departure if they plan to travel to the tropics, with organized tourist groups at any time of year, or to the Southern Hemisphere from April through September.

No information is available about the benefits of revaccinating people before summer travel who already were vaccinated during the preceding fall, and revaccination is not recommended. People at higher risk for influenza complications should consult with their health care provider to discuss the risk for influenza or other travel-related diseases before embarking on travel during the summer.

Seasonal influenza vaccines are not expected to provide protection against human infection with animal-origin influenza viruses, including avian influenza viruses H5N1 and A H7N9.

Vaccine Safety and Adverse Reactions
Inactivated influenza vaccine (IIV)

The most frequent side effects of vaccination with intramuscular and intradermal IIV in adults are soreness and redness at the vaccination site. These local reactions are slightly more common with vaccine administered intradermally and with high-dose IIV. They generally are mild and rarely interfere with the ability to conduct usual activities. Fever, malaise, myalgia, and other systemic symptoms sometimes occur after vaccination; these may be more frequent in people with no previous exposure to the influenza virus antigens in the vaccine (such as young children) and are generally short-lived.

Guillain-Barré syndrome (GBS) was associated with the 1976 swine influenza vaccine, with an increased risk of 1 additional case of GBS per 100,000 people vaccinated. None of the studies of influenza vaccines other than the 1976 influenza vaccine have demonstrated a similar increase in GBS. Currently, the estimated risk for vaccine-related GBS is low, approximately 1 additional case per 1 million people vaccinated.

Live attenuated influenza vaccine (LAIV)

The most frequent side effects of LAIV reported in healthy adults include minor upper respiratory symptoms, runny nose, and sore throat, which are generally well tolerated. Some children and adolescents have reported fever, vomiting, myalgia, and wheezing. These symptoms, particularly fever, are more often associated with the first administered LAIV dose and are self-limited.

LAIV should not be administered to any child aged <2 years or adult aged ≥50 years. Children aged 2–4 years who have a history of wheezing in the past year or who have a diagnosis of asthma should not receive LAIV. Children and adults aged 2–49 years who have conditions that increase the risk of severe influenza, including pregnancy, should receive IIV or RIV and not LAIV.

Recombinant influenza vaccine (RIV)

The first RIV was licensed in the United States in January 2013. Postmarketing safety data have not yet accumulated; however, prelicensure safety data indicate that the most common reactions were headache, fatigue, and myalgia. Safety and effectiveness of RIV have not been established in pregnant women, nursing mothers, children, or adults ≥50 years of age.

Precautions and Contraindications

Influenza vaccine is contraindicated in people who have had a previous severe allergic reaction to influenza vaccine, regardless of which vaccine component was responsible for the reaction. Immediate hypersensitivity reactions (such as hives, angioedema, allergic asthma, and systemic anaphylaxis) rarely occur after influenza vaccination. These reactions likely result from hypersensitivity to vaccine components, one of which is residual egg protein. Vaccine options are available for people with a history of egg allergy who have experienced only hives after exposure to egg, people with a history of severe reaction to egg, and people with no known history of egg allergy but who are suspected of being egg-allergic; these are outlined at www.cdc.gov/flu/professionals/vaccination/vax-summary.htm#egg-allergy.

Personal Protection Measures

Measures that may help prevent influenza virus infection and other infections during travel include avoiding close contact with sick people, washing hands often with soap and water (where soap and a safe source of water are not available, use of an alcohol-based hand sanitizer containing ≥60% alcohol is recommended), and avoiding touching one's eyes, nose, and mouth. If you are ill, you can help prevent the spread of illness to others by covering your nose and mouth when coughing and sneezing and avoiding close contact with others.

The best way to prevent infection with animal-origin influenza viruses, including H5N1 and H7N9, is to follow standard travel safety precautions: follow good hand hygiene and food safety practices and avoid contact with sources of exposure. Most human infections with avian influenza viruses have occurred after direct or close contact with infected poultry. In countries where avian influenza virus outbreaks are occurring, travelers or those living abroad should avoid markets and farms where live animals are sold or raised, avoid contact with sick or dead animals, not eat undercooked or raw animal products (including eggs), and not eat or drink foods or beverages that contain animal blood.

CDC website: www.cdc.gov/flu

BIBLIOGRAPHY

1. CDC. Evaluation of 11 commercially available rapid influenza diagnostic tests—United States, 2011–2012. MMWR Morb Mortal Wkly Rep. 2012 Nov 2;61(43):873–6.

2. CDC. Prevention and control of influenza with vaccines: recommendations of the Advisory Committee on Immunization Practices (ACIP), 2013. MMWR Morb Mortal Wkly Rep. 2013 May 10;62(18):356.

3. Donnelly CA, Finelli L, Cauchemez S, Olsen SJ, Doshi S, Jackson ML, et al. Serial intervals and the temporal distribution of secondary infections within households of 2009 pandemic influenza A (H1N1): implications for influenza control recommendations. Clin Infect Dis. 2011 Jan 1;52 Suppl 1:S123–30.

4. Jain S, Kamimoto L, Bramley AM, Schmitz AM, Benoit SR, Louie J, et al. Hospitalized patients with 2009 H1N1 influenza in the United States, April–June 2009. N Engl J Med. 2009 Nov 12;361(20):1935–44.

5. Jhung MA, Epperson S, Biggerstaff M, Allen D, Balish A, Barnes N, et al. Outbreak of variant influenza A(H3N2) virus in the United States. Clin Infect Dis. 2013 Dec;57(12):1703–12.

6. Li Q, Zhou L, Zhou M, Chen Z, Li F, Wu H, et al. Epidemiology of human infections with avian influenza A(H7N9) virus in China. N Engl J Med. 2014 Feb 6;370(6):520–32.

7. McGeer A, Green KA, Plevneshi A, Shigayeva A, Siddiqi N, Raboud J, et al. Antiviral therapy and outcomes of influenza requiring hospitalization in Ontario, Canada. Clin Infect Dis. 2007 Dec 15;45(12):1568–75.

8. Pabbaraju K, Tellier R, Wong S, Li Y, Bastien N, Tang JW, et al. Full-genome analysis of avian influenza A(H5N1) virus from a human, North America, 2013. Emerg Infect Dis. 2014 May;20(5):887–91.

9. Siston AM, Rasmussen SA, Honein MA, Fry AM, Seib K, Callaghan WM, et al. Pandemic 2009 influenza A(H1N1) virus illness among pregnant women in the United States. JAMA. 2010 Apr 21;303(15):1517–25.

10. Writing Committee of the WHO Consultation on Clinical Aspects of Pandemic Influenza. Clinical aspects of pandemic 2009 influenza A (H1N1) virus infection. N Engl J Med. 2010 May 6;362(18):1708–19.

JAPANESE ENCEPHALITIS
Susan L. Hills, Ingrid B. Rabe, Marc Fischer

INFECTIOUS AGENT

Japanese encephalitis (JE) virus is a single-stranded RNA virus that belongs to the genus *Flavivirus* and is closely related to West Nile and Saint Louis encephalitis viruses.

TRANSMISSION

JE virus is transmitted to humans through the bite of an infected mosquito, primarily *Culex* species. The virus is maintained in an enzootic cycle between mosquitoes and amplifying vertebrate hosts, primarily pigs and wading birds. Humans are incidental or dead-end hosts, because they usually do not develop a level or duration of viremia sufficient to infect mosquitoes.

EPIDEMIOLOGY

JE virus is the most common vaccine-preventable cause of encephalitis in Asia, occurring throughout most of Asia and parts of the western Pacific (Map 3-8). Local transmission of JE virus has not been detected in Africa, Europe, or the Americas. Transmission principally occurs in rural agricultural areas, often associated with rice cultivation and flood irrigation. In some areas of Asia, these ecologic conditions may occur near, or occasionally within, urban centers. In temperate areas of Asia, transmission is seasonal, and human disease usually peaks in summer and fall. In the subtropics and tropics, seasonal transmission varies with monsoon rains and irrigation practices and may be prolonged or even occur year-round.

In endemic countries, where adults have acquired immunity through natural infection, JE is primarily a disease of children. However, travel-associated JE can occur among people of any age. For most travelers to Asia, the risk for JE is extremely low but varies based on destination, duration, season, and activities.

From 1973 through 2013, 68 JE cases among travelers or expatriates from nonendemic countries were published or reported to CDC. From the time JE vaccine became available in the United States in 1993–2013, only 8 JE cases among US travelers were reported to CDC.

The overall incidence of JE among people from nonendemic countries traveling to Asia is estimated to be <1 case per 1 million travelers. However, expatriates and travelers who stay for prolonged periods in rural areas with active JE virus transmission are likely at similar risk as the susceptible resident population (5–50 cases per 100,000 children per year). Travelers on even brief trips might be at increased risk if they have extensive outdoor or nighttime exposure in rural areas during periods of active transmission. Short-term (<1 month) travelers whose visits are restricted to major urban areas are at minimal risk for JE. In some endemic areas there are few human cases among residents because of natural immunity among older people or vaccination; however, JE virus is usually still maintained in these areas in an enzootic cycle between animals and mosquitoes. Therefore, susceptible visitors may be at risk for infection.

CLINICAL PRESENTATION

Most human infections with JE virus are asymptomatic; <1% of people infected with JE virus develop clinical disease. Acute encephalitis is the most commonly recognized clinical manifestation of JE virus infection. Milder forms of disease, such as aseptic meningitis or undifferentiated febrile illness, can also occur. The incubation period is 5–15 days. Illness usually begins with sudden onset of fever, headache, and vomiting. Mental status changes, focal neurologic deficits, generalized weakness, and movement disorders may develop over the next few days. The classical description of JE includes a parkinsonian syndrome with masklike facies, tremor, cogwheel rigidity, and choreoathetoid movements. Acute flaccid paralysis, with clinical and pathological features similar to those of poliomyelitis, has also been

MAP 3-8. GEOGRAPHIC DISTRIBUTION OF JAPANESE ENCEPHALITIS

INFECTIOUS DISEASES RELATED TO TRAVEL

associated with JE virus infection. Seizures are common, especially among children. The case-fatality ratio is approximately 20%–30%. Among survivors, 30%–50% have serious neurologic, cognitive, or psychiatric sequelae.

Common clinical laboratory findings include moderate leukocytosis, mild anemia, and hyponatremia. Cerebrospinal fluid (CSF) typically has a mild to moderate pleocytosis with a lymphocytic predominance, slightly elevated protein, and normal ratio of CSF to plasma glucose.

DIAGNOSIS

JE should be suspected in a patient with evidence of a neurologic infection (such as encephalitis, meningitis, or acute flaccid paralysis) who has recently traveled to or resided in an endemic country in Asia or the western Pacific. Laboratory diagnosis of JE virus infection should be performed by using a JE virus–specific IgM-capture ELISA on CSF or serum. JE virus–specific IgM can be measured in the CSF of most patients by 4 days after onset of symptoms and in serum by 7 days after onset. Plaque reduction neutralization tests can be performed to confirm the presence of JE virus–specific neutralizing antibodies and discriminate between cross-reacting antibodies from closely related flaviviruses (such as dengue and West Nile viruses). A ≥4-fold rise in JE virus–specific neutralizing antibodies between acute- and convalescent-phase serum specimens may be used to confirm recent infection. Vaccination history, date of onset of symptoms, and information regarding other flaviviruses known to circulate in the geographic area that may cross-react in serologic assays need to be considered when interpreting results.

Humans have low levels of transient viremia and usually have neutralizing antibodies by the time distinctive clinical symptoms are recognized. Virus isolation and nucleic-acid amplification tests are insensitive in detecting JE virus or viral RNA in blood or CSF and should not be used for ruling out a diagnosis of JE. Clinicians should contact their state or local health department or CDC at 970-221-6400 for assistance with diagnostic testing.

TREATMENT

There is no specific antiviral treatment for JE; therapy consists of supportive care and management of complications.

PREVENTION
Personal Protection Measures

The best way to prevent mosquitoborne diseases, including JE, is to avoid mosquito bites (see Chapter 2, Protection against Mosquitoes, Ticks, & Other Arthropods).

Vaccine

One JE vaccine is licensed and available in the United States—an inactivated Vero cell culture–derived vaccine, Ixiaro (Table 3-6).

Table 3-6. Vaccine to prevent Japanese encephalitis (JE)

VACCINE	TRADE NAME (MANUFACTURER)	AGE	DOSE	ROUTE	SCHEDULE	BOOSTER[1]
JE vaccine, inactivated	Ixiaro (Valneva)	≥17 y	0.5 mL	IM	0, 28 d	≥1 y after primary series
		3–16 y	0.5 mL	IM	0, 28 d	Data not available
		2 mo–2 y	0.25 mL	IM	0, 28 d	Data not available

Abbreviation: IM, intramuscular.
[1]If potential for JE virus exposure continues.

Ixiaro is manufactured by Valneva Scotland Limited and distributed by Novartis Vaccines. It was approved in March 2009 for use in people aged ≥17 years and in May 2013 for use in children aged 2 months through 16 years. Other inactivated and live attenuated JE vaccines are manufactured and used in other countries but are not licensed for use in the United States.

Indications for Use of JE Vaccine for Travelers

When making recommendations regarding the use of JE vaccine for travelers, clinicians must weigh the overall low risk of travel-associated JE, the high rate of death and disability when JE occurs, the low probability of serious adverse events after immunization, and the cost of the vaccine. Evaluation of a traveler's risk should take into account the planned itinerary, including travel location, duration, activities, and seasonal patterns of disease in the areas to be visited (Table 3-7). The data in the table should be interpreted cautiously, because JE virus transmission activity varies within countries and from year to year.

The Advisory Committee on Immunization Practices recommends JE vaccine for travelers who plan to spend ≥1 month in endemic areas during the JE virus transmission season. This includes long-term travelers, recurrent travelers, or expatriates who will be based in urban areas but are likely to visit endemic rural or agricultural areas during a high-risk period of JE virus transmission. Vaccine should also be considered for the following:

- Short-term (<1 month) travelers to endemic areas during the JE virus transmission season, if they plan to travel outside an urban area and their activities will increase the risk of JE virus exposure. Examples of higher-risk activities or itineraries include 1) spending substantial time outdoors in rural or agricultural areas, especially during the evening or night; 2) participating in extensive outdoor activities (such as camping, hiking, trekking, biking, fishing, hunting, or farming); and 3) staying in accommodations without air conditioning, screens, or bed nets.

- Travelers to an area with an ongoing JE outbreak.
- Travelers to endemic areas who are uncertain of specific destinations, activities, or duration of travel.

JE vaccine is not recommended for short-term travelers whose visits will be restricted to urban areas or times outside a well-defined JE virus transmission season.

Vaccine Efficacy and Immunogenicity

There are no efficacy data for Ixiaro. The vaccine was licensed in the United States on the basis of its ability to induce JE virus neutralizing antibodies as a surrogate for protection, as well as safety evaluations in almost 5,000 adults. In pivotal immunogenicity studies, 96% of adults and 100% of children aged 2 months through 17 years developed protective neutralizing antibodies after receiving a primary immunization series of 2 doses administered 28 days apart.

The full duration of protection after primary immunization with Ixiaro is unknown. In a clinical trial assessing duration of protection, 83% of adults who received 2 doses of Ixiaro maintained protective levels of antibodies at 12 months after the first vaccine dose. In a second study, 58% and 48% of adults had protective antibodies at 12 and 24 months, respectively, and in a third, 69% of adults had protective antibodies at 15 months.

Vaccine Administration

The primary immunization schedule for Ixiaro is 2 doses administered intramuscularly on days 0 and 28 (Table 3-6). For children aged 2 months through 2 years, each dose is 0.25 mL, and for adults and children aged ≥3 years, each dose is 0.5 mL. To administer a 0.25-mL dose, health care providers must expel and discard half of the volume from the 0.5-mL prefilled syringe by pushing the plunger stopper up to the edge of the red line on the syringe barrel before injection. The 2-dose series should be completed ≥1 week before travel.

Booster Doses

For adults, if the primary series of Ixiaro was administered ≥1 year previously, a booster dose should be given before potential

Table 3-7. Risk for Japanese encephalitis (JE), by country[1]

COUNTRY	AFFECTED AREAS	TRANSMISSION SEASON	COMMENTS
Australia	Outer Torres Strait islands	December–May; all human cases reported February–April	1 human case reported from north Queensland mainland
Bangladesh	Presumed widespread	Most human cases reported May–October	Sentinel surveillance has identified human cases in Chittagong, Dhaka, Khulna, Rajshahi, Ranjpur, and Sylhet Divisions; highest incidence reported from Rajshahi Division; outbreak reported from Tangail District, Dhaka Division, in 1977
Bhutan	Very rare reports; probably endemic in nonmountainous areas	No data	Proximity to other endemic areas and presence of vectors suggests virus transmission is likely
Brunei	Very rare reports; presumed to be endemic countrywide	Unknown; presumed year-round	Proximity to other endemic areas suggests virus transmission is likely
Burma (Myanmar)	Limited data; presumed to be endemic countrywide	Unknown; most human cases reported May–October	Outbreaks of human disease documented in Shan State; antibodies documented in animals and humans in other areas
Cambodia	Presumed to be endemic countrywide	Year-round with peak season May–October	Sentinel surveillance has identified human cases in at least 15 of 23 provinces, including Phnom Penh, Takeo, Kampong Cham, Battambang, Svay Rieng, and Siem Reap; 1 case reported in 2010 in a traveler who visited Phnom Penh and Angkor Wat/Siem Reap only
China	Human cases reported from all provinces except Xizang (Tibet), Xinjiang, and Qinghai	Most human cases reported June–October	Highest rates reported from Guizhou, Shaanxi, Sichuan, and Yunnan Provinces, and Chongqing City; vaccine not routinely recommended for travel limited to Beijing, Shanghai, Hong Kong City/Kowloon, Macau, or other major cities

continued

COUNTRY	AFFECTED AREAS	TRANSMISSION SEASON	COMMENTS
India	Human cases reported from all states except Dadra, Daman, Diu, Gujarat, Himachal Pradesh, Jammu and Kashmir, Lakshadweep, Meghalaya, Nagar Haveli, Punjab, Rajasthan, and Sikkim	Most human cases reported May–October, especially in northern India; the season may be extended or year-round in some areas, especially in southern India	Highest rates of human disease reported from the states of Andhra Pradesh, Assam, Bihar, Goa, Haryana, Karnataka, Kerala, Tamil Nadu, Uttar Pradesh, and West Bengal
Indonesia	Presumed to be endemic countrywide	Year-round; peak season varies by island	Sentinel surveillance has identified human cases in Bali, Kalimantan, Java, Nusa Tenggara, Papua, and Sumatra
Japan[2]	Rare sporadic human cases on all islands except Hokkaido; enzootic activity ongoing	Most human cases reported July–October	Large number of human cases reported until JE vaccination program introduced in late 1960s; most recent small outbreak reported from Chugoku district in 2002; enzootic transmission without human cases observed on Hokkaido; vaccine not routinely recommended for travel limited to Tokyo or other major cities
Korea, North	Limited data; presumed to be endemic countrywide	No data; proximity to South Korea suggests peak season is likely to be May–October	
Korea, South[2]	Rare sporadic human cases countrywide; enzootic activity ongoing	Most human cases reported May–October	Large number of human cases reported until routine JE vaccination program introduced in mid-1980s; last major outbreak reported in 1982; vaccine not routinely recommended for travel limited to Seoul or other major cities
Laos	Limited data; presumed to be endemic countrywide	Year-round, with peak season June–September	Sentinel surveillance has identified human cases in north, central, and southern Laos

continued

COUNTRY	AFFECTED AREAS	TRANSMISSION SEASON	COMMENTS
Malaysia	Endemic in Sarawak; sporadic cases reported from all other states; occasional outbreaks reported	Year-round; in Sarawak, peak season October–December	Most human cases reported from Sarawak; vaccine not routinely recommended for travel limited to Kuala Lumpur or other major cities
Nepal	Endemic in southern lowlands (Terai); cases also reported from hill and mountain districts, including the Kathmandu valley	Most human cases reported June–October	Highest rates of human disease reported from western Terai districts, including Banke, Bardiya, Dang, and Kailali; vaccine not routinely recommended for those trekking in high-altitude areas
Pakistan	Limited data; human cases reported from around Karachi	Unknown	
Papua New Guinea	Limited data; probably widespread	Unknown; probably year-round	Sporadic human cases reported from Western Province; serologic evidence of disease from Gulf and Southern Highland Provinces; a case of JE was reported from near Port Moresby in 2004
Philippines	Limited data; presumed to be endemic on all islands	Year-round with peak season July–September	Outbreaks reported in Nueva Ecija and Manila; sentinel surveillance has identified human cases in other areas of Luzon and the Visayas
Russia	Rare human cases reported from the Far Eastern maritime areas south of Khabarovsk	Most human cases reported July–September	
Singapore	Rare sporadic human cases reported	Year-round	Vaccine not routinely recommended

continued

TABLE 3-7. RISK FOR JAPANESE ENCEPHALITIS (JE), BY COUNTRY[1] (continued)

COUNTRY	AFFECTED AREAS	TRANSMISSION SEASON	COMMENTS
Sri Lanka	Endemic countrywide except in mountainous areas	Year-round with variable peaks based on monsoon rains	Highest rates of human disease reported from Anuradhapura, Gampaha, Kurunegala, Polonnaruwa, and Puttalam districts
Taiwan[2]	Rare sporadic human cases islandwide	Most human cases reported May–October	Large number of human cases reported until routine JE vaccination introduced in 1968; vaccine not routinely recommended for travel limited to Taipei or other major cities
Thailand	Endemic countrywide; seasonal epidemics in the northern provinces	Year-round with peak season May–October, especially in the north	Highest rates of human disease reported from the Chiang Mai Valley; sporadic human cases reported from Bangkok suburbs; several cases reported recently in travelers who visited resort or coastal areas of southern Thailand
Timor-Leste	Sporadic human cases reported; presumed to be endemic countrywide	No data; cases reported year-round in neighboring West Timor	
Vietnam	Endemic countrywide; seasonal epidemics in the northern provinces	Year-round with peak season May–October, especially in the north	Highest rates of disease in the northern provinces around Hanoi and northwestern and northeastern provinces bordering China
Western Pacific Islands	Outbreaks of human disease reported in Guam in 1947–1948 and Saipan in 1990	Unknown; most human cases reported October–March	Enzootic cycle might not be sustainable; outbreaks may follow introductions of virus; vaccine not recommended

[1]Data are based on published reports and personal correspondence. Risk assessments should be performed cautiously, because risk can vary within areas and from year to year, and surveillance data regarding human cases and JE virus transmission are incomplete.
[2]In some endemic areas, human cases among residents are limited because of natural immunity among older people or vaccination. However, because JE virus is maintained in an enzootic cycle between animals and mosquitoes, susceptible visitors to these areas still may be at risk for infection.

reexposure or if there is a continued risk for JE virus infection. Data on the response to a booster dose administered ≥2 years after the primary series are not available. Data on the need for and timing of additional booster doses, and on the need for a booster dose in children, are also not available.

There are limited data on the use of Ixiaro as a booster dose after a primary series with the mouse brain–derived inactivated JE vaccine. Two studies have been conducted, 1 in US military personnel and the other at 2 travel clinics in Europe. Both studies demonstrated that in adults who had previously received at least a primary series of mouse brain–derived inactivated JE vaccine, a single dose of Ixiaro adequately boosted neutralizing antibody levels and provided at least short-term protection. In addition, seroprotective titers against both vaccine virus strains persisted in all participants who could be followed up at 2 years in the European study (N = 18). However, additional data are needed on the duration of protection after a single dose of Ixiaro in prior recipients of a mouse brain–derived vaccine. Until those data are available, people who have received JE-Vax, the mouse brain–derived vaccine formerly used in the United States, and require further vaccination against JE virus, should receive a 2-dose primary series of Ixiaro.

BIBLIOGRAPHY

Vaccine Safety and Adverse Reactions

Local symptoms of pain and tenderness were the most commonly reported symptoms in a safety study with 1,993 adult participants who received 2 doses of Ixiaro. Headache, myalgia, fatigue, and an influenzalike illness were each reported at a rate of >10%. In children, fever was the most commonly reported systemic reaction in studies.

Precautions and Contraindications

A severe allergic reaction after a previous dose of Ixiaro or any other JE vaccine, or to any component of Ixiaro, is a contraindication to administration of Ixiaro. Ixiaro contains protamine sulfate, a compound known to cause hypersensitivity reactions in some people. No studies of Ixiaro in pregnant women have been conducted. Therefore, administration of Ixiaro to pregnant women usually should be deferred. However, pregnant women who must travel to an area where risk for JE virus infection is high should be vaccinated when the theoretical risk of immunization is outweighed by the risk of infection.

CDC website: www.cdc.gov/japaneseencephalitis/

1. CDC. Japanese encephalitis vaccines: recommendations of the Advisory Committee on Immunization Practices (ACIP). MMWR Recomm Rep. 2010 Mar 12;59(RR-1):1–27.

2. CDC. Recommendations for use of a booster dose of inactivated Vero cell culture–derived Japanese encephalitis vaccine: advisory committee on immunization practices, 2011. MMWR Morb Mortal Wkly Rep. 2011 May 27;60(20):661–3.

3. CDC. Use of Japanese encephalitis vaccine in children: recommendations of the advisory committee on immunization practices, 2013. MMWR Morb Mortal Wkly Rep. 2013 Nov 15;62(45):898–900.

4. Hills SL, Griggs AC, Fischer M. Japanese encephalitis in travelers from non-endemic countries, 1973–2008. Am J Trop Med Hyg. 2010 May;82(5):930–6.

5. Hills SL, Stoltey J, Martinez D, Kim PY, Sheriff H, Zangeneh A, et al. A case series of three US adults with Japanese encephalitis, 2010–2012. J Travel Med. 2014 Sep;21(5):310–3.

6. Schuller E, Klingler A, Dubischar-Kastner K, Dewasthaly S, Muller Z. Safety profile of the Vero cell–derived Japanese encephalitis virus (JEV) vaccine IXIARO®. Vaccine. 2011 Nov 3;29(47):8669–76.

7. Tauber E, Kollaritsch H, Korinek M, Rendi-Wagner P, Jilma B, Firbas C, et al. Safety and immunogenicity of a Vero-cell-derived, inactivated Japanese encephalitis vaccine: a non-inferiority, phase III, randomised controlled trial. Lancet. 2007 Dec 1;370(9602):1847–53.

8. Tauber E, Kollaritsch H, von Sonnenburg F, Lademann M, Jilma B, Firbas C, et al. Randomized, double-blind, placebo-controlled phase 3 trial of the safety and tolerability of IC51, an inactivated Japanese encephalitis vaccine. J Infect Dis. 2008 Aug 15;198(4):493–9.

9. Woolpert T, Staples JE, Faix DJ, Nett RJ, Kosoy OI, Biggerstaff BJ, et al. Immunogenicity of one dose of Vero cell culture–derived Japanese encephalitis (JE) vaccine in adults previously vaccinated with mouse brain–derived JE vaccine. Vaccine. 2012 Apr 26;30(20):3090–6.

LEGIONELLOSIS (LEGIONNAIRES' DISEASE & PONTIAC FEVER)

Laurel E. Garrison, Preeta K. Kutty

INFECTIOUS AGENT

Gram-negative bacteria of the genus *Legionella*. Most cases of legionellosis are caused by *Legionella pneumophila,* but all species of *Legionella* can cause disease.

TRANSMISSION

Inhalation of a water aerosol containing the bacteria. The bacterium grows in warm freshwater environments. Person-to-person transmission does not occur with either Legionnaires' disease or Pontiac fever.

EPIDEMIOLOGY

Legionellae are ubiquitous worldwide. Disease occurs after exposure to aquatic settings that promote bacterial growth—the aquatic environment is somewhat stagnant, the water is warm (77°F–108°F [25°C–42°C]), and the water must be aerosolized so that the bacteria can be inhaled into the lungs. These 3 conditions are met almost exclusively in developed or industrialized settings. Disease does not occur in association with natural freshwater settings such as waterfalls, lakes, or streams.

Legionellosis has been reported worldwide. The largest outbreak (449 cases) ever reported was traced to a cooling tower on the roof of a city hospital in Murcia, Spain, in 2001. Travel-associated outbreaks are commonly recognized.

Despite the presence of *Legionella* bacteria in many aquatic environments, the risk of developing legionellosis for most people is low. Travelers who are exposed to aerosolized, warm water containing *Legionella* are at risk for infection. Travelers who are aged >50 years, are current or former smokers, have chronic lung conditions, or are immunocompromised are at higher risk. Many outbreaks have been associated with exposure to cruise ships, hotels, and resorts. Exposures can occur when a person is in or near a whirlpool spa, showering in a hotel, standing near a decorative fountain, or touring in cities with buildings that have cooling towers. Patients often do not recall specific water exposures, as they frequently occur during normal activities.

CLINICAL PRESENTATION

Legionnaires' disease typically presents with pneumonia, which usually requires hospitalization and can be fatal in 10%–15% of cases. Symptom onset occurs 2–14 days after exposure. In outbreak settings, <5% of people exposed to the source of the outbreak develop Legionnaires' disease.

Pontiac fever is milder than Legionnaires' disease and presents as an influenzalike illness, with fever, headache, and muscle aches, but no signs of pneumonia. Pontiac fever can affect healthy people, as well as those with underlying illnesses, and symptoms occur within 72 hours of exposure. Most patients fully recover. Up to 95% of people exposed in outbreak settings can develop symptoms of Pontiac fever.

DIAGNOSIS

Isolation of *Legionella* from respiratory secretions, lung tissue, pleural fluid, or a normally sterile site is an important method for diagnosis of Legionnaires' disease. Clinical isolates are often necessary to interpret the findings of an investigation through comparison with isolates obtained from environmental sources. Because of differences in mechanism of disease, *Legionella* cannot be isolated in people who have Pontiac fever.

The most used diagnostic method is the *Legionella* urinary antigen assay. However, the assay can only detect *L. pneumophila* serogroup 1, the most common cause of legionellosis. Paired serology showing a 4-fold rise in antibody titer between acute- and convalescent-phase specimens also confirms the diagnosis. A single antibody titer of any level is not diagnostic of legionellosis. Other diagnostic tests include direct fluorescent antibody and PCR.

TREATMENT

For travelers with suspected Legionnaires' disease, specific antibiotic treatment is necessary and should be administered promptly while diagnostic tests are being processed. Appropriate antibiotics include fluoroquinolones and macrolides. Treatment may be necessary for up to 3 weeks. In severe cases, patients may have prolonged stays in intensive care units. Consultation with an infectious disease specialist is advised. Pontiac fever is a self-limited illness that requires supportive care only; antibiotics have no benefit.

PREVENTION

There is no vaccine for legionellosis, and antibiotic prophylaxis is not effective. Travelers at increased risk for infection, such as the elderly or those with immunocompromising conditions such as cancer or diabetes, may choose to avoid high-risk areas, such as whirlpool spas. If exposure cannot be avoided, travelers should be advised to seek medical attention promptly if they develop symptoms of Legionnaires' disease or Pontiac fever.

CDC website: www.cdc.gov/legionella

BIBLIOGRAPHY

1. Burnsed LJ, Hicks LA, Smithee LM, Fields BS, Bradley KK, Pascoe N, et al. A large, travel-associated outbreak of legionellosis among hotel guests: utility of the urine antigen assay in confirming Pontiac fever. Clin Infect Dis. 2007 Jan 15;44(2):222–8.
2. CDC. Surveillance for travel-associated Legionnaires' disease—United States, 2005–2006. MMWR Morb Mortal Wkly Rep. 2007 Dec 7;56(48):1261–3.
3. de Jong B, Payne Hallstrom L, Robesyn E, Ursut D, Zucs P, Eldsnet. Travel-associated Legionnaires' disease in Europe, 2010. Euro Surveill. 2013;18(23):1–8.
4. Fields BS, Benson RF, Besser RE. *Legionella* and Legionnaires' disease: 25 years of investigation. Clin Microbiol Rev. 2002 Jul;15(3):506–26.
5. Garcia-Fulgueiras A, Navarro C, Fenoll D, Garcia J, Gonzalez-Diego P, Jimenez-Bunuales T, et al. Legionnaires' disease outbreak in Murcia, Spain. Emerg Infect Dis. 2003 Aug;9(8):915–21.
6. Guyard C, Low DE. *Legionella* infections and travel associated legionellosis. Travel Med Infect Dis. 2011 Jul;9(4):176–86.
7. Silk BJ, Moore MR, Bergtholdt M, Gorwitz RJ, Kozak NA, Tha MM, et al. Eight years of Legionnaires' disease transmission in travellers to a condominium complex in Las Vegas, Nevada. Epidemiol Infect. 2012 Nov;140(11):1993–2002.

LEISHMANIASIS, CUTANEOUS

Barbara L. Herwaldt, Alan J. Magill

Leishmaniasis is a parasitic disease found in parts of the tropics, subtropics, and southern Europe. Leishmaniasis has several different forms. This section focuses on cutaneous leishmaniasis (CL), the most common form, both in general and in travelers.

INFECTIOUS AGENT

Leishmaniasis is caused by obligate intracellular protozoan parasites; approximately 20 *Leishmania* species cause CL.

TRANSMISSION

CL is transmitted through the bite of an infected female phlebotomine sand fly. CL also can occur after accidental occupational (laboratory) exposures to *Leishmania* parasites.

EPIDEMIOLOGY

In the Old World (Eastern Hemisphere), CL is found in parts of the Middle East, Asia (particularly southwest and central Asia), Africa (particularly the tropical region and North Africa), and southern Europe. In the New World (Western Hemisphere), CL is found in parts of Mexico, Central America, and South America. Occasional cases have been reported in Texas and Oklahoma. CL is not found in Chile, Uruguay, or Canada. Overall, CL is found in focal areas of >90 countries.

The geographic distribution of cases of CL evaluated in countries such as the United States reflects travel and immigration patterns. More than 75% of the cases diagnosed in US civilians have been acquired in Latin America, including popular tourist destinations such as Costa Rica. Cases in US service personnel have reflected military activities (such as in Afghanistan and Iraq). CL is usually more common in rural than urban areas, but it is found in some periurban and urban areas (such as in Kabul, Afghanistan). The ecologic settings range from rainforests to arid regions.

The risk is highest from dusk to dawn because sand flies typically feed (bite) at night and during twilight hours. Although sand flies are less active during the hottest time of the day, they may bite if they are disturbed (for example, if hikers brush against tree trunks or other sites where sand flies are resting). Vector activity can easily be overlooked: sand flies do not make noise, they are small (approximately one-third the size of mosquitoes), and their bites might not be noticed.

Examples of types of travelers who might have an increased risk for CL include ecotourists, adventure travelers, bird watchers, Peace Corps volunteers, missionaries, military personnel, construction workers, and people who do research outdoors at night or twilight. However, even short-term travelers in endemic areas have developed CL.

CLINICAL PRESENTATION

CL is characterized by skin lesions (open or closed sores), which typically develop within several weeks or months after exposure. In some people, the sores first appear months or years later, in the context of trauma (such as skin wounds or surgery). The sores can change in size and appearance over time. They typically progress from small papules to nodular plaques, and often lead to open sores with a raised border and central crater

(ulcer), which can be covered with scales or crust. The lesions usually are painless but can be painful, particularly if open sores become infected with bacteria. Satellite lesions, regional lymphadenopathy and nodular lymphangitis can be noted. The sores usually heal eventually, even without treatment. However, they can last for months or years and typically result in scarring.

A potential concern applies to some of the *Leishmania* species in South and Central America: some parasites can spread from the skin to the mucosal surfaces of the nose or mouth and cause sores there. This form of leishmaniasis, mucosal leishmaniasis (ML), might not be noticed until years after the original skin sores appear to have healed. Although ML is uncommon, it has occurred in travelers and expatriates whose cases of CL were not treated or were inadequately treated. The initial clinical manifestations typically involve the nose (chronic stuffiness, bleeding, and inflamed mucosa or sores) and less often the mouth; in advanced cases, ulcerative destruction of the nose, mouth, and pharynx can be noted (such as perforation of the nasal septum).

DIAGNOSIS

Clinicians should consider CL in people with chronic (nonhealing) skin lesions who have been in areas where leishmaniasis is found. Laboratory confirmation of the diagnosis is achieved by detecting *Leishmania* parasites (or DNA) in infected tissue, through light-microscopic examination of stained specimens, culture techniques, or molecular methods.

CDC can assist in all aspects of the diagnostic evaluation. Identification of the *Leishmania* species can be important, particularly if >1 species is found where the patient traveled and if the species can have different clinical and prognostic implications. Serologic testing generally is not useful for CL but can provide supportive evidence for the diagnosis of ML.

For consultative services, contact CDC Parasitic Diseases Inquiries (404-718-4745; parasites@cdc.gov).

TREATMENT

Decisions about whether and how to treat CL should be individualized, including whether to use a systemic (oral or parenteral) medication rather than a local or topical approach. All cases of ML should be treated with systemic therapy. Clinicians may consult with CDC staff about the relative merits of various approaches to treat CL and ML (see the Diagnosis section above for contact information). The response to a particular regimen may vary not only among *Leishmania* species but also for the same species in different geographic regions.

In March 2014, the Food and Drug Administration (FDA) approved the oral agent miltefosine to treat New World CL caused by 3 species in the *Viannia* subgenus [*Leishmania* (V.) *braziliensis*, *L.* (V.) *panamensis*, and *L.* (V.) *guyanensis*] and ML caused by *L.* (V.) *braziliensis* in adults and adolescents ≥12 years of age who weigh ≥30 kg and who are not pregnant or breastfeeding.

Various parenteral options (such as liposomal amphotericin B) are commercially available, although not FDA-approved to treat CL or ML. The pentavalent antimonial compound sodium stibogluconate (Pentostam) is available to US-licensed physicians through the CDC Drug Service (404-639-3670) for intravenous or intramuscular administration under an investigational new drug protocol (see www.cdc.gov/laboratory/drugservice/index.html).

PREVENTION

No vaccines or drugs to prevent infection are available. Preventive measures are aimed at reducing contact with sand flies by using personal protective measures (see Chapter 2, Protection against Mosquitoes, Ticks, & Other Arthropods). Travelers should be advised to

- Avoid outdoor activities, to the extent possible, especially from dusk to dawn, when sand flies generally are the most active.
- Wear protective clothing and apply insect repellent to exposed skin and under the edges of clothing, such as sleeves and pant legs, according to the manufacturer's instructions.
- Sleep in air-conditioned or well-screened areas. Spraying the quarters with insecticide might provide some protection. Fans or ventilators might inhibit the movement of sand flies, which are weak fliers.

Sand flies are so small (approximately 2–3 mm, less than one-eighth of an inch) that they can pass through the holes in ordinary bed nets. Although closely woven nets are available, they may be uncomfortable in hot climates. The effectiveness of bed nets can be enhanced by treatment with a pyrethroid-containing insecticide. The same treatment can be applied to window screens, curtains, bed sheets, and clothing.

C.DC website: www.cdc.gov/parasites/leishmaniasis

BIBLIOGRAPHY

1. Blum J, Buffet P, Visser L, Harms G, Bailey MS, Caumes E, et al. LeishMan recommendations for treatment of cutaneous and mucosal leishmaniasis in travelers, 2014. J Travel Med. 2014 Mar–Apr;21(2):116–29.
2. Blum J, Lockwood DN, Visser L, Harms G, Bailey MS, Caumes E, et al. Local or systemic treatment for New World cutaneous leishmaniasis? Re-evaluating the evidence for the risk of mucosal leishmaniasis. Int Health. 2012 Sep;4(3):153–63.
3. Magill AJ. Cutaneous leishmaniasis in the returning traveler. Infect Dis Clin North Am. 2005 Mar;19(1): x–xi, 241–66.
4. Murray HW. Leishmaniasis in the United States: treatment in 2012. Am J Trop Med Hyg. 2012 Mar;86(3):434–40.
5. Murray HW, Berman JD, Davies CR, Saravia NG. Advances in leishmaniasis. Lancet. 2005 Oct 29–Nov 4;366(9496):1561–77.
6. Schwartz E, Hatz C, Blum J. New World cutaneous leishmaniasis in travellers. Lancet Infect Dis. 2006 Jun;6(6):342–9.
7. World Health Organization. Control of the leishmaniases. Geneva: World Health Organization; 2010 [cited 2014 Sep 21]. Available from: http://whqlibdoc.who.int/trs/WHO_TRS_949_eng.pdf.

LEISHMANIASIS, VISCERAL

Barbara L. Herwaldt, Alan J. Magill

Leishmaniasis is a parasitic disease found in parts of the tropics, subtropics, and southern Europe. Leishmaniasis has several different forms. This section focuses on visceral leishmaniasis (VL), which affects some of the internal organs of the body (such as the spleen, liver, and bone marrow).

INFECTIOUS AGENT

VL is caused by obligate intracellular protozoan parasites, particularly by the species *Leishmania donovani* and *L. infantum/L. chagasi*.

TRANSMISSION

VL is predominantly transmitted through the bite of an infected female phlebotomine sand fly, although congenital and parenteral transmission (through blood transfusions and needle sharing) have been reported.

EPIDEMIOLOGY

VL is usually more common in rural than urban areas, but it is found in some periurban areas (such as in northeastern Brazil). In the Old World (Eastern Hemisphere), VL is found in parts of Asia (particularly the Indian subcontinent and southwest and central Asia), the Middle East, Africa (particularly East Africa), and southern Europe. In the New World (Western Hemisphere), most cases occur in Brazil; some cases occur in scattered foci elsewhere in Latin America. Overall, VL is found in focal areas of >60 countries. Most (>90%) of the world's cases of VL occur in the Indian subcontinent (India and Bangladesh; also Nepal), East Africa (Sudan, South Sudan, and Ethiopia), and Brazil; none of the affected areas in these 7 countries are common tourist destinations.

The geographic distribution of cases of VL evaluated in countries such as the United States reflects travel and immigration patterns. VL is uncommon in US travelers and expatriates. Occasional cases have been diagnosed in short-term travelers (tourists) to southern Europe and also in longer-term travelers (such as expatriates and deployed soldiers) to the Mediterranean region and other areas where VL is found.

CLINICAL PRESENTATION

Among symptomatic people, the incubation period typically ranges from weeks to months. The onset of illness can be abrupt or gradual. Stereotypical manifestations of VL include fever, weight loss, hepatosplenomegaly (especially splenomegaly), and pancytopenia (anemia, leukopenia, and thrombocytopenia). If untreated, severe (advanced) cases of VL typically are fatal. Latent infection can become clinically manifest years to decades after exposure in people who become immunocompromised for other medical reasons (such as HIV infection).

DIAGNOSIS

Clinicians should consider VL in people with a relevant travel history (even in the distant past) and a persistent, unexplained febrile illness, especially if accompanied by other suggestive manifestations (such as splenomegaly and pancytopenia). Laboratory confirmation of the diagnosis is achieved by detecting *Leishmania* parasites (or DNA) in infected tissue (such as in bone marrow, liver, lymph node, or blood), through light-microscopic examination of stained specimens, culture techniques, or molecular methods. Serologic testing can provide supportive evidence for the diagnosis.

CDC can assist in all aspects of the diagnostic evaluation, including species identification. For consultative services, contact CDC Parasitic Diseases Inquiries (404-718-4745; parasites@cdc.gov) or see www.dpd.cdc.gov/dpdx.

TREATMENT

Infected travelers should be advised to consult an infectious disease or tropical medicine specialist. Therapy for VL should be individualized with expert consultation. The relative merits of various approaches can be discussed with CDC staff (see the Diagnosis section above for contact information).

Liposomal amphotericin B (AmBisome) is approved by the Food and Drug Administration (FDA) to treat VL and generally constitutes the drug of choice for US patients. In March 2014, FDA approved the oral agent miltefosine to treat VL in patients who are infected with *L. donovani*, are ≥12 years of age, weigh ≥30 kg, and are not pregnant or breastfeeding. The pentavalent antimonial compound sodium stibogluconate (Pentostam) is available to US-licensed physicians through the CDC Drug Service (404-639-3670) under an investigational new drug protocol (see www.cdc.gov/laboratory/drugservice/index.html).

PREVENTION

No vaccines or drugs to prevent infection are available. Preventive measures are aimed at reducing contact with sand flies (see Chapter 2, Protection against Mosquitoes, Ticks, & Other Arthropods; and Prevention in the previous section, Cutaneous Leishmaniasis). Preventive measures include minimizing outdoor activities, to the extent possible, especially from dusk to dawn, when sand flies generally are the most active; wearing protective clothing; applying insect repellent to exposed skin; using bed nets treated with a pyrethroid-containing insecticide; and spraying dwellings with residual-action insecticides.

CDC website: www.cdc.gov/parasites/leishmaniasis

BIBLIOGRAPHY

1. Malik AN, John L, Bryceson AD, Lockwood DN. Changing pattern of visceral leishmaniasis, United Kingdom, 1985–2004. Emerg Infect Dis. 2006 Aug;12(8):1257–9.
2. Murray HW. Leishmaniasis in the United States: treatment in 2012. Am J Trop Med Hyg. 2012 Mar;86(3):434–40.
3. Murray HW, Berman JD, Davies CR, Saravia NG. Advances in leishmaniasis. Lancet. 2005 Oct 29–Nov 4;366(9496):1561–77.
4. Myles O, Wortmann GW, Cummings JF, Barthel RV, Patel S, Crum-Cianflone NF, et al. Visceral leishmaniasis: clinical observations in 4 US army soldiers deployed to Afghanistan or Iraq, 2002–2004. Arch Intern Med. 2007 Sep 24;167(17):1899–901.
5. Pavli A, Maltezou HC. Leishmaniasis, an emerging infection in travelers. Int J Infect Dis. 2010 Dec;14(12):e1032–9.
6. Weisser M, Khanlari B, Terracciano L, Arber C, Gratwohl A, Bassetti S, et al. Visceral leishmaniasis: a threat to immunocompromised patients in non-endemic areas? Clin Microbiol Infect. 2007 Aug;13(8):751–3.
7. World Health Organization. Control of the leishmaniases. Geneva: World Health Organization; 2010 [cited 2014 Sep 21]. Available from: http://whqlibdoc.who.int/trs/WHO_TRS_949_eng.pdf.

LEPTOSPIROSIS

Robyn A. Stoddard, Renee L. Galloway, Marta A. Guerra

INFECTIOUS AGENT

Obligate aerobic spirochete bacteria in the genus *Leptospira*.

TRANSMISSION

Infection occurs through abrasions or cuts in the skin, or through the conjunctiva and mucous membranes. Humans may be infected by direct contact with urine or reproductive fluids from infected animals, or with water or soil contaminated with those fluids. Prolonged immersion in contaminated water increases the risk for infection. Infection rarely occurs through animal bites or human-to-human contact.

EPIDEMIOLOGY

Leptospirosis has worldwide distribution, with a higher incidence in tropical climates, especially after heavy rainfall or flooding due to hurricanes. Outbreaks of leptospirosis have occurred in the United States after flooding in Hawaii and Puerto Rico. Travelers participating in recreational water activities are at increased risk, particularly after heavy rainfall or flooding.

CLINICAL PRESENTATION

The incubation period is 2 days to 3 weeks. The acute phase (approximately 7 days) presents as an acute febrile illness with symptoms including headache (can be severe and include retroorbital pain and photophobia), fever, chills, myalgia, nausea, diarrhea, abdominal pain, uveitis, conjunctival suffusion, and occasionally, a skin rash. The second or immune phase is characterized by antibody production and the presence of leptospires in the urine. The icteric or severe form of the disease (Weil disease) occurs in 5%–10% of patients with leptospirosis. Symptoms include jaundice, renal failure, hemorrhage (especially pulmonary), cardiac arrhythmias, pneumonitis, and hemodynamic collapse.

DIAGNOSIS

Diagnosis of leptospirosis is usually based on clinical recognition and serology; microscopic agglutination test is the gold standard. Culture is relatively insensitive, but detection of the organism using real-time PCR can provide a more timely diagnosis.

TREATMENT

Doxycycline is effective in decreasing the severity and duration of leptospirosis and should be initiated early, without waiting for confirmatory test results, if leptospirosis is suspected. Intravenous penicillin is a drug of choice for patients with severe leptospirosis. Patients with severe leptospirosis may require hospitalization, supportive therapy, and close monitoring.

PREVENTION

No vaccine is available in the United States. Travelers who might be at an increased risk for infection should be advised to consider preventive measures such as chemoprophylaxis; wearing protective clothing, especially footwear; and covering cuts and abrasions with occlusive dressings. Until further data become available, CDC recommends chemoprophylaxis with doxycycline (200 mg orally, weekly), begun 1–2 days before and continuing through the period of exposure for people at high risk of leptospirosis. Doxycycline is not recommended for pregnant women or children aged <8 years.

CDC website: www.cdc.gov/leptospirosis

BIBLIOGRAPHY

1. Bajani MD, Ashford DA, Bragg SL, Woods CW, Aye T, Spiegel RA, et al. Evaluation of four commercially available rapid serologic tests for diagnosis of leptospirosis. J Clin Microbiol. 2003 Feb;41(2):803–9.
2. CDC. Outbreak of leptospirosis among white-water rafters—Costa Rica, 1996. MMWR Morb Mortal Wkly Rep. 1997 Jun 27;46(25):577–9.
3. Haake DA, Dundoo M, Cader R, Kubak BM, Hartskeerl RA, Sejvar JJ, et al. Leptospirosis, water sports, and chemoprophylaxis. Clin Infect Dis. 2002 May 1;34(9):e40–3.
4. Jensenius M, Han PV, Schlagenhauf P, Schwartz E, Parola P, Castelli F, et al. Acute and potentially life-threatening tropical diseases in western travelers—a GeoSentinel multicenter study, 1996–2011. Am J Trop Med Hyg. 2013 Feb;88(2):397–404.
5. Katz AR, Sasaki DM, Mumm AH, Escamilla J, Middleton CR, Romero SE. Leptospirosis on Oahu: an outbreak among military personnel associated with recreational exposure. Mil Med. 1997 Feb;162(2):101–4.
6. Levett PN. Leptospirosis. Clin Microbiol Rev. 2001 Apr;14(2):296–326.
7. Pappas G, Cascio A. Optimal treatment of leptospirosis: queries and projections. Int J Antimicrob Agents. 2006 Dec;28(6):491–6.
8. Sejvar J, Bancroft E, Winthrop K, Bettinger J, Bajani M, Bragg S, et al. Leptospirosis in "Eco-Challenge" athletes, Malaysian Borneo, 2000. Emerg Infect Dis. 2003 Jun;9(6):702–7.
9. Stoddard RA, Gee JE, Wilkins PP, McCaustland K, Hoffmaster AR. Detection of pathogenic *Leptospira* spp. through TaqMan polymerase chain reaction targeting the LipL32 gene. Diagn Microbiol Infect Dis. 2009 Jul;64(3):247–55.
10. van de Werve C, Perignon A, Jaureguiberry S, Bricaire F, Bourhy P, Caumes E. Travel-related leptospirosis: a series of 15 imported cases. J Travel Med. 2013 Jul–Aug;20(4):228–31.

LYME DISEASE

Paul S. Mead

INFECTIOUS AGENT

Spirochetes belonging to the *Borrelia burgdorferi* sensu lato complex, including B. *afzelii*, B. *burgdorferi* sensu stricto, and B. *garinii*.

TRANSMISSION

Through the bite of *Ixodes* ticks; infected people are often unaware that they have been bitten.

EPIDEMIOLOGY

In Europe, endemic from southern Scandinavia into the northern Mediterranean countries of Italy, Spain, and Greece and eastward from the British Isles into central Russia. Incidence is highest in central and Eastern European countries. In Asia, infected ticks occur from western Russia through Mongolia, northeastern China, and in Japan; human infection appears to be uncommon in most of these areas. In North America, highly endemic areas are the northeastern and north-central United States. Transmission has not been documented in the tropics. Lyme disease is rarely reported in returning travelers but should be considered in those with consistent symptoms and a history of hiking or camping.

CLINICAL PRESENTATION

Incubation period is typically 3–30 days. Approximately 80% of people infected with B. *burgdorferi* develop a characteristic rash, erythema migrans (EM), within 30 days of exposure. EM is a red, expanding rash, with or without central clearing, that is often accompanied by symptoms of fatigue, fever, headache, mild stiff neck, arthralgia, or myalgia. Within days or weeks, infection can spread to other parts of the body, causing more serious neurologic conditions (meningitis, radiculopathy, and facial palsy) or cardiac abnormalities (myocarditis with atrioventricular heart block). Untreated, infection can progress over a period of months to cause monoarticular or oligoarticular arthritis, peripheral neuropathy, or encephalopathy. These long-term sequelae can be typically observed over a number of months, ranging from 1 week to a few years.

DIAGNOSIS

Observation of an EM rash with a history of recent travel to an endemic area (with or without history of tick bite) is sufficient. For patients with evidence of disseminated infection (musculoskeletal, neurologic, or cardiac manifestations), 2-tiered serologic testing, consisting of an ELISA/IFA and confirmatory Western blot, is recommended. Patients suspected of acquiring Lyme disease overseas should be tested by using a C6-based ELISA, as other serologic tests may not detect infection with European species of *Borrelia*.

TREATMENT

Most patients can be treated with either oral doxycycline or intravenous ceftriaxone.

PREVENTION

Avoid tick habitats, use insect repellent on exposed skin and clothing, and carefully check every day for attached ticks. Minimize areas of exposed skin by wearing long-sleeved shirts, long pants, and closed shoes; tucking shirts in and tucking pants into socks may also reduce risk (see Chapter 2, Protection against Mosquitoes, Ticks, & Other Arthropods).

CDC website: www.cdc.gov/lyme

BIBLIOGRAPHY

1. Hao Q, Hou X, Geng Z, Wan K. Distribution of *Borrelia burgdorferi* sensu lato in China. J Clin Microbiol. 2011 Feb;49(2):647–50.
2. Hubalek Z. Epidemiology of lyme borreliosis. Curr Probl Dermatol. 2009;37:31–50.
3. Masuzawa T. Terrestrial distribution of the Lyme borreliosis agent *Borrelia burgdorferi* sensu lato in East Asia. Jpn J Infect Dis. 2004 Dec;57(6):229–35.
4. O'Connell S. Lyme borreliosis: current issues in diagnosis and management. Curr Opin Infect Dis. 2010 Jun;23(3):231–5.
5. Stanek G, Strle F. Lyme disease: European perspective. Infect Dis Clin North Am. 2008 Jun;22(2):327–39.
6. Steere AC. Lyme disease. N Engl J Med. 2001 Jul 12;345(2):115–25.
7. Wormser GP, Dattwyler RJ, Shapiro ED, Halperin JJ, Steere AC, Klempner MS, et al. The clinical assessment, treatment, and prevention of Lyme disease, human granulocytic anaplasmosis, and babesiosis: clinical practice guidelines by the Infectious Diseases Society of America. Clin Infect Dis. 2006 Nov 1;43(9):1089–134.

MALARIA

Paul M. Arguin, Kathrine R. Tan

INFECTIOUS AGENT

Malaria in humans is caused by protozoan parasites of the genus *Plasmodium: Plasmodium falciparum*, *P. vivax*, *P. ovale*, or *P. malariae*. In addition, *P. knowlesi*, a parasite of Old World (Eastern Hemisphere) monkeys, has been documented as a cause of human infections and some deaths in Southeast Asia.

TRANSMISSION

All species are transmitted by the bite of an infective female *Anopheles* mosquito. Occasionally, transmission occurs by blood transfusion, organ transplantation, needle sharing, or congenitally from mother to fetus.

EPIDEMIOLOGY

Malaria is a major international public health problem, causing an estimated 207 million infections worldwide and 627,000 deaths in 2012, according to the World Health Organization (WHO) World Malaria report 2013. Although these numbers are decreasing, the numbers of cases of malaria in travelers has been increasing steadily for the past 4 years. Despite the apparent progress in reducing the global prevalence of malaria, many areas remain malaria endemic, and the use of prevention measures by travelers is still inadequate. Information about malaria transmission in specific countries (see Yellow Fever & Malaria Information, by Country later in this chapter) is derived from various sources, including WHO. The information presented herein was accurate at the time of publication; however, factors that can change rapidly and from year to year (such as local weather conditions, mosquito vector density, and prevalence of infection) can markedly affect local malaria transmission patterns. Updated information may be found on the CDC website at www.cdc.gov/malaria. Tools such as the Malaria Map Application can assist in locating more unusual destinations and determining if malaria transmission occurs there (www.cdc.gov/malaria/map).

Malaria transmission occurs in large areas of Africa, Latin America, parts of the Caribbean, Asia (including South Asia, Southeast Asia, and the Middle East), Eastern Europe, and the South Pacific (Maps 3-9 and 3-10).

The risk for acquiring malaria differs substantially from traveler to traveler and from region to region, even within a single country. This variability is a function of the intensity of transmission within the various regions and the itinerary, duration, season, and type of travel. In 2012, almost 1,700 cases of malaria (including 6 deaths)

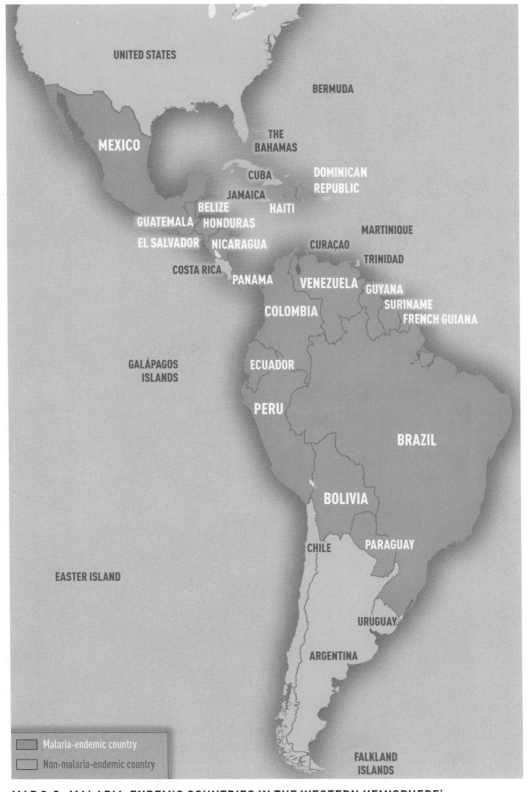

MAP 3-9. MALARIA-ENDEMIC COUNTRIES IN THE WESTERN HEMISPHERE[1]

[1] In this map, countries with areas endemic for malaria are shaded completely even if transmission occurs only in a small part of the country. For more specific within-country malaria transmission information, see the Yellow Fever & Malaria Information, by Country section in this chapter.

 MALARIA | 237

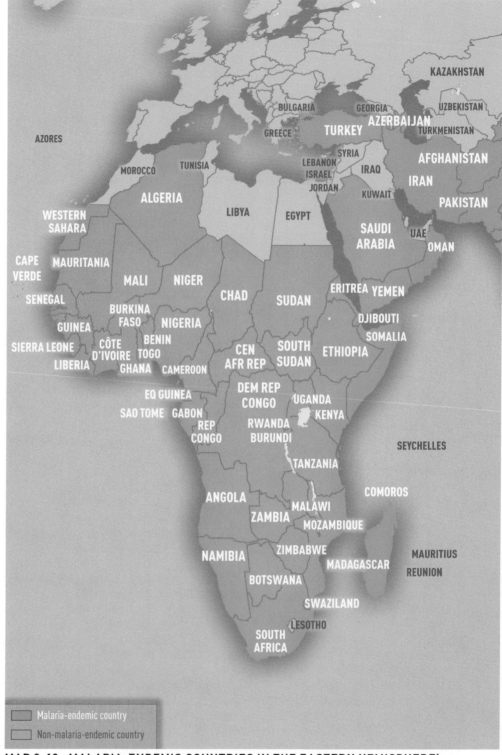

MAP 3-10. MALARIA-ENDEMIC COUNTRIES IN THE EASTERN HEMISPHERE[1]

[1] In this map, countries with areas endemic for malaria are shaded completely even if transmission occurs only in a small part of the country. For more specific within-country malaria transmission information, see the Yellow Fever & Malaria Information, by Country section in this chapter.

BOX 3-2. CLINICAL HIGHLIGHTS FOR MALARIA

- Overdose of antimalarial drugs, particularly chloroquine, can be fatal. Medication should be stored in childproof containers out of the reach of infants and children.
- Chemoprophylaxis can be started earlier if there are particular concerns about tolerating a medication. For example, mefloquine can be started 3–4 weeks in advance to allow potential adverse events to occur before travel. If unacceptable side effects develop, there would be time to change the medication before the traveler's departure.
- The drugs used for antimalarial chemoprophylaxis are generally well tolerated. However, side effects can occur. Minor side effects usually do not require stopping the drug. Travelers who have serious side effects should see a clinician who can determine if their symptoms are related to the medicine and make a medication change.
- In comparison with drugs with short half-lives, which are taken daily, drugs with longer half-lives, which are taken weekly, offer the advantage of a wider margin of error if the traveler is late with a dose. For example, if a traveler is 1–2 days late with a weekly drug, prophylactic blood levels can remain adequate; if the traveler is 1–2 days late with a daily drug, protective blood levels are less likely to be maintained.
- In those who are glucose-6-phosphate dehydrogenase (G6PD) deficient, primaquine can cause hemolysis, which can be fatal. Be sure to document a normal G6PD level before prescribing primaquine.
- Travelers should be informed that malaria could be fatal if treatment is delayed. Medical help should be sought promptly if malaria is suspected, and a blood sample should be taken and examined for malaria parasites on 1 or more occasions.
- Travelers should also be informed that malaria could be fatal even when treated, which is why it is always preferable to prevent malaria cases rather than rely on treating infections after they occur.
- Malaria smear results or a rapid diagnostic test must be available immediately (within a few hours). Sending specimens to offsite laboratories where results are not available for extended periods of time (days) is not acceptable. If a patient has an illness suggestive of severe malaria and a compatible travel history in an area where malaria transmission occurs, it is advisable to start treatment as soon as possible, even before the diagnosis is established. CDC recommendations for malaria treatment can be found at www.cdc.gov/malaria/diagnosis_treatment/index.html.

diagnosed in the United States and its territories were reported to CDC. Of these, 79% were acquired in Africa, 13% in Asia, 7% in the Caribbean and the Americas, and <1% in Oceania. These absolute numbers of cases should be considered in the context of the volume of travel to these locations. Travelers with the highest estimated relative risk for infection are those going to West Africa and Oceania. Travelers going to other parts of Africa, South Asia, and South America have a moderate estimated relative risk for infection. Travelers with lower estimated relative risk are those going to Mexico, Central America, and other parts of Asia.

CLINICAL PRESENTATION

Malaria is characterized by fever and influenzalike symptoms, including chills, headache, myalgias, and malaise; these symptoms can occur at intervals. Uncomplicated disease may be associated with anemia and jaundice. In severe disease, seizures, mental confusion, kidney failure, acute respiratory distress syndrome, coma, and death may occur. Malaria symptoms can develop as early as 7 days (usually ≥14 days) after initial exposure in a malaria-endemic area and as late as several months or more after departure. Suspected or confirmed malaria, especially *P. falciparum*, is a medical emergency, requiring urgent intervention as clinical deterioration can occur rapidly and unpredictably. See Box 3-2 detailing some clinical highlights for malaria.

DIAGNOSIS

Travelers who have symptoms of malaria should seek medical evaluation **as soon as possible**. Clinicians should consider malaria in any patient with a febrile illness who has recently returned from a malaria-endemic country.

Smear microscopy remains the gold standard for malaria diagnosis. Microscopy can also be used to determine the species of malaria parasite, identify the parasite life-cycle stages present, and quantify the parasitemia—all of which are necessary for providing the most appropriate treatment. Microscopy results should ideally be available within a few hours. It is an unacceptable practice to send these tests to an offsite laboratory or batch them for results to be provided days later.

Various test kits are available to detect antigens derived from malaria parasites. Such immunologic (immunochromatographic) tests most often use a dipstick or cassette format and provide results in 2–15 minutes. These rapid diagnostic tests (RDTs) offer a useful alternative to microscopy in situations where reliable microscopic diagnosis is not immediately available. Although RDTs can detect malaria antigens within minutes, they cannot determine the species, are less sensitive for diagnosis, and cannot quantify parasitemia. In addition, CDC recommends that positive and negative results always be confirmed by microscopy. Although confirmation does not have to occur simultaneously with the RDT, the information from microscopy, including the actual presence of malaria parasites, the species, life-cycle stages (asexual vs sexual blood-stage forms), and parasitemia will be most useful if it is available as soon as possible. The Food and Drug Administration (FDA) has approved 1 RDT for use in the United States by hospital and commercial laboratories, not by individual clinicians or by patients themselves. This RDT is called BinaxNOW Malaria test. Laboratories that do not provide in-house on-the-spot microscopy services should maintain a stock of malaria RDTs so that they will be able to perform malaria diagnostic testing when needed.

PCR tests are also available for detecting malaria parasites. Although these tests are more sensitive than routine microscopy, results are not usually available as quickly as microscopy results should be, thus limiting the utility of this test for acute diagnosis. PCR testing is most useful for definitively identifying the species of malaria parasite and detecting mixed infections. Species confirmation by PCR is available at the CDC malaria laboratory.

In sub-Saharan Africa, clinical overdiagnosis and the rate of false-positive microscopy for malaria may be high. Travelers to this region should be warned they may be diagnosed with malaria incorrectly, even though they are taking a reliable antimalarial regimen. In such cases, acutely ill travelers should be advised to seek the best available medical services and follow the treatment offered locally (except the use of halofantrine, which is not recommended; see below) but *not* to stop their chemoprophylaxis regimen.

TREATMENT

Malaria can be treated effectively early in the course of the disease, but delay of therapy can have serious or even fatal consequences. Travelers who have symptoms of malaria should be advised to seek medical evaluation **as soon as possible**. Specific treatment options depend on the species of malaria, the likelihood of drug resistance (based on where the infection was acquired), the age of the patient, pregnancy status, and the severity of infection.

Detailed CDC recommendations for malaria treatment can be found at www.cdc.gov/malaria/diagnosis_treatment/treatment.html. Clinicians who require assistance with the diagnosis or treatment of malaria should call the CDC Malaria Hotline (770-488-7788 or toll-free at 855-856-4713) from 9 AM to 5 PM Eastern Time. After hours or on weekends and holidays, clinicians requiring assistance should call the CDC Emergency Operations Center at 770-488-7100 and ask the operator to page the person on call for the Malaria Branch. In addition, it is advisable to consult with a clinician who has specialized travel or tropical medicine expertise or with an infectious disease physician.

Medications that are not used in the United States for the treatment of malaria, such as halofantrine, are widely available overseas. CDC does not recommend halofantrine for treatment because of cardiac adverse events, including deaths, which have been documented after treatment. These adverse events have occurred in people with and without preexisting cardiac problems and both in the presence and absence of other antimalarial drugs (such as mefloquine).

Travelers who reject the advice to take prophylaxis, who choose a suboptimal drug regimen (such as chloroquine in an area with chloroquine-resistant *P. falciparum*), or who require a less-than-optimal drug regimen for medical reasons are at increased risk for acquiring malaria and needing prompt treatment while overseas. In addition, some travelers who are taking effective prophylaxis but who will be in remote areas may decide, in consultation with their travel health provider, to take along a reliable supply of a full course of an approved malaria treatment regimen (see Box 3-3 for a definition of *reliable supply*). In the event that they are diagnosed with malaria, they will have immediate access to this treatment regimen, which if acquired in the United States is unlikely to be counterfeit and will not deplete local resources. In rare instances when access to medical care is not available and the traveler develops a febrile illness consistent with malaria, the reliable supply medication can be self-administered presumptively. **Travelers should be advised that this self-treatment of a possible malarial infection is only a temporary measure and that prompt medical evaluation is imperative.**

Two malaria treatment regimens available in the United States can be prescribed as a reliable supply: atovaquone-proguanil and artemether-lumefantrine. The use of the same or related drugs that have been taken for prophylaxis is not recommended to treat malaria. For example, atovaquone-proguanil may be used as a reliable supply medication by travelers not taking atovaquone-proguanil for prophylaxis. See Table 3-8 for the dosing recommendation.

PREVENTION

The goal of these malaria prevention guidelines is to prevent malaria caused by all species, not only *P. falciparum*. These guidelines apply to both short-term and long-term travelers. Malaria prevention consists of a combination of mosquito avoidance measures and chemoprophylaxis. Although efficacious, the recommended interventions are not 100% effective. For details about how CDC determines malaria prevention recommendations for travelers, see Box 3-4.

Preventing malaria involves striking a balance between ensuring that all people at risk for infection use the recommended prevention measures, while preventing rare occurrences of adverse effects of these interventions among people using them unnecessarily. An individual risk assessment should be conducted for every traveler, taking into account not only the destination country but also the detailed itinerary, including specific cities, types of accommodation, season, and style of travel. In addition, conditions such as pregnancy or antimalarial drug resistance at the destination may modify the risk assessment.

Depending on the level of risk, it may be appropriate to recommend no specific interventions, mosquito avoidance measures only, or mosquito avoidance measures plus chemoprophylaxis. For areas of intense transmission, such as West Africa, exposure for even short periods of time can result in transmission, so travelers to this area should be considered at high risk for infection. Malaria transmission is not distributed

---

BOX 3-3. WHAT IS A RELIABLE SUPPLY?

A reliable supply is a complete course of an approved malaria treatment regimen obtained in the United States before travel. A reliable supply

- Is not counterfeit or substandard
- Will not interact adversely with the patient's other medicines, including chemoprophylaxis
- Will not deplete local resources in the destination country

Table 3-8. Reliable supply regimens for the treatment of malaria

DRUG[1]	ADULT DOSE	PEDIATRIC DOSE	COMMENTS
ATOVAQUONE-PROGUANIL The adult tablet contains 250 mg atovaquone and 100 mg proguanil. The pediatric tablet contains 62.5 mg atovaquone and 25 mg proguanil.	4 adult tablets, orally as a single daily dose for 3 consecutive days	Daily dose to be taken for 3 consecutive days: 5–8 kg: 2 pediatric tablets 9–10 kg: 3 pediatric tablets 11–20 kg: 1 adult tablet 21–30 kg: 2 adult tablets 31–40 kg: 3 adult tablets >41 kg: 4 adult tablets	Contraindicated in people with severe renal impairment (creatinine clearance <30 mL/min) Not recommended for people on atovaquone-proguanil prophylaxis Not recommended for children weighing <5 kg, pregnant women, and women breastfeeding infants weighing <5 kg
ARTEMETHER-LUMEFANTRINE One tablet contains 20 mg artemether and 120 mg lumefantrine.	A 3-day treatment schedule with a total of 6 oral doses is recommended for both adult and pediatric patients based on weight. The patient should receive the initial dose, followed by the second dose 8 hours later, then 1 dose twice per day for the following 2 days. 5 to <15 kg: 1 tablet per dose 15 to <25 kg: 2 tablets per dose 25 to <35 kg: 3 tablets per dose ≥35 kg: 4 tablets per dose	Not for people on mefloquine prophylaxis Not recommended for children weighing <5 kg, pregnant women, and women breastfeeding infants weighing <5 kg

[1] If used for presumptive self-treatment, medical care should be sought as soon as possible.

homogeneously throughout all countries. Some destinations have malaria transmission occurring only in certain areas. If travelers are going to high-transmission areas during peak transmission times, even though the country as a whole may have relatively low malaria transmission, they may be at high risk for infection while there.

Geography is just a part of determining a traveler's risk for infection. Risk can differ substantially for different travelers as their behaviors and circumstances differ. For example, travelers staying in air-conditioned hotels may be at lower risk than backpackers or adventure travelers. Similarly, long-term residents living in screened and air-conditioned housing are less likely to be exposed than are people living without such amenities. The highest risk is associated with first- and second-generation immigrants living in non-endemic countries who return to their countries of origin to visit friends and relatives (VFRs). VFR travelers often consider themselves to be at no risk, because they grew up in a malarious country and consider themselves immune. However, acquired immunity is lost quickly, and VFRs should be considered to have the same risk as other nonimmune travelers (see Chapter 8, Immigrants Returning Home to Visit Friends & Relatives [VFRs]). Travelers should also be reminded that even if a person has had malaria before, he or she can get it again, and preventive measures are still necessary.

Mosquito Avoidance Measures
Because of the nocturnal feeding habits of *Anopheles* mosquitoes, malaria transmission

BOX 3-4. HOW CDC ARRIVES AT RECOMMENDATIONS FOR PREVENTING MALARIA AMONG TRAVELERS

Countries are not required to submit malaria surveillance data to CDC. On an ongoing basis, we actively solicit data from multiple sources, including World Health Organization (main and regional offices); national malaria control programs; international organizations, such as the International Society of Travel Medicine; CDC overseas staff; US military; academic, research, and aid organizations; and published records from the medical literature. We also make judgments about the reliability and accuracy of those data. When possible, we assess trends and consider the data in the context of what we know about the malaria control activities within that country or other mitigating factors, such as natural disasters, wars, and other events that may be affecting the ability to control malaria or accurately count and report it. We consider factors such as the volume of travel to that country and the number of acquired cases reported in the US surveillance system. Based on all those considerations, we then try to accurately describe areas of that country where transmission occurs, substantial occurrences of antimalarial drug resistance, the proportions of species present, and the recommended chemoprophylaxis options.

occurs primarily between dusk and dawn. Contact with mosquitoes can be reduced by remaining in well-screened areas, using mosquito bed nets (preferably insecticide-treated nets), using an effective insecticide spray in living and sleeping areas during evening and nighttime hours, and wearing clothes that cover most of the body.

All travelers should use an effective mosquito repellent (see Chapter 2, Protection against Mosquitoes, Ticks, & Other Arthropods). Repellents should be applied to exposed parts of the skin when mosquitoes are likely to be present. If travelers are also wearing sunscreen, sunscreen should be applied first and insect repellent second. In addition to using a topical insect repellent, a permethrin-containing product may be applied to bed nets and clothing for additional protection against mosquitoes.

Chemoprophylaxis

All recommended primary chemoprophylaxis regimens involve taking a medicine before, during, and after travel to an area with malaria. Beginning the drug before travel allows the antimalarial agent to be in the blood before the traveler is exposed to malaria parasites. In choosing a chemoprophylaxis regimen before travel, the traveler and the travel health provider should consider several factors. The travel itinerary should be reviewed in detail and compared with information on where malaria

transmission occurs within a given country, to determine whether the traveler will be traveling in a part of the country where malaria occurs and if antimalarial drug resistance has been reported in that location (see the Yellow Fever & Malaria Information, by Country section later in this chapter). Additional factors to consider are the patient's other medical conditions, medications being taken (to assess potential drug interactions), the cost of the medicines, and the potential side effects. Table 3-9 lists some of the benefits and limitations of medicines used for malaria chemoprophylaxis; additional information about choosing a malaria chemoprophylaxis regimen can be found at www.cdc.gov/malaria/travelers/drugs.html.

The resistance of P. falciparum to chloroquine has been confirmed in all areas with P. falciparum malaria except the Caribbean, Central America west of the Panama Canal, and some countries in the Middle East. In addition, resistance to sulfadoxine-pyrimethamine is widespread in the Amazon River Basin area of South America, much of Southeast Asia, other parts of Asia, and in large parts of Africa. Resistance to mefloquine has been confirmed on the borders of Thailand with Burma (Myanmar) and Cambodia, in the western provinces of Cambodia, in the eastern states of Burma on the border between Burma and China, along the borders of Laos and Burma, the adjacent parts of the Thailand–Cambodia

Table 3-9. Considerations when choosing a drug for malaria prophylaxis

DRUG	REASONS TO CONSIDER USE OF THIS DRUG	REASONS TO CONSIDER AVOIDING USE OF THIS DRUG
Atovaquone-proguanil	• Good for last-minute travelers because the drug is started 1–2 days before travel. • Some people prefer to take a daily medicine. • Good choice for shorter trips because the traveler takes the medicine for only 7 days after traveling rather than 4 weeks. • Well tolerated—side effects uncommon. • Pediatric tablets are available and may be more convenient.	• Cannot be used by women who are pregnant or breastfeeding a child that weighs <5 kg. • Cannot be taken by people with severe renal impairment. • Tends to be more expensive than some of the other options (especially for long trips). • Some people (including children) would rather not take a medicine every day.
Chloroquine	• Some people would rather take medicine weekly. • Good choice for long trips because it is taken only weekly. • Some people are already taking hydroxychloroquine chronically for rheumatologic conditions; in those instances, they may not have to take an additional medicine. • Can be used in all trimesters of pregnancy.	• Cannot be used in areas with chloroquine or mefloquine resistance. • May exacerbate psoriasis. • Some people would rather not take a weekly medication. • For short trips, some people would rather not take medication for 4 weeks after travel. • Not a good choice for last-minute travelers, because drug needs to be started 1–2 weeks before travel.
Doxycycline	• Some people prefer to take a daily medicine. • Good for last-minute travelers because the drug is started 1–2 days before travel. • Tends to be the least expensive antimalarial. • People who are already taking doxycycline chronically to prevent acne do not have to take an additional medicine. • Doxycycline also can prevent some additional infections (such as rickettsial infections and leptospirosis), so it may be preferred by people planning to hike, camp, and swim in fresh water.	• Cannot be used by pregnant women and children aged <8 years. • Some people would rather not take a medicine every day. • For short trips, some people would rather not take medication for 4 weeks after travel. • Women prone to getting vaginal yeast infections when taking antibiotics may prefer taking a different medicine. • People may want to avoid the increased risk of sun sensitivity. • Some people are concerned about the potential of getting an upset stomach from doxycycline.
Mefloquine	• Some people would rather take medicine weekly. • Good choice for long trips because it is taken only weekly. • Can be used in all trimesters of pregnancy.	• Cannot be used in areas with mefloquine resistance. • Cannot be used in patients with certain psychiatric conditions. • Cannot be used in patients with a seizure disorder. • Not recommended for people with cardiac conduction abnormalities. • Not a good choice for last-minute travelers because drug needs to be started ≥2 weeks before travel. • Some people would rather not take a weekly medication. • For short trips, some people would rather not take medication for 4 weeks after travel.

continued

MALARIA | 245

DRUG	REASONS TO CONSIDER USE OF THIS DRUG	REASONS TO CONSIDER AVOIDING USE OF THIS DRUG
Primaquine.	• It is the most effective medicine for preventing *P. vivax*, so it is a good choice for travel to places with >90% *P. vivax*. • Good choice for shorter trips because the traveler takes the medicine for 7 days after traveling rather than 4 weeks. • Good for last-minute travelers because the drug is started 1–2 days before travel. • Some people prefer to take a daily medicine.	• Cannot be used in patients with G6PD deficiency. • Cannot be used in patients who have not been tested for G6PD deficiency. • There are costs and delays associated with getting a G6PD test; however, it only has to be done once. Once a normal G6PD level is verified and documented, the test does not have to be repeated the next time primaquine is considered. • Cannot be used by pregnant women. • Cannot be used by women who are breastfeeding, unless the infant has also been tested for G6PD deficiency. • Some people (including children) would rather not take a medicine every day. • Some people are concerned about the potential of getting an upset stomach from primaquine.

Abbreviation: G6PD, glucose-6-phosphate dehydrogenase.

border, and in southern Vietnam. The resistance of P. vivax to chloroquine has been confirmed in Papua New Guinea and Indonesia.

In addition to primary prophylaxis, presumptive antirelapse therapy (also known as terminal prophylaxis) uses a medication toward the end of the exposure period (or immediately thereafter) to prevent relapses or delayed-onset clinical presentations of malaria caused by hypnozoites (dormant liver stages) of P. vivax or P. ovale. Because most malarious areas of the world (except the Caribbean) have at least 1 species of relapsing malaria, travelers to these areas have some risk for acquiring either P. vivax or P. ovale, although the actual risk for an individual traveler is difficult to define. Presumptive antirelapse therapy is generally indicated only for people who have had prolonged exposure in malaria-endemic areas (such as missionaries, military personnel, or Peace Corps volunteers).

The medications recommended for chemoprophylaxis of malaria may also be available at overseas destinations. However, combinations of these medications and additional drugs that are not recommended may be commonly prescribed and used in other countries. Travelers should be strongly discouraged from obtaining chemoprophylaxis medications while abroad. The quality of these products is not known; they may not be protective and could be dangerous. These medications may have been produced by substandard manufacturing practices, may be counterfeit, or may contain contaminants. Additional information on this topic can be found in Chapter 2, *Perspectives*: Pharmaceutical Quality & Counterfeit Drugs, and on the FDA website (www.fda.gov/Drugs/ResourcesForYou/Consumers/BuyingUsingMedicineSafely/BuyingMedicinefromOutsidetheUnitedStates/default.htm).

Medications Used for Chemoprophylaxis
Atovaquone-Proguanil

Atovaquone-proguanil is a fixed combination of the drugs atovaquone and proguanil. Prophylaxis should begin 1–2 days before travel to malarious areas and should be taken daily, at the same time each day, while in the malarious areas, and daily for 7 days after leaving the areas (see Table 3-10 for recommended dosages). Atovaquone-proguanil is well tolerated, and side effects are rare.

Table 3-10. Drugs used in the prophylaxis of malaria

DRUG	USAGE	ADULT DOSE	PEDIATRIC DOSE	COMMENTS
Atovaquone-proguanil	Prophylaxis in all areas	Adult tablets contain 250 mg atovaquone and 100 mg proguanil hydrochloride. 1 adult tablet orally, daily	Pediatric tablets contain 62.5 mg atovaquone and 25 mg proguanil hydrochloride. 5–8 kg: 1/2 pediatric tablet daily >8–10 kg: 3/4 pediatric tablet daily >10–20 kg: 1 pediatric tablet daily >20–30 kg: 2 pediatric tablets daily >30–40 kg: 3 pediatric tablets daily >40 kg: 1 adult tablet daily	Begin 1–2 days before travel to malarious areas. Take daily at the same time each day while in the malarious area and for 7 days after leaving such areas. Contraindicated in people with severe renal impairment (creatinine clearance <30 mL/min). Atovaquone-proguanil should be taken with food or a milky drink. Not recommended for prophylaxis for children weighing <5 kg, pregnant women, and women breastfeeding infants weighing <5 kg. Partial tablet doses may need to be prepared by a pharmacist and dispensed in individual capsules, as described in the text.
Chloroquine phosphate	Prophylaxis only in areas with chloroquine-sensitive malaria	300 mg base (500 mg salt) orally, once/week	5 mg/kg base (8.3 mg/kg salt) orally, once/week, up to a maximum adult dose of 300 mg base	Begin 1–2 weeks before travel to malarious areas. Take weekly on the same day of the week while in the malarious area and for 4 weeks after leaving such areas. May exacerbate psoriasis.
Doxycycline	Prophylaxis in all areas	100 mg orally, daily	≥8 years of age: 2.2 mg/kg up to adult dose of 100 mg/day	Begin 1–2 days before travel to malarious areas. Take daily at the same time each day while in the malarious area and for 4 weeks after leaving such areas. Contraindicated in children aged <8 years and pregnant women.
Hydroxy-chloroquine sulfate	An alternative to chloroquine for prophylaxis only in areas with chloroquine-sensitive malaria	310 mg base (400 mg salt) orally, once/week	5 mg/kg base (6.5 mg/kg salt) orally, once/week, up to a maximum adult dose of 310 mg base	Begin 1–2 weeks before travel to malarious areas. Take weekly on the same day of the week while in the malarious area and for 4 weeks after leaving such areas.

continued

MALARIA | 247

TABLE 3-10. DRUGS USED IN THE PROPHYLAXIS OF MALARIA (continued)

DRUG	USAGE	ADULT DOSE	PEDIATRIC DOSE	COMMENTS
Mefloquine	Prophylaxis in areas with mefloquine-sensitive malaria	228 mg base (250 mg salt) orally, once/week	≤9 kg: 4.6 mg/kg base (5 mg/kg salt) orally, once/week >9–19 kg: 1/4 tablet once/week >19–30 kg: 1/2 tablet once/week >30–45 kg: 3/4 tablet once/week >45 kg: 1 tablet once/week	Begin ≥2 weeks before travel to malarious areas. Take weekly on the same day of the week while in the malarious area and for 4 weeks after leaving such areas. Contraindicated in people allergic to mefloquine or related compounds (quinine, quinidine) and in people with active depression, a recent history of depression, generalized anxiety disorder, psychosis, schizophrenia, other major psychiatric disorders, or seizures. Use with caution in people with psychiatric disturbances or a previous history of depression. Not recommended for people with cardiac conduction abnormalities.
Primaquine[1]	Prophylaxis for short-duration travel to areas with principally *P. vivax*	30 mg base (52.6 mg salt) orally, daily	0.5 mg/kg base (0.8 mg/kg salt) up to adult dose orally, daily	Begin 1–2 days before travel to malarious areas. Take daily at the same time each day while in the malarious area and for 7 days after leaving such areas. Contraindicated in people with G6PD deficiency. Also contraindicated during pregnancy and lactation, unless the infant being breastfed has a documented normal G6PD level.
	Used for presumptive antirelapse therapy (terminal prophylaxis) to decrease the risk for relapses of *P. vivax* and *P. ovale*	30 mg base (52.6 mg salt) orally, daily for 14 days after departure from the malarious area	0.5 mg/kg base (0.8 mg/kg salt) up to adult dose orally, daily for 14 days after departure from the malarious area	Indicated for people who have had prolonged exposure to *P. vivax*, *P. ovale*, or both. Contraindicated in people with G6PD deficiency. Also contraindicated during pregnancy and lactation, unless the infant being breastfed has a documented normal G6PD level.

Abbreviation: G6PD, glucose-6-phosphate dehydrogenase.
[1] All people who take primaquine should have a documented normal G6PD level before starting the medication.

The most common adverse effects reported in people using atovaquone-proguanil for prophylaxis or treatment are abdominal pain, nausea, vomiting, and headache. Atovaquone-proguanil is not recommended for prophylaxis in children weighing <5 kg (11 lb), pregnant women, or patients with severe renal impairment (creatinine clearance <30 mL/min). Proguanil may increase the effect of warfarin, so international normalized ratio monitoring or dosage adjustment may be needed.

Chloroquine and Hydroxychloroquine

Chloroquine phosphate or hydroxychloroquine sulfate can be used for prevention of malaria only in destinations where chloroquine resistance is not present (see Maps 3-9 and 3-10 and the Yellow Fever & Malaria Information, by Country section later in this chapter). Prophylaxis should begin 1–2 weeks before travel to malarious areas. It should be continued by taking the drug once a week, on the same day of the week, during travel in malarious areas and for 4 weeks after a traveler leaves these areas (see Table 3-10 for recommended dosages). Reported side effects include gastrointestinal disturbance, headache, dizziness, blurred vision, insomnia, and pruritus, but generally these effects do not require that the drug be discontinued. High doses of chloroquine, such as those used to treat rheumatoid arthritis, have been associated with retinopathy; this serious side effect appears to be extremely unlikely when chloroquine is used for routine weekly malaria prophylaxis. Chloroquine and related compounds have been reported to exacerbate psoriasis. People who experience uncomfortable side effects after taking chloroquine may tolerate the drug better by taking it with meals. As an alternative, the related compound hydroxychloroquine sulfate may be better tolerated.

Doxycycline

Doxycycline prophylaxis should begin 1–2 days before travel to malarious areas. It should be continued once a day, at the same time each day, during travel in malarious areas and daily for 4 weeks after the traveler leaves such areas. Insufficient data exist on the antimalarial prophylactic efficacy of related compounds such as minocycline (commonly prescribed for the treatment of acne). People on a long-term regimen of minocycline who need malaria prophylaxis should stop taking minocycline 1–2 days before travel and start doxycycline instead. Minocycline can be restarted after the full course of doxycycline is completed (see Table 3-10 for recommended dosages).

Doxycycline can cause photosensitivity, usually manifested as an exaggerated sunburn reaction. The risk for such a reaction can be minimized by avoiding prolonged, direct exposure to the sun and by using sunscreen. In addition, doxycycline use is associated with an increased frequency of vaginal yeast infections. Gastrointestinal side effects (nausea or vomiting) may be minimized by taking the drug with a meal or by specifically prescribing doxycycline monohydrate or the enteric-coated doxycycline hyclate, rather than the generic doxycycline hyclate, which is often less expensive. To reduce the risk for esophagitis, travelers should be advised to swallow the medicine with sufficient fluids and not to take doxycycline before going to bed. Doxycycline is contraindicated in people with an allergy to tetracyclines, during pregnancy, and in infants and children aged <8 years. Vaccination with the oral typhoid vaccine Ty21a should be delayed for ≥24 hours after taking a dose of doxycycline.

Mefloquine

Mefloquine prophylaxis should begin ≥2 weeks before travel to malarious areas. It should be continued once a week, on the same day of the week, during travel in malarious areas and for 4 weeks after a traveler leaves such areas (see Table 3-10 for recommended dosages). Mefloquine has been associated with rare but serious adverse reactions (such as psychoses or seizures) at prophylactic doses; these reactions are more frequent with the higher doses used for treatment. Other side effects that have occurred in chemoprophylaxis studies include gastrointestinal disturbance, headache, insomnia, abnormal dreams, visual disturbances, depression, anxiety disorder, and dizziness. Other more severe neuropsychiatric disorders occasionally reported during postmarketing surveillance include sensory and motor neuropathies (including paresthesia, tremor, and ataxia), agitation or restlessness, mood changes, panic attacks, forgetfulness, confusion, hallucinations, aggression, paranoia, and encephalopathy. On occasion, psychiatric symptoms have been reported to continue long after mefloquine has been stopped. FDA also includes a boxed warning about rare reports of persistent dizziness after mefloquine use. Mefloquine is contraindicated for use by travelers with a known hypersensitivity to mefloquine or related compounds (such as quinine or quinidine) and in people with active depression, a recent history of depression, generalized anxiety disorder, psychosis, schizophrenia, other major psychiatric disorders, or seizures. It should be used with caution in people with psychiatric disturbances or a history of depression. A review of available data suggests that mefloquine may be used safely in people concurrently on β-blockers, if they have no underlying arrhythmia. However, mefloquine is not recommended for people with cardiac conduction abnormalities. Any traveler receiving a prescription for mefloquine must also receive a copy of the FDA medication guide, which can be found at www.accessdata.fda.gov/drugsatfda_docs/label/2008/019591s023lbl.pdf.

Primaquine

Primaquine phosphate has 2 distinct uses for malaria prevention: primary prophylaxis in areas with primarily P. vivax and presumptive antirelapse therapy (terminal prophylaxis).

When taken for primary prophylaxis, primaquine should be taken 1–2 days before travel to malarious areas, daily, at the same time each day, while in the malarious areas, and daily for 7 days after leaving the areas (see Table 3-10 for recommended dosages). Primary prophylaxis with primaquine obviates the need for presumptive antirelapse therapy.

When used for presumptive antirelapse therapy, primaquine is administered for 14 days after the traveler has left a malarious area. When chloroquine, doxycycline, or mefloquine is used for primary prophylaxis, primaquine is usually taken during the last

2 weeks of postexposure prophylaxis. When atovaquone-proguanil is used for prophylaxis, primaquine may be taken during the final 7 days of atovaquone-proguanil, and then for an additional 7 days. Primaquine should be given concurrently with the primary prophylaxis medication. However, if that is not feasible, the primaquine course should still be administered after the primary prophylaxis medication has been completed.

The most common adverse event in people with normal glucose-6-phosphate dehydrogenase (G6PD) levels is gastrointestinal upset if primaquine is taken on an empty stomach. This problem is minimized or eliminated if primaquine is taken with food. In G6PD-deficient people, primaquine can cause hemolysis that can be fatal. **Before primaquine is used, G6PD deficiency MUST be ruled out by laboratory testing.**

Travel to Areas with Limited Malaria Transmission

For destinations where malaria cases occur sporadically and risk for infection to travelers is assessed as being low, CDC recommends that travelers use mosquito avoidance measures only, and no chemoprophylaxis should be prescribed (see the Yellow Fever & Malaria Information, by Country section later in this chapter).

Travel to Areas with Mainly P. vivax Malaria

For destinations where the main species of malaria present is P. vivax, in addition to mosquito avoidance measures, primaquine is a good choice for primary prophylaxis for travelers who are not G6PD deficient. Its use for this indication is considered off-label in the United States. The predominant species of malaria and the recommended chemoprophylaxis medicines are listed in the Yellow Fever & Malaria Information, by Country section later in this chapter. For people unable to take primaquine, other drugs can be used as described below, depending on the presence of antimalarial drug resistance.

Travel to Areas with Chloroquine-Sensitive Malaria

For destinations where chloroquine-sensitive malaria is present, in addition to mosquito avoidance measures, the many effective chemoprophylaxis options include chloroquine, atovaquone-proguanil, doxycycline, mefloquine, and in some instances, primaquine for travelers who are not G6PD deficient. Longer-term travelers may prefer the convenience of weekly chloroquine, while shorter-term travelers may prefer the shorter course of atovaquone-proguanil or primaquine.

Travel to Areas with Chloroquine-Resistant Malaria

For destinations where chloroquine-resistant malaria is present, in addition to mosquito avoidance measures, chemoprophylaxis options are atovaquone-proguanil, doxycycline, and mefloquine.

Travel to Areas with Mefloquine-Resistant Malaria

For destinations where mefloquine-resistant malaria is present, in addition to mosquito avoidance measures, chemoprophylaxis options are either atovaquone-proguanil or doxycycline.

Chemoprophylaxis for Infants, Children, and Adolescents

Infants of any age or weight or children and adolescents of any age can contract malaria. Therefore, all children traveling to malaria-endemic areas should use the recommended prevention measures, which often include taking an antimalarial drug. In the United States, antimalarial drugs are available only in oral formulations and may taste bitter. Pediatric doses should be carefully calculated according to body weight but should never exceed adult dose. Pharmacists can pulverize tablets and prepare gelatin capsules for each measured dose. If the child is unable to swallow the capsules or tablets, parents should prepare the child's dose of medication by breaking open the gelatin capsule and mixing the drug with a small amount of something sweet, such as applesauce, chocolate syrup, or jelly, to ensure the entire dose is delivered to the child. Giving the dose on a full stomach may minimize stomach upset and vomiting.

Chloroquine and mefloquine are options for use in infants and children of all ages and weights, depending on drug resistance at their destination. Primaquine can be used for children who are not G6PD deficient traveling to areas with principally *P. vivax*. Doxycycline may be used for children who are aged ≥8 years. Atovaquone-proguanil may be used for prophylaxis for infants and children weighing ≥5 kg (11 lb). Prophylactic dosing for children weighing <11 kg (24 lb) constitutes off-label use in the United States. Pediatric dosing regimens are contained in Table 3-10.

Chemoprophylaxis during Pregnancy and Breastfeeding

Malaria infection in pregnant women can be more severe than in non-pregnant women. Malaria increases the risk for adverse pregnancy outcomes, including prematurity, spontaneous abortion, and stillbirth. For these reasons, and because no chemoprophylaxis regimen is completely effective, women who are pregnant or likely to become pregnant should be advised to avoid travel to areas with malaria transmission if possible (see Chapter 8, Pregnant Travelers). If travel to a malarious area cannot be deferred, use of an effective chemoprophylaxis regimen is essential.

Pregnant women traveling to areas where chloroquine-resistant *P. falciparum* has not been reported may take chloroquine prophylaxis. Chloroquine has not been found to have any harmful effects on the fetus when used in the recommended doses for malaria prophylaxis; therefore, pregnancy is not a contraindication for malaria prophylaxis with chloroquine phosphate or hydroxychloroquine sulfate.

For travel to areas where chloroquine resistance is present, mefloquine is the only medication recommended for malaria chemoprophylaxis during pregnancy. In 2011, the FDA reviewed available data for mefloquine use during pregnancy and reclassified it from category C (animal reproduction studies have shown an adverse effect on the fetus and there are no adequate and well-controlled studies in humans, but potential benefits may warrant use of the drug in pregnant women despite potential risks) to category B (animal reproduction studies have failed to demonstrate a risk to the fetus and there are no adequate and well-controlled studies in pregnant women).

Experts are investigating ways to examine the safety of atovaquone-proguanil use during pregnancy. Proguanil has been used for decades in pregnant women; however, until such time as these data are fully evaluated, atovaquone-proguanil is not recommended for use during pregnancy. Doxycycline is contraindicated for malaria prophylaxis during pregnancy because of the risk for adverse effects seen with tetracycline, a related drug, on the fetus, which include discoloration and dysplasia of the teeth and inhibition of bone growth. Primaquine should not be used during pregnancy because the drug may be passed transplacentally to a G6PD-deficient fetus and cause hemolytic anemia in utero.

Very small amounts of antimalarial drugs are excreted in the breast milk of lactating women. Because the quantity of antimalarial drugs transferred in breast milk is insufficient to provide adequate protection against malaria, infants who require chemoprophylaxis must receive the recommended dosages of antimalarial drugs listed in Table 3-10. Because chloroquine and mefloquine may be safely prescribed to infants, it is also safe for infants to be exposed to the small amounts excreted in breast milk. Although data are very limited about the use of doxycycline in lactating women, most experts consider the theoretical possibility of adverse events to the infant to be remote.

Although no information is available on the amount of primaquine that enters human breast milk, the mother and infant should be tested for G6PD deficiency before primaquine is given to a woman who is breastfeeding. Because data are not yet available on the safety of atovaquone-proguanil prophylaxis in infants weighing <5 kg (11 lb), CDC does not recommend it to prevent malaria in women breastfeeding infants weighing <5 kg. However, it can be used to treat women who are breastfeeding infants of any weight when the potential benefit outweighs the potential risk to the infant (such as treating a breastfeeding woman who has acquired *P. falciparum* malaria in an area of multidrug-resistant strains and who cannot tolerate other treatment options).

Choosing a Drug to Prevent Malaria

Recommendations for drugs to prevent malaria differ by country of travel and can be found in the Yellow Fever & Malaria Information, by Country section later in this chapter. Recommended drugs for each country are listed in alphabetical order and have comparable efficacy in that country. No antimalarial drug is 100% protective; therefore, prophylaxis must be combined with the use of personal protective measures (such as insect repellent, long sleeves, long pants, sleeping in a mosquito-free setting or using an insecticide-treated bed net). When several different drugs are recommended for an area, Table 3-9 may help in the decision-making process.

Changing Medications as a Result of Side Effects during Chemoprophylaxis

Medications recommended for prophylaxis against malaria have different modes of action that affect the parasites at different stages of the life cycle. Thus, if the medication needs to be changed because of side effects before a full course has been completed, there are some special considerations (see Table 3-11).

BLOOD DONATION AFTER TRAVEL TO MALARIOUS AREAS

People who have been in an area where malaria transmission occurs should be deferred from donating blood in the United States for a period of time after returning from the malarious area to prevent transmission of malaria through blood transfusion (Table 3-12).

Risk assessments may differ between travel health providers and blood banks. A travel health provider advising a traveler going to a country with relatively low malaria transmission for a short period of time and engaging in low-risk behaviors may choose insect avoidance only and no chemoprophylaxis for the traveler. However, upon the traveler's return, a blood bank may still choose to defer that traveler for 1 year because of the travel to an area where transmission occurs.

CDC website: www.cdc.gov/malaria

Table 3-11. Changing medications as a result of side effects during chemoprophylaxis

DRUG BEING STOPPED	DRUG BEING STARTED	COMMENTS
Mefloquine	Doxycycline	Begin doxycycline, continue daily while in malaria-endemic area, and continue for 4 weeks after leaving malaria-endemic area.
	Atovaquone-proguanil	• If the switch occurs ≥3 weeks before departure from the endemic area, atovaquone-proguanil should be taken daily for the rest of the stay in the endemic area and for 1 week thereafter. • If the switch occurs <3 weeks before departure from the endemic area, atovaquone-proguanil should be taken daily for 4 weeks after the switch. • If the switch occurs after departure from the endemic area, atovaquone-proguanil should be taken daily until 4 weeks after the date of departure.
	Chloroquine	Not recommended
	Primaquine	This switch would be unlikely as primaquine is only recommended for primary prophylaxis in areas with mainly *P. vivax* for people with normal G6PD activity. Should that be the case, begin primaquine, continue daily while in malaria-endemic area, and continue for 7 days after leaving malaria-endemic area.
Doxycycline	Mefloquine	Not recommended
	Atovaquone-proguanil	• If the switch occurs ≥3 weeks before departure from the endemic area, atovaquone-proguanil should be taken daily for the rest of the stay in the endemic area and for 1 week thereafter. • If the switch occurs <3 weeks before departure from the endemic area, atovaquone-proguanil should be taken daily for 4 weeks after the switch. • If the switch occurs after departure from the endemic area, atovaquone-proguanil should be taken daily until 4 weeks after the date of departure.
	Chloroquine	Not recommended
	Primaquine	This switch would be unlikely as primaquine is only recommended for primary prophylaxis in areas with mainly *P. vivax* for people with normal G6PD activity. Should that be the case, begin primaquine, continue daily while in malaria-endemic area, and continue for 7 days after leaving malaria-endemic area.
Atovaquone-proguanil	Doxycycline	Begin doxycycline, continue daily while in malaria-endemic area, and continue for 4 weeks after leaving malaria-endemic area.
	Mefloquine	Not recommended
	Chloroquine	Not recommended
	Primaquine	This switch would be unlikely as primaquine is only recommended for primary prophylaxis in areas with mainly *P. vivax* for people with normal G6PD activity. Should that be the case, begin primaquine, continue daily while in malaria-endemic area, and continue for 7 days after leaving malaria-endemic area.

continued

TABLE 3-11. CHANGING MEDICATIONS AS A RESULT OF SIDE EFFECTS DURING CHEMOPROPHYLAXIS (continued)

DRUG BEING STOPPED	DRUG BEING STARTED	COMMENTS
Chloroquine	Doxycycline	Begin doxycycline, continue daily while in malaria-endemic area, and continue for 4 weeks after leaving malaria-endemic area.
	Atovaquone-proguanil	• If the switch occurs ≥3 weeks before departure from the endemic area, atovaquone-proguanil should be taken daily for the rest of the stay in the endemic area and for 1 week thereafter. • If the switch occurs <3 weeks before departure from the endemic area, atovaquone-proguanil should be taken daily for 4 weeks after the switch. • If the switch occurs following departure from the endemic area, atovaquone-proguanil should be taken daily until 4 weeks after the date of departure.
	Mefloquine	Not recommended
	Primaquine	Primaquine is only recommended for primary prophylaxis in areas with mainly *P. vivax* for people with normal G6PD activity. Should that be the case, begin primaquine, continue daily while in malaria-endemic area, and continue for 7 days after leaving malaria-endemic area.
Primaquine	Doxycycline	Begin doxycycline, continue daily while in malaria-endemic area, and continue for 4 weeks after leaving malaria-endemic area.
	Atovaquone-proguanil	Begin atovaquone-proguanil, continue daily while in malaria-endemic area, and continue for 7 days after leaving malaria-endemic area.
	Chloroquine	Not recommended
	Mefloquine	Not recommended

Abbreviation: G6PD, glucose-6-phosphate dehydrogenase.

Table 3-12. Food and Drug Administration recommendations for deferring blood donation in people returning from malarious areas

GROUP	BLOOD DONATION DEFERRAL
Travelers to malaria-endemic areas	May not donate blood for 1 year after travel.
Former residents of malaria-endemic areas	May not donate blood for 3 years after departing. If they return to a malaria-endemic area within that 3-year period, they are deferred for an additional 3 years.
People diagnosed with malaria	May not donate for 3 years after treatment.

BIBLIOGRAPHY

1. Baird JK, Fryauff DJ, Hoffman SL. Primaquine for prevention of malaria in travelers. Clin Infect Dis. 2003 Dec 15;37(12):1659–67.

2. Boggild AK, Parise ME, Lewis LS, Kain KC. Atovaquone-proguanil: report from the CDC expert meeting on malaria chemoprophylaxis (II). Am J Trop Med Hyg. 2007 Feb;76(2):208–23.

3. CDC. Malaria surveillance—United States, 2011. MMWR Surveill Summ. 2013 Nov 1;62(5):1–17.

4. Fradin MS, Day JF. Comparative efficacy of insect repellents against mosquito bites. N Engl J Med. 2002 Jul 4;347(1):13–8.

5. Hill DR, Baird JK, Parise ME, Lewis LS, Ryan ET, Magill AJ. Primaquine: report from CDC expert meeting on malaria chemoprophylaxis I. Am J Trop Med Hyg. 2006 Sep;75(3):402–15.

6. Leder K, Black J, O'Brien D, Greenwood Z, Kain KC, Schwartz E, et al. Malaria in travelers: a review of the GeoSentinel surveillance network. Clin Infect Dis. 2004 Oct 15;39(8):1104–12.

7. Newman RD, Parise ME, Barber AM, Steketee RW. Malaria-related deaths among US travelers, 1963–2001. Ann Intern Med. 2004 Oct 5;141(7):547–55.

8. Reyburn H, Mbatia R, Drakeley C, Carneiro I, Mwakasungula E, Mwerinde O, et al. Overdiagnosis of malaria in patients with severe febrile illness in Tanzania: a prospective study. BMJ. 2004 Nov 20;329(7476):1212.

9. Steinhardt LC, Magill AJ, Arguin PM. Review: Malaria chemoprophylaxis for travelers to Latin America. Am J Trop Med Hyg. 2011 Dec;85(6):1015–24.

10. Tan KR, Magill AJ, Parise ME, Arguin PM. Doxycycline for malaria chemoprophylaxis and treatment: report from the CDC expert meeting on malaria chemoprophylaxis. Am J Trop Med Hyg. 2011 Apr;84(4):517–31.

3

For the Record

A HISTORY OF MALARIA CHEMOPROPHYLAXIS
Alan J. Magill

Among the many dreaded fevers that plague man, "marsh fever" was distinguished by its periodicity, enlarged spleen, and pattern of attacking those exposed to wet, warm, boggy areas. In the mid-1700s, it became known by its Italian name, *mal'aria* ("bad air"), referring to bad or foul air emanating from swampy lands. The discovery and development of drugs to treat and prevent malaria have been driven for centuries by the desire and need to protect travelers, military personnel, explorers, and the commercial interest of imperial powers when they went into the malaria-endemic tropics.

HISTORICAL MILESTONES IN ANTIMALARIAL CHEMOPROPHYLAXIS

- 1620s: Jesuit missionaries living in Peru learned of the healing power of powdered bark, often known as "Jesuits' bark," from the cinchona trees growing in the high forests of Peru and Bolivia.

- 1768: James Lind, a British naval surgeon, recommended that "every man receives a daily ration of cinchona powder" as long as a ship lay at anchor in any tropical port. His advice, however, was not widely accepted, and it would be almost 100 years before the concept of chemoprophylaxis would be accepted.
- Early 1800s: Crews of the British Royal Navy manning the blockade of the West African coast to suppress the Atlantic slave trade were decimated by malaria.
- 1820: French chemists isolated quinine, the most active compound in cinchona bark, which allowed for quinine's expanded availability and use.
- 1854: The Scottish surgeon William Balfour Baikie gave 6–8 grains (1 grain = 65 mg) of quinine, half in the morning and half in the evening, dissolved in sherry, to all the ship's crew during a 118-day expedition up the river Benue in modern-day Nigeria. No men died. This unprecedented accomplishment gradually led to acceptance that malaria could be prevented by chemoprophylaxis.
- 1861: Quinine first saw widespread use as a prophylactic agent in the American Civil War when both the Union and Confederate Armies, plagued with malaria, used massive quantities to prevent the disease.
- 1880: A French military physician working in Algeria, Alphonse Laveran, discovered parasites in the blood of a French soldier. The identification of the infectious agent and its life cycle was an essential step in opening the way to the development of effective prophylactic agents.
- 1914–1918: During World War I, both Allied and Axis militaries suffered terribly from malaria. German armies were denied access to quinine, as most was held by a monopoly of Dutch growers on the island of Java.
- 1920s: German chemists pursued a synthetic route to new antimalarial drugs to circumvent the Dutch monopoly, achieving spectacular success with the introduction of pamaquine and mepacrine during the 1930s.
- 1941: With America's entry into World War II, trade between the United States and Germany ceased, and mepacrine was no longer available to the Allies.
- 1942: Japanese armies overran the Dutch cinchona plantations on Java, cutting off the supply of quinine and leaving the Allies with no antimalarial drugs.
- 1943: American scientists quickly devised a manufacturing process for mepacrine, and the drug was given as a treatment and as a prophylactic under the name Atabrine. Meanwhile, the Allies, especially the Americans, launched the largest antimalarial drug discovery and development program the world had seen. By 1945, several new antimalarial drugs had been introduced, including chloroquine and proguanil. Chloroquine went on to assume a role both in prophylaxis for travelers and as a treatment drug for endemic areas.
- 1959: Chloroquine-resistant *Plasmodium falciparum* malaria was first reported.
- 1965: Large-scale American military involvement began in South Vietnam, reaching almost 200,000 soldiers by the end of 1965. Chloroquine-resistant malaria caused illness and death in US forces.
- 1967: A second massive US government–sponsored antimalarial drug discovery effort centered at the Walter Reed Army Institute of Research began and led to the discovery of mefloquine.

- 1971: During studies of volunteers with experimentally induced malaria infections, it was observed that tetracycline, administered to treat inter-current bacterial infections, appeared to exert blood schizontocidal activity against chloroquine-resistant *P. falciparum*. A few additional studies were performed with tetracycline, doxycycline, and minocycline, but no formal development of the drug as an antimalarial was pursued.
- Early 1980s: The Wellcome Research Laboratories developed atovaquone as an antimalarial drug. Clinical trials in uncomplicated *P. falciparum* malaria as monotherapy were disappointing, with early treatment failures due to the emergence of atovaquone-resistant parasites. However, combining atovaquone with proguanil led to an efficacious combination therapy.
- 1982: The fixed combination of pyrimethamine and sulfadoxine (Fansidar) became available in the United States and was recommended by CDC for prophylactic use in travelers at risk of acquiring chloroquine-resistant *P. falciparum*.
- 1985: Pyrimethamine-sulfadoxine as weekly malaria chemoprophylaxis was abruptly withdrawn because of fatal cases of Stevens-Johnson syndrome. Since no alternative drugs were licensed to prevent chloroquine-resistant *P. falciparum* malaria, CDC recommended daily doxycycline for antimalarial prophylaxis.
- Late 1980s: The US Army conducted several field and human challenge clinical trials demonstrating the efficacy of doxycycline as malaria prophylaxis.
- 1989: The Food and Drug Administration (FDA) approved mefloquine (Lariam).
- 1992: Pfizer, at the request of FDA, submitted a supplemental new drug application for doxycycline for malaria chemoprophylaxis.
- 2000: Combination of fixed dose atovaquone-proguanil (Malarone) approved by FDA.

The 3 largest antimalarial drug development efforts of modern times occurred during and after major conflicts of the 20th century—World War I, World War II, and the Vietnam War. The modern history of developing drugs to prevent malaria grew almost entirely from the need to protect military personnel and keep them healthy to conduct combat operations in malaria-endemic areas. Those massive government-funded efforts produced the drugs now used to keep modern civilian travelers safe from the sickness and death that mark malaria's march through time.

BIBLIOGRAPHY

1. Greenwood D. Conflicts of interest: the genesis of synthetic antimalarial agents in peace and war. J Antimicrob Chemother. 1995 Nov;36(5):857–72.
2. Kitchen LW, Vaughn DW, Skillman DR. Role of US military research programs in the development of US Food and Drug Administration—approved antimalarial drugs. Clin Infect Dis. 2006 Jul 1;43(1):67–71.
3. Smith DC. Quinine and fever: The development of the effective dosage. J Hist Med Allied Sci. 1976 Jul;31(3):343–67.
4. Smith DC, Sanford LB. Laveran's germ: the reception and use of a medical discovery. Am J Trop Med Hyg. 1985 Jan;34(1):2–20.
5. Sweeney AW. Wartime research on malaria chemotherapy. Parassitologia. 2000 Jun;42(1–2):33–45.

MEASLES (RUBEOLA)

Amy Parker Fiebelkorn, James L. Goodson

INFECTIOUS AGENT

Measles virus is a member of the genus *Morbillivirus* of the family Paramyxoviridae.

TRANSMISSION

Measles is transmitted primarily from person to person by large respiratory droplets but can also spread by the airborne route as aerosolized droplet nuclei. Infected people are usually contagious from 4 days before until 4 days after rash onset. Measles is among the most contagious viral diseases known; secondary attack rates are >90% in susceptible household and institutional contacts. Humans are the only natural host for sustaining measles virus transmission, which makes global eradication of measles feasible.

EPIDEMIOLOGY

The number of reported measles cases in the United States has declined from nearly 900,000 annually in the early 1940s to 37–220 cases annually from 2001 through 2013. As a result of high vaccination coverage and better measles control in the Americas, in 2000, measles in the United States was declared eliminated (defined as the absence of endemic measles virus transmission in a defined geographic area for ≥12 months in the presence of a well-performing surveillance system). In 2002, indigenous measles virus circulation was interrupted in the entire Western Hemisphere, and measles elimination has been maintained in the region through high vaccination coverage. However, measles virus continues to be imported into the region, including into the United States, from other parts of the world. Globally, an estimated 20 million people are infected with measles each year. Given the large global incidence and high communicability of the disease, travelers may be exposed to the virus in almost any country they visit, particularly those outside the Western Hemisphere, where measles is endemic or where large outbreaks are

occurring. In recent years, measles has been imported into the United States from frequently visited countries, including England, France, Germany, India, and the Philippines, where large outbreaks have been reported. Most measles cases imported into the United States have come from unvaccinated US residents who became infected while traveling abroad, became symptomatic after returning to the United States, and in some cases infected others in their communities, causing outbreaks. Additional information on global measles control efforts is available on the Measles & Rubella Initiative website at www.measlesrubellainitiative.org.

CLINICAL PRESENTATION

The incubation period ranges from 7 to 21 days from exposure to onset of fever; rash usually appears about 14 days after exposure. Symptoms include prodromal fever that can rise as high as 105°F (40.6°C), conjunctivitis, coryza (runny nose), cough, and small spots with white or bluish-white centers on an erythematous base on the buccal mucosa (Koplik spots). A characteristic red, blotchy (maculopapular) rash appears on the third to seventh day after the prodromal symptoms appear. The rash begins on the face, becomes generalized, and lasts 4–7 days. Common complications include diarrhea (8%), middle ear infection (7%–9%), and pneumonia (1%–6%). Encephalitis, which can result in permanent brain damage, occurs in approximately 1 per 1,000–2,000 cases of measles.

Subacute sclerosing panencephalitis (SSPE), a rare but serious degenerative central nervous system disease caused by a persistent infection with a defective measles virus, is estimated to occur in 4–11 per 100,000 cases. However, among people who became infected with measles during the 1989–1991 measles resurgence in the United States, the estimated risk of SSPE was 22 per 100,000 reported measles cases. SSPE is manifested by mental and motor deterioration that starts an average of 7–10 years after measles virus infection (most frequently in children who were infected at age <2 years), progressing to coma and death. The risk of serious complications and death is highest for children aged ≤5 years and adults aged ≥20 years. It is also higher in populations with poor nutritional status.

DIAGNOSIS

Laboratory criteria for diagnosis include any of the following: a positive serologic test for measles IgM, IgG seroconversion, a significant rise in measles IgG level by any standard serologic assay, isolation of measles virus, or identification by PCR of measles virus RNA from a clinical specimen.

A clinical case of measles illness is characterized by all of the following:

- Generalized maculopapular rash lasting ≥3 days
- Temperature of ≥101°F (38.3°C)
- Cough, coryza, or conjunctivitis

A confirmed case is one with an acute febrile rash illness with laboratory confirmation or direct epidemiologic linkage to a laboratory confirmed case. In a laboratory-confirmed case, the temperature does not need to reach ≥101°F(38.3°C) and the rash does not need to last ≥3 days.

TREATMENT

Treatment is supportive. The World Health Organization recommends vitamin A for all children with acute measles, regardless of their country of residence, to reduce the risk of complications. Vitamin A is administered once a day for 2 days at the following doses:

- 50,000 IU for infants aged <6 months
- 100,000 IU for infants aged 6–11 months
- 200,000 IU for children aged ≥12 months

An additional (third) age-specific dose of vitamin A should be given 2–4 weeks later to children with clinical signs and symptoms of vitamin A deficiency. Parenteral and oral formulations of vitamin A are available in the United States.

PREVENTION

Measles has been preventable since 1963 through vaccination. People who do not have

evidence of measles immunity should be considered at risk for measles, particularly during international travel. Acceptable presumptive evidence of immunity to measles for international travelers includes meeting any of the following criteria:

- Documentation of age-appropriate vaccination with a live measles-containing vaccine (MMR or MMRV):
  > For infants aged 6–11 months, documented administration of 1 dose of MMR or MMRV
  > For people aged ≥12 months, 2 doses of MMR or MMRV (the first dose should be administered at age ≥12 months; the second dose should be administered no earlier than 28 days after the first dose)
- Laboratory evidence of immunity
- Laboratory confirmation of disease
- Birth before 1957

Vaccine

Measles vaccine contains live, attenuated measles virus. In the United States, it is available only in combination formulations, such as measles-mumps-rubella (MMR) and measles-mumps-rubella-varicella (MMRV) vaccines. MMRV vaccine is licensed for children aged 12 months to 1–12 years and may be used in place of MMR vaccine if vaccination for measles, mumps, rubella, and varicella is needed.

International travelers, including people traveling to industrialized countries, who do not have presumptive evidence of measles immunity and who have no contraindications to MMR or MMRV, should receive MMR or MMRV before travel according to the following guidelines:

- Infants aged 6–11 months should receive 1 MMR or MMRV dose. Infants vaccinated before age 12 months must be revaccinated on or after the first birthday with 2 doses of MMR or MMRV separated by ≥28 days. MMRV is not licensed for children aged <12 months.
- Preschool and school-age children (aged ≥12 months) should be given 2 MMR or MMRV doses separated by ≥28 days.
- Adults born in or after 1957 should be given 2 MMR or MMRV doses separated by ≥28 days.

 MEASLES (RUBEOLA)

One dose of MMR or MMRV is approximately 85% effective when administered at age 9 months and 93% effective when administered at age ≥1 year. More than 99% of people who receive 2 doses of MMR or MMRV develop serologic evidence of measles immunity.

Measles-containing vaccine and immune globulin (IG) may be effective as postexposure prophylaxis. MMR or MMRV, if administered within 72 hours after initial exposure to measles virus, may provide some protection. If the exposure does not result in infection, the vaccine should induce protection against subsequent measles virus infection. IG can be used to prevent or mitigate measles in a susceptible person when administered within 6 days of exposure. However, any immunity conferred is temporary unless modified or typical measles occurs, and the person should receive MMR or MMRV 6 months after intramuscularly administered IG or 8 months after intravenously administered IG, provided the person is then aged ≥12 months and the vaccine is not otherwise contraindicated.

Vaccine Safety and Adverse Reactions

In rare circumstances, MMR vaccination has been associated with the following adverse events:

- Anaphylaxis (approximately 1–3.5 occurrences per million doses administered)
- Thrombocytopenia (a rate of 1 case in every 25,000 doses during the 6 weeks after immunization)
- Febrile seizures (The risk of febrile seizures increases approximately 3-fold 8–14 days after receipt of MMR vaccine, but overall, the rate of febrile seizure after measles-containing vaccine is much lower than the rate with measles disease.)
- Joint symptoms (Arthralgia develops among approximately 25% of susceptible postpubertal women from the rubella component of the MMR vaccination. Approximately 10% have acute arthritis-like signs and symptoms that generally persist for 1 day to 3 weeks and rarely recur. Chronic joint symptoms are rare, if they occur at all.)

Evidence does not support a causal link between MMR vaccination and any of the following: hearing loss, retinopathy, optic neuritis, ocular palsies, Guillain-Barré syndrome, cerebellar ataxia, Crohn disease, or autism. A published report on MMR vaccination and inflammatory bowel disease and pervasive developmental disorders (such as autism) has never been replicated by other studies, and has subsequently been widely discredited and retracted by the journal.

Compared with use of MMR and varicella vaccines at the same visit, use of MMRV vaccine is associated with a higher risk for fever and febrile seizures 5–12 days after the first dose among children aged 12–23 months, and approximately 1 additional febrile seizure for every 2,300–2,600 MMRV vaccine doses administered. Use of separate MMR and varicella vaccines avoids this increased risk for fever and febrile seizures.

Precautions and Contraindications
Allergy

People with severe allergy (hives, swelling of the mouth or throat, difficulty breathing, hypotension, and shock) to gelatin or neomycin, or who have had a severe allergic reaction to a prior dose of MMR or MMRV vaccine, should not be revaccinated. MMR or MMRV vaccine may be administered to people who are allergic to eggs without prior routine skin testing or the use of special protocols.

Immunosuppression

Enhanced replication of live vaccine viruses can occur in people who have immune deficiency disorders. Death related to vaccine-associated measles virus infection has been reported among severely immunocompromised people. Therefore, severely immunosuppressed people should not be vaccinated with MMR or MMRV vaccine (for a thorough discussion of recommendations for immunocompromised travelers, see Chapter 8, Immunocompromised Travelers):

- People with leukemia in remission, and off chemotherapy, who were not immune to measles when diagnosed with leukemia, may receive MMR vaccine. At least 3 months should elapse after termination of chemotherapy before administration of the first dose.

- MMR vaccination is recommended for all people aged ≥12 months with HIV infection who do not have evidence of measles, rubella, and mumps immunity or evidence of severe immunosuppression. Absence of severe immunosuppression is defined as CD4 percentages ≥15% for ≥6 months for people aged ≤5 years and CD4 percentages ≥15% and CD4 count ≥200 cells/mm³ for ≥6 months for people aged >5 years. When only CD4 counts or CD4 percentages are available for those aged >5 years, the assessment of severe immunosuppression can be on the basis of the CD4 values (count or percentage) that are available.
- People who have received high-dose corticosteroid therapy (in general, considered to be >20 mg prednisone or equivalent daily or on alternate days for an interval of ≥14 days) should avoid vaccination with MMR or MMRV for ≥1 month after cessation of steroid therapy.
- People who have received high-dose corticosteroid therapy daily or on alternate days for an interval of <14 days generally can be vaccinated with MMR or MMRV immediately after cessation of treatment, although some experts prefer waiting until 2 weeks after completion of therapy.
- Other immunosuppressive therapy: in general, MMR or MMRV vaccine should be withheld for ≥3 months after cessation of the immunosuppressive therapy and remission of the underlying disease. This interval is based on the assumptions that the immune response will have been restored in 3 months and the underlying disease for which the therapy was given remains in remission.

Thrombocytopenia

The benefits of primary immunization are usually greater than the potential risks of thrombocytopenia. However, avoiding a subsequent dose of MMR or MMRV vaccine may be prudent if an episode of thrombocytopenia occurred within approximately 6 weeks after a previous dose of vaccine.

CDC website: www.cdc.gov/measles

BIBLIOGRAPHY

1. American Academy of Pediatrics. Measles. In: Pickering LK, editor. Red Book: 2012 Report of the Committee on Infectious Diseases. 29th ed. Elk Grove Village, IL: American Academy of Pediatrics; 2012. p. 489–99.

2. Bellini WJ, Rota JS, Lowe LE, Katz RS, Dyken PR, Zaki SR, et al. Subacute sclerosing panencephalitis: more cases of this fatal disease are prevented by measles immunization than was previously recognized. J Infect Dis. 2005 Nov 15;192(10):1686–93.

3. CDC. General recommendations on immunization—recommendations of the Advisory Committee on Immunization Practices (ACIP). MMWR Recomm Rep. 2011;60(RR-02):1–60.

4. CDC. Prevention of measles, rubella, congenital rubella syndrome, and mumps, 2013: summary recommendations of the Advisory Committee on Immunization Practices (ACIP). MMWR Recomm Rep. 2013 Jun 14;62(RR-04):1–34.

5. CDC. Use of combination measles, mumps, rubella, and varicella vaccine: recommendations of the Advisory Committee on Immunization Practices (ACIP). MMWR Recomm Rep. 2010 May 7;59(RR-03):1–12.

6. King GE, Markowitz LE, Patriarca PA, Dales LG. Clinical efficacy of measles vaccine during the 1990 measles epidemic. Pediatr Infect Dis J. 1991 Dec;10(12):883–8.

7. Measles & Rubella Initiative [Internet]. Washington, DC: American Red Cross; 2014 [cited 2014 Sep 22]. Available from: http://www.measlesrubellainitiative.org.

8. National Notifiable Diseases Surveillance System. Measles (rubeola): 2013 case definition. Atlanta: CDC; 2013 [cited 2014 Sep 22]. Available from: http://wwwn.cdc.gov/NNDSS/script/casedef.aspx?CondYrID=908&DatePub=1/1/2013.

9. Perry RT, Halsey NA. The clinical significance of measles: a review. J Infect Dis. 2004 May 1;189 Suppl 1:S4–16.

10. World Health Organization. Measles [fact sheet no. 286]. Geneva: World Health Organization; 2014 [cited 2014 Sep 22]. Available from: http://www.who.int/mediacentre/factsheets/fs286/en.

MELIOIDOSIS

David D. Blaney, Jay E. Gee, Tina J. Benoit

INFECTIOUS AGENT

Burkholderia pseudomallei, a saprophytic gram-negative bacillus, is the causative agent of melioidosis. The bacteria are found in soil and water, widely distributed in tropical and subtropical countries.

TRANSMISSION

Through subcutaneous inoculation, ingestion, or inhalation; person-to-person transmission is extremely rare but may occur through contact with the blood or body fluids of an infected person.

EPIDEMIOLOGY

Melioidosis is endemic in Southeast Asia, Papua New Guinea, much of the Indian subcontinent, southern China, Hong Kong, and Taiwan and is considered highly endemic in northeast Thailand, Malaysia, Singapore, and northern Australia. Sporadic cases have been reported among residents of or travelers to Aruba, Colombia, Costa Rica, El Salvador, Guatemala, Guadeloupe, Honduras, Martinique, Mexico, Panama, Venezuela, and many other countries in the Americas, as well as Puerto Rico. In northern Brazil, clusters of melioidosis have been reported and are associated with periods of heavy rainfall. The risk is highest for adventure travelers, ecotourists, military personnel, construction and resource extraction workers, and other people whose contact with contaminated soil or water may expose them to the bacteria; infections have been reported in people who have spent less than a week in an endemic area. Risk factors for systemic melioidosis include diabetes, excessive alcohol use, chronic renal disease, chronic lung disease (such as associated with cystic fibrosis or chronic obstructive pulmonary disease), thalassemia, and malignancy or other non-HIV-related immune suppression.

CLINICAL PRESENTATION

Incubation period is generally 1–21 days, although it may extend for months or years; with a high inoculum, symptoms can develop in a few hours. Melioidosis may occur as a subclinical infection, localized infection (such as cutaneous abscess), pneumonia, meningoencephalitis, sepsis, or chronic suppurative infection. The latter may mimic tuberculosis, with fever, weight loss, productive cough, and upper lobe infiltrate, with or without cavitation. More than 50% of cases present with pneumonia.

DIAGNOSIS

Culture of *B. pseudomallei* from blood, sputum, pus, urine, synovial fluid, peritoneal fluid, or pericardial fluid is diagnostic. Indirect hemagglutination assay is a widely used serologic test but is not considered confirmatory. Diagnostic assistance is available through CDC (http://www.cdc.gov/ncezid/dhcpp/bacterial_special/zoonoses_lab.html).

TREATMENT

Ceftazidime, imipenem, or meropenem is used for initial treatment of 10–14 days, followed by 20–24 weeks of trimethoprim-sulfamethoxazole. Relapse may be seen, especially in patients who received a shorter-than-recommended course of therapy.

PREVENTION

Travelers should use personal protective equipment such as waterproof boots and gloves to protect against contact with contaminated soil and water and thoroughly clean skin lacerations, abrasions, or burns that have been contaminated with soil or surface water.

CDC website: www.cdc.gov/melioidosis

BIBLIOGRAPHY

1. Brilhante RS, Bandeira TJ, Cordeiro RA, Grangeiro TB, Lima RA, Ribeiro JF, et al. Clinical-epidemiological features of 13 cases of melioidosis in Brazil. J Clin Microbiol. 2012 Oct;50(10):3349–52.

2. Currie BJ, Dance DA, Cheng AC. The global distribution of *Burkholderia pseudomallei* and melioidosis: an update. Trans R Soc Trop Med Hyg. 2008 Dec;102 Suppl 1:S1–4.

3. Inglis TJ, Rolim DB, Sousa Ade Q. Melioidosis in the Americas. Am J Trop Med Hyg. 2006 Nov;75(5):947–54.

4. Limmathurotsakul D, Kanoksil M, Wuthiekanun V, Kitphati R, deStavola B, Day NP, et al. Activities of daily living associated with acquisition of melioidosis in northeast Thailand: a matched case-control study. PLoS Negl Trop Dis. 2013;7(2):e2072.

5. O'Sullivan BP, Torres B, Conidi G, Smole S, Gauthier C, Stauffer KE, et al. *Burkholderia pseudomallei* infection in a child with cystic fibrosis: acquisition in the Western Hemisphere. Chest. 2011 Jul;140(1):239–42.

6. Wiersinga WJ, Currie BJ, Peacock SJ. Melioidosis. N Engl J Med. 2012 Sep 13;367(11):1035–44.

MENINGOCOCCAL DISEASE

Jessica R. MacNeil, Sarah A. Meyer

INFECTIOUS AGENT

Neisseria meningitidis is a gram-negative diplococcus. Meningococci are classified into serogroups on the basis of the composition of the capsular polysaccharide. The 6 major meningococcal serogroups associated with disease are A, B, C, W, X, and Y.

TRANSMISSION

Person-to-person transmission occurs by close contact with respiratory secretions or saliva.

EPIDEMIOLOGY

N. meningitidis is found worldwide, but the highest incidence is in the "meningitis belt" of sub-Saharan Africa (Map 3-11). Meningococcal disease is hyperendemic in this region, and periodic epidemics during the dry season (December–June) reach up to 1,000 cases per 100,000 population. By contrast, rates of disease in the United States, Europe, Australia, and South America range from 0.3 to 3 cases per 100,000 population per year. Although most common in the African meningitis belt, meningococcal outbreaks can occur anywhere in the world. Serogroup A predominates in the meningitis belt, although serogroups C, X, and W are also found. At any time, 5%–10% of the population may be carriers of *N. meningitidis*.

Outside the meningitis belt, infants have the highest rates of disease. In meningitis belt countries, high attack rates are seen up to 30 years of age. Risk for travelers is highest in people visiting meningitis belt countries who have prolonged contact with local populations during an epidemic. The Hajj pilgrimage to Saudi Arabia has also been associated with outbreaks of meningococcal disease in returning pilgrims and their contacts.

CLINICAL PRESENTATION

Meningococcal disease generally occurs 1–10 days after exposure and presents as meningitis in ≥50% of cases. Meningococcal meningitis is characterized by sudden onset of headache, fever, and stiffness of the neck, sometimes accompanied by nausea, vomiting, photophobia, or altered mental status. Up to 20% of people with meningococcal disease present with meningococcal sepsis, known as meningococcemia. Meningococcemia is characterized by an abrupt onset of fever and a petechial or purpuric rash. The rash may progress to purpura fulminans. Meningococcemia often involves hypotension, acute adrenal hemorrhage, and multiorgan failure. Among infants and children aged <2 years, meningococcal disease may have nonspecific symptoms. Neck stiffness,

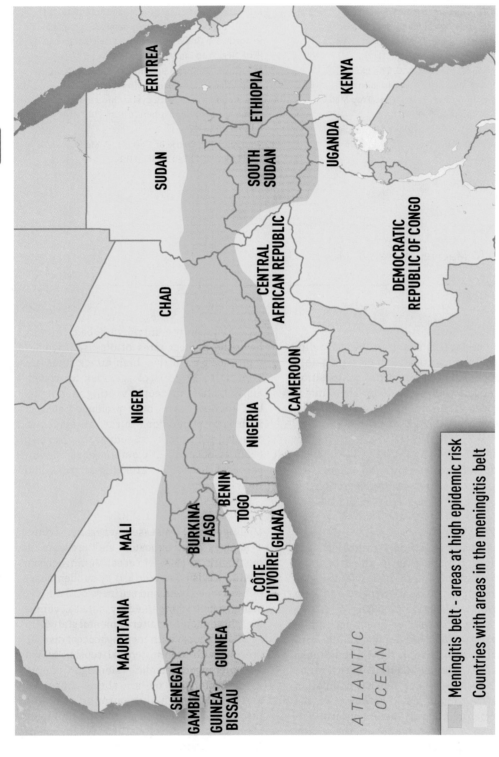

Meningitis belt - areas at high epidemic risk

Countries with areas in the meningitis belt

MAP 3-11. AREAS WITH FREQUENT EPIDEMICS OF MENINGOCOCCAL MENINGITIS

usually seen in people with meningitis, may be absent in this age group.

DIAGNOSIS

Early diagnosis and treatment are critical. A lumbar puncture should be done to examine the cerebrospinal fluid (CSF) and perform a Gram stain. If possible, the lumbar puncture should be done before starting antibiotic therapy to ensure that bacteria, if present, can be cultured from CSF. Diagnosis is generally made by isolating N. meningitidis from blood or CSF through culture, by detecting meningococcal antigen in CSF by latex agglutination, or by evidence of N. meningitidis DNA by PCR.

The signs and symptoms of meningococcal meningitis are similar to those of other causes of bacterial meningitis, such as Haemophilus influenzae and Streptococcus pneumoniae. The causative organism should be identified so that the correct antibiotics can be used for treatment and prophylaxis.

TREATMENT

Meningococcal disease is potentially fatal and should always be viewed as a medical emergency. Antibiotic treatment must be started early in the course of the disease, and empirically prior to the diagnostic test results. Several antibiotic choices are available, including third-generation cephalosporins.

PREVENTION
Vaccine
Indications for Use

The Advisory Committee on Immunization Practices (ACIP) recommends vaccination against meningococcal disease for people aged 11–18 years, people with certain underlying medical conditions, and for people who travel to or reside in countries where N. meningitidis is hyperendemic or epidemic, particularly if contact with the local population will be prolonged. Hyperendemic regions include the meningitis belt of Africa during the dry season (December–June). Advisories for travelers to other countries are issued when epidemics of meningococcal disease caused by vaccine-preventable serogroups are recognized (see the CDC Travelers' Health website at www.cdc.gov/travel). Note that proof of receipt of quadrivalent vaccination against meningococcal disease is required for people traveling to Mecca during the annual Hajj and Umrah pilgrimages.

Vaccine Administration

Four meningococcal vaccines are licensed in the United States: 3 polysaccharide–protein conjugate vaccines and 1 polysaccharide vaccine. The quadrivalent (serogroups A, C, W, and Y) conjugate vaccines are Menactra (MenACWY-D, Sanofi Pasteur) and Menveo (MenACWY-CRM, Novartis). A bivalent (serogroups C and Y) conjugate vaccine MenHibrix (HibMenCY-TT, GSK) is also licensed. MPSV4 is the only licensed meningococcal vaccine for adults aged ≥56 years and is immunogenic in older adults. Currently no licensed vaccine is available in the United States to prevent serogroup B meningococcal disease, although serogroup B vaccines have recently been licensed in Europe, Australia, and Canada. A monovalent serogroup A vaccine (MenAfriVac, Serum Institute of India) has progressively been introduced into meningitis belt countries since 2010. This vaccine is not licensed outside the meningitis belt and is not available outside national and subnational immunization campaigns in meningitis belt countries. Approximately 7–10 days are required after vaccination for development of protective antibody levels. Refer to Table 3-13 for more information about available meningococcal vaccines.

Routine Immunization

CDC recommends routine administration of a quadrivalent meningococcal conjugate vaccine MenACWY for all people aged 11–18 years. A single dose of vaccine should be administered at age 11 or 12 years, and a booster dose should be administered at age 16 years. Routine immunization is not recommended for other age groups in the United States, with the exception of people at increased risk for meningococcal disease. Those at increased risk for meningococcal disease include people who have a persistent complement component deficiency (C3, C5-9, properdin, factor D, or factor H), people who have functional or anatomic asplenia, or travelers to or residents of countries where meningococcal disease is hyperendemic or epidemic. Vaccine, product, number of doses, and booster dose recommendations are based

Table 3-13. Vaccines to prevent meningococcal disease

VACCINE	TRADE NAME (MANUFACTURER)	AGE	DOSE	ROUTE	INTERVAL BETWEEN DOSES	BOOSTER
Meningococcal polysaccharide diphtheria toxoid conjugate vaccine (MenACWY-D)[1]	Menactra (Sanofi Pasteur)	9–23 mo	0.5 mL	IM	0, 3 mo	If at continued risk[2]
		2–55 y	0.5 mL	IM	1 dose	
Meningococcal oligosaccharide diphtheria CRM$_{197}$ conjugate vaccine (MenACWY-CRM)[1]	Menveo (Novartis)	2–12 mo	0.5 mL	IM	0, 2, 4, 10–13 mo	If at continued risk[2]
		7–23 mo	0.5 mL	IM	0, 3 mo (2nd dose administered in 2nd year of life)	
		2–55 y	0.5 mL	IM	1 dose	
Meningococcal and *Haemophilus influenzae* type B polysaccharide tetanus toxoid conjugated vaccine[3]	MenHibrix (GSK)	6 wk–18 mo	0.5 mL	IM	0, 2, 4, 10–13 mo	If at continued risk[2]
Meningococcal polysaccharide vaccine (MPSV4)	Menomune (Sanofi Pasteur)	≥2 y	0.5 mL	SC	1 dose	If at continued risk[4]

Abbreviations: IM, intramuscular; SC, subcutaneous.

[1] In an infant is receiving the vaccine before travel, 2 doses may be administered as early as 8 weeks apart.

[2] Revaccination with meningococcal conjugate vaccine (MenACWY-D or MenACWY-CRM) is recommended after 3 years for children who were previously vaccinated at ages 9 months through 6 years. Revaccination with meningococcal conjugate vaccine is recommended after 5 years for people who were previously vaccinated at ages 7–55 years, and every 5 years thereafter for people who are at continued risk.

[3] Infants and children who received HibMenCY-TT and are traveling to areas with high endemic rates of meningococcal disease such as the African meningitis belt are not protected against serogroups A and W and should receive a quadrivalent meningococcal vaccine before travel.

[4] Revaccination with meningococcal polysaccharide vaccine is recommended for adults aged >55 years who remain at increased risk 5 years after the last dose.

on age and risk factor and are described in detail for each risk group in the 2013 ACIP Meningococcal Disease Recommendations (www.cdc.gov/mmwr/preview/mmwrhtml/rr6202a1.htm).

Immunization for Travelers

Travelers who visit or reside in countries where meningococcal disease is hyperendemic or epidemic, including the meningitis belt of sub-Saharan Africa during the dry season (December–June), should receive vaccination with a quadrivalent

meningococcal vaccine, either MenACWY vaccine (people aged 2 months through 55 years and meningococcal vaccine non-naïve people aged ≥ 56 years) or MPSV4 (meningococcal vaccine-naïve people aged ≥56 years) before travel. Infants and children who received Hib-MenCY-TT are not protected against serogroups A and W and should receive a quadrivalent vaccine before travel if traveling to areas with high endemic rates of meningococcal disease.

In children initiating vaccination at 2 months of age, MenACWY-CRM should be administered as a 4-dose series at 2, 4, 6, and 12 months of age. In children initiating vaccination at 7–9 months through 23 months of age, MenACWY-CRM or MenACWY-D should be administered as a 2-dose series. Children aged 7–23 months can receive the second dose as early as 8 weeks after the first dose before travel. For people aged 2–55 years, 1 dose of a MenACWY vaccine is recommended. For people aged ≥56 years who have never received meningococcal vaccine, MPSV4 is recommended. However, for people aged ≥56 years who were previously vaccinated with MenACWY or for whom multiple doses are anticipated, MenACWY is preferred, although it is not licensed for this age group.

Travelers aged ≥2 years to the Kingdom of Saudi Arabia for Umrah or Hajj are required by the Saudi government to provide documentation of quadrivalent vaccine receipt in the 3 years before the date of travel. Travelers aged 3 months through 2 years are required to show documentation of 2 doses of a meningococcal vaccine against serogroup A.

International travelers at risk for meningococcal disease who were previously vaccinated with a quadrivalent vaccine should receive a booster dose: for children who received their last dose at <7 years of age, an additional dose of MenACWY should be administered 3 years after the last dose. For people who received their last dose at ≥7 years of age, a booster dose should be administered 5 years after the last dose.

Vaccine Safety and Adverse Reactions
Low-grade fevers and local reactions, such as injection site pain, arm swelling, and pain that limits movement of the injected arm, are side effects seen after both conjugate and polysaccharide meningococcal vaccines but occur more commonly after conjugate vaccine. Symptoms are generally mild to moderate and resolve within 48–72 hours. Severe adverse events, such as high fever, chills, joint pain, rash, or seizures are rare (<5% of vaccinees) with either type of vaccine.

Although no clinical trials of meningococcal vaccines have been conducted in pregnant or lactating women, postlicensure safety data have not identified any serious safety concerns to the mother or fetus. Pregnancy or lactation should not preclude vaccination with MenACWY or MPSV4 if indicated.

Precautions and Contraindications
People with moderate or severe acute illness should defer vaccination until their condition improves. Vaccination is contraindicated for people who have a severe allergic reaction to any component of the vaccines. All meningococcal vaccines are inactivated and may be given to immunosuppressed people.

Antibiotic Chemoprophylaxis
In the United States and most industrialized countries, antibiotic chemoprophylaxis is recommended for close contacts of a patient with invasive meningococcal disease to prevent secondary cases. Chemoprophylaxis ideally should be initiated within 24 hours after the index patient is identified; prophylaxis given >2 weeks after exposure has little value. Antibiotic regimens for prophylaxis include rifampin, ciprofloxacin, and ceftriaxone. Ceftriaxone is recommended for pregnant women.

CDC website: www.cdc.gov/meningitis/bacterial.html

BIBLIOGRAPHY

1. American Academy of Pediatrics. Meningococcal infections. In: Pickering LK, editor. Red Book: 2012 Report of the Committee on Infectious Diseases. 29th ed. Elk Grove Village, IL: American Academy of Pediatrics; 2012. p. 500–9.
2. Bilukha OO, Rosenstein N. Prevention and control of meningococcal disease. Recommendations of the Advisory Committee on Immunization Practices (ACIP). MMWR Recomm Rep. 2005 May 27;54(RR-7):1–21.
3. CDC. Prevention and control of meningococcal disease: recommendations of the Advisory Committee on Immunization Practices (ACIP). MMWR Morb Mortal Wkly Rep. 2013;62(2):1–28.
4. Greenwood B. Manson Lecture. Meningococcal meningitis in Africa. Trans R Soc Trop Med Hyg. 1999 Jul–Aug;93(4):341–53.
5. Halperin SA, Bettinger JA, Greenwood B, Harrison LH, Jelfs J, Ladhani SN, et al. The changing

and dynamic epidemiology of meningococcal disease. Vaccine. 2012 May 30;30 Suppl 2: B26–36.

6. Rosenstein NE, Perkins BA, Stephens DS, Popovic T, Hughes JM. Meningococcal disease. N Engl J Med. 2001 May 3;344(18):1378–88.

7. Stephens DS, Greenwood B, Brandtzaeg P. Epidemic meningitis, meningococcaemia, and *Neisseria meningitidis*. Lancet. 2007 Jun 30;369(9580):2196–210.

8. Wilder-Smith A. Meningococcal disease: risk for international travellers and vaccine strategies. Travel Med Infect Dis. 2008 Jul;6(4):182–6.

MIDDLE EAST RESPIRATORY SYNDROME (MERS)

John T. Watson, Susan I. Gerber

INFECTIOUS AGENT

The MERS coronavirus, a single-stranded, positive-sense RNA virus that belongs to the family Coronaviridae, genus *Betacoronavirus*.

TRANSMISSION

Transmission dynamics are not well understood. The MERS coronavirus is genetically similar to bat coronaviruses and has been detected in camels in North Africa and the Arabian Peninsula. Although a zoonotic reservoir of MERS has been speculated, little is known about the specific exposures that result in primary human cases. Evidence suggests that MERS can be spread from person to person among close contacts, resulting in outbreaks in families and in health care settings. Sustained community transmission of MERS has not been shown.

EPIDEMIOLOGY

MERS coronavirus is an emerging novel coronavirus that causes severe acute respiratory illness, and approximately 40% of confirmed cases have been fatal. MERS was first reported in September 2012, but illnesses with onsets as early as April 2012 were subsequently documented. The risk is ongoing in the area of the Arabian Peninsula. Index cases have lived in or recently traveled to Iran, Jordan, Kuwait, Lebanon, Oman, Qatar, Saudi Arabia, United Arab Emirates, or Yemen. MERS has also been identified in travelers from these countries returning to North America, Europe, Asia, and North Africa.

CLINICAL PRESENTATION

MERS is associated with severe acute respiratory failure, multiple organ dysfunction, and high mortality, although the spectrum of illness and clinical course are not fully defined. Mild or asymptomatic cases have been documented among contacts of cases. For people who develop symptomatic illness, the incubation period is approximately 2–14 days; median incubation period is slightly more than 5 days. Disease is most often characterized by fever, cough, and shortness of breath. Other symptoms may include chills, sore throat, myalgia, arthralgia, diarrhea, and vomiting. Initial nonspecific symptoms can progress to pneumonia. Chest radiographs have shown variable pulmonary involvement.

In addition to acute and often severe respiratory compromise, serious complications of MERS include cardiovascular collapse and acute renal injury. Abnormal laboratory findings can include thrombocytopenia, lymphopenia, and elevated liver function tests. Older age and comorbidities are associated with poor outcomes.

DIAGNOSIS

Several diagnostic assays have been developed to detect acute infection with MERS coronavirus, including real-time RT-PCR. Lower respiratory specimens (sputum, bronchoalveolar lavage, endotracheal aspirates) are the priority respiratory specimens for testing, although upper and lower respiratory, stool, and serum specimens should also be collected if possible. To increase the likelihood of detecting the virus, multiple specimens from these sites should be collected over the course of the illness. In the United States, most state laboratories are approved to test for MERS by using CDC's RT-PCR assay. Testing should be coordinated through state and local health departments and CDC.

In coordination with state and local health departments, health care providers should evaluate patients for MERS if they develop fever and pneumonia or acute respiratory distress syndrome within 14 days after traveling from countries in or near the Arabian Peninsula or have had close contact with a recent traveler from this area who has fever and acute respiratory illness.

TREATMENT

No specific antiviral treatment is available. Treatment is limited to supportive care. Standard, contact, and airborne infection control precautions are recommended for hospitalized patients with known or suspected MERS.

PREVENTION

No vaccine or preventive drug is available. CDC recommends that travelers practice general hygiene precautions such as frequent handwashing; avoiding touching the eyes, nose, and mouth; and avoiding contact with sick people. The World Health Organization (WHO) considers certain groups to be at high risk for severe MERS, including people with diabetes, kidney failure, chronic lung disease, or immunocompromised people. WHO recommends that these groups take additional precautions: avoid contact with camels, do not drink raw camel milk or raw camel urine, and do not eat undercooked meat, particularly camel meat. For more information, see www.who.int/csr/disease/coronavirus_infections/faq/en/.

CDC website: www.cdc.gov/coronavirus/mers

BIBLIOGRAPHY

1. Arabi YM, Arifi AA, Balkhy HH, Najm H, Aldawood AS, Ghabashi A, et al. Clinical course and outcomes of critically ill patients with Middle East respiratory syndrome coronavirus infection. Ann Intern Med. 2014 Mar 18;160(6):389–97.
2. Assiri A, McGeer A, Perl TM, Price CS, Al Rabeeah AA, Cummings DA, et al. Hospital outbreak of Middle East respiratory syndrome coronavirus. N Engl J Med. 2013 Aug 1;369(5):407–16.
3. CDC. Interim infection prevention and control recommendations for hospitalized patients with Middle East respiratory syndrome coronavirus (MERS-CoV). [updated 2014 Jul 11; cited 2014 Aug 11].

Available from: http://www.cdc.gov/coronavirus/mers/infection-prevention-control.html.
4. Memish ZA, Zumla AI, Al-Hakeem RF, Al-Rabeeah AA, Stephens GM. Family cluster of Middle East respiratory syndrome coronavirus infections. N Engl J Med. 2013 Jun 27;368(26):2487–94.
5. WHO MERS-CoV Research Group. State of knowledge and data gaps of Middle East respiratory syndrome coronavirus (MERS-CoV) in humans. PLoS Curr. 2013;5.
6. World Health Organization. Coronavirus infections. [cited 2014 Aug 11]. Available from: http://www.who.int/csr/disease/coronavirus_infections/en/.

MUMPS

Paul A. Gastañaduy, Gregory S. Wallace

INFECTIOUS AGENT

An enveloped, negative-strand RNA virus (a paramyxovirus) of the genus *Rubulavirus*.

TRANSMISSION

By respiratory droplets, saliva, or contact with contaminated fomites.

EPIDEMIOLOGY

Endemic in many countries throughout the world. Mumps vaccine is routinely used in 61% of countries in the world, and the risk of exposure among travelers is high in many countries, including industrialized countries.

CLINICAL PRESENTATION

Incubation period is 16–18 days (range, 12–25 days). Mumps is characterized by parotitis (swelling of the parotid salivary glands), either unilateral or bilateral. Onset of illness is usually nonspecific, with symptoms of fever, headache, malaise, myalgia, and anorexia. Complications may occur such as orchitis, aseptic meningitis, encephalitis, and pancreatitis. Approximately 20% of cases are asymptomatic.

DIAGNOSIS

Usually clinical, defined as illness with acute onset of unilateral or bilateral tender, self-limited swelling of the parotid glands, other salivary glands, or both, lasting ≥2 days, and without other apparent cause. Laboratory confirmation of mumps involves virus isolation with RT-PCR or culture. For further information on laboratory testing, see www.cdc.gov/mumps/lab/index.html.

TREATMENT

Supportive care.

PREVENTION

Travelers aged ≥6 months who do not have acceptable evidence of mumps immunity (as documented by 2 doses of live mumps virus vaccine ≥28 days apart on or after the first birthday, laboratory evidence of immunity, laboratory confirmation of disease, or birth before 1957) should be vaccinated with measles-mumps-rubella (MMR) vaccine. Before departure from the United States, infants aged 6–11 months should receive 1 dose of MMR vaccine (for measles protection), and children aged ≥12 months and adults should receive 2 doses of MMR vaccine ≥28 days apart on or after the first birthday.

CDC website: www.cdc.gov/mumps

BIBLIOGRAPHY

1. CDC. Manual for the surveillance of vaccine-preventable diseases. Atlanta: CDC; 2012 [cited 2014 Sep 18]. Available from: http://www.cdc.gov/vaccines/pubs/surv-manual/index.html.

2. CDC. Prevention of measles, rubella, congenital rubella syndrome, and mumps, 2013: summary recommendations of the Advisory Committee on Immunization Practices (ACIP). MMWR Recomm Rep. 2013 Jun 14;62(RR-04):1–34.

3. CDC. Update: mumps outbreak—New York and New Jersey, June 2009–January 2010. MMWR Morb Mortal Wkly Rep. 2010 Feb 12; 59(5):125–9.

4. Dayan GH, Quinlisk MP, Parker AA, Barskey AE, Harris ML, Schwartz JM, et al. Recent resurgence of mumps in the United States. N Engl J Med. 2008 Apr 10;358(15):1580–9.

NOROVIRUS

Aron J. Hall, Ben Lopman

INFECTIOUS AGENT

Norovirus infection is caused by non-enveloped, single-stranded RNA viruses of the genus *Norovirus*, which have also been referred to as "Norwalk-like viruses," Norwalk viruses, and small round-structured viruses. Norovirus gastroenteritis is sometimes incorrectly referred to as "stomach flu"; however, there is no biologic association with influenza or influenza viruses.

TRANSMISSION

Transmission occurs primarily through the fecal-oral route, either through direct person-to-person contact or indirectly via contaminated food or water. Norovirus is also spread through aerosols of vomitus and contaminated environmental surfaces and objects.

EPIDEMIOLOGY

Norovirus infections are common throughout the world, and globally most children will have experienced ≥1 infection by the age of 5 years. Norovirus infections can occur year round, but in temperate climates, norovirus activity peaks during the winter. Noroviruses are common in both developing and developed countries. In the United States, norovirus is the leading cause of sporadic cases and outbreaks of gastroenteritis, estimated to cause 19–21 million illnesses a year and approximately 50% of all foodborne outbreaks.

Norovirus is a cause of travelers' diarrhea; prevalence ranges from 3% to 17% of travelers returning with diarrhea. However, coinfection and asymptomatic infection with norovirus are common, so focused studies are needed to determine exactly how frequently norovirus is the cause of disease. Risk for infection is present anywhere food is prepared in an unsanitary manner and may become contaminated, or where drinking water is inadequately treated. Of particular risk are "ready-to-eat" cold foods, such as sandwiches and salads. Raw shellfish, especially oysters, are also a frequent source of infection, because virus from contaminated water concentrates in the gut of these filter feeders. Contaminated ice has also been implicated in outbreaks.

Large norovirus outbreaks are associated with settings where people live in close quarters and can easily infect each other, such as hotels, cruise ships, camps, dormitories, and hospitals. Viral contamination of inanimate objects or environmental surfaces (fomites) may persist during and after outbreaks and be a source of infection. On cruise ships, for instance, such environmental contamination has caused recurrent norovirus outbreaks on successive cruises with newly boarded passengers. Transmission of norovirus on airplanes has been reported during both domestic and international flights and likely results from contamination of lavatories or from symptomatic passengers in the cabin.

CLINICAL PRESENTATION

Infected people usually have an acute onset of vomiting with nonbloody diarrhea. The incubation period is 12–48 hours. Other symptoms include abdominal cramps, nausea, and sometimes a low-grade fever. Illness is generally self-limited, and full recovery can be expected in 1–3 days. In some cases, dehydration, especially in patients who are very young or elderly, may require medical attention.

DIAGNOSIS

Norovirus infection is generally diagnosed based on symptoms. No laboratory tests have been approved by the Food and Drug Administration to guide clinical management of individual patients, but laboratory testing is used during outbreak investigations by public health agencies. Norovirus diagnostic testing is usually not available in developing countries.

The most common diagnostic test used at state public health laboratories and CDC is RT-PCR, which rapidly and reliably detects the virus in stool specimens. Several commercial EIAs are available to detect the virus in stool specimens. The specificity and sensitivity of these assays are poor compared with RT-PCR.

TREATMENT

Supportive care is the mainstay of treatment of norovirus disease, especially oral or intravenous rehydration. Antimotility agents should be avoided in children aged <3 years, but may be a useful adjunct to rehydration in older children and adults. Antiemetic agents should generally be reserved for adults. Antibiotics are not useful in treating patients with norovirus disease.

PREVENTION

No vaccine is currently available, although vaccine development efforts are advancing. Noroviruses are common and highly contagious, but the risk for infection can be minimized by frequent and proper handwashing and avoiding possibly contaminated food and water. Washing hands with soap and water for at least 20 seconds is considered the most effective way to reduce norovirus contamination; alcohol-based hand sanitizers might be useful between handwashings but should not be considered a substitute for soap and water.

In addition to handwashing, measures to prevent transmission of noroviruses between people traveling together include carefully cleaning up fecal material or vomit and disinfecting contaminated surfaces and toilet areas. Products should be approved by the Environmental Protection Agency for norovirus disinfection; alternatively, a solution of domestic bleach (5–25 table-spoons bleach per gallon of water) may be used. Soiled articles of clothing should be washed at the maximum available cycle length and machine-dried at high heat.

To help prevent the spread of noroviruses, ill people have been isolated on cruise ships and in institutional settings.

CDC website: www.cdc.gov/norovirus

BIBLIOGRAPHY

1. Ajami NJ, Kavanagh OV, Ramani S, Crawford SE, Atmar RL, Jiang ZD, et al. Seroepidemiology of norovirus-associated travelers' diarrhea. J Travel Med. 2014 Jan–Feb;21(1):6–11.
2. Apelt N, Hartberger C, Campe H, Loscher T. The prevalence of norovirus in returning international travelers with diarrhea. BMC Infect Dis. 2010;10:131.
3. Atmar RL, Bernstein DI, Harro CD, Al-Ibrahim MS, Chen WH, Ferreira J, et al. Norovirus vaccine against experimental human Norwalk virus illness. N Engl J Med. 2011 Dec 8;365(23):2178–87.
4. Glass RI, Parashar UD, Estes MK. Norovirus gastroenteritis. N Engl J Med. 2009 Oct 29;361(18):1776–85.
5. Hall AJ, Eisenbart VG, Etingue AL, Gould LH, Lopman BA, Parashar UD. Epidemiology of foodborne norovirus outbreaks, United States, 2001–2008. Emerg Infect Dis. 2012 Oct;18(10):1566–73.
6. Hall AJ, Lopman BA, Payne DC, Patel MM, Gastanaduy PA, Vinje J, et al. Norovirus disease in the United States. Emerg Infect Dis. 2013 Aug;19(8):1198–205.
7. Hall AJ, Vinjé J, Lopman B, Park GW, Yen C, Gregoricus N, et al. Updated norovirus outbreak management and disease prevention guidelines. MMWR Recomm Rep. 2011 Mar 4;60(RR-3):1–18.
8. Koo HL, Ajami NJ, Jiang ZD, Neill FH, Atmar RL, Ericsson CD, et al. Noroviruses as a cause of diarrhea in travelers to Guatemala, India, and Mexico. J Clin Microbiol. 2010 May;48(5):1673–6.
9. Patel MM, Widdowson MA, Glass RI, Akazawa K, Vinje J, Parashar UD. Systematic literature review of role of noroviruses in sporadic gastroenteritis. Emerg Infect Dis. 2008 Aug;14(8):1224–31.
10. Thornley CN, Emslie NA, Sprott TW, Greening GE, Rapana JP. Recurring norovirus transmission on an airplane. Clin Infect Dis. 2011 Sep;53(6):515–20.

ONCHOCERCIASIS (RIVER BLINDNESS)
Paul T. Cantey

INFECTIOUS AGENT
Onchocerca volvulus, a filarial nematode.

TRANSMISSION
Through female blackflies (genus *Simulium*), which typically bite during the day and breed near rapidly flowing rivers and streams.

EPIDEMIOLOGY
Endemic in much of sub-Saharan Africa. Small endemic foci are also present in the Arabian Peninsula (Yemen) and in the Americas (Brazil and Venezuela). Foci center around blackfly breeding sites, which are located near rapidly flowing water. Most infections, outside those in endemic populations, occur in expatriate groups, such as missionaries, field scientists, and Peace Corps volunteers, though infection may sometimes occur in short-term travelers (<31 days).

CLINICAL PRESENTATION
Highly pruritic, papular dermatitis; subcutaneous nodules; lymphadenitis; and ocular lesions, which can progress to visual loss and blindness. Symptoms begin after patent infections are established, which may take 18 months. Symptoms in travelers are primarily dermatologic (rash and pruritus) and may occur years after departure from endemic areas. Nodules are more common in endemic populations.

DIAGNOSIS
Presence of microfilariae in superficial skin shavings or punch biopsy, adult worms in

histologic sections of excised nodules, or characteristic eye lesions. Serologic testing is most useful for detecting infection when microfilariae are not identifiable. Determination of serum antifilarial IgG is available through the National Institutes of Health (301-496-5398) or CDC (www.dpd.cdc.gov/dpdx; 404-718-4745; parasites @cdc.gov).

TREATMENT
Ivermectin is the drug of choice. Repeated annual or semiannual doses may be required, as the drug kills the microfilariae but not the adult worms. Some experts recommend treating patients with 1 dose of ivermectin followed by 6 weeks of doxycycline to kill *Wolbachia*, an endosymbiotic rickettsialike bacterium that appears to be required for the survival of the *O. volvulus* macrofilariae and for embryogenesis. Diethylcarbamazine is contraindicated in onchocerciasis, because it has been associated with severe and fatal posttreatment reactions. An expert in tropical medicine should be consulted to help manage these patients.

PREVENTION
Avoid blackfly habitats (free-flowing rivers and streams) and use protection measures against biting insects (see Chapter 2, Protection against Mosquitoes, Ticks, & Other Arthropods).

CDC website: www.cdc.gov/parasites/onchocerciasis

BIBLIOGRAPHY
1. Hoerauf A. Filariasis: new drugs and new opportunities for lymphatic filariasis and onchocerciasis. Curr Opin Infect Dis. 2008 Dec;21(6):673–81.
2. Lipner EM, Law MA, Barnett E, Keystone JS, von Sonnenburg F, Loutan L, et al. Filariasis in travelers presenting to the GeoSentinel Surveillance Network. PLoS Negl Trop Dis. 2007;1(3):e88.
3. McCarthy JS, Ottesen EA, Nutman TB. Onchocerciasis in endemic and nonendemic populations: differences in clinical presentation and immunologic findings. J Infect Dis. 1994 Sep;170(3):736–41.
4. Tielsch JM, Beeche A. Impact of ivermectin on illness and disability associated with onchocerciasis. Trop Med Int Health. 2004 Apr;9(4):A45–56.
5. WHO Expert Committee. Onchocerciasis and its control. Report of a WHO Expert Committee on Onchocerciasis Control. World Health Organ Tech Rep Ser. 1995;852:1–104.

PERTUSSIS
Tami H. Skoff, Jennifer L. Liang

INFECTIOUS AGENT
Fastidious gram-negative coccobacillus, *Bordetella pertussis*.

TRANSMISSION
Person-to-person transmission via aerosolized respiratory droplets or by direct contact with respiratory secretions.

EPIDEMIOLOGY
Pertussis is endemic worldwide, even in areas with high vaccination rates. In recent years, pertussis has resurged in a number of countries with successful vaccination programs, including the United States. In 2012, >48,000 cases of pertussis were reported nationally, the largest number in the United States since 1955. Disease rates are highest among young children in countries where vaccination coverage is low, which is primarily in the developing world. In developed countries, the incidence of pertussis is highest among infants too young to be vaccinated.

Immunity from childhood vaccination and natural disease wanes with time; therefore, adolescents and adults who have not received a tetanus-diphtheria-pertussis

(Tdap) booster vaccination can become infected or reinfected. US travelers are not at increased risk for disease specifically because of international travel, but they are at risk if they come in close contact with infected people. Infants too young to be protected by a complete vaccination series are at highest risk for severe illness and death from pertussis.

CLINICAL PRESENTATION

In classic disease, mild upper respiratory tract symptoms begin 7–10 days (range, 6–21 days) after exposure, followed by a cough that becomes paroxysmal. Coughing paroxysms can vary in frequency and are often followed by vomiting. Fever is absent or minimal. The clinical case definition for pertussis includes cough for ≥2 weeks with paroxysms, whoop, or posttussive vomiting.

Disease in infants aged <6 months can be atypical, with a short catarrhal stage, gagging, gasping, or apnea as early manifestations. Among infants aged <2 months, the case-fatality ratio is approximately 1%. Recently immunized children who develop disease may have mild cough illness; older children and adults may have prolonged cough with or without paroxysms. The cough gradually wanes over several weeks to months.

DIAGNOSIS

Factors such as prior vaccination status, stage of disease, antibiotic use, specimen collection and transport conditions, and use of nonstandardized tests may affect the sensitivity, specificity, and interpretation of available diagnostic tests for B. *pertussis*. CDC guidelines for the laboratory confirmation of pertussis cases include culture and PCR (when the above clinical case definition is met); serology and direct fluorescent antibody tests are not confirmatory tests included in the current case definition for reporting purposes.

TREATMENT

Macrolide antibiotics (azithromycin, clarithromycin, and erythromycin) are recommended for the treatment of pertussis in people aged ≥1 month; for infants aged <1 month, azithromycin is the preferred antibiotic. Antimicrobial therapy with a macrolide antibiotic administered <3 weeks after cough onset can limit transmission to others. Postexposure prophylaxis is recommended for all household contacts of cases and for people at high risk of developing severe disease (such as infants and women in the third trimester of pregnancy) or those who will have contact with a person at high risk of severe illness. The recommended agents and dosing regimens for prophylaxis are the same as for the treatment of pertussis.

PREVENTION
Vaccine

Travelers should be up-to-date with pertussis vaccinations before departure. Multiple pertussis vaccines are available in the United States for infants and children, and 2 vaccines are available for adolescents and adults. A complete listing of licensed vaccines can be found at www.fda.gov/BiologicsBloodVaccines/Vaccines/ApprovedProducts/ucm093833.htm.

Infants and Children

In the United States, all infants and children should receive 5 doses of acellular pertussis vaccine in combination with diphtheria and tetanus toxoids (DTaP) at ages 2, 4, 6, and 15–18 months and 4–6 years. An accelerated schedule of doses may be used to complete the DTaP series.

Children aged 7–10 years who are not fully vaccinated against pertussis and for whom no contraindication to pertussis vaccine exists should receive a single dose of tetanus toxoid, reduced diphtheria toxoid, and acellular pertussis vaccine (Tdap) to provide protection against pertussis. If additional doses of tetanus and diphtheria toxoid-containing vaccines are needed, then they should be vaccinated according to catch-up guidance, with Tdap preferred as the first dose.

Adolescents and Adults

Adolescents aged 11–18 years who have completed the recommended childhood DTwP/DTaP vaccination series and who have not previously received Tdap and adults aged ≥19 years who have not previously received Tdap should receive a single dose of Tdap instead of tetanus and diphtheria toxoids (Td) vaccine for booster immunization against tetanus, diphtheria, and pertussis. To provide pertussis protection before travel, Tdap can be given regardless of the interval from the last Td, except to people for whom pertussis vaccination is contraindicated or for people who have previously received Tdap. Adolescents and adults who have never been immunized against pertussis, tetanus, or diphtheria; who have incomplete immunization; or whose immunity is uncertain should follow the catch-up schedule established for Td/Tdap.

Pregnant Women

Pregnant Women

Women should have a dose of Tdap during each pregnancy, irrespective of her history of receiving Tdap. Although Tdap may be given at any time during pregnancy, to maximize the maternal antibody response and passive antibody transfer to the infant, optimal timing for Tdap administration is at 27–36 weeks' gestation.

CDC website: www.cdc.gov/pertussis

BIBLIOGRAPHY

1. American Academy of Pediatrics. Pertussis (whooping cough). In: Pickering LK, editor. Red Book: 2012 Report of the Committee on Infectious Diseases. 29th ed. Elk Grove Village, IL: American Academy of Pediatrics; 2012. p. 553–66.
2. Broder KR, Cortese MM, Iskander JK, Kretsinger K, Slade BA, Brown KH, et al. Preventing tetanus, diphtheria, and pertussis among adolescents: use of tetanus toxoid, reduced diphtheria toxoid and acellular pertussis vaccines. Recommendations of the Advisory Committee on Immunization Practices (ACIP). MMWR Recomm Rep. 2006 Dec 15;55(RR-17):1–33.
3. CDC. Updated recommendations for use of tetanus toxoid, reduced diphtheria toxoid and acellular pertussis (Tdap) vaccine from the Advisory Committee on Immunization Practices, 2010. MMWR Morb Mortal Wkly Rep. 2011 Jan 14;60(1):13–5.
4. CDC. Updated recommendations for use of tetanus toxoid, reduced diphtheria toxoid, and acellular pertussis vaccine (Tdap) in pregnant women—Advisory Committee on Immunization Practices (ACIP), 2012. MMWR Morb Mortal Wkly Rep. 2013;62(7):131–5.
5. Edwards KM, Decker MD. Pertussis vaccines. In: Plotkin SA, Orenstein WA, Offit PA, editors. Vaccines. 6th ed. Philadelphia: Saunders Elsevier; 2012. p. 447–92.
6. Tiwari T, Murphy TV, Moran J. Recommended antimicrobial agents for the treatment and postexposure prophylaxis of pertussis: 2005 CDC Guidelines. MMWR Recomm Rep. 2005 Dec 9;54 (RR-14):1–16.

PINWORM (ENTEROBIASIS, OXYURIASIS, THREADWORM)

Christine Dubray

INFECTIOUS AGENT

The intestinal nematode (roundworm) *Enterobius vermicularis*.

TRANSMISSION

Egg transmission occurs by the fecal-oral route, either directly or indirectly via contaminated hands or objects such as clothes, toys, and bedding.

EPIDEMIOLOGY

Pinworm is endemic worldwide and commonly clusters within families. Those most likely to be infected with pinworm are school-age children, people who take care of infected children, and people who are institutionalized. Travelers are at risk if staying in crowded conditions with infected people.

CLINICAL PRESENTATION

Incubation period is usually 1–2 months, but successive reinfections may be needed before symptoms appear. The most common symptom is an itchy anal region, which can disturb sleep. Adult worms can migrate from the anal area to other sites, including the vulva, vagina, and urethra. Secondary bacterial infection can occur from skin irritation.

DIAGNOSIS

The first option is to look for adult worms near the anus 2–3 hours after the infected person is asleep. The second option is microscopic identification of worm eggs collected by touching transparent tape to the anal area when the person first awakens in the morning. This method should be conducted on 3 consecutive mornings and before washing. The third option is microscopic examination of samples taken from under fingernails; samples should be taken before handwashing. Examining stool samples is not recommended because pinworm eggs are sparse.

TREATMENT

Drugs of choice are mebendazole, albendazole, or pyrantel pamoate (which is available without prescription). Each is given as a single dose and repeated in 2 weeks. In households where >1 member is infected or where repeated, symptomatic infections occur, all household members should be treated at the same time. For children younger than 2 years of age, in whom experience with these drugs is limited, risks and benefits should be considered by a physician before drug administration. Infected people should also bathe in the morning and change underwear and bedclothes frequently. Infected people should also practice personal hygiene measures such as washing hands before eating or preparing food, keeping fingernails short, not scratching the perianal region, and not biting nails.

PREVENTION

Hand hygiene is the most effective method of prevention. Bed linen and underclothing of infected children should be handled carefully, should not be shaken (to avoid contaminating the environment), and should be laundered promptly.

CDC website: www.cdc.gov/parasites/pinworm

BIBLIOGRAPHY

1. American Academy of Pediatrics. Pinworm infection (*Enterobius vermicularis*). In: Pickering LK, editor. Red Book: 2012 Report of the Committee on Infectious Diseases. 29th ed. Elk Grove Village, IL: American Academy of Pediatrics; 2012. p. 566–7.
2. American Public Health Association. Enterobiasis. In: Heyman DL, editor. Control of Communicable Diseases Manual. 19th ed. Washington, DC: American Public Health Association; 2008. p. 223–5.
3. Kucik CJ, Martin GL, Sortor BV. Common intestinal parasites. Am Fam Physician. 2004 Mar 1;69(5):1161–8.

PLAGUE (BUBONIC, PNEUMONIC, SEPTICEMIC)

Paul S. Mead

INFECTIOUS AGENT

The gram-negative bacterium *Yersinia pestis*.

TRANSMISSION

Usually through the bite of infected rodent fleas. Less common exposures include handling infected animal tissues (hunters, wildlife personnel), inhalation of infectious droplets from cats or dogs with plague, and, rarely, contact with a pneumonic plague patient.

EPIDEMIOLOGY

Endemic in rural areas in central and southern Africa (especially eastern Democratic Republic of Congo, northwestern Uganda, and Madagascar), central Asia and the Indian subcontinent, the northeastern part of South America, and parts of the south-western United States. Overall risk to travelers is low.

CLINICAL PRESENTATION

Incubation period is typically 1–6 days. Symptoms and signs of the 3 clinical presentations of plague illness are as follows:

- Bubonic (most common)—rapid onset of fever; painful, swollen, and tender lymph nodes, usually inguinal, axillary, or cervical
- Pneumonic—high fever, overwhelming pneumonia, cough, bloody sputum, chills
- Septicemic—fever, prostration, hemorrhagic or thrombotic phenomena, progressing to acral gangrene

DIAGNOSIS

Y. pestis can be isolated from bubo aspirates, blood cultures, or sputum culture if pneumonic. Diagnosis can be confirmed in public health laboratories by culture or serologic tests for the *Y. pestis* F1 antigen.

TREATMENT

Parenteral antibiotic therapy with streptomycin or gentamicin appears to be equally effective. Levofloxacin was recently approved by the Food and Drug Administration for treatment and is highly effective in animal studies. Second-line agents include doxycycline, tetracycline, and chloramphenicol.

PREVENTION

Reduce contact with fleas and potentially infected rodents and other wildlife.

CDC website: www.cdc.gov/plague

BIBLIOGRAPHY

1. Neerinckx S, Bertherat E, Leirs H. Human plague occurrences in Africa: an overview from 1877 to 2008. Trans R Soc Trop Med Hyg. 2010 Feb;104(2):97–103.
2. Perry RD, Fetherston JD. *Yersinia pestis*—etiologic agent of plague. Clin Microbiol Rev. 1997 Jan;10(1):35–66.
3. World Health Organization. Human plague: review of regional morbidity and mortality, 2004–2009. Wkly Epidemiol Rec. 2009 Feb 5;85(6):40–5.

PNEUMOCOCCAL DISEASE

Ronnie Henry

INFECTIOUS AGENT

The gram-positive coccus *Streptococcus pneumoniae.*

TRANSMISSION

Person to person through close contact via respiratory droplets.

EPIDEMIOLOGY

Streptococcus pneumoniae is the most common cause of community-acquired pneumonia worldwide. The prevalence is higher in developing than in industrialized countries. Risk is highest in young children, the elderly, and those with chronic illnesses or immune suppression.

CLINICAL PRESENTATION

Pneumococcal pneumonia classically presents with sudden onset of fever and malaise, cough, pleuritic chest pain, or purulent or blood-tinged sputum. In the elderly, fever, shortness of breath, or altered mental status may be initial symptoms. Pneumococcal meningitis may present as a stiff neck, headache, lethargy, or seizures.

DIAGNOSIS

Isolation from blood or cerebrospinal fluid, but most patients do not have detectable bacteremia. Pneumococcal urine antigen test may be useful but is not routinely recommended for diagnosis, as per the Infectious

Diseases Society of America and American Thoracic Society guidelines (www.idsociety.org). Infection can be suspected if a sputum specimen contains gram-positive diplococci, polymorphonuclear leukocytes, and few epithelial cells. High white blood cell counts should raise suspicion for bacterial infection.

TREATMENT

Therapy depends on the syndrome, but patients who present with community-acquired pneumonia should be empirically treated for pneumococcal infection. Many strains are resistant to penicillin, cephalosporins, and macrolides. In the United States and other countries where β-lactam resistance is common, the initial regimen for pneumococcal meningitis might include vancomycin or a fluoroquinolone, plus a third-generation cephalosporin.

PREVENTION

The 13-valent pneumococcal conjugate vaccine (PCV13) is recommended for all children aged <5 years and children aged <72 months with chronic medical conditions; the vaccine is also recommended for children aged <18 years with immunocompromising conditions. A 23-valent pneumococcal polysaccharide vaccine (PPSV23) is recommended for adults aged ≥65 years and people aged 2–64 years with underlying medical conditions. Adults with immunocompromising conditions, functional or anatomic asplenia, cerebrospinal fluid leaks, or cochlear implants should receive PCV13 followed by PPSV23. See www.cdc.gov/vaccines/pubs/ACIP-list.htm#pcv.

CDC website: http://www.cdc.gov/pneumococcal/index.html

BIBLIOGRAPHY

1. CDC. Licensure of a 13-valent pneumococcal conjugate vaccine (PCV13) and recommendations for use among children—Advisory Committee on Immunization Practices (ACIP), 2010. MMWR Morb Mortal Wkly Rep. 2010 Mar 12;59(9):258–61.
2. CDC. Updated recommendations for prevention of invasive pneumococcal disease among adults using the 23-valent pneumococcal polysaccharide vaccine (PPSV23). MMWR Morb Mortal Wkly Rep. 2010;59(34):1102–6.
3. CDC. Use of 13-valent pneumococcal conjugate vaccine and 23-valent pneumococcal polysaccharide vaccine among children aged 6–18 years with immunocompromising conditions: recommendations of the Advisory Committee on Immunization Practices (ACIP). MMWR Morb Mortal Wkly Rep. 2013 June 28; 62(25):521–4.
4. CDC. Use of 13-valent pneumococcal conjugate vaccine and 23-valent pneumococcal polysaccharide vaccine for adults with immunocompromising conditions: recommendations of the Advisory Committee on Immunization Practices (ACIP). MMWR Morb Mortal Wkly Rep. 2012;61(40):816–9.
5. World Health Organization. Pneumococcal vaccines WHO position paper—2012—Recommendations. Vaccine. 2012;30(32):4717–8.

POLIOMYELITIS

James P. Alexander, Gregory S. Wallace, Steven G. F. Wassilak

INFECTIOUS AGENT

Poliovirus (genus *Enterovirus*) types 1, 2, and 3. Polioviruses are small (27–30 nm), non-enveloped viruses with capsids enclosing a single-stranded, positive-sense RNA genome about 7,500 nucleotides long. Most of the properties of polioviruses are shared with the other enteroviruses.

TRANSMISSION

Fecal-oral or oral transmission. Acute infection involves the oropharynx, gastrointestinal tract, and occasionally the central nervous system.

EPIDEMIOLOGY

Before a vaccine was available, infection with poliovirus was common worldwide, with seasonal peaks and epidemics in the summer and fall in temperate areas. The incidence of poliomyelitis in the United States declined rapidly after the licensure of inactivated polio vaccine (IPV) in 1955 and live oral polio vaccine (OPV) in the 1960s. The last cases of indigenously acquired polio in the United States occurred in 1979. The Global Polio Eradication Initiative (GPEI) subsequently eliminated polio in the Americas, where the last wild poliovirus (WPV)–associated polio case was detected in 1991. In January 2000, a change in vaccination policy in the United States from use of live OPV to exclusive use of IPV eliminated the 8–10 vaccine-associated paralytic poliomyelitis (VAPP) cases that had occurred annually since the introduction of OPV in the 1960s.

GPEI has built upon the success in the Americas and made great progress in eradicating WPVs, reducing the number of reported polio cases worldwide by more than 99% since the mid-1980s. As of April 2014, WPV circulation has never been interrupted in only 3 countries: Afghanistan, Nigeria, and Pakistan. Because of polio eradication efforts, the number of countries where travelers are at risk for polio has decreased dramatically. The last documented case of WPV-associated paralysis in a US resident traveling abroad occurred in 1986 in a 29-year-old vaccinated adult who had been traveling in South and Southeast Asia. In 2005, an unvaccinated US adult traveling abroad acquired VAPP after contact with an infant recently vaccinated with OPV.

In spite of progress made in eradicating WPVs globally, polio-free countries remain at risk for imported cases and outbreaks, and travelers to some countries are at risk for exposure to WPV. In 2012 and 2013, WPV outbreaks from importations occurred in 7 countries in Africa and the Middle East, with a total of 262 cases. A "WPV importation belt" extends across sub-Saharan Africa from the west coast to the Horn of Africa in the east, where WPV importation and outbreaks have occurred in a number of countries since 2003. From 2012 through early 2014, imported WPV from Pakistan was found in some sewage samples taken in Egypt, Israel, and the West Bank and Gaza (without any identified polio cases) and caused outbreaks in Iraq and Syria.

For additional information on the status of polio eradication efforts, countries or areas with active WPV circulation, and vaccine recommendations, consult the travel notices on the CDC Travelers' Health website (www.cdc.gov/travel) or the GPEI website (www.polioeradication.org).

CLINICAL PRESENTATION
Clinical manifestations of poliovirus infection range from asymptomatic (most infections) to symptomatic, including acute flaccid paralysis of a single limb to quadriplegia, respiratory failure, and rarely, death.

DIAGNOSIS
The diagnosis is made by identifying poliovirus in clinical specimens (usually stool) obtained from an acutely ill patient. Poliovirus may be detected by culture of cell lines followed by identification using neutralization tests or PCR. Poliovirus may also be identified by direct amplification from stool specimens followed by genomic sequencing to identify the possible source of the virus. Shedding in fecal specimens can be intermittent, but usually poliovirus can be detected for up to 4 weeks after onset of illness. During the first 3–10 days of the illness, poliovirus can also be detected from oropharyngeal specimens. Poliovirus is rarely detected in the blood or cerebrospinal fluid.

TREATMENT
Only treatment for symptoms is available, ranging from pain and fever relief to intubation and mechanical ventilation for patients with respiratory insufficiency.

PREVENTION
Vaccine
Recommendations for Health Protection
In the United States, infants and children should be vaccinated against polio as part of a routine immunization series (see Infants and Children below). Polio vaccination is recommended for all travelers to countries with WPV circulation. Countries are considered to have WPV circulation if they have evidence during the previous 12 months of ongoing endemic circulation, a polio outbreak, or environmental evidence (through sewage sampling) of WPV circulation. For additional information on countries with

WPV circulation and vaccine recommendations, consult the travel notices on the CDC Travelers' Health website (www.cdc.gov/travel) or the weekly update of reported WPV cases at the GPEI website (www.polioeradication.org/Dataandmonitoring/Poliothisweek.aspx).

Before traveling to areas where that have WPV circulation, travelers should ensure that they have completed the recommended age-appropriate polio vaccine series and that adults have received a single lifetime IPV booster dose. In addition, CDC recommends a single lifetime IPV booster dose for certain adult travelers to some countries that border areas with WPV circulation. These recommendations are based on evidence of historical cross-border transmission. These recommendations apply only to travelers with a high risk of exposure to someone with imported WPV infection. These travelers would include those working in health care settings, refugee camps, or other humanitarian aid settings. Since the situation is dynamic, refer to the CDC Travelers' Health website destination pages for the most up-to-date polio vaccine recommendations (wwwnc.cdc.gov/travel/destinations/list).

To eliminate the risk for VAPP, IPV has been the only polio vaccine available in the United States since 2000; however, OPV continues to be used in many countries and for global polio eradication activities. For complete information on recommendations for poliomyelitis vaccination, consult the Advisory Committee on Immunization Practices recommendations website (www.cdc.gov/vaccines/hcp/acip-recs/vacc-specific/polio.html).

Country Requirements

In May 2014, the World Health Organization (WHO) declared the international spread of polio to be a public health emergency of international concern under the authority of the International Health Regulations (2005). To prevent further spread of disease, WHO issued temporary polio vaccine recommendations for long-term travelers (staying >4 weeks) and residents departing from countries with WPV transmission ("exporting WPV" or "infected with WPV"). Clinicians should be aware that long-term travelers and residents may be required to show proof of polio vaccination when departing from these countries. All polio vaccination administration should be documented on an International Certificate of Vaccination or Prophylaxis (ICVP). The polio vaccine must be received between 4 weeks and 12 months before the date of departure from the polio-affected country. Country requirements may change, so clinicians should check for updates on the CDC Travelers' Health website. Refer to the Clinical Update: Interim CDC Guidance for Travel to and from Countries Affected by the New Polio Vaccine Requirements (wwwnc.cdc.gov/travel/news-announcements/polio-guidance-new-requirements) for a list of affected countries, guidance on meeting the vaccination requirements, and instructions on how to order and fill out the ICVP.

Infants and Children

In the United States, all infants and children should receive 4 doses of IPV at ages 2, 4, and 6–18 months and 4–6 years. The final dose should be administered at age ≥4 years, regardless of the number of previous doses, and should be given ≥6 months after the previous dose. A fourth dose in the routine IPV series is not necessary if the third dose was administered at age ≥4 years and ≥6 months after the previous dose. If the routine series cannot be administered within the recommended intervals before protection is needed, the following alternatives are recommended:

- The first dose should be given to infants ≥6 weeks old.
- The second and third doses should be administered ≥4 weeks after the previous doses.
- The minimum interval between the third and fourth doses is 6 months.

If the age-appropriate series is not completed before departure, the remaining IPV doses to complete a full series should be administered when feasible, at the intervals recommended above.

Adults

Adults who are traveling to areas where WPV is actively circulating and who are unvaccinated, incompletely vaccinated, or whose vaccination status is unknown should receive a series of 3 doses: 2 doses of IPV administered at an interval of 4–8 weeks; a third dose should be administered 6–12 months after the second. If 3 doses of IPV cannot be administered within the recommended intervals before protection is needed, the following alternatives are recommended:

- If >8 weeks is available before protection is needed, 3 doses of IPV should be administered ≥4 weeks apart.
- If <8 weeks but >4 weeks is available before protection is needed, 2 doses of IPV should be administered ≥4 weeks apart.
- If <4 weeks is available before protection is needed, a single dose of IPV is recommended.

If <3 doses are administered, the remaining IPV doses to complete a 3-dose series should be administered when feasible, at the intervals recommended above, if the person remains at increased risk for poliovirus exposure.

Adults who have completed a routine series of polio vaccine are considered to have lifelong immunity to poliomyelitis, but data on duration of immunity are lacking. As a precaution, adults (≥18 years of age) who are traveling to areas where WPV is actively circulating and who have received a routine series with either IPV or OPV in childhood should receive another dose of IPV before departure. For adults, available data do not indicate the need for more than a single lifetime booster dose with IPV.

International Adoption of Children

The international adoption of children from countries or areas where WPV is actively circulating is a special situation. International adoptees might not have completed a primary vaccination series against polio and might not have received a dose of polio vaccine before departure. Thus, there is a small risk that they might be infected with WPV and remain infectious upon entry into the United States and potentially transmit to US household members and caregivers. So as a measure of prudence, the polio vaccination status of all household members and caregivers of international adoptees whose origin is a country with active WPV circulation should be assessed before the entry of the child into the United States. Those who are unvaccinated, incompletely vaccinated, or whose vaccination status is unknown should be brought up-to-date. Adults who have completed the primary series should consider a one-time booster of IPV as well.

Vaccine Safety and Adverse Reactions

Minor local reactions (pain and redness) can occur after IPV administration. No serious adverse reactions to IPV have been documented. IPV should not be administered to people who have experienced a severe allergic reaction (such as anaphylaxis) after a previous dose of IPV or after receiving streptomycin, polymyxin B, or neomycin, which IPV contains in trace amounts; hypersensitivity reactions can occur after IPV administration among people sensitive to these 3 antibiotics.

Pregnancy and Breastfeeding

If a pregnant woman is unvaccinated or incompletely vaccinated and requires immediate protection against polio because of planned travel to a country or area where WPV is actively circulating, IPV can be administered as recommended for adults. Breastfeeding is not a contraindication to administration of polio vaccine to an infant or mother.

Precautions and Contraindications

IPV may be administered to people with diarrhea. Minor upper respiratory illnesses with or without fever, mild to moderate local reactions to a previous dose of IPV, current antimicrobial therapy, and the convalescent phase of acute illness are not contraindications for vaccination.

Immunosuppression

IPV may be administered safely to immunocompromised travelers and their household contacts. Although a protective immune response cannot be ensured, IPV might confer some protection to the immunocompromised person. People with certain primary immunodeficiency diseases should not be given OPV and should avoid contact with excreted OPV virus (such as exposure to a child vaccinated with OPV in the previous 6 weeks); however, this situation no longer occurs in the United States unless a child receives OPV overseas.

BIBLIOGRAPHY

1. CDC. Assessing the risks for poliovirus outbreaks in polio-free countries—Africa, 2012–2013. MMWR Morb Mortal Wkly Rep. 2013 Sep 20;62(37):768–72.

2. CDC. Immunization schedules. Atlanta: CDC; 2014 [cited 2014 Apr 14]. Available from: http://www.cdc.gov/vaccines/schedules/index.html.

3. CDC. Progress toward eradication of polio—worldwide, January 2011–March 2013. MMWR Morb Mortal Wkly Rep. 2013 May 3;62(17):335–8.

4. CDC. Update on vaccine-derived polioviruses—worldwide, July 2012–December 2013. MMWR Morb Mortal Wkly Rep. 2014 Mar 21;63(11):242–8.

5. CDC. Updated recommendations of the Advisory Committee on Immunization Practices (ACIP) regarding routine poliovirus vaccination. MMWR Morb Mortal Wkly Rep. 2009 Aug 7;58(30):829–30.

6. Prevots DR, Burr RK, Sutter RW, Murphy TV. Poliomyelitis prevention in the United States. Updated recommendations of the Advisory Committee on Immunization Practices (ACIP). MMWR Recomm Rep. 2000 May 9;49(RR-5):1–22.

7. Sutter RW, Kew OM, Cochi SL, Aylward RB. Poliovirus vaccine—live. In: Plotkin SA, Orenstein WA, Offit PA, editors. Vaccines. 6th ed. Philadelphia: Saunders Elsevier; 2012. p. 598–645.

8. Vidor E, Plotkin SA. Poliovirus vaccine—inactivated. In: Plotkin SA, Orenstein WA, Offit PA, editors. Vaccines. 6th ed. Philadelphia: Saunders Elsevier; 2012. p. 573–97.

9. World Health Organization. Polio vaccines: WHO position paper, January 2014—Recommendations. Vaccine. 2014 Jul 16;32(33):4117–8.

10. World Health Organization. Wild poliovirus weekly update. World Health Organization; 2014 [cited 2014 Aug 11]. Available from: http://www.polioeradication.org/Dataandmonitoring/Poliothisweek.aspx.

CDC website: http://www.cdc.gov/vaccines/vpd-vac/polio/in-short-both.htm

For the Record

A HISTORY OF POLIO ERADICATION

Gregory L. Armstrong, MD

Before licensing of the inactivated (1955) and live attenuated (1961) polio vaccines, poliomyelitis was ubiquitous and distributed globally. Poliovirus infected most people in childhood, causing paralysis in approximately 1 in 200. Where vaccine was introduced, it had a rapid effect on the disease. In the United States, reported paralytic cases fell from approximately 20,000 per year in the early 1950s to 2,525 in 1960 and 61 in 1965.

By the early 1980s, the feasibility of globally eradicating polio was already being discussed. Several characteristics of poliovirus made it an ideal candidate for eradication, including the lack of an animal reservoir and the availability of an effective, inexpensive, easily administered oral polio vaccine

(OPV). Furthermore, experience in Cuba and Brazil had demonstrated the ability of mass vaccination campaigns to interrupt poliovirus transmission. In 1988, the World Health Assembly formally resolved to eradicate poliomyelitis by 2000, giving birth to the Global Polio Eradication Initiative (GPEI).

Much progress toward eradication was achieved in the 1990s: the number of cases globally dropped by >99%, polio was eliminated from the Americas, and 1 of the 3 types of wild poliovirus (type 2) was eradicated globally. However, the goal of eradication by 2000 was not achieved, and the program entered into a decade-long period where progress appeared to have stalled, with 1,000–2,000 cases annually. Critics began to question whether polio eradication was feasible or even ethical. However, during this period there was another trend in the program—one of determined innovation. In India, for example, where nothing seemed to be successful at bringing down case counts, the program underwent a major transformation, with innovations to improve supervision and accountability in the field and other innovations to identify and reach chronically undervaccinated groups—groups that were often outside the reach of the formal public health system. In addition, technical advances were brought to fruition, most importantly the division of OPV into its individual components ([monovalent] mOPV1 and mOPV3) for the first time since they had been combined into the trivalent vaccine in the 1960s. These monovalent vaccines and, later on, the bivalent (types 1 and 3) vaccine greatly increased immunogenicity because interference by the more robust type 2 component was removed.

In late 2011, the program found itself at a crossroads. It was becoming increasingly likely that transmission had been interrupted in India in early 2011, with the last reported case in January. This success seemed to answer the question of feasibility—if polio could be eradicated in India, it could be eradicated anywhere. However, in the 3 remaining "endemic" countries—Nigeria, Pakistan, and Afghanistan, where wild poliovirus transmission had never been interrupted—case counts were increasing, and multiple outbreaks were occurring in countries that had previously been polio free. In October 2011, GPEI's independent monitoring board issued a critical report, stating bluntly that the program was "not on track to interrupt polio transmission" and that "polio eradication needs to be treated as a global health emergency" if the ultimate goal of the program was ever to be achieved. This report initiated a new era in the program, one in which the GPEI partnership has scaled up activities, particularly in the 3 remaining endemic countries, in order to complete eradication.

The strategy of wild poliovirus eradication is organized around 4 "pillars":

- Strengthening routine immunization programs
- "Supplementary immunization activities" (SIAs) in the form of mass vaccination campaigns, either at the national or subnational level
- Surveillance for acute flaccid paralysis (AFP) and confirmation of polio by laboratory testing of stool samples
- Targeted "mop-up" campaigns around any confirmed cases of polio

In endemic countries and other countries with active wild poliovirus transmission, SIAs, the most visible aspect of the program, are typically conducted every 4–8 weeks until transmission has been stopped. AFP surveillance is a critical component in countries both with and without polio, where the surveillance system is expected to detect nonpolio cases of AFP at a rate of at least 1 per 100,000 per year in industrialized countries and 2 per 100,000 per year in developing countries. Environmental surveillance—the testing of sewage for polioviruses—is also a sensitive tool for poliovirus detection and plays an increasing role in surveillance for poliovirus.

The polio eradication program will not end with the last case of polio. In addition to interrupting wild poliovirus, the program will also need to interrupt circulation of vaccine-derived polioviruses (VDPVs). These viruses emerge usually from the type 2 component of OPV in locations where childhood vaccination coverage is exceptionally low and are eliminated by increasing vaccination coverage or conducting SIAs with the trivalent vaccine. To prevent further VDPV2 emergence, inactivated poliovirus vaccine is being introduced in countries where it is not in use, and trivalent OPV is being replaced with bivalent OPV. At the same time, GPEI will gradually transition its resources toward supporting other public health objectives ("legacy"), and laboratories with samples containing poliovirus will need to destroy or consolidate and safely store those samples ("containment"). The plan for carrying out this massive set of tasks is documented in the GPEI *Polio Eradication and Endgame Strategic Plan, 2013–2018*.

BIBLIOGRAPHY

1. Dowdle WR, Cochi SL. Global eradication of poliovirus: history and rationale. In: Selmer BL, Wimmer E, editors. Molecular Biology of Picornaviruses. Washington, DC: ASM Press; 2002. p. 473–80.
2. Global Polio Eradication Initiative. Polio eradication and endgame strategic plan, 2013–2018. Geneva: World Health Organization; 2013 [cited 2014 Jun 23]. Available from: http://www.polioeradication.org/resourcelibrary/strategyandwork.aspx.
3. Independent Monitoring Board (Global Polio Eradication Intiative). Report October 2011. Geneva: Global Polio Eradication Initiative; 2011 [cited 2014 Sep 18]. Available from: http://www.polioeradication.org/Portals/0/Document/Aboutus/Governance/IMB/4IMBMeeting/IMBReportOctober2011.pdf.

Q FEVER

Alicia Anderson, Jennifer McQuiston

INFECTIOUS AGENT

The gram-negative intracellular bacterium *Coxiella burnetii*.

TRANSMISSION

Most commonly, through inhalation of aerosols or dust contaminated with dried birth fluids or excreta from infected animals (usually cattle, sheep, or goats). *C. burnetii* is highly infectious and persists in the environment. Infections via ingestion of contaminated, unpasteurized dairy products and human-to-human transmission via sexual contact have been rarely reported.

EPIDEMIOLOGY

Distributed worldwide; the prevalence is highest in African and Middle Eastern countries. More than 200 cases have been reported since 2003 in US military personnel deployed to Iraq. Reported rates of human infection are higher in France and Australia than in the United States. The largest known reported Q fever outbreak to date involved approximately 4,000 human cases and occurred during 2007–2010 in the Netherlands. Travelers who visit rural areas or farms with cattle, sheep, goats, or other livestock may be exposed to Q fever. Occupational exposure to infected animals (such as in farmers, veterinarians, butchers, meat packers, and seasonal or migrant farm workers), particularly during parturition, poses a high risk for disease transmission.

CLINICAL PRESENTATION

Approximately half of acute infections are mild or asymptomatic. Incubation period is typically 2–3 weeks but may be shorter after exposure to large numbers of organisms. The most common presentation of acute infection is a self-limiting influenzalike illness, with pneumonia or hepatitis in more severe acute infections. Chronic infections occur primarily in patients with preexisting cardiac valvulopathies, vascular abnormalities, or immunosuppression. Women infected during pregnancy are at high risk for adverse pregnancy outcomes unless treated. The most common manifestations of chronic disease are endocarditis and endovascular infections.

DIAGNOSIS

Serologic evidence of a 4-fold rise in phase II IgG by indirect immunofluorescent assay (IFA) between paired sera taken 3–4 weeks apart is the gold standard for diagnosis of acute infection. A single high serum phase II IgG titer (>1:128) by IFA in conjunction with clinical evidence of infection may be considered evidence of probable infection. *C. burnetii* may be detected in infected tissues by using immunohistochemical staining or DNA detection methods or by direct isolation of the agent via culture. PCR assays may be used on whole blood or serum samples in the early stages of illness and before initiation of antibiotic therapy.

TREATMENT

Doxycycline is the treatment of choice for acute Q fever. Pregnant women, children aged <8 years with mild illness, and patients allergic to doxycycline may be treated with alternative antibiotics such as trimethoprim-sulfamethoxazole. Treatment for acute Q fever is not recommended for asymptomatic people or for those whose symptoms have resolved. Chronic *C. burnetii* infections require long-term combination therapy with agents such as doxycycline, hydroxychloroquine, trimethoprim-sulfamethoxazole, fluoroquinolones, and rifampin.

PREVENTION

Avoid areas where potentially infected animals are kept, and avoid consumption of unpasteurized dairy products. A human vaccine for Q fever has been developed and used in Australia, but it is not available in the United States.

CDC website: www.cdc.gov/qfever

BIBLIOGRAPHY

1. Anderson A, Bijlmer H, Fournier PE, Graves S, Hartzell J, Kersh GJ, et al. Diagnosis and management of Q fever—United States, 2013: recommendations from CDC and the Q Fever Working Group. MMWR Recomm Rep. 2013 Mar 29;62(RR-03):1–30.

2. Kobbe R, Kramme S, Gocht A, Werner M, Lippert U, May J, et al. Travel-associated *Coxiella burnetii* infections: three cases of Q fever with different clinical manifestation. Travel Med Infect Dis. 2007 Nov;5(6):374–9.

3. Maurin M, Raoult D. Q fever. Clin Microbiol Rev. 1999 Oct;12(4):518–53.

4. McQuiston JH, Childs JE, Thompson HA. Q fever. J Am Vet Med Assoc. 2002 Sep 15;221(6):796–9.

5. Million M, Thuny F, Richet H, Raoult D. Long-term outcome of Q fever endocarditis: a 26-year personal survey. Lancet Infect Dis. 2010 Aug;10(8):527–35.

6. Roest HI, Tilburg JJ, van der Hoek W, Vellema P, van Zijderveld FG, Klaassen CH, et al. The Q fever epidemic in The Netherlands: history, onset, response and reflection. Epidemiol Infect. 2011 Jan;139(1):1–12.

7. Ta TH, Jimenez B, Navarro M, Meije Y, Gonzalez FJ, Lopez-Velez R. Q Fever in returned febrile travelers. J Travel Med. 2008 Mar–Apr;15(2):126–9.

RABIES

Cathleen A. Hanlon, David R. Shlim

INFECTIOUS AGENTS

Rabies is an acute, fatal, progressive encephalomyelitis caused by neurotropic viruses in the family Rhabdoviridae, genus *Lyssavirus*. Numerous and diverse variants of lyssaviruses are found throughout the world, all of which may cause fatal human rabies cases. Tens of millions of human exposures and tens of thousands of deaths may occur each year.

TRANSMISSION

The most natural and successful mode of transmission is through the bite of a rabid animal. Virus at the wound site may remain undetectable during a variable incubation period; there is no viremia. Clinical illness begins following invasion of the peripheral and then central nervous system and culminates in acute fatal encephalitis. Exposure of highly innervated tissue and close proximity to the brain increases the risk of successful infection and may result in postexposure prophylaxis (PEP) failure if there is a delay in administration. Rarely, virus has been transmitted by exposures other than bites, such as introducing the agent into open wounds (such as through scratches) or mucous membranes and transplantation of tissues from undiagnosed rabid donors.

All mammals are believed to be susceptible to infection, but major reservoirs are carnivores and bats. Although dogs are the main reservoir in developing countries, the epidemiology of the disease differs from one region or country to another, so that all patients with mammal bites should be medically evaluated. **Bat bites anywhere in the world are a cause of concern and an indication to consider prophylaxis.**

EPIDEMIOLOGY

Rabies is found on all continents, except Antarctica. Regionally, different viral variants are adapted to various mammalian hosts and perpetuate in dogs and wildlife, such as bats and some carnivores, including foxes, jackals, mongooses, raccoons, and skunks. In certain areas of the world, canine rabies remains enzootic, including parts of Africa, Asia, and Central and South America. Table 3-14 lists countries that have reported no cases of rabies during the most recent period for which information is available (formerly referred to as "rabies-free" countries).

Timely and specific information about the global occurrence of rabies is often difficult to find. Surveillance levels vary, and reporting status can change suddenly as a result of disease reintroduction or emergence. The rate of rabies exposures in travelers is at best an estimate and may range from 16 to 200 per 100,000 travelers.

CLINICAL PRESENTATION

After infection, the incubation period is variable, but clinical illness most commonly develops in several weeks to several months after exposure. The disease progresses rapidly from a nonspecific, prodromal phase with fever and vague symptoms to an acute, progressive encephalitis. The neurologic phase may be characterized by anxiety, paresis, paralysis, and other signs of encephalitis; spasms of swallowing muscles can be stimulated by the sight, sound, or perception of water (hydrophobia); and delirium and convulsions can develop, followed rapidly by coma and death. Once clinical signs manifest, patients die quickly, but with intensive supportive care may succumb in 7–14 days.

DIAGNOSIS

The diagnosis may be relatively simple in a patient with a compatible history and a classic clinical presentation. However, clinical suspicion and prioritization of differential diagnoses may be complicated by variations in clinical presentation and a lack of exposure history. The exposure history is especially evasive if the risk of exposure to rabies was not recognized, the exposure was not discussed with friends and family, and several weeks to months have elapsed since the exposure.

Table 3-14. Countries and political units that reported no indigenous cases of rabies during 2013[1]

REGION	COUNTRIES/LOCALITIES
Africa	Cape Verde, Mauritius, Réunion, São Tomé and Príncipe, and Seychelles
Americas	North: Bermuda and Saint Pierre and Miquelon Caribbean: Antigua and Barbuda, Aruba, The Bahamas, Barbados, Cayman Islands, Dominica, Guadeloupe, Jamaica, Martinique, Montserrat, Netherlands Antilles, Saint Kitts (Saint Christopher) and Nevis, Saint Lucia, Saint Martin, Saint Vincent and Grenadines, Turks and Caicos, and the British and US Virgin Islands
Asia and the Middle East	Hong Kong, Japan, Kuwait, Malaysia (Sabah), Qatar, Singapore and United Arab Emirates
Europe[2]	Albania, Austria, Belgium, Corsica, Cyprus, Czech Republic, Denmark, Finland, France, Germany, Gibraltar, Greece, Hungary, Iceland, Ireland, Isle of Man, Liechtenstein, Luxembourg, Monaco, Netherlands, Norway (except Svalbard), Portugal, Slovakia, Slovenia, Spain (except Ceuta and Melilla), Sweden, Switzerland, and United Kingdom
Oceania[3]	Australia, Cook Islands, Fiji, French Polynesia, Guam, Hawaii, Kiribati, Micronesia, New Caledonia, New Zealand, Northern Mariana Islands, Palau, Papua New Guinea, Samoa, Solomon Islands, and Vanuatu

[1] Global surveillance efforts and reporting standards differ dramatically, conditions may change rapidly because of animal translocation, and bat rabies may exist in some areas that are reportedly "free" of rabies in other mammals.
[2] Bat lyssaviruses have been reported throughout Europe, including areas that are reportedly free of rabies in other wild mammals.
[3] Most of Pacific Oceania is reportedly "rabies free," with the exception of Australia, where lyssaviruses in bats have been reported, as well as fatal human rabies cases.

Definitive antemortem diagnosis requires high-complexity experimental test methods on multiple samples (such as serum, cerebrospinal fluid [CSF], saliva, and skin biopsy from the nape of the neck), which are best collected sequentially if initial testing is negative. Additional detailed information on diagnostic testing may be obtained from CDC (http://www.cdc.gov/rabies/specific_groups/doctors/ante_mortem.html). Rising levels of rabies virus–neutralizing antibodies, particularly in the CSF, is diagnostic in an unvaccinated, encephalitic patient.

TREATMENT

There is not yet an evidence-based "best practices" medical approach to treating patients with rabies; most patients are managed with symptomatic and palliative supportive care. An experimental approach, known as the Milwaukee protocol, involves inducing coma and treating with antiviral drugs, but it remains controversial (www.chw.org/display/PPF/DocID/33223/router.asp). Rabies is still considered 100% fatal for practical purposes, and preventive measures are the only way to optimize survival after a bite from a rabid animal.

PREVENTION

Rabies in travelers is best prevented by having a comprehensive strategy. This consists of 1) education about risks and the need to avoid bites from mammals, especially high-risk rabies reservoir species; 2) knowing how to prevent rabies after a bite; and 3) being able to obtain PEP, which may involve urgent international travel to where PEP is available. No traveler is known to have died while trying to obtain PEP. Travelers who have died of rabies either did not seek PEP or received inadequate care when they did.

Avoiding Animal Bites

Travelers to rabies-enzootic countries should be warned about the risk of rabies exposure and educated in avoiding animal bites. Travelers should avoid free-ranging mammals, be aware of their surroundings so that they do not accidentally surprise a dog, and avoid contact with bats and other wildlife. Although nonhuman primates are rarely rabid, they are a common source of bites, mainly on the Indian subcontinent. Awareness of this risk and simple prevention is particularly effective. Travelers should be advised to not approach or otherwise interact with monkeys or carry food while monkeys are near, especially those habituated to tourists. Entering caves where bats may be found is usually not a concern for rabies (although bat caves may be a source of Marburg or other viruses [see Viral Hemorrhagic Fevers later in this chapter]), but travelers should be educated to not handle bats or other wildlife. Many bats have tiny teeth, and not all wounds may be apparent. Any suspected or documented bite or wound from a bat should be grounds for seeking PEP.

Children are at higher risk for rabies exposure and subsequent illness because of their smaller stature, which makes severe bites to high-risk areas, such as the face and head, more likely. Also contributing to the higher risk is their natural curiosity and attraction to animals and the possibility that they may not report an exposure.

Preexposure Vaccination

Preexposure rabies vaccination may be recommended for certain international travelers, based on the occurrence of animal rabies in the destination country; the availability of antirabies biologics; intended activities, especially in remote areas; and duration of stay. A decision to receive preexposure rabies immunization may also be based on the likelihood of repeat travel to at-risk destinations or long-term travel to a high-risk destination. Preexposure vaccination may be recommended for veterinarians, animal handlers, field biologists, cavers, missionaries, and certain laboratory workers. Table 3-15 provides criteria for preexposure vaccination. The level of rabies virus neutralizing antibodies is typically used to dictate the need for booster vaccination. Globally, few laboratories perform the rapid fluorescent focus inhibition test, which is the gold standard test method for measuring rabies antibody levels. Those in the United States are listed on the CDC website (http://www.cdc.gov/rabies/specific_groups/doctors/serology.html). Regardless of whether preexposure vaccine is administered, travelers going to areas where the risk of rabies is high should be encouraged to purchase medical evacuation insurance (see Chapter 2, Travel Insurance, Travel Health Insurance, & Medical Evacuation Insurance).

In the United States, preexposure vaccination consists of a series of 3 intramuscular injections in the deltoid with human diploid cell rabies vaccine (HDCV) or purified chick embryo cell (PCEC) vaccine. The schedule for this series is given in Table 3-16. Travelers should receive all 3 preexposure immunizations before travel. If 3 doses of rabies vaccine cannot be completed before travel, the traveler should not start the series, as few data exist to guide PEP after a partial immunization series.

Preexposure vaccination does not eliminate the need for additional medical attention after a rabies exposure, but it simplifies PEP. Preexposure vaccination may also provide some protection when an exposure to rabies virus is unrecognized and PEP might be delayed. Travelers who have completed a 3-dose preexposure rabies immunization series or have received full PEP are considered preexposure immunized and do not require routine boosters. Periodic serum testing for rabies virus–neutralizing antibody is not necessary in most international travelers.

Wound Management

Any animal bite or scratch should be thoroughly cleaned with copious amounts of soap and water. All travelers should be informed that immediately cleaning bites as soon as possible substantially reduces the risk of infection, especially when followed by timely administration of PEP. For previously unvaccinated patients, wounds that might require

Table 3-15. Criteria for preexposure immunization for rabies

RISK CATEGORY	NATURE OF RISK	TYPICAL POPULATIONS	PREEXPOSURE REGIMEN
Continuous	Virus present continuously, often in high concentrations Specific exposures likely to go unrecognized Bite, nonbite, or aerosol exposure	Rabies research laboratory workers,[1] rabies biologics production workers	Primary course; serologic testing every 6 months; booster vaccination if antibody titer is below acceptable level[2]
Frequent	Exposure usually episodic with source recognized, but exposure might also be unrecognized Bite, nonbite, or aerosol exposure possible	Rabies diagnostic laboratory workers,[1] cavers, veterinarians and staff, and animal control and wildlife workers in rabies-epizootic areas	Primary course; serologic testing every 2 years; booster vaccination if antibody titer is below acceptable level[2]
Infrequent (more than general population)	Exposure nearly always episodic with source recognized Bite or nonbite exposure	Veterinarians, animal control, and wildlife workers in areas with low rabies rates; veterinary students; and travelers visiting areas where rabies is enzootic and immediate access to medical care, including biologics, is limited	Primary course; no serologic testing or booster vaccination
Rare (general population)	Exposure always episodic, with source recognized	US population at large, including people in rabies-epizootic areas	No preexposure immunization necessary

[1] Judgment of relative risk and extra monitoring of vaccination status of laboratory workers are the responsibility of the laboratory supervisor (see www.cdc.gov/biosafety/publications/bmbl5 for more information).
[2] Preexposure booster immunization consists of 1 dose of human diploid cell (rabies) vaccine or purified chick embryo cell vaccine, 1.0-mL dose, intramuscular (deltoid area). Per Advisory Committee on Immunization Practices recommendations, minimum acceptable antibody level is complete virus neutralization at a 1:5 serum dilution by the rapid fluorescent focus inhibition test, which is equivalent to approximately 0.1 IU/mL. A booster dose should be administered if titer falls below this level in populations that remain at risk.

Table 3-16. Preexposure immunization for rabies[1]

VACCINE	DOSE (mL)	NUMBER OF DOSES	SCHEDULE (DAYS)	ROUTE
HDCV, Imovax (Sanofi)	1.0	3	0, 7, and 21 or 28	IM
PCEC, RabAvert (Novartis)	1.0	3	0, 7, and 21 or 28	IM

Abbreviations: HDCV, human diploid cell vaccine; IM, intramuscular; PCEC, purified chick embryo cell.
[1] Patients who are immunosuppressed by disease or medications should postpone preexposure vaccinations and consider avoiding activities for which rabies preexposure prophylaxis is indicated. If this is not possible, immunosuppressed people who are at risk for rabies should have their antibody titers checked after vaccination.

suturing should have the suturing delayed for a few days. If suturing is necessary to control bleeding or for functional or cosmetic reasons, rabies immune globulin (RIG) should be injected into all wounded tissues before suturing. The use of local anesthetic is not contraindicated in wound management.

Postexposure Prophylaxis
In Travelers Who Received Preexposure Vaccination
PEP for someone previously immunized consists of 2 doses of modern cell culture vaccine given on days 0 and 3 after the exposure. The booster doses do not have to be the same brand as the one in the original preexposure immunization series.

In Travelers Who Did Not Receive Preexposure Vaccination
PEP for a previously unvaccinated patient consists of injections of RIG (20 IU/kg) and a series of 4 injections of rabies vaccine over 14 days or 5 doses over a 1-month period in immunosuppressed patients (Table 3-17). After wound cleansing, as much of the dose-appropriate

volume of RIG (Table 3-17) as is anatomically feasible should be injected at the wound site, striving to put the RIG in the areas where the animal's teeth have wounded the tissue. If the wound is small and on a distal extremity such as a finger or toe, the health care provider will have to use judgment as to how much to inject at the wound to avoid local tissue compression and complications. Any remaining dose should be administered intramuscularly. If the wounds are extensive, the dose-appropriate volume of RIG must not be exceeded. If the volume is inadequate to inject all the wounds, the RIG may be diluted with normal saline so that some can be injected in each of the wounds. This is a particular issue in children, whose body weight may be small in relation to the size and number of wounds.

RIG is difficult to access in many countries. If modern cell culture vaccine is available but access to RIG is delayed, the vaccine series should be started as soon as possible, and RIG may be added to the regimen up to and including day 7. After day 7, RIG is contraindicated because it may compromise the patient's adaptive immunity to the vaccination series.

Table 3-17. Postexposure immunization for rabies[1]

IMMUNIZATION STATUS	VACCINE/ PRODUCT	DOSE	NUMBER OF DOSES	SCHEDULE (DAYS)	ROUTE
Not previously immunized	RIG plus	20 IU/kg body weight	1	0	Infiltrated at bite site (if possible); remainder IM
	HDCV or PCEC	1.0 mL	4[2]	0, 3, 7, 14 (28 if immuno-compromised[3])	IM
Previously immunized[4,5]	HDCV or PCEC	1.0 mL	2	0, 3	IM

Abbreviations: RIG, rabies immune globulin; IM, intramuscular; HDCV, human diploid cell vaccine; PCEC, purified chick embryo cell.
[1] All postexposure prophylaxis should begin with immediate, thorough cleansing of all wounds with soap and water.
[2] Five vaccine doses for the immunosuppressed patient. The first 4 vaccine doses are given on the same schedule as for an immunocompetent patient, and the fifth dose is given on day 28; patient follow-up should include monitoring antibody response. See http://www.cdc.gov/mmwr/preview/mmwrhtml/rr5902a1.htm for more information. The World Health Organization recommends this fifth dose for all patients, not just those who are immunocompromised.
[3] CDC recommends 4 postexposure vaccine doses, on days 0, 3, 7, and 14, unless the patient is immunocompromised in some way, in which case a fifth dose is given at day 28.
[4] Preexposure immunization with HDCV or PCEC, prior postexposure prophylaxis with HDCV or PCEC, or people previously immunized with any other type of rabies vaccine and a documented history of positive rabies virus neutralizing antibody response to the prior vaccination.
[5] RIG should not be administered.

Because rabies virus can persist in tissue for a long time before gaining access to a peripheral nerve, a traveler who has sustained a bite that is suspicious for rabies should receive full PEP, including RIG, even if a considerable length of time has passed since the initial exposure. If there is a scar, or the patient remembers where the bite occurred, an appropriate amount of RIG should be injected in that area.

Human RIG is manufactured by plasmapheresis of blood from hyperimmunized volunteers. The quantity of commercially produced human RIG falls short of worldwide demand, and it is not available in many developing countries. Equine RIG or purified fractions of equine RIG may be available in some developing countries where human RIG might not be available. If necessary, such heterologous products are preferable to no RIG.

The incidence of adverse events after the use of modern equine-derived RIG is low (0.8%–6.0%), and most reactions are minor. However, such products are not evaluated by US standards or regulated by the Food and Drug Administration, and their use cannot unequivocally be recommended. In addition, unpurified antirabies serum of equine origin might still be used in some countries where neither human nor equine RIG is available. The use of this antirabies serum is associated with higher rates of serious adverse reactions, including anaphylaxis.

Different PEP schedules, alternative routes of administration, and other rabies vaccines besides HDCV and PCEC may be used abroad. For example, commercially available purified Vero cell rabies vaccine and purified duck embryo cell vaccine are acceptable alternatives if available. Assistance in managing complicated PEP scenarios may be obtained from experienced travel medicine professionals, health departments, and CDC.

Rabies vaccine was once manufactured from viruses grown in animal brains, and some of these vaccines are still in use in developing countries. Typically, the brain-derived vaccines can be identified if the traveler is offered a large-volume injection (5 mL) daily for approximately 14–21 days. Because of variability of potency in these preparations, which may limit effectiveness, and the risk of adverse reactions, the traveler should not accept these vaccines but travel to where acceptable vaccines and RIG are available.

Rabies Vaccine
Vaccine Safety and Adverse Reactions
Travelers should be advised that they may experience local reactions after vaccination, such as pain, erythema, swelling, or itching at the injection site, or mild systemic reactions, such as headache, nausea, abdominal pain, muscle aches, and dizziness. Approximately 6% of people receiving booster vaccinations with HDCV may experience an immune complex–like reaction characterized by urticaria, pruritus, and malaise. The likelihood of these reactions may be less with PCEC. Once initiated, rabies PEP should not be interrupted or discontinued because of local or mild systemic reactions to rabies vaccine.

Precautions and Contraindications
Pregnancy is not a contraindication to PEP. In infants and children, the dose of HDCV or PCEC for preexposure or PEP is the same as that recommended for adults. The dose of RIG for PEP is based on body weight (Table 3-17).

CDC website: www.cdc.gov/rabies

BIBLIOGRAPHY

1. Gautret P, Parola P. Rabies vaccination for international travelers. Vaccine. 2012 Jan 5;30(2):126–33.
2. Gautret P, Tantawichien T, Vu Hai V, Piyaphanee W. Determinants of pre-exposure rabies vaccination among foreign backpackers in Bangkok, Thailand. Vaccine. 2011 May 23;29(23):3931–4.
3. Malerczyk C, Detora L, Gniel D. Imported human rabies cases in Europe, the United States, and Japan, 1990 to 2010. J Travel Med. 2011 Nov–Dec;18(6):402–7.
4. Mills DJ, Lau CL, Weinstein P. Animal bites and rabies exposure in Australian travellers. Med J Aust. 2011 Dec 19;195(11–12):673–5.
5. Rupprecht CE, Briggs D, Brown CM, Franka R, Katz SL, Kerr HD, et al. Use of a reduced (4-dose) vaccine schedule for postexposure prophylaxis to prevent human rabies: recommendations of the advisory committee on immunization practices. MMWR Recomm Rep. 2010 Mar 19;59(RR-2):1–9.

6. Rupprecht CE, Gibbons RV. Clinical practice. Prophylaxis against rabies. N Engl J Med. 2004 Dec 16;351(25):2626–35.

7. Smith A, Petrovic M, Solomon T, Fooks A. Death from rabies in a UK traveller returning from India. Euro Surveill. 2005 Jul;10(30):pii=2761.

8. van Thiel PP, de Bie RM, Eftimov F, Tepaske R, Zaaijer HL, van Doornum GJ, et al. Fatal human rabies due to Duvenhage virus from a bat in Kenya: failure of treatment with coma-induction, ketamine, and antiviral drugs. PLoS Negl Trop Dis. 2009;3(7):e428.

9. Warrell MJ, Warrell DA. Rabies and other lyssavirus diseases. Lancet. 2004 Mar 20;363(9413):959–69.

10. World Health Organization. WHO expert consultation on rabies. World Health Organ Tech Rep Ser. 2005;931:1–88.

Perspectives

INTRADERMAL RABIES PREEXPOSURE IMMUNIZATION

David R. Shlim

Few topics in travel medicine prompt more concern and persistent questions than the prevention of rabies in travelers. Although we understand the basics of rabies prevention for travelers, the logistics of providing this care in a timely fashion remain a challenge. Unimmunized travelers who are exposed to rabies and other lyssaviruses require proper wound care, infiltration of human rabies immune globulin (RIG), and a series of 4 or 5 doses of rabies vaccine intramuscularly over a 2- to 4-week period. Travelers who receive 3 doses of rabies vaccine before travel need to receive 2 more doses of rabies vaccine, 3 days apart, after a viral exposure. Notably, human RIG and equine RIG are often unavailable in developing countries, although modern cell culture rabies vaccines are increasingly available. Thus, preexposure rabies immunization can facilitate the traveler's access to adequate postexposure rabies prophylaxis.

One limiting factor in the use of preexposure rabies immunization is the cost of the vaccine. In the United States, rabies vaccine may cost more than $250 per dose, resulting in a cost to the patient in excess of $750 for three 1.0-mL intramuscular injections. As a way of decreasing the cost of preexposure immunization, some practitioners have used a 0.1-mL dose of rabies vaccine administered intradermally.

Perspectives sections are written as editorial discussions aiming to add depth and clinical perspective to the official recommendations contained in the book. The views and opinions expressed in this section are those of the author and do not necessarily represent the official position of CDC.

At approximately $45 per dose in the early 1980s, many people already considered the vaccine too expensive. Thus, intradermal rabies immunization began almost as soon as the intramuscular human diploid cell vaccine (HDCV) was manufactured. By reconstituting the 1.0 mL of vaccine in the vial, practitioners could draw up approximately eight 0.1-mL doses. One problem was that the entire vial had to be used within a few hours of reconstituting, meaning that a provider had to either be in a busy clinic or line up groups of people, such as families, for rabies immunization at the same time.

Early studies of the immune response to intradermal rabies vaccine, using HDCV and later other rabies vaccines, were uniformly encouraging. Virtually 100% of vaccinees seroconverted. A 1982 statement by the US Advisory Committee on Immunization Practices (ACIP) reviewed data on >1,500 vaccinees and declared, "It appears that, with this vaccine, the 0.1-mL intradermal (ID) regimen is an acceptable alternative to the currently approved 1.0-mL intramuscular (IM) regimen for preexposure prophylaxis." They called upon manufacturers to produce a product with appropriate packaging and labeling.

In 1986, the Mérieux Institute (now Sanofi Pasteur) received approval to market a 0.1-mL dose in an individual syringe. Sharing reconstituted vials of 1.0 mL between patients remained off-label. Although the new product solved the logistical problem of providing individual travelers with an ID dose, the cost of the prepackaged ID dose was 75% of the full 1.0-mL IM dose.

As ID rabies immunization was being implemented, a death from rabies in an American Peace Corps volunteer in Kenya brought the enthusiasm for ID immunization to a temporary halt. The 23-year-old female volunteer died of rabies after a bite from a stray puppy that she had adopted. She had received 3 doses of ID rabies vaccine in Kenya, finishing 6 months before the bite. She did not suspect that the dog had rabies, even though it died shortly after biting her. As a result, she did not seek postexposure boosters. Serum drawn at the onset of her symptoms revealed she did not have an adequate antibody response. The Peace Corps medical personnel wondered why the recent ID immunization had not been effective. Concerned that she may have had an atypical response to immunization, they tested serum specimens from 11 other Peace Corps volunteers in Kenya who had been immunized at the same time. To their surprise, 9 of 11 also had an inadequate immunologic response. As a control group, Peace Corps volunteers who had received rabies ID preexposure immunization in Nepal and Morocco were also tested, and 31 (39%) of 79 had an inadequate antibody response.

Studies were undertaken to confirm the potency of the vaccine lot, maintenance of the cold chain, the method of administration, and the effect of concomitant medication. None of these factors proved to be an entirely adequate explanation. For example, chloroquine taken as an antimalarial medication during ID rabies immunization reduced the levels of antibody induced. However, the seroconversion rate on chloroquine was still adequate, and the volunteers in Morocco and Nepal were not taking chloroquine. After the investigation, it was recommended that people using ID preexposure immunization should complete the course before starting chloroquine and traveling abroad or else use the IM regimen.

ACIP continued to endorse the concept of ID preexposure rabies immunization in a 1999 statement on rabies prevention. However, 3 lots of a prepackaged rabies ID vaccine were recalled during 2000 for having a potency that fell below the specification level before the expiration date. In 2001, the

ID rabies vaccine was withdrawn from the market. Since then, authorities in the United States have not recommended sharing 1.0-mL vials for ID rabies immunization, as the manufacturer has not applied for the appropriate packaging and labeling to the Food and Drug Administration (FDA). This lack of endorsement of ID preexposure immunization has frustrated some travel medicine professionals.

Based on recent data, the World Health Organization has recommended the use of ID preexposure rabies immunization as an alternative to IM immunization. In a recent study of 420 Australian travelers given a modified ID rabies preexposure immunization (2 doses on day 0, 2 doses on day 7, and 1 dose on day 21–28), a seroconversion rate of 98.3% was documented. Although a potential savings might accrue from use of only 0.5 mL of vaccine total, this does not alleviate the problem of needing to identify several travelers in a few hours or use multiple doses from a single-use vial.

Neither ACIP nor FDA are likely to endorse the use of 1.0-mL vials of rabies vaccine for multiple-dose ID use unless the manufacturer requests that indication. Until then, the use of ID rabies vaccine will remain off-label in the United States. The current status of ID rabies immunization in the United States reflects a regulatory situation and ACIP opinion and is not a comment on the effectiveness of ID rabies preexposure immunization for travelers elsewhere.

BIBLIOGRAPHY

1. Bernard KW, Fishbein DB, Miller KD, Parker RA, Waterman S, Sumner JW, et al. Pre-exposure rabies immunization with human diploid cell vaccine: decreased antibody responses in persons immunized in developing countries. Am J Trop Med Hyg. 1985 May;34(3):633–47.
2. CDC. Recommendation of the Immunization Practices Advisory Committee (ACIP). Supplementary statement on pre-exposure rabies prophylaxis by the intradermal route. MMWR Morb Mortal Wkly Rep. 1982 Jun 4;31(21):279–80, 85.
3. Mills DJ, Lau CL, Fearnley EJ, Weinstein P. The immunogenicity of a modified intradermal pre-exposure rabies vaccination schedule—a case series of 420 travelers. J Travel Med. 2011 Sep–Oct;18(5):327–32.

RICKETTSIAL (SPOTTED & TYPHUS FEVERS) & RELATED INFECTIONS (ANAPLASMOSIS & EHRLICHIOSIS)

Jennifer McQuiston

INFECTIOUS AGENTS

Rickettsial infections are caused by a variety of bacteria from the genera *Rickettsia*, *Orientia*, *Ehrlichia*, *Neorickettsia*, *Neoehrlichia*, and *Anaplasma* (Table 3-18). *Rickettsia* spp. are classically divided into the typhus group and spotted fever group (SFG). *Orientia* spp. make up the scrub typhus group. The rickettsial pathogens most likely to be encountered during travel outside the United States

Table 3-18. Classification, primary vector, and reservoir occurrence of rickettsiae known to cause disease in humans

ANTIGENIC GROUP	DISEASE	SPECIES	VECTOR	ANIMAL RESERVOIR(S)	GEOGRAPHIC DISTRIBUTION
Anaplasma	Human anaplasmosis	*Anaplasma phagocytophilum*	Tick	Small mammals, rodents, deer	Primarily United States, worldwide
Ehrlichia	Human ehrlichiosis	*Ehrlichia chaffeensis* E. muris E. ewingii	Tick	Deer, wild and domestic dogs, domestic ruminants, rodents	Common in United States, possibly worldwide
Neoehrlichia	Human neoehrlichiosis	*Neoehrlichia mikurensis*	Tick	Rodents	Europe, Asia
Neorickettsia	Sennetsu fever	*Neorickettsia sennetsu*	Trematode	Fish	Japan, Malaysia, possibly other parts of Asia
Scrub typhus	Scrub typhus	*Orientia tsutsugamushi*	Larval mite (chigger)	Rodents	Asia-Pacific region from maritime Russia and China to Indonesia and North Australia to Afghanistan
Spotted fever	Rickettsiosis	*Rickettsia aeschlimannii*	Tick	Unknown	South Africa, Morocco, Mediterranean littoral
	African tick-bite fever	R. africae	Tick	Ruminants	Sub-Saharan Africa, West Indies
	Rickettsialpox	R. akari	Mite	House mice, wild rodents	Countries of the former Soviet Union, South Africa, Korea, Turkey, Balkan countries, North and South America
	Queensland tick typhus	R. australis	Tick	Rodents	Australia, Tasmania
	Mediterranean spotted fever or Boutonneuse fever	R. conorii[1]	Tick	Dogs, rodents	Southern Europe, southern and western Asia, Africa, India
	Cat flea rickettsiosis	R. felis	Flea	Domestic cats, rodents, opossums	Europe, North and South America, Africa, Asia
	Far Eastern spotted fever	R. heilongjiangensis	Tick	Rodents	Far East of Russia, Northern China, eastern Asia
	Aneruptive fever	R. Helvetica	Tick	Rodents	Central and northern Europe, Asia
	Flinders Island spotted fever, Thai tick typhus	R. honei, including strain "marmionii"	Tick	Rodents, reptiles	Australia, Thailand

continued

TABLE 3-18. CLASSIFICATION, PRIMARY VECTOR, AND RESERVOIR OCCURRENCE OF RICKETTSIAE KNOWN TO CAUSE DISEASE IN HUMANS (continued)

ANTIGENIC GROUP	DISEASE	SPECIES	VECTOR	ANIMAL RESERVOIR(S)	GEOGRAPHIC DISTRIBUTION
	Japanese spotted fever	*R. japonica*	Tick	Rodents	Japan
	Mediterranean spotted fever–like disease	*R. massiliae*	Tick	Unknown	France, Greece, Spain, Portugal, Switzerland, Sicily, central Africa, and Mali
	Mediterranean spotted fever–like illness	*R. monacensis*	Tick	Lizards, possibly birds	Europe, North Africa
	Maculatum infection	*R. parkeri*	Tick	Rodents	North and South America
	Tickborne lymphadenopathy, *Dermacentor*-borne necrosis and lymphadenopathy	*R. raoultii*	Tick	Unknown	Europe, Asia
	Rocky Mountain spotted fever, Brazilian spotted fever, febre maculosa, São Paulo exanthematic typhus, Minas Gerais exanthematic typhus	*R. rickettsii*	Tick	Rodents	North, Central, and South America
	North Asian tick typhus, Siberian tick typhus	*R. sibirica*	Tick	Rodents	Russia, China, Mongolia
	Lymphangitis-associated rickettsiosis	*R. sibirica mongolotimonae*	Tick	Rodents	Southern France, Portugal, China, Africa
	Tickborne lymphadenopathy [TIBOLA], *Dermacentor*-borne necrosis and lymphadenopathy [DEBONEL]	*R. slovaca*	Tick	Lagomorphs, rodents	Southern and eastern Europe, Asia
Typhus fever	Epidemic typhus, sylvatic typhus	*R. prowazekii*	Human body louse, flying squirrel ectoparasites, possibly some ticks	Humans, flying squirrels	Central Africa; Asia; Central, North, and South America
	Murine typhus	*R. typhi*	Flea	Rodents	Tropical and subtropical areas worldwide

[1] Includes 4 different subspecies that can be distinguished serologically and by PCR assay and that are the etiologic agents of Boutonneuse fever and Mediterranean tick fever in southern Europe and Africa (*R. conorii* subsp. *conorii*), Indian tick typhus in south Asia (*R. conorii* subsp. *indica*), Israeli tick typhus in southern Europe and Middle East (*R. conorii* subsp. *israelensis*), and Astrakhan spotted fever in the North Caspian region of Russia (*R. conorii* subsp. *caspiae*), respectively.

include R. *africae* (African tick-bite fever), R. *conorii* (Mediterranean spotted fever), R. *rickettsii* (known as both Rocky Mountain spotted fever and Brazilian spotted fever), O. *tsutsugamushi* (scrub typhus), and R. *typhi* (murine typhus).

TRANSMISSION

Most rickettsial pathogens are transmitted by ectoparasites such as fleas, lice, mites, and ticks. Organisms can be transmitted by bites from these ectoparasites or by the inoculation of infectious fluids or feces from the ectoparasites into the skin. Inhaling or inoculating conjunctiva with infectious material may also cause infection for some of these organisms. The specific vectors that transmit each form of rickettsiae are listed in Table 3-18. Transmission of some rickettsial diseases after transfusion or organ transplantation is rare but has been reported.

EPIDEMIOLOGY

All age groups are at risk for rickettsial infections during travel to endemic areas. Both short and long-term travelers are at risk for infection. Transmission is increased during outdoor activities in the spring and summer months when ticks and fleas are most active. However, infection can occur throughout the year. Because of the 5- to 14-day incubation period for most rickettsial diseases, tourists may not necessarily experience symptoms during their trip, and onset may coincide with their return home or develop within a week after returning. Although the most commonly diagnosed rickettsial diseases in travelers are usually in the spotted fever or typhus groups, travelers may acquire a wide range of rickettsioses, including emerging and newly recognized species (Table 3-18).

Tickborne spotted fever rickettsioses are the most frequently reported travel-associated rickettsial infections. Game hunting and traveling to southern Africa from November through April are risk factors for African tick-bite fever, and this consistently remains the most commonly reported rickettsial infection acquired during travel. Mediterranean spotted fever infections are less commonly reported but occur over an even larger region, including (but not limited to) much of Europe, Africa, India, and the Middle East. Rocky Mountain spotted fever (also known as Brazilian spotted fever, as well as other local names) is reported throughout much of the Western Hemisphere, including Canada, the United States, Mexico, and various countries in Central and South America. Contact with dogs (in both rural and urban settings) and outdoor activities such as hiking, hunting, fishing, and camping increase the risk of infection.

Scrub typhus, which is transmitted by mites encountered in high grass and brush, is endemic in northern Japan, Southeast Asia, the western Pacific Islands, eastern Australia, China, maritime areas and several parts of south-central Russia, India, and Sri Lanka. More than 1 million cases occur annually. Most travel-acquired cases of scrub typhus occur during visits to rural areas in endemic countries for activities such as camping, hiking, or rafting, but urban cases have also been described.

R. *typhi* and R. *felis*, which are transmitted by fleas, are widely distributed, especially throughout the tropics and subtropics and in port cities and coastal regions with rodents. Humans exposed to flea-infested cats, dogs, and peridomestic animals while traveling in endemic regions, or who enter or sleep in areas infested with rodents, are at most risk for fleaborne rickettsioses. Murine typhus has been reported among travelers returning from Asia, Africa, and the Mediterranean Basin and has also been reported from Hawaii, California, and Texas in the United States.

R. *akari*, the causative agent of rickettsialpox, is transmitted by house-mouse mites, and circulates in mainly urban centers in Ukraine, South Africa, Korea, the Balkan states, and the United States. Outbreaks of rickettsialpox most often occur after contact with infected rodents and their mites, especially during natural die-offs or exterminations of infected rodents that cause the mites to seek out new hosts, including humans. The agent may spill over and occasionally be found in other wild rodent populations.

Epidemic typhus is rarely reported among tourists but can occur in communities and refugee populations where body lice are prevalent. Outbreaks often occur during the colder months when infested clothing is not laundered. Travelers at most risk for epidemic typhus include those who may work with or visit areas with large homeless populations, impoverished areas, refugee camps, and regions that have recently experienced war or natural disasters. Active foci of epidemic typhus are known in the Andes regions of South America and some parts of Africa (including but not limited to Burundi, Ethiopia, and Rwanda). Louseborne epidemic typhus does not regularly occur in the United States, but a zoonotic reservoir occurs in the southern flying squirrel, and sporadic sylvatic epidemic typhus cases are reported. Tick-associated reservoirs of *R. prowazekii* have been described in Ethiopia, Mexico, and Brazil, but documented human cases are rare.

Ehrlichiosis and anaplasmosis are tickborne infections most commonly reported in the United States. A variety of species are implicated in infection, but *E. chaffeensis* and *A. phagocytophilum* are most common. Infections with various *Ehrlichia* and *Anaplasma* spp. have also been reported in Europe, Asia, and South America. *Neoehrlichia mikurensis* is a tickborne pathogen that occurs in Europe and Asia. Sennetsu fever, caused by *Neorickettsia sennetsu*, occurs in Japan, Malaysia, and possibly other parts of Asia. This disease can be contracted from eating raw infected fish.

CLINICAL PRESENTATION

Rickettsioses are difficult to diagnose, even by health care providers experienced with these diseases. Most symptomatic rickettsial diseases cause moderate illness, but some Rocky Mountain and Brazilian spotted fevers, Mediterranean spotted fever, scrub typhus, and epidemic typhus may be fatal in 20%–60% of untreated cases, so prompt treatment is essential.

Clinical presentations vary with the causative agent and patient; however, common symptoms that typically develop within 1–2 weeks of infection include fever, headache, malaise, rash, nausea, and vomiting. Many rickettsioses are accompanied by a maculopapular, vesicular, or petechial rash or sometimes an eschar at the site of the tick bite. African tick-bite fever is typically milder than some other rickettsioses, but recovery is improved with treatment. It should be suspected in a patient who presents with fever, headache, myalgia, and an eschar (tache noir) after recent travel to southern Africa. Mediterranean spotted fever is a potentially life-threatening rickettsial infection and should be suspected in patients with rash, fever, and eschar after recent travel to northern Africa or the Mediterranean. Rocky Mountain and Brazilian spotted fever are characterized by fever, headache, nausea, abdominal pain, and cough; a rash is commonly reported, but eschars are not. Scrub typhus should be suspected in patients with a fever, headache, and myalgia after recent travel to Asia; eschar, lymphadenopathy, cough, and encephalitis may be present. Patients with murine or epidemic typhus usually present with a severe but nonspecific febrile illness, and approximately half will also present with a rash. Ehrlichiosis and anaplasmosis should be suspected in febrile patients with leukopenia with an exposure history.

DIAGNOSIS

Diagnosis is usually based on clinical recognition and serology; the latter requires comparison of acute- to convalescent-phase serology, so is only helpful in retrospect. Etiologic agents can generally only be identified to the genus level by serologic testing. PCR and immunohistochemical analyses may also be helpful. If ehrlichiosis or anaplasmosis is suspected, a buffy coat may be examined to identify characteristic intraleukocytic morulae. Contact the CDC Rickettsial Zoonoses Branch at 404-639-1075 for further information.

TREATMENT

Treatment of patients with possible rickettsioses should be started early and should never await confirmatory testing, which may take weeks when serology is used. Immediate empiric treatment with a tetracycline is recommended, most commonly doxycycline. Broad-spectrum antibiotics are not usually helpful. Chloramphenicol may be an alternative in some cases, but its use is associated with more deaths, particularly for *R. rickettsii*. Expert advice should be sought if alternative agents are being considered.

PREVENTION

No vaccine is available for preventing rickettsial infections. Antibiotics are not recommended for prophylaxis of rickettsial diseases.

Travelers should be instructed to minimize exposure to infectious arthropods during travel (including lice, fleas, ticks, mites) and animal reservoirs (particularly dogs) when traveling in endemic areas. The proper use of insect or tick repellents, self-examination after visits to vector-infested areas, and wearing protective clothing are ways to reduce risk. These precautions are especially important for people with underlying conditions that may compromise their immune systems, as these people may be more susceptible to severe disease. For more detailed information, see Chapter 2, Protection against Mosquitoes, Ticks, & Other Arthropods.

CDC website: www.cdc.gov/ticks

BIBLIOGRAPHY

1. Angelakis E, Botelho E, Socolovschi C, Sobas CR, Piketty C, Parola P, et al. Murine typhus as a cause of fever in travelers from Tunisia and Mediterranean areas. J Travel Med. 2010 Sep–Oct;17(5):310–5.

2. Demeester R, Claus M, Hildebrand M, Vlieghe E, Bottieau E. Diversity of life-threatening complications due to Mediterranean spotted fever in returning travelers. J Travel Med. 2010 Mar–Apr;17(2):100–4.

3. Dobler G, Wolfel R. Typhus and other rickettsioses: emerging infections in Germany. Dtsch Arztebl Int. 2009 May;106(20):348–54.

4. Hendershot EF, Sexton DJ. Scrub typhus and rickettsial diseases in international travelers: a review. Curr Infect Dis Rep. 2009 Jan;11(1):66–72.

5. Jensenius M, Davis X, von Sonnenburg F, Schwartz E, Keystone JS, Leder K, et al. Multicenter GeoSentinel analysis of rickettsial diseases in international travelers, 1996–2008. Emerg Infect Dis. 2009 Nov;15(11):1791–8.

6. Leshem E, Meltzer E, Schwartz E. Travel-associated zoonotic bacterial diseases. Curr Opin Infect Dis. 2011 Oct;24(5):457–63.

7. Nachega JB, Bottieau E, Zech F, Van Gompel A. Travel-acquired scrub typhus: emphasis on the differential diagnosis, treatment, and prevention strategies. J Travel Med. 2007 Sep–Oct;14(5):352–5.

8. Raoult D, Parola P, editors. Rickettsial Diseases. New York: Informa Healthcare USA, Inc; 2007.

9. Rar V, Golovljova I. *Anaplasma, Ehrlichia*, and "*Candidatus* Neoehrlichia" bacteria: pathogenicity, biodiversity, and molecular genetic characteristics, a review. Infect Genet Evol. 2011 Dec;11(8):1842–61.

10. Roch N, Epaulard O, Pelloux I, Pavese P, Brion JP, Raoult D, et al. African tick bite fever in elderly patients: 8 cases in French tourists returning from South Africa. Clin Infect Dis. 2008 Aug 1;47(3):e28–35.

RUBELLA

Emmaculate J. Lebo, Susan E. Reef

INFECTIOUS AGENT

Rubella virus (family Togaviridae, genus *Rubivirus*).

TRANSMISSION

Person-to-person contact or droplets shed from the respiratory secretions of infected people. People may shed virus from 7 days before the onset of the rash to approximately 5–7 days after rash onset. Transmission from mother to fetus can also occur, with the highest risk of congenital rubella syndrome (CRS) if infection occurs in the first trimester. Infants with CRS can transmit virus for up to 1 year after birth.

EPIDEMIOLOGY

Even though endemic rubella virus transmission has been interrupted in the Americas, rubella virus continues to circulate widely, especially in Africa, the Eastern Mediterranean, and Southeast Asia regions. In 2013, 2 large outbreaks were reported in Poland and Japan; cases were mostly among adolescent boys and adult men, but pregnant women were also affected, and their children subsequently developed CRS. In the United States, endemic rubella virus transmission has been eliminated since 2001, but cases continue to be imported. From 2004 to 2013, a median of 10 (range, 4–18) imported cases were reported annually in the United States, and 6 CRS cases were reported during the same period.

CLINICAL PRESENTATION
Average incubation period is 14 days (range, 12–23 days). Usually presents as a nonspecific, maculopapular, generalized rash that lasts ≤3 days with generalized lymphadenopathy. Rash may be preceded by low-grade fever, malaise, anorexia, mild conjunctivitis, runny nose, and sore throat. Adolescents and adults, especially women, can also present with transient arthritis. Asymptomatic rubella virus infections are common. Infection during early pregnancy can lead to miscarriage, fetal death, or CRS with severe birth defects.

DIAGNOSIS
Demonstration of specific rubella IgM or significant increase in rubella IgG in acute- and convalescent-phase specimens. RT-PCR can be used to detect virus infection; viral culture is also acceptable but is time-consuming and expensive.

TREATMENT
Supportive care.

PREVENTION
All travelers aged ≥12 months should have evidence of immunity to rubella, as documented by ≥1 dose of rubella-containing vaccine on or after the first birthday, laboratory evidence of immunity, or birth before 1957. Unlike measles, there is no recommendation for rubella vaccination for infants aged <12 months before international travel. Health care providers should also ensure that all women of childbearing age and recent immigrants are up-to-date on their immunization status or have evidence of immunity to rubella, because these groups are at the highest risk for maternal-fetal transmission of rubella virus.

CDC website: www.cdc.gov/rubella

BIBLIOGRAPHY
1. CDC. Summary of notifiable diseases—United States, 2011. MMWR Morb Mortal Wkly Rep. 2013 Jul 5;60(53):1–117.
2. CDC. Rubella. In: Atkinson W, Wolfe S, Hamborsky J, editors. Epidemiology and Prevention of Vaccine-Preventable Diseases. 12th ed. Washington, DC: Public Health Foundation; 2012. p. 275–89.
3. Papania MJ, Wallace GS, Rota PA, Icenogle JP, Fiebelkorn AP, Armstrong GL, et al. Elimination of endemic measles, rubella, and congenital rubella syndrome from the Western hemisphere: the US experience. JAMA Pediatr. 2014 Feb;168(2):148–55.
4. Reef SE, Plotkin SA. Rubella vaccine. In: Plotkin SA, Orenstein WA, Offit PA, editors. Vaccines. 6th ed. Philadelphia: Saunders Elsevier; 2012. p. 688–717.
5. Reef SE, Redd SB, Abernathy E, Kutty PK, Icenogle JP. Evidence used to support the achievement and maintenance of elimination of rubella and congenital rubella syndrome in the United States. J Infect Dis. 2011 Sep 1;204(Suppl 2):S593–7.
6. World Health Organization. Rubella vaccines: WHO position paper. Wkly Epidemiol Rec. 2011 July 15; 86(29):301–16.

SALMONELLOSIS (NONTYPHOIDAL)
Martha Iwamoto

INFECTIOUS AGENT
Salmonella enterica subspecies *enterica* is a gram-negative, rod-shaped bacillus. More than 2,500 *Salmonella* serotypes have been identified. Nontyphoidal salmonellosis refers to illnesses caused by all serotypes of *Salmonella* except for Typhi, Paratyphi A, Paratyphi B (tartrate negative), and Paratyphi C.

TRANSMISSION

Usually through the consumption of food or water contaminated with animal feces. Transmission can also occur through direct contact with infected animals or their environment and directly between humans.

EPIDEMIOLOGY

Nontyphoidal salmonellae are a leading cause of bacterial diarrhea worldwide; they are estimated to cause 94 million cases of gastroenteritis and 115,000 deaths globally each year. The risk of *Salmonella* infection among travelers returning to the United States varies by region of the world visited. In one analysis, the incidence of laboratory-confirmed infections from 2004 through 2009 was 7.1 cases per 100,000 among travelers to Latin American and Caribbean, 5.8 cases per 100,000 among travelers to Asia, and 25.8 cases per 100,000 among travelers to Africa. The true number of illnesses is much higher, because most ill people do not have a stool specimen tested. Travelers with salmonellosis were most likely to report visiting the following countries: Mexico (38% of travel-associated salmonellosis), India (9%), Jamaica (7%), the Dominican Republic (4%), China (3%), and the Bahamas (2%). *Salmonella* infection and carriage has been reported among internationally adopted children.

CLINICAL PRESENTATION

Gastroenteritis is the most common clinical presentation of nontyphoidal *Salmonella* infection. The incubation period of nontyphoidal salmonellosis is 6–72 hours, but illness usually occurs within 12–36 hours after exposure. Illness is commonly manifested by acute diarrhea, abdominal pain, fever, and sometimes vomiting. The illness usually lasts 4–7 days, and most people recover without treatment. Approximately 5% of people develop bacteremia or focal infection (such as meningitis or osteomyelitis). Salmonellosis outcomes differ by serotype. Infections with some serotypes, including Dublin and Choleraesuis, are more likely to result in invasive infections. Rates of invasive infections and death are generally higher among infants, older adults, and people with immunosuppressive conditions (including HIV), hemoglobinopathies, and malignant neoplasms.

DIAGNOSIS

Diagnosis is based on isolation of *Salmonella* organisms. About 90% of isolates are obtained from routine stool culture, but isolates are also obtained from blood, urine, and material from sites of infection. Isolates of salmonellae are needed for serotyping and antimicrobial susceptibility testing.

TREATMENT

Current recommendations are to treat most patients with uncomplicated *Salmonella* infection with supportive therapy and no antimicrobial agents. Antimicrobial therapy should be considered for patients who are severely ill (for example, those with severe diarrhea, high fever, or manifestations of extraintestinal infection) and for gastroenteritis caused by *Salmonella* species in people at increased risk of invasive disease (infants aged <3 months, older adults aged ≥60 years, and the debilitated or immunosuppressed). Fluoroquinolones are often employed for empiric treatment of patients with moderate to severe travelers' diarrhea; azithromycin and rifaximin are also commonly used. Resistance to antimicrobial agents varies by serotype and geographic region. Resistance to older antimicrobial agents (chloramphenicol, ampicillin, and trimethoprim-sulfamethoxazole) has been present for many years, and resistance to both fluoroquinolones and third-generation cephalosporins has increased.

PREVENTION

No vaccine is available against nontyphoidal *Salmonella* infection. Preventive measures are aimed at avoiding foods and drinks at high risk for contamination; frequent handwashing, especially after contacting animals or their environment; and taking additional food and water precautions while traveling (see Chapter 2, Food & Water Precautions).

CDC website: www.cdc.gov/salmonella

BIBLIOGRAPHY

1. American Academy of Pediatrics. *Salmonella* infections. In: Pickering LK, editor. Red Book: 2012 Report of the Committee on Infectious Diseases. 29th ed. Elk Grove Village, IL: American Academy of Pediatrics; 2012. p. 635–40.

2. American Public Health Association. Salmonellosis. In: Heymann DL, editor. Control of Communicable Diseases Manual. 19th ed. Washington, DC: American Public Health Association; 2008. p. 534–40.

3. CDC. National enteric disease surveillance: *Salmonella* annual report, 2011. Atlanta: CDC; 2011 [cited 2014 Sep 24]. Available from: http://www.cdc.gov/ncezid/dfwed/PDFs/salmonella-annual-report-2011-508c.pdf.

4. Galanis E, Lo Fo Wong DM, Patrick ME, Binsztein N, Cieslik A, Chalermchikit T, et al. Web-based surveillance and global *Salmonella* distribution, 2000–2002. Emerg Infect Dis. 2006 Mar;12(3):381–8.

5. Johnson LR, Gould LH, Dunn JR, Berkelman R, Mahon BE, FoodNet Travel Working Group. *Salmonella* infections associated with international travel: a Foodborne Diseases Active Surveillance Network (FoodNet) study. Foodborne Pathog Dis. 2011 Sep;8(9):1031–7.

6. Jones TF, Ingram LA, Cieslak PR, Vugia DJ, Tobin-D'Angelo M, Hurd S, et al. Salmonellosis outcomes differ substantially by serotype. J Infect Dis. 2008 Jul 1;198(1):109–14.

7. Kendall ME, Crim S, Fullerton K, Han PV, Cronquist AB, Shiferaw B, et al. Travel-associated enteric infections diagnosed after return to the United States, Foodborne Diseases Active Surveillance Network (FoodNet), 2004–2009. Clin Infect Dis. 2012 Jun;54 Suppl 5:S480–7.

8. Majowicz SE, Musto J, Scallan E, Angulo FJ, Kirk M, O'Brien SJ, et al. The global burden of nontyphoidal *Salmonella* gastroenteritis. Clin Infect Dis. 2010 Mar 15;50(6):882–9.

9. Medalla F, Hoekstra RM, Whichard JM, Barzilay EJ, Chiller TM, Joyce K, et al. Increase in resistance to ceftriaxone and nonsusceptibility to ciprofloxacin and decrease in multidrug resistance among *Salmonella* strains, United States, 1996–2009. Foodborne Pathog Dis. 2013 Apr;10(4):302–9.

10. Paredes-Paredes M, Flores-Figueroa J, Dupont HL. Advances in the treatment of travelers' diarrhea. Curr Gastroenterol Rep. 2011 Oct;13(5):402–7.

SCABIES

Diana L. Martin

INFECTIOUS AGENT

The human itch mite, *Sarcoptes scabiei* var. *hominis*.

TRANSMISSION

Through prolonged skin-to-skin contact with a person with conventional scabies. Crusted scabies (formerly called Norwegian scabies) is a more severe form of scabies in which a person is infested with a large number of mites and is more highly contagious. Indirect transmission may occur through contact with objects contaminated by a person with crusted scabies but is rare if the person has conventional scabies.

EPIDEMIOLOGY

Scabies occurs worldwide. It is transmitted most easily in settings where skin contact is common. Crusted scabies most commonly occurs among elderly, disabled, debilitated, or immunosuppressed people, often in institutional settings. Skin conditions are some of the most common complaints among European travelers to tropical countries, and scabies is a more common skin infection among travelers participating in missionary or volunteer work and long-term (>8 weeks) travelers.

CLINICAL PRESENTATION

Symptoms occur 2–6 weeks after a person is first infested. However, if someone has had scabies before, symptoms appear much sooner (1–4 days after exposure). Conventional scabies is characterized by intense itching, particularly at night, and by a papular or papulovesicular, erythematous rash. Crusted scabies is characterized by widespread crusts and scales that contain large numbers of mites, although itching may be less than in conventional scabies.

DIAGNOSIS

Scabies is generally diagnosed by identifying burrows in a patient with itching and by observing the characteristic rash. Diagnosis can be confirmed by microscopically identifying mites, mite eggs, or mite feces; however, microscopic identification of mites is far less sensitive than clinical diagnosis. Crusted scabies is often misdiagnosed as psoriasis but can be accurately diagnosed by using skin scrapings because of the high number of mites in the sores.

TREATMENT

Permethrin (5%) cream is considered by many to be the drug of choice. Ivermectin is reported to be safe and effective to treat scabies. Ivermectin is not FDA-approved for scabies but should be considered for off-label use in patients in whom treatment has failed or who cannot tolerate other approved medications. Crusted scabies must be treated more aggressively; a combination of permethrin and ivermectin is recommended.

PREVENTION

Avoid prolonged skin-to-skin contact with people who have conventional scabies and even brief skin-to-skin contact with people who have crusted scabies. Contact with items such as clothing and bed linens that have been used by an infested person should be avoided, especially if the person has crusted scabies.

CDC website: www.cdc.gov/parasites/scabies

BIBLIOGRAPHY

1. American Academy of Pediatrics. Scabies. In: Pickering LK, editor. Red Book: 2012 Report of the Committee on Infectious Diseases. 29th ed. Elk Grove Village, IL: American Academy of Pediatrics; 2012. p. 641–3.
2. Ansart S, Perez L, Vergely O, Danis M, Bricaire F, Caumes E. Illnesses in travelers returning from the tropics: a prospective study of 622 patients. J Travel Med. 2005 Nov–Dec;12(6):312–8.
3. Bouvresse S, Chosidow O. Scabies in healthcare settings. Curr Opin Infect Dis. 2010 Apr;23(2):111–8.
4. Chosidow O. Clinical practices. Scabies. N Engl J Med. 2006 Apr 20;354(16):1718–27.
5. Currie BJ, McCarthy JS. Permethrin and ivermectin for scabies. N Engl J Med. 2010 Feb 25;362(8):717–25.
6. Hengge UR, Currie BJ, Jager G, Lupi O, Schwartz RA. Scabies: a ubiquitous neglected skin disease. Lancet Infect Dis. 2006 Dec;6(12):769–79.
7. Heukelbach J, Feldmeier H. Scabies. Lancet. 2006 May 27;367(9524):1767–74.
8. O'Brien BM. A practical approach to common skin problems in returning travellers. Travel Med Infect Dis. 2009 May;7(3):125–46.

SCHISTOSOMIASIS
Susan Montgomery

INFECTIOUS AGENT

Schistosomiasis is caused by helminth parasites of the genus *Schistosoma*. Other helminth infections are discussed in the Helminths, Soil-Transmitted section earlier in this chapter.

TRANSMISSION

Waterborne transmission occurs when larval cercariae, found in contaminated bodies of freshwater, penetrate the skin.

EPIDEMIOLOGY

An estimated 85% of the world's cases of schistosomiasis are in Africa, where prevalence rates can exceed 50% in local populations. *Schistosoma mansoni* and *S. haematobium* are distributed throughout Africa; only *S. haematobium* is found in areas of the Middle East; and *S. japonicum* is found in Indonesia and parts of China and Southeast Asia (Map 3-12). Two other species can infect

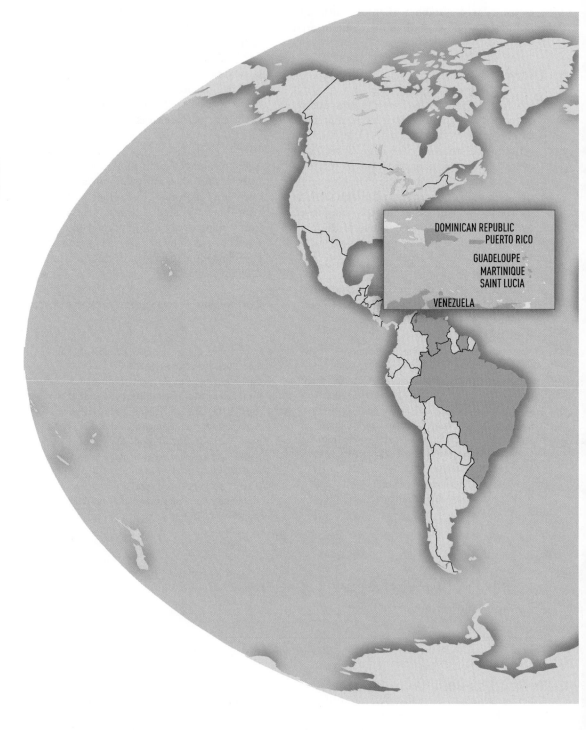

MAP 3-12. GEOGRAPHIC DISTRIBUTION OF SCHISTOSOMIASIS[1]

[1] The distribution of schistosomiasis is very focal; however, surveillance for schistosomiasis is limited in most countries. Therefore, this map shades entire countries where schistosomiasis transmission has been reported.

3

Schistosomiasis-Endemic Areas

- Hepatic-Intestinal
- Both Hepatic-Intestinal and Urinary
- Not Endemic
- Low Risk for Urinary
- Low Risk for Hepatic-Intestinal
- Low Risk for both Hepatic-Intestinal and Urinary

humans: *S. mekongi*, found in Cambodia and Laos, and *S. intercalatum*, found in parts of Central and West Africa. These 2 species are rarely reported causes of human infection. Many countries endemic for schistosomiasis have established control programs, but others have not. Countries where development has led to widespread improvements in sanitation and water safety, as well as successful schistosomiasis control programs, may have eliminated this disease. However, there are currently no international guidelines for certification of elimination.

All ages are at risk for infection with freshwater exposure in endemic areas. Swimming, bathing, and wading in contaminated freshwater can result in infection. Human schistosomiasis is not acquired by contact with saltwater (oceans or seas). The distribution of schistosomiasis is very focal and determined by the presence of competent snail vectors, inadequate sanitation, and infected humans. The geographic distribution of cases of schistosomiasis acquired by travelers reflects travel and immigration patterns. Most travel-associated cases of schistosomiasis are acquired in sub-Saharan Africa. Sites in Africa frequently visited by travelers are common sites of infection. These sites include rivers and water sources in the Banfora region (Burkina Faso) and areas populated by the Dogon people (Mali), Lake Malawi, Lake Tanganyika, Lake Victoria, the Omo River (Ethiopia), the Zambezi River, and the Nile River. However, as visitors travel to more uncommon sites, it is important to remember that most freshwater surface water sources in Africa are potentially contaminated and can be sources of infection. A local claim that there is no schistosomiasis in a body of freshwater is not necessarily reliable.

The specific snail vectors can be difficult to identify, and infection of snails with human schistosome species must be determined in the laboratory. The types of travelers and expatriates potentially at increased risk for infection include adventure travelers, Peace Corps volunteers, missionaries, soldiers, and ecotourists. Outbreaks of schistosomiasis have occurred among adventure travelers on river trips in Africa.

CLINICAL PRESENTATION

The incubation period is typically 14–84 days for acute schistosomiasis (Katayama syndrome), but chronic infection can remain asymptomatic for years. Penetration of cercariae can be associated with a rash that develops within hours or up to a week after contaminated water exposures. Acute schistosomiasis is characterized by fever, headache, myalgia, diarrhea, and respiratory symptoms. Eosinophilia is present, as well as often painful hepatomegaly or splenomegaly.

The clinical manifestations of chronic schistosomiasis are the result of host immune responses to schistosome eggs. Eggs secreted by adult worm pairs enter the circulation and lodge in organs and cause granulomatous reactions. Eosinophilia may be present. *S. mansoni* and *S. japonicum* eggs most commonly lodge in the blood vessels of the liver or intestine and can cause diarrhea, constipation, and blood in the stool. Chronic inflammation can lead to bowel wall ulceration, hyperplasia, and polyposis and, with heavy infections, to periportal liver fibrosis. *S. haematobium* eggs typically lodge in the urinary tract and can cause dysuria and hematuria. Calcifications in the bladder may appear late in the disease. *S. haematobium* infection can also cause genital symptoms and has been associated with increased risk of bladder cancer.

Rarely, central nervous system schistosomiasis may develop; this form is thought to result from aberrant migration of adult worms or eggs depositing in the spinal cord or brain. Signs and symptoms are related to ectopic granulomas in the central nervous system and can present as transverse myelitis.

DIAGNOSIS

Diagnosis is made by microscopic identification of parasite eggs in stool (*S. mansoni* or *S. japonicum*) or urine (*S. haematobium*). Serologic tests are useful to diagnose light infections where egg shedding may not be consistent in travelers and in others who have not had schistosomiasis previously. Antibody tests do not distinguish between past and current infection. Test sensitivity and specificity vary, depending on the antigen preparation used and how the test is performed. Health care providers should consider screening asymptomatic people who may have been exposed during travel and may benefit from treatment.

More detailed information and assistance with diagnosis may be obtained from CDC (www.cdc.gov/parasites/schistosomiasis or CDC Parasitic Diseases Inquiries, 404-718-4745).

TREATMENT

Schistosomiasis is uncommon in the United States, and the inexperienced clinician should consult an infectious disease or tropical medicine specialist for diagnosis and treatment. Praziquantel is used to treat schistosomiasis. Praziquantel is most effective against adult forms of the parasite and requires an immune response to the adult worm to be fully effective.

PREVENTION

No vaccine is available. No drugs for preventing infection are available. Preventive measures are primarily avoiding wading, swimming, or other contact with freshwater in disease-endemic countries. Untreated piped water coming directly from freshwater sources may contain cercariae, but filtering with fine-mesh filters, heating bathing water to 122°F (50°C) for 5 minutes, or allowing water to stand for ≥24 hours before exposure can eliminate risk for infection.

Swimming in adequately chlorinated swimming pools is virtually always safe, even in disease-endemic countries. Vigorous towel-drying after accidental exposure to water has been suggested as a way to remove cercariae before they can penetrate, but this may only prevent some infections and should not be recommended as a preventive measure. Topical applications of insect repellents such as DEET can block penetrating cercariae, but the effect depends on the repellent formulation, may be short-lived, and cannot reliably prevent infection.

CDC website: www.cdc.gov/parasites/schistosomiasis

BIBLIOGRAPHY

1. Bierman WF, Wetsteyn JC, van Gool T. Presentation and diagnosis of imported schistosomiasis: relevance of eosinophilia, microscopy for ova, and serology. J Travel Med. 2005 Jan–Feb;12(1): 9–13.

2. Clerinx J, Van Gompel A. Schistosomiasis in travellers and migrants. Travel Med Infect Dis. 2011 Jan;9(1):6-24.

3. Corachan M. Schistosomiasis and international travel. Clin Infect Dis. 2002 Aug 15;35(4):446–50.

4. Grobusch MP, Muhlberger N, Jelinek T, Bisoffi Z, Corachan M, Harms G, et al. Imported schistosomiasis in Europe: sentinel surveillance data from TropNetEurop. J Travel Med. 2003 May–Jun;10(3): 164–9.

5. Meltzer E, Artom G, Marva E, Assous MV, Rahav G, Schwartzt E. Schistosomiasis among travelers: new aspects of an old disease. Emerg Infect Dis. 2006 Nov;12(11):1696–700.

6. Nicolls DJ, Weld LH, Schwartz E, Reed C, von Sonnenburg F, Freedman DO, et al. Characteristics of schistosomiasis in travelers reported to the GeoSentinel Surveillance Network 1997–2008. Am J Trop Med Hyg. 2008 Nov;79(5):729–34.

7. Ross AG, Bartley PB, Sleigh AC, Olds GR, Li Y, Williams GM, et al. Schistosomiasis. N Engl J Med. 2002 Apr 18;346(16):1212–20.

8. Ross AG, Vickers D, Olds GR, Shah SM, McManus DP. Katayama syndrome. Lancet Infect Dis. 2007 Mar;7(3):218–24.

9. World Health Organization Expert Committee. Prevention and control of schistosomiasis and soil-transmitted helminthiasis. World Health Organ Tech Rep Ser. 2002;912:1–57.

SEXUALLY TRANSMITTED DISEASES

Sarah E. Kidd, Kimberly Workowski

INFECTIOUS AGENT

Sexually transmitted diseases (STDs) are the infections and resulting clinical syndromes caused by approximately 30 infectious organisms.

TRANSMISSION

Sexual activity is the predominant mode of transmission, through genital, anal, or oral mucosal contact.

EPIDEMIOLOGY

STDs are among the most common infectious diseases. Annually, an estimated 19.7 million sexually transmitted infections occur in the United States alone. Worldwide, an estimated 499 million cases of chlamydia, gonorrhea, syphilis, and trichomoniasis occur each year. Some STDs are more prevalent in developing countries (chancroid, lymphogranuloma venereum [LGV], granuloma inguinale [donovanosis]) or in specific regions (gonorrhea with treatment failure and decreased susceptibility to cephalosporins in Asia) and may be imported into other countries by travelers returning from such locales.

Casual sexual relationships occur frequently during travel to foreign countries. In a systematic review published in 2010, the pooled prevalence of travel-associated casual sex among foreign travelers was 20.4%. In addition, commercial sex in various destinations, such as Southeast Asia, attracts many foreign travelers. Commercial sex workers in some regions have high rates of STDs, including HIV, and travelers who have sex with them risk acquiring these infections.

Knowledge of the clinical presentation, frequency of infection, and antimicrobial resistance patterns is needed to manage STDs that occur in travelers. Assessing risk for men who have sex with men is important because of the recent increased rates of infectious syphilis, gonorrhea with treatment failure and decreased susceptibility to cephalosporins, and lymphogranuloma venereum in various geographic locations.

CLINICAL PRESENTATION

Many infections may be asymptomatic (chlamydia, gonorrhea), so screening for these infections at anatomic sites of contact and serologic testing for syphilis should be encouraged among travelers who present in clinic concerned they may have acquired an STD. Any traveler who might have been exposed and who develops vaginal, urethral, or rectal discharge, an unexplained rash or genital lesion, or genital or pelvic pain should be advised to cease sexual activity and promptly seek medical evaluation.

Some systemic infections are acquired through sexual transmission (hepatitis A, hepatitis B, hepatitis C, HIV, syphilis). Human papillomavirus (HPV) infection is usually subclinical and asymptomatic and most often clears spontaneously within 2 years. However, persistent HPV infection can lead to genital warts, cervical and other anogenital cancers, and oropharyngeal cancer. Because many travelers do not volunteer a history of sexual contact during travel, clinicians should inquire about sexual exposures when caring for returned travelers.

DIAGNOSIS

Genital ulcer evaluation should include a serologic test for syphilis and a culture or PCR testing for genital herpes. If exposure occurred in areas where chancroid is more common (Africa, Asia, and Latin America), a test for *Haemophilus ducreyi* should also be performed. Lymphadenopathy can accompany genital ulceration with chancroid infections, as well as with LGV and donovanosis. If painful perianal ulcers are present or mucosal ulcers are detected on anoscopy, presumptive therapy should include a regimen for anogenital herpes. LGV should be suspected in a traveler with tender unilateral inguinal or femoral lymphadenopathy or proctocolitis. Presumptive treatment for LGV should be considered for men who have sex with men and who have proctitis and perianal or mucosal ulcers, after obtaining specific testing for *Chlamydia trachomatis* (culture, direct immunofluorescence, or nucleic acid testing) from relevant specimens (genital lesions, rectal, or lymph node). Donovanosis is endemic in India, Papua New Guinea, central Australia, and southern Africa and is diagnosed with a crush tissue preparation from the lesion.

Testing specimens from the anatomic site of exposure with nucleic acid amplification testing can detect *C. trachomatis* and *Neisseria gonorrhoeae*. Culture and antibiotic susceptibility testing should be considered when gonorrhea is suspected, because of geographic differences in antimicrobial susceptibility. Various diagnostic methods are available to identify the cause of an abnormal vaginal discharge, including microscopic evaluation and pH testing of vaginal secretions, DNA probe-based testing, nucleic acid amplification testing, and culture.

Diagnosis of anogenital warts is made by visual inspection, with confirmation by biopsy if clinically indicated.

Anyone who seeks evaluation for STDs, or is diagnosed with an STD, should be screened for HIV infection.

TREATMENT

Evaluation, management, and follow-up of STDs should be based on standard guidelines (CDC and the World Health Organization). The prevalence of antimicrobial resistance in different areas should be considered when selecting treatment regimens. Early detection and treatment are important, as many STDs are asymptomatic. STDs can often result in serious and long-term complications, including pelvic inflammatory disease, infertility, stillbirths and neonatal infections, anogenital and other cancers, and an increased risk for HIV acquisition and transmission.

PREVENTION

The prevention and control of STDs are based on accurate risk assessment, education, counseling, early identification of asymptomatic infection, and effective treatment of patients and their sex partners. Pre-travel advice should include specific messages about the need to avoid acquiring or transmitting STDs. Abstinence or mutual monogamy with an uninfected partner is the most reliable way to avoid acquiring and transmitting STDs.

For people whose sexual behaviors place them at risk for STDs, correct and consistent use of the male latex condom can reduce the risk of HIV infection and other STDs, including chlamydia, gonorrhea, and trichomoniasis. Preventing lower genital tract infections might reduce the risk of pelvic inflammatory disease in women. Correct and consistent use of male latex condoms also reduces the risk of HPV infection, genital herpes, syphilis, and chancroid, although data are limited. Only water-based lubricants (such as K-Y Jelly or glycerin) should be used with latex condoms because oil-based lubricants (such as petroleum jelly, shortening, mineral oil, or massage oil) can weaken latex condoms. Spermicides containing nonoxynol-9 are not recommended for STD/HIV prevention, as nonoxynol-9 may disrupt genital or rectal epithelium and has been associated with an increased risk of HIV transmission. Contraceptive methods that are not mechanical barriers do not protect against HIV or other STDs.

Prompt evaluation of sexual partners is necessary to prevent reinfection and disrupt transmission of many STDs. Preexposure vaccination is among the most effective methods for preventing some STDs. Two HPV vaccines are available and licensed for girls and women aged 9–26 years to prevent cervical precancers and cancers: the quadrivalent HPV and the bivalent HPV vaccine. The quadrivalent vaccine also prevents genital warts and is recommended for boys and men aged 9–26 years as well as girls and women. All travelers should be considered candidates for both hepatitis A and hepatitis B vaccines, as these infections can be sexually transmitted. Hepatitis B vaccine is recommended for all people being evaluated or treated for an STD. In addition, hepatitis A and hepatitis B vaccines are recommended for men who have sex with men and injection drug users. Travelers, particularly those at high risk for acquiring HIV infection, may consider discussing preexposure prophylaxis with their health care providers (see www.cdc.gov/hiv/prep and HIV section in this chapter).

CDC website: www.cdc.gov/std

SEXUALLY TRANSMITTED DISEASES

BIBLIOGRAPHY

1. CDC. Condoms and STDs: factsheet for public health personnel. Atlanta: CDC; 2011 [cited 2014 Jun 23]. Available from: http://www.cdc.gov/condomeffectiveness/latex.htm.

2. CDC. Recommendations on the use of quadrivalent human papillomavirus vaccine in males—Advisory Committee on Immunization Practices (ACIP), 2011. MMWR Morb Mortal Wkly Rep. 2011;60(50):1705–8.

3. Lahra MM, Lo YR, Whiley DM. Gonococcal antimicrobial resistance in the Western Pacific Region. Sex Transm Infect. 2013 Dec;89 Suppl 4:iv19–23.

4. Peterman TA, Heffelfinger JD, Swint EB, Groseclose SL. The changing epidemiology of syphilis. Sex Transm Dis. 2005 Oct;32(10 Suppl):S4–10.

5. Satterwhite CL, Torrone E, Meites E, Dunne EF, Mahajan R, Ocfemia MC, et al. Sexually transmitted infections among US women and men: prevalence and incidence estimates, 2008. Sex Transm Dis. 2013 Mar;40(3):187–93.

6. Unemo M, Nicholas RA. Emergence of multidrug-resistant, extensively drug-resistant and untreatable gonorrhea. Future Microbiol. 2012 Dec;7(12):1401–22.

7. Vivancos R, Abubakar I, Hunter PR. Foreign travel, casual sex, and sexually transmitted infections: systematic review and meta-analysis. Int J Infect Dis. 2010 Oct;14(10):e842–51.

8. Ward H, Martin I, Macdonald N, Alexander S, Simms I, Fenton K, et al. Lymphogranuloma venereum in the United Kingdom. Clin Infect Dis. 2007 Jan 1;44(1):26–32.

9. Workowski KA, Berman S. Sexually transmitted diseases treatment guidelines, 2010. MMWR Recomm Rep. 2010 Dec 17;59(RR-12):1–110.

10. World Health Organization. Global incidence and prevalence of selected curable sexually transmitted infections—2008. Geneva: World Health Organization; 2012 [cited 2014 Jun. 23]. Available from: http://www.who.int/reproductivehealth/publications/rtis/stisestimates/en/.

Perspectives

SEX & TOURISM

Elissa Meites

TRAVEL AND SEXUAL HEALTH

Whether or not sex is the purpose of a trip, sex with a new partner is common during travel of any length. An estimated 5%–50% of international travelers have sex with a new partner while abroad, and the risk of developing a sexually transmitted disease (STD) may be up to 3 times higher in people who experience casual travel sex. Travelers may be unaware of the high prevalence of HIV and STDs in some other countries. For example, antibiotic-resistant

Perspectives sections are written as editorial discussions aiming to add depth and clinical perspective to the official recommendations contained in the book. The views and opinions expressed in this section are those of the author and do not necessarily represent the official position of CDC.

gonorrhea has been considered a public health threat since it was first identified internationally.

The mainstays of sexually transmitted infection prevention (condoms and vaccinations against hepatitis A, hepatitis B, and human papillomavirus), contraception, and other prescription medications may not be subject to US quality control standards in manufacturing, storage, or distribution when obtained in other countries. Condoms that are low quality, stored improperly, or past their expiration date are more likely to break. Clinicians seeing travelers at high risk for acquiring HIV infection should consider discussing preexposure prophylaxis with them (see www.cdc.gov/hiv/prep and HIV section in this chapter).

All people who have sex with a new partner should consult a clinician about recommended screening tests to check for HIV and treatable STDs. Travelers should also be alert to attempts at coercion or fraud from previously unknown partners professing romantic interest, especially in relationships beginning exclusively online. People who have experienced a high-risk sexual encounter should consider taking medications for postexposure prophylaxis of HIV or unintended pregnancy within 72 hours. These and other prescription medications can be costly or difficult to obtain overseas, but US consular officers may be able to assist in locating needed medical services. See Box 3-5 for a summary of sexual health recommendations for travelers.

SEX TOURISM

"Sex tourism" has been defined as travel planned specifically to procure sex. Sex tourism commonly involves male tourists traveling to economically disadvantaged countries to pay for sex with female sex workers. In certain regions, commercial sex work is legal and culturally acceptable. However, travelers should be aware that HIV and STD infections are common among commercial sex workers. Also, sex tourism helps to support sex trafficking, among the largest criminal industries in the world, in which victims are forced to perform sex work. Travelers should be familiar with applicable US and local laws and should report known or suspected violations promptly to the authorities. The regional security officer at the local US embassy or foreign law enforcement officials can assist.

SEXUAL ABUSE AND THE LAW

Although commercial sex work may be legal in some countries, sex trafficking, sex with a minor, and child pornography are always criminal activities according to US law and can be prosecuted in the United States even if the behavior occurred abroad. The Trafficking Victims Protection Act makes it illegal to recruit, entice, or obtain a person of any age to engage in commercial sex acts or to benefit from such activities. Federal law also bars US residents from engaging in sexual or pornographic activities with a child aged <18 years anywhere in the world, regardless of local age of consent, or to travel abroad for the purpose of having sex with a minor. In addition, child pornography, including sexual photographs or videos of minors in foreign countries, is illegal in the United States. These crimes are subject to prosecution with penalties of up to 30 years in prison.

Nearly 2 million children around the world are victims of commercial sexual exploitation, and roughly 1 million children are victims of trafficking. Children abused by sex tourists suffer not only sexual abuse but also poverty,

BOX 3-5. SUMMARY OF SEXUAL HEALTH RECOMMENDATIONS FOR TRAVELERS

Before travel

1. Obtain recommended vaccinations, including those that protect against sexually transmitted infections.
2. Get recommended tests for HIV and treatable STDs. Be aware of STD symptoms in case any develop.
3. Pack sufficient quantities of needed prescription medications and supplies. Check condom expiration dates.
4. Review local laws and contact information for medical and law enforcement services.

During travel

5. Use good judgment in choosing consensual adult sex partners.
6. Condoms, used consistently and correctly, can decrease the risk of HIV and STDs.
7. If indicated, be prepared to start taking medications for HIV postexposure prophylaxis or unintended pregnancy within 72 hours after a high-risk sexual encounter.
8. Never engage in sex with a minor (<18 years old), child pornography, or trafficking activities, in any country.
9. Report suspicious activity to US and local authorities as soon as it occurs.

After travel

10. To avoid exposing sex partners at home, get recommended tests for HIV and treatable STDs.

homelessness, and physical, emotional, and psychological abuse, as well as health problems including illnesses, addictions, malnourishment, infections, physical injuries, and STDs.

If you suspect child sexual exploitation occurring overseas, you can report tips anonymously by using the Operation Predator smartphone app (https://itunes.apple.com/us/app/operation-predator/id695130859?mt=8), calling the Immigration and Customs Enforcement hotline toll-free at 866-347-2423, or submitting the information online at www.ice.gov/tips. In the United States, the National Center for Missing & Exploited Children's Cybertipline collects reports of child prostitution and other crimes against children (toll-free at 800-843-5678, www.cybertipline.com). At least 8,000 Americans have been arrested for child sex exploitation and 99 Americans have been convicted for child sex tourism since 2003, when the federal PROTECT Act was passed to strengthen the US government's prosecution of crimes related to sex tourism.

Americans and US permanent residents account for an estimated 25% of child sex tourists worldwide and up to 80% in Latin America. These are typically Caucasian men aged ≥40 and have been traced visiting Mexico, Central and South America (Brazil, Colombia, Costa Rica, Dominican Republic), Southeast Asia (Cambodia, India, Laos, Philippines, Thailand), Eastern Europe (Estonia, Latvia, Lithuania, Russia), and other regions.

To combat child sexual abuse, some international hotels and other tourism services have voluntarily adopted a code of conduct that includes training and reporting suspicious activities. Tourist establishments supporting this initiative to protect children from sex tourism are listed online (www.thecode.org). For more ways you can help, see the Department of State list of 20 ways to fight human trafficking (www.state.gov/j/tip/id/help).

BIBLIOGRAPHY

1. Abdullah AS, Ebrahim SH, Fielding R, Morisky DE. Sexually transmitted infections in travelers: implications for prevention and control. Clin Infect Dis. 2004 Aug 15;39(4):533–8.
2. Marrazzo JM. Sexual tourism: implications for travelers and the destination culture. Infect Dis Clin North Am. 2005 Mar;19(1):103–20.
3. Newman WJ, Holt BW, Rabun JS, Phillips G, Scott CL. Child sex tourism: extending the borders of sexual offender legislation. Int J Law Psychiatry. 2011 Mar–Apr;34(2):116–21.
4. Vivancos R, Abubakar I, Hunter PR. Foreign travel, casual sex, and sexually transmitted infections: systematic review and meta-analysis. Int J Infect Dis. 2010 Oct;14(10):e842–51.
5. Workowski KA, Berman S. Sexually transmitted diseases treatment guidelines, 2010. MMWR Recomm Rep. 2010 Dec 17;59(RR-12):1–110.

SHIGELLOSIS

Anna Bowen

INFECTIOUS AGENT

Shigellosis is an acute infection of the intestine caused by bacteria in the genus *Shigella*. There are 4 species of *Shigella*: *Shigella dysenteriae*, *S. flexneri*, *S. boydii*, and *S. sonnei* (also referred to as group A, B, C, and D, respectively). Several distinct serotypes are recognized within the first 3 species.

TRANSMISSION

Transmission occurs via the fecal-oral route, through direct person-to-person contact, or indirectly through contaminated food, water, or fomites. Since as few as 10 organisms can cause infection, shigellosis is easily transmitted and can be acquired during short-term travel. Only humans and higher primates carry *Shigella*. In the United States, *S. sonnei* infection is usually transmitted through interpersonal contact, particularly among young children and their caregivers. Foodborne outbreaks have been linked to contaminated foods commonly consumed raw, as well as infected food handlers. Outbreaks have also been traced to contaminated drinking water, swimming in contaminated water, and sexual contact between men.

EPIDEMIOLOGY

Worldwide, *Shigella* is estimated to cause 80–165 million cases of disease and 600,000 deaths annually. *Shigella* spp. are endemic in temperate and tropical climates. Transmission of *Shigella* spp. is most likely when hygiene and sanitation are insufficient. Shigellosis is predominantly caused by *S. sonnei* in industrialized countries, whereas *S. flexneri* prevails in the developing world. Infections caused by *S. boydii* and *S. dysenteriae* are less common globally but can make up a substantial proportion of *Shigella* spp. isolated in sub-Saharan Africa and South Asia. *Shigella* spp. are detected in the stools of 5%–18% of patients with travelers' diarrhea. In a study of travel-associated enteric infections diagnosed after return to the United States, *Shigella* was the third most common bacterial pathogen isolated by clinical laboratories (of note, these laboratories did not test for enterotoxigenic *Escherichia coli*, a common cause of travelers' diarrhea). Many infections caused by *S. dysenteriae* (56%) and *S. boydii* (44%) were travel-associated, but infections caused by *S. flexneri* and *S. sonnei* were less often associated with travel (24%

and 12%, respectively). In this study, the risk of infection caused by *Shigella* spp. was highest for people traveling to Africa, followed by Central America, South America, and Asia. Outbreaks of infections caused by multidrug-resistant *Shigella*, including isolates resistant to azithromycin or ciprofloxacin, have been reported in Australia, Europe, and North America among men who have sex with men.

CLINICAL PRESENTATION
Illness typically begins 12–96 hours after exposure. The symptoms of shigellosis range from mild to severe and typically last 4–7 days. Disease severity varies according to species; serotype *S. dysenteriae* serotype 1 (Sd1) is the agent of epidemic dysentery, while *S. sonnei* commonly causes milder diarrheal illness. However, *Shigella* of any species can cause severe illness among people with compromised immune systems. Shigellosis is characterized by watery, bloody, or mucoid diarrhea; fever; stomach cramps; and nausea. Occasionally, patients experience vomiting, seizures (young children), or postinfectious arthritis. Hemolytic uremic syndrome can occur after infection with Sd1.

DIAGNOSIS
Rapid diagnostic tests for shigellosis are used in some US laboratories; however, shigellosis should be confirmed through culture of a stool specimen or rectal swab. *Shigella* isolates may then be speciated and

serotyped and their antimicrobial susceptibilities determined to help guide treatment. Fecal specimens should be processed rapidly because *Shigella* often does not survive for long outside the body.

TREATMENT
Although antimicrobial treatment, when given early in the course of illness, can slightly shorten the duration of symptoms and of carriage, shigellosis can be mild and typically resolves within 4–7 days without treatment. When treatment is required for shigellosis associated with travel outside the United States, a fluoroquinolone or ceftriaxone may be used empirically until antimicrobial susceptibility data are available. However, clinicians should be aware that rates of multidrug resistance among *Shigella* spp. are high globally, including resistance to fluoroquinolones, azithromycin, and third- and fourth-generation cephalosporins, particularly in South and East Asia.

PREVENTION
No vaccines are available for *Shigella*. The best defense against shigellosis is thorough, frequent handwashing; strict adherence to standard food and water safety precautions (see Chapter 2, Food & Water Precautions); and minimizing fecal-oral exposures during sexual contact.

CDC website: www.cdc.gov/shigella/

BIBLIOGRAPHY

1. American Academy of Pediatrics. *Shigella* infections. In: Pickering LK, editor. Red Book: 2012 Report of the Committee on Infectious Diseases. 29th ed. Elk Grove Village, IL: American Academy of Pediatrics; 2012. p. 645–7.

2. Bardhan P, Faruque AS, Naheed A, Sack DA. Decrease in shigellosis-related deaths without *Shigella* spp.-specific interventions, Asia. Emerg Infect Dis. 2010 Nov;16(11):1718–23.

3. Heiman KE, Karlsson M, Grass J, Howie B, Kirkcaldy RD, Mahon B, et al. Notes from the field: *Shigella* with decreased susceptibility to azithromycin among men who have sex with men—United States, 2002–2013. MMWR Morb Mortal Wkly Rep. 2014 Feb 14;63(6):132–3.

4. Hoffmann C, Sahly H, Jessen A, Ingiliz P, Stellbrink HJ, Neifer S, et al. High rates of quinolone-resistant

strains of *Shigella sonnei* in HIV-infected MSM. Infection. 2013 Oct;41(5):999–1003.

5. Kendall ME, Crim S, Fullerton K, Han PV, Cronquist AB, Shiferaw B, et al. Travel-associated enteric infections diagnosed after return to the United States, Foodborne Diseases Active Surveillance Network (FoodNet), 2004–2009. Clin Infect Dis. 2012 Jun;54 Suppl 5:S480–7.

6. Nygren BL, Schilling KA, Blanton EM, Silk BJ, Cole DJ, Mintz ED. Foodborne outbreaks of shigellosis in the USA, 1998–2008. Epidemiol Infect. 2013 Feb;141(2):233–41.

7. Tajbakhsh M, Garcia Migura L, Rahbar M, Svendsen CA, Mohammadzadeh M, Zali MR, et al. Antimicrobial-resistant *Shigella* infections from Iran: an overlooked problem? J Antimicrob Chemother. 2012 May;67(5):1128–33.

8. von Seidlein L, Kim DR, Ali M, Lee H, Wang X, Thiem VD, et al. A multicentre study of *Shigella* diarrhoea in six Asian countries: disease burden, clinical manifestations, and microbiology. PLoS Med. 2006 Sep;3(9):e353.

9. Wong MR, Reddy V, Hanson H, Johnson KM, Tsoi B, Cokes C, et al. Antimicrobial resistance trends of *Shigella* serotypes in New York City, 2006–2009. Microb Drug Resist. 2010 Jun;16(2):155–61.

10. Zhang W, Luo Y, Li J, Lin L, Ma Y, Hu C, et al. Wide dissemination of multidrug-resistant *Shigella* isolates in China. J Antimicrob Chemother. 2011 Nov;66(11):2527–35.

SMALLPOX & OTHER ORTHOPOXVIRUS-ASSOCIATED INFECTIONS

Mary G. Reynolds

INFECTIOUS AGENT

Smallpox is caused by variola virus, genus *Orthopoxvirus*. Other members of this genus that cause infection in humans are vaccinia virus, monkeypox virus, and cowpox virus. In 1980, the World Health Organization officially declared smallpox to be eradicated.

TRANSMISSION

Smallpox

Person to person, principally respiratory; less commonly through contact with infectious skin lesions or scabs.

Monkeypox

Person to person, principally respiratory; less commonly through contact with infectious skin lesions or scabs. African rodents and primates may harbor the virus and could infect humans, but the reservoir host is unknown.

Vaccinia

Vaccinia virus is the live-virus component of contemporary smallpox vaccines. Rarely, social contacts of people recently vaccinated for smallpox develop infections with vaccinia virus when their skin comes into contact with fluid from the inoculation lesion. Zoonotic infections with vaccinialike viruses have been reported in Brazil and India.

Cowpox

Contact with infected animals; transmission between humans has not been observed.

EPIDEMIOLOGY

Smallpox

Eradicated globally. A single confirmed case of smallpox would be the result of an intentional act (bioterrorism) and would be considered an emergency.

Monkeypox

Endemic in tropical forested regions of West and Central Africa, notably the Congo Basin. Rodents imported from West Africa were the source of a 2003 outbreak of human monkeypox in the United States. Monkeypox is endemic in the Democratic Republic of the Congo (DRC) and occurs sporadically in neighboring countries (Republic of the Congo, Central African Republic, Sudan). Refugees and immigrants who have recently left DRC may harbor monkeypox virus infection, but reports of this are rare. Short-term travelers to monkeypox-endemic areas would not generally be at risk.

Vaccinia

Infections with wild vaccinialike viruses have been reported among cattle and buffalo herders in India and among dairy workers in southern Brazil. Travelers who have direct (hands-on) contact with affected bovines may be at risk for acquiring cutaneous infection.

Cowpox

Human infections with cowpox and cowpox-like viruses have been reported in Europe and the Caucasus (Georgia). Travelers who have direct (hands-on) contact with affected bovines, felines, rodents, or captive exotics (zoo animals) may be at risk for cutaneous infection.

CLINICAL PRESENTATION
Smallpox

Infections present with acute onset of fever >101°F (38.3°C), malaise, head and body aches, and sometimes vomiting. This phase is followed by a rash characterized by firm, deep-seated vesicles or pustules in the same stage of development. Clinically, the most common rash illness likely to be confused with smallpox is varicella (chickenpox). A detailed explanation of the clinical signs and symptoms of smallpox can be found at www.bt.cdc.gov/agent/smallpox/overview/disease-facts.asp.

Monkeypox

Clinically identical to smallpox, with fever and widespread vesiculopustular rash involving the palms and soles. One feature distinctive to monkeypox is marked lymphadenopathy.

Vaccinia and Cowpox

Human infections with vaccinia, wild vac-cinialike viruses, and cowpox virus are most often self-limited, characterized by localized pustular (and in cowpox, occasionally ulcerative) lesions. Fever and other constitutional symptoms may occur briefly after lesions first appear. Lesions can be painful and can persist for weeks. People who are immunocompromised or who have exfoliative skin conditions (such as eczema or atopic dermatitis) are at higher risk of severe illness or death.

DIAGNOSIS

Orthopoxvirus infection is confirmed by PCR or virus isolation. Health care providers can refer to the CDC smallpox website (www.bt.cdc.gov/agent/smallpox/diagnosis) for guidance in the application of a clinical algorithm designed to aid in distinguishing orthopoxvirus infections from other disseminated rash illnesses, namely chickenpox.

TREATMENT

Mainly supportive, to include hydration, nutritional supplementation, and prevention of secondary infections. Vaccinia lesions should remain covered until the scab detaches to diminish chances of spreading virus to other parts of the body or to another person. Health care providers managing orthopoxvirus infection in a patient who is at high risk for severe outcome (such as a patient who is immunocompromised or has an underlying skin condition) should consult with CDC to explore investigational treatment options (770-488-7100). Investigational use of antivirals could be considered.

PREVENTION

Smallpox vaccine is not recommended for international travelers. Smallpox vaccination is recommended only for laboratory workers who handle variola virus (the agent of smallpox) or closely related viruses and health care and public health officials who would be designated first responders in the event of an intentional release of variola virus. In addition, members of the US military may be required to receive the vaccine.

For other orthopoxvirus infections, avoid contact with rodents and sick or dead animals, including pets and domestic ruminants (cattle, buffalo). For more information about monkeypox and other orthopoxviruses, contact the CDC Poxvirus Inquiry Line (404-639-4129).

CDC websites: http://emergency.cdc.gov/agent/smallpox and www.cdc.gov/ncidod/monkeypox

BIBLIOGRAPHY

1. Baxby D, Bennett M, Getty B. Human cowpox 1969–93: a review based on 54 cases. Br J Dermatol. 1994 Nov;131(5):598–607.
2. Levine RS, Peterson AT, Yorita KL, Carroll D, Damon IK, Reynolds MG. Ecological niche and geographic distribution of human monkeypox in Africa. PLoS One. 2007; 2(1):e176.
3. Nakazawa Y, Emerson GL, Carroll DS, Zhao H, Li Y, Reynolds MG, et al. Phylogenetic and ecologic perspectives of a monkeypox outbreak,

southern Sudan, 2005. Emerg Infect Dis. 2013 Feb;19(2):237–45.

4. Reynolds MG, Emerson GL, Pukuta E, Karhemere S, Muyembe JJ, Bikindou A, et al. Detection of human monkeypox in the Republic of the Congo following intensive community education. Am J Trop Med Hyg. 2013 May;88(5):982–5.

5. Trindade GS, Guedes MI, Drumond BP, Mota BE, Abrahao JS, Lobato ZI, et al. Zoonotic vaccinia virus: clinical and immunological characteristics in a naturally infected patient. Clin Infect Dis. 2009 Feb 1; 48(3):e37–40.

STRONGYLOIDIASIS
LeAnne M. Fox

INFECTIOUS AGENT

An intestinal nematode, *Strongyloides stercoralis*.

TRANSMISSION

Filariform larvae found in contaminated soil penetrate human skin. Person-to-person transmission is rare but documented.

EPIDEMIOLOGY

Endemic in the tropics and subtropics and in limited foci in the southeastern United States, Europe, Australia, and Japan. Estimates of global prevalence vary between 3 million and 100 million. Most documented infections in the United States occur in immigrants, refugees, and military veterans who have lived in endemic areas for long periods of time. Risk for short-term travelers is low, but infections can occur.

CLINICAL PRESENTATION

Most infections are asymptomatic. With acute infections, a localized, pruritic, erythematous papular rash can develop at the site of skin penetration, followed by pulmonary symptoms (a Löffler-like pneumonitis), diarrhea, abdominal pain, and eosinophilia. Migrating larvae in the skin cause larva currens, a serpiginous urticarial rash.

Immunocompromised people, especially those receiving systemic corticosteroids, those with human T-cell lymphotropic virus type 1 infection, those with hematologic malignancies, or who have had organ transplants, are at risk for hyperinfection or disseminated disease, characterized by abdominal pain, diffuse pulmonary infiltrates, and septicemia or meningitis from enteric gram-negative bacilli. The death rate from untreated disseminated strongyloidiasis is very high. Unexplained eosinophilia may be a presenting sign.

DIAGNOSIS

Rhabditiform larvae on microscopic examination of stool, either directly or by culture on agar plates. Repeated stool examinations or examination of duodenal contents may be necessary. Hyperinfection and disseminated strongyloidiasis are diagnosed by examining stool, sputum, cerebrospinal fluid, and other body fluids and tissues, which typically contain high numbers of larvae. Serologic testing is available through commercial laboratories and through the National Institutes of Health and CDC (www.dpd.cdc.gov/dpdx; 404-718-4745; parasites@cdc.gov).

TREATMENT

Treatment of choice for both chronic and disseminated disease or hyperinfection is ivermectin. The alternative is albendazole, although associated with slightly lower cure rates. Prolonged or repeated treatment may be necessary in patients with hyperinfection and disseminated disease, and relapse can occur.

PREVENTION

No vaccine or preventative drugs are available. Protective measures include wearing shoes when walking in areas where humans may have defecated. It may be reasonable to perform serologic testing on patients who have been at high risk for *Strongyloides* infection and who will either be placed on immunosuppressive drug regimens or who will undergo procedures that involve immunosuppression such as transplantation. If indicated, these patients should be treated before immunosuppression. Further information may be found on the CDC website.

CDC website: www.cdc.gov/parasites/strongyloides

BIBLIOGRAPHY

1. Angheben A, Mistretta M, Gobbo M, Bonafini S, Iacovazzi T, Sepe A, et al. Acute strongyloidiasis in Italian tourists returning from Southeast Asia. J Travel Med. 2011 Mar–Apr;18(2):138–40.
2. Arthur RP, Shelley WB. Larva currens; a distinctive variant of cutaneous larva migrans due to *Strongyloides stercoralis*. AMA Arch Derm. 1958 Aug;78(2):186–90.
3. Genta RM, Weesner R, Douce RW, Huitger-O'Connor T, Walzer PD. Strongyloidiasis in US veterans of the Vietnam and other wars. JAMA. 1987 Jul 3;258(1):49–52.
4. Keiser PB, Nutman TB. *Strongyloides stercoralis* in the immunocompromised population. Clin Microbiol Rev. 2004 Jan;17(1):208–17.
5. Seybolt LM, Christiansen D, Barnett ED. Diagnostic evaluation of newly arrived asymptomatic refugees with eosinophilia. Clin Infect Dis. 2006 Feb 1;42(3):363–7.
6. Siddiqui AA, Berk SL. Diagnosis of *Strongyloides stercoralis* infection. Clin Infect Dis. 2001 Oct 1;33(7):1040–7.

TAENIASIS

Paul T. Cantey, Jeffrey L. Jones

INFECTIOUS AGENT
Taenia solium (pork tapeworm) and *T. saginata* or *T. asiatica* (beef tapeworm).

TRANSMISSION
Eating raw or undercooked contaminated pork or beef.

EPIDEMIOLOGY
The highest prevalences are in Latin America, Africa, and South and Southeast Asia. Taeniasis has been reported at lower rates in Eastern Europe, Spain, and Portugal. Tapeworm infections are unusual in travelers.

CLINICAL PRESENTATION
The incubation period is 8–10 weeks for *T. solium* and 10–14 weeks for *T. saginata*. Symptoms may include abdominal discomfort, weight loss, anorexia, nausea, insomnia, weakness, perianal pruritus, and nervousness.

DIAGNOSIS
Presence of eggs, proglottids (segments), or tapeworm antigens in the feces or on anal swabs. Differentiation of *T. solium* from *T. saginata* and *T. asiatica* is based on morphology of the scolex and gravid proglottids.

TREATMENT
Praziquantel is the drug of choice, except in the setting of symptomatic neurocysticercosis (see Cysticercosis in this chapter). Niclosamide is an alternative but is not as widely available.

PREVENTION
Avoid undercooked meat.

CDC website: www.cdc.gov/parasites/taeniasis

BIBLIOGRAPHY

1. Garcia HH, Gonzalez AE, Evans CA, Gilman RH, Cysticercosis Working Group in Peru. *Taenia solium* cysticercosis. Lancet. 2003 Aug 16;362(9383):547–56.
2. Wittner M, White AC Jr, Tanowitz HB. *Taenia* and other tapeworm infections. In: Guerrant RL, Walker DH, Weller PF, editors. Tropical Infectious Diseases: Principles, Pathogens, and Practice. 3rd ed. Philadelphia: Sanders Elsevier; 2011. p. 839–47.

3

TETANUS

Tejpratap S. P. Tiwari

INFECTIOUS AGENT

Clostridium tetani, a spore-forming, anaerobic, gram-positive bacterium. Bacteria are ubiquitous in the environment.

TRANSMISSION

Contact with nonintact skin, usually via injuries from contaminated objects. "Tetanus-prone" wounds include those contaminated with dirt, human or animal excreta, or saliva; punctures; burns; crush injuries; or injuries with necrotic tissue.

EPIDEMIOLOGY

Distributed worldwide; more common in rural and agricultural regions, areas where contact with soil or animal excreta is likely, and areas where immunization is inadequate. Tetanus can affect any age group.

CLINICAL PRESENTATION

Incubation period is 10 days (range, 3–21 days). Acute symptoms typically include muscle rigidity and spasms, often in the jaw and neck. Symptoms of less common forms of tetanus (localized or cephalic) can include muscle spasms confined to the injury site, head or face lesions, and flaccid cranial nerve palsies. Progression from these forms to generalized tetanus may occur. Severe tetanus can lead to respiratory failure and death. Case-fatality ratios are high even where modern intensive care is available.

DIAGNOSIS

Diagnosis is made clinically; no confirmatory laboratory tests are available.

TREATMENT

Tetanus requires hospitalization, treatment with human tetanus immune globulin (TIG), a tetanus toxoid booster, agents to control muscle spasm, aggressive wound care, and antibiotics. Metronidazole is the most appropriate antibiotic. The wound should be debrided widely and excised if possible.

PREVENTION

Ensure adequate immunity to tetanus by completing the childhood primary vaccine series with tetanus toxoid, a booster dose during adolescence, and at 10-year intervals thereafter during adulthood. For heavily contaminated wounds, a booster dose may be given if more than 5 years have elapsed since the last dose. For detailed information regarding the tetanus vaccine, visit www.cdc.gov/vaccines/vpd-vac/tetanus. Additional tetanus prophylaxis with TIG may be required in wounded patients.

CDC website: www.cdc.gov/tetanus/

BIBLIOGRAPHY

1. CDC. Updated recommendations for use of tetanus toxoid, reduced diphtheria toxoid and acellular pertussis (Tdap) vaccine from the Advisory Committee on Immunization Practices, 2010. MMWR Morb Mortal Wkly Rep. 2011 Jan 14;60(1):13–5.

2. Farrar JJ, Yen LM, Cook T, Fairweather N, Binh N, Parry J, et al. Tetanus. J Neurol Neurosurg Psychiatry. 2000 Sep;69(3):292–301.

3. World Health Organization. Tetanus vaccine. Wkly Epidemiol Rec. 2006 May 19;81(20):198–208.

TICKBORNE ENCEPHALITIS

Marc Fischer, Ingrid B. Rabe, Pierre E. Rollin

INFECTIOUS AGENT

Tickborne encephalitis (TBE) virus is a single-stranded RNA virus that belongs to the genus *Flavivirus*. TBE virus has 3 subtypes: European, Siberian, and Far Eastern.

TRANSMISSION

TBE virus is transmitted to humans through the bite of an infected tick of the *Ixodes* species, primarily *I. ricinus* (European subtype) or *I. persulcatus* (Siberian and Far Eastern subtypes). The virus is maintained in discrete areas of deciduous forests. Ticks act as both vector and virus reservoir, and small rodents are the primary amplifying host. TBE can also be acquired by ingesting unpasteurized dairy products (such as milk and cheese) from infected goats, sheep, or cows. TBE virus transmission has infrequently been reported through laboratory exposure and slaughtering viremic animals. Direct person-to-person spread of TBE virus occurs only rarely, through blood transfusion or breastfeeding.

EPIDEMIOLOGY

TBE is endemic in focal areas of Europe and Asia, extending from eastern France to northern Japan and from northern Russia to Albania. Approximately 5,000–13,000 TBE cases are reported each year, with large annual fluctuations. Russia has the largest number of reported cases. The highest disease incidence has been reported from western Siberia and the Baltic States (Estonia, Latvia, Lithuania). Other European countries with reported cases or known endemic areas include Albania, Austria, Belarus, Bosnia, Croatia, Czech Republic, Denmark, Finland, France, Germany, Hungary, Italy, Norway, Poland, Romania, Serbia, Slovakia, Slovenia, Sweden, Switzerland, and Ukraine. Asian countries with reported TBE cases or virus activity include China, Japan, Kazakhstan, Kyrgyzstan, Mongolia, and South Korea.

Most cases occur from April through November, with peaks in early and late summer when ticks are active. The incidence and severity of disease are highest in people aged ≥50 years. Most cases occur in areas <2,500 ft (750 m). In the last 30 years, the geographic range of TBE virus appears to have expanded to new areas, and the virus has been found at altitudes up to and above 5,000 ft (1,500 m). These trends are likely due to a complex combination of changes in diagnosis and surveillance, human activities and socioeconomic factors, and ecology and climate.

The overall risk of acquiring TBE for an unvaccinated visitor to a highly endemic area during the TBE virus transmission season has been estimated at 1 case per 10,000 person-months of exposure. Most TBE virus infections result from tick bites acquired in forested areas through activities such as camping; hiking; fishing; bicycling; collecting mushrooms, berries, or flowers; and outdoor occupations such as forestry or military training. The risk is negligible for people who remain in urban or unforested areas and who do not consume unpasteurized dairy products.

Vector tick population density and infection rates in TBE virus-endemic foci are highly variable. For example, TBE virus infection rates in *I. ricinus* in central Europe vary from <0.1% to approximately 5%, depending on geographic location and time of year, while rates of up to 40% have been reported in *I. persulcatus* in Siberia. The number of TBE cases reported from a country depends on the ecology and geographic distribution of TBE virus, the intensity of diagnosis and surveillance, and the vaccine coverage in the population. Therefore, the number of human TBE cases reported from an area may not be a reliable predictor of a traveler's risk for infection. The same ticks that transmit TBE virus can also transmit other pathogens, including *Borrelia burgdorferi* (the agent for Lyme disease), *Anaplasma phagocytophilum* (anaplasmosis), and *Babesia* spp. (babesiosis), and simultaneous infection with multiple organisms has been described.

From 2000 through 2011, 5 cases of TBE among US travelers to Europe and China were reported. TBE is not a nationally notifiable disease in the United States, and additional cases may have occurred.

CLINICAL PRESENTATION

Approximately two-thirds of infections are asymptomatic. The median incubation period for TBE is 8 days (range, 4–28 days). The incubation period for milkborne exposure is usually shorter (3–4 days). Acute neuroinvasive disease is the most commonly recognized clinical manifestation of TBE virus infection. However, TBE disease often presents with milder forms of the disease or a biphasic course:

- First phase: nonspecific febrile illness with headache, myalgia, and fatigue. Usually lasts for several days and may be followed by an afebrile and relatively asymptomatic period. Up to two-thirds of patients may recover without any further illness.
- Second phase: central nervous system involvement resulting in aseptic meningitis, encephalitis, or myelitis. Findings include meningeal signs, altered mental status, cognitive dysfunction, ataxia, rigidity, seizures, tremors, cranial nerve palsies, and limb paresis.

Disease severity increases with age. Although TBE tends to be less severe in children, residual symptoms and neurologic deficits have been described. Clinical course and long-term outcome also vary by TBE virus subtype:

- The European subtype is associated with milder disease, a case-fatality ratio of <2%, and neurologic sequelae in up to 30% of patients.
- The Far Eastern subtype is often associated with a more severe disease course, including a case-fatality ratio of 20%–40% and higher rates of severe neurologic sequelae.
- The Siberian subtype is more frequently associated with chronic or progressive disease and has a case-fatality ratio of 2%–3%.

DIAGNOSIS

TBE should be suspected in travelers who develop a nonspecific febrile illness that progresses to neuroinvasive disease within 4 weeks of arriving from an endemic area. A history of tick bite may be a clue to this diagnosis; however, approximately 30% of TBE patients do not recall a tick bite.

Serology is typically used for laboratory diagnosis. IgM-capture ELISA performed on serum or cerebrospinal fluid is virtually always positive during the neuroinvasive phase of the illness. Vaccination history, date of onset of symptoms, and information regarding other flaviviruses known to circulate in the geographic area that may cross-react in serologic assays need to be considered when interpreting results. During the first phase of the illness, TBE virus or viral RNA can sometimes be detected in serum samples by virus isolation or RT-PCR. However, by the time neurologic symptoms are recognized, the virus or viral RNA is usually undetectable. Therefore, virus isolation and RT-PCR should not be used to rule out a diagnosis of TBE. Clinicians should contact their state or local health department, the CDC Viral Special Pathogens Branch (404-639-1115), or CDC Division of Vector-Borne Diseases (970-221-6400) for assistance with diagnostic testing.

TREATMENT

There is no specific antiviral treatment for TBE; therapy consists of supportive care and management of complications.

PREVENTION

Personal Protection Measures

Travelers should avoid consuming unpasteurized dairy products and use all measures to avoid tick bites (see Chapter 2, Protection against Mosquitoes, Ticks, & Other Arthropods).

Vaccine

No TBE vaccines are licensed or available in the United States. Two inactivated cell culture-derived TBE vaccines are available in Europe, in adult and pediatric formulations: FSME-IMMUN (Baxter, Austria) and Encepur (Novartis, Germany). The adult formulation of FSME-IMMUN is also licensed in Canada. Two other inactivated TBE vaccines are available in Russia: TBE-Moscow (Chumakov Institute, Russia) and EnceVir (Microgen, Russia). Immunogenicity studies suggest that the European and Russian vaccines should provide cross-protection against all 3 TBE virus subtypes. At least 1 other TBE vaccine is produced in China, but information regarding this vaccine is not available in the English literature.

For both FSME-IMMUN and Encepur, the primary vaccination series consists of 3 doses. The specific recommended intervals between doses vary by country and vaccine (Table 3-19). Although no formal efficacy trials of these vaccines have been conducted, indirect evidence suggests that their efficacy is >95%. Vaccine failures have been reported, particularly in people aged ≥50 years.

Because the routine primary vaccination series requires ≥6 months for completion, most travelers to TBE-endemic areas will find avoiding tick bites to be more practical than vaccination. However, an accelerated vaccination schedule has been evaluated for both European vaccines, and results in seroconversion rates are similar to those observed with the standard vaccination

Table 3-19. Tickborne encephalitis (TBE) vaccines licensed in Canada, Europe, and Russia[1]

TRADE NAME (MANUFACTURER, LOCATION)	AGE (Y)	DOSE	ROUTE	PRIMARY SERIES	FIRST BOOSTER (Y)	SUBSEQUENT BOOSTERS (Y)
FSME-IMMUN (Baxter, Austria)	≥16	0.5 mL	IM	3 doses (0, 1–3 mo, 6–15 mo)[2]	3	5[3]
FSME-IMMUN Junior (Baxter, Austria)	1–15	0.25 mL	IM	3 doses (0, 1–3 mo, 6–15 mo)[2]	3	5
Encepur-Adults (Novartis, Germany)	≥17	0.5 mL	IM	3 doses (0, 1–3 mo, 9–12 mo)[4]	3	5[3]
Encepur-Children (Novartis, Germany)	1–11	0.25 mL	IM	3 doses (0, 1–3 mo, 9–12 mo)[4]	3	5
EnceVir (Microgen, Russia)	≥3	0.5 mL	IM	2 doses (0, 5–7 mo)[5]	1	3
TBE-Moscow (Chumakov Institute, Russia)	≥3	0.5 mL	IM	2 doses (0, 1–7 mo)	1	3

Abbreviation: IM, intramuscular.

[1] No TBE vaccines are licensed or available in the United States. FSME-IMMUN is licensed in Canada and Europe; FSME-IMMUN Junior, Encepur-Adults, and Encepur-Children are licensed in Europe; and EnceVir and TBE-Moscow are licensed in Russia.

[2] If a rapid immune response is required, the second dose can be administered 2 weeks after the first dose.

[3] Booster doses recommended every 3 years for people aged ≥50 years.

[4] An accelerated schedule has been used with 3 doses given on days 0, 7, and 21. After the primary series, the first booster dose is administered at 12–18 months.

[5] For emergency situations, there is a rapid primary series schedule of 0 and 1–2 months.

schedule. Travelers anticipating high-risk exposures, such as working or camping in forested areas or farmland, adventure travel, or living in TBE-endemic countries for an extended period of time, may wish to be vaccinated in Canada or Europe.

CDC website: www.cdc.gov/vhf/tbe

BIBLIOGRAPHY

1. CDC. Tick-borne encephalitis among US travelers to Europe and Asia—2000–2009. MMWR Morb Mortal Wkly Rep. 2010 Mar 26;59(11):335–8.

2. Committee to Advise on Tropical Medicine and Travel (CATMAT). Statement on tick-borne encephalitis. An Advisory Committee Statement (ACS). Can Commun Dis Rep. 2006 Apr 1;32(ACS-3):1–18.

3. Donoso Mantke O, Escadafal C, Niedrig M, Pfeffer M, Working Group For Tick-Borne Encephalitis Virus. Tick-borne encephalitis in Europe, 2007 to 2009. Euro Surveill. 2011 Sep;16(39):7–18.

4. Kollaritsch H, Paulke-Korinek M, Holzmann H, Hombach J, Bjorvatn B, Barrett A. Vaccines and vaccination against tick-borne encephalitis. Expert Rev Vaccines. 2012 Sep;11(9):1103–19.

5. Lindquist L, Vapalahti O. Tick-borne encephalitis. Lancet. 2008 May 31;371(9627):1861–71.

6. Lu Z, Broker M, Liang G. Tick-borne encephalitis in mainland China. Vector Borne Zoonotic Dis. 2008 Oct;8(5):713–20.

7. Ruzek D, Dobler G, Donoso Mantke O. Tick-borne encephalitis: pathogenesis and clinical implications. Travel Med Infect Dis. 2010 Jul;8(4):223–32.

8. Stefanoff P, Polkowska A, Giambi C, Levy-Bruhl D, O'Flanagan D, Dematte L, et al. Reliable surveillance of tick-borne encephalitis in European countries is necessary to improve the quality of vaccine recommendations. Vaccine. 2011 Feb 1;29(6):1283–8.

9. Suss J. Tick-borne encephalitis 2010: epidemiology, risk areas, and virus strains in Europe and Asia—an overview. Ticks Tick Borne Dis. 2011 Mar;2(1):2–15.

10. World Health Organization. Vaccines against tick-borne encephalitis: WHO position paper. Wkly Epidemiol Rec. 2011 Jun 10;86(24):241–56.

TOXOPLASMOSIS

Jeffrey L. Jones

INFECTIOUS AGENT

Toxoplasma gondii, an intracellular coccidian protozoan parasite.

TRANSMISSION

Ingestion of soil, water, or food contaminated with cat feces, ingestion of undercooked meat, congenital transmission when a woman becomes infected during pregnancy, and contaminated blood transfusion and organ transplantation.

EPIDEMIOLOGY

T. gondii is endemic throughout most of the world. Risk is higher in developing and tropical countries, especially when people eat undercooked meat, drink untreated water, or are extensively exposed to soil.

CLINICAL PRESENTATION

Incubation period is 5–23 days. Symptoms may include influenzalike symptoms or a mononucleosis syndrome with prolonged fever, lymphadenopathy, elevated liver enzymes, lymphocytosis, and weakness. Rarely, chorioretinitis or disseminated disease can occur in immunocompetent people. In severely immunocompromised people, severe and even fatal toxoplasmic encephalitis, pneumonitis, and other systemic illnesses can occur, most often from reactivation of a previous infection. Infants with congenital toxoplasmosis are often asymptomatic, but eye disease, neurologic disease, or other systemic symptoms can occur, and learning disabilities, mental retardation, or visual impairments may develop later in life.

DIAGNOSIS

Serologic testing for *T. gondii* antibodies. Eye disease is diagnosed by ocular examination. Diagnosis of toxoplasmic encephalitis in immunocompromised people (mostly seen in people with AIDS) can be based on typical clinical course and identification of ≥1 mass lesion by CT, MRI, or other radiographic testing. Biopsy may be needed to make a definitive diagnosis.

TREATMENT
Pyrimethamine and sulfadiazine are the mainstays of treatment.

BIBLIOGRAPHY
1. Anand R, Jones CW, Ricks JH, Sofarelli TA, Hale DC. Acute primary toxoplasmosis in travelers returning from endemic countries. J Travel Med. 2012 Jan–Feb;19(1):57–60.
2. Bottieau E, Clerinx J, Van den Enden E, Van Esbroeck M, Colebunders R, Van Gompel A, et al. Infectious mononucleosis-like syndromes in febrile travelers returning from the tropics. J Travel Med. 2006 Jul–Aug;13(4):191–7.
3. Montoya JG, Liesenfeld O. Toxoplasmosis. Lancet. 2004 Jun 12;363(9425):1965–76.
4. Montoya JG, Remington JS. Management of *Toxoplasma gondii* infection during pregnancy. Clin Infect Dis. 2008 Aug 15;47(4):554–66.

PREVENTION
Food and water precautions (see Chapter 2, Food & Water Precautions). Avoid direct contact with soil or sand. If caring for a cat, change the litter box daily. If pregnant or immunocompromised, avoid changing cat litter if possible, and do not adopt or handle stray cats.

CDC website: www.cdc.gov/parasites/toxoplasmosis

TRYPANOSOMIASIS, AFRICAN (SLEEPING SICKNESS)
Dana M. Woodhall

INFECTIOUS AGENT
Two subspecies of the protozoan parasite *Trypanosoma brucei* (*T. b. rhodesiense* and *T. b. gambiense*).

TRANSMISSION
The bite of an infected tsetse fly (*Glossina* spp.). Bloodborne and congenital transmission are rare.

EPIDEMIOLOGY
Endemic in rural sub-Saharan Africa. *T. b. rhodesiense* is found in eastern and southeastern Africa, mainly Tanzania, Uganda, Malawi, Zambia, and Zimbabwe. *T. b. gambiense* is found in central Africa and in limited areas of West Africa, primarily in Democratic Republic of the Congo, Angola, Sudan, Central African Republic, Guinea, Republic of the Congo, Chad, and northern Uganda. In 2012, 7,197 sleeping sickness cases were reported to the World Health Organization; *T. b. gambiense* accounted for >98% of cases.

Tsetse flies inhabit rural, densely vegetated areas; people who only travel to urban areas are not at risk. Flies bite during the day, and <1% are infected. Risk of infection increases with the number of fly bites, which is not always directly correlated with duration of travel.

CLINICAL PRESENTATION
T. b. rhodesiense
Symptoms generally appear within 1–3 weeks of the infective bite and may include high fever, a chancre at the bite site, skin rash, headache, myalgia, thrombocytopenia, and less commonly, splenomegaly, renal failure, or cardiac dysfunction. Central nervous system involvement can occur within a month of infection and results in mental deterioration and eventually, death.

T. b. gambiense
Nonspecific but may include fever, headache, malaise, myalgia, facial edema, pruritus,

lymphadenopathy, and weight loss. Central nervous system involvement occurs after months to years of infection and is characterized by somnolence, severe headache, and a range of neurologic manifestations, including mood disorders, behavior change, focal deficits, and endocrine disorders. The clinical course of disease caused by T. b. gambiense is generally less severe than that caused by T. b. rhodesiense, but both are fatal if not treated.

DIAGNOSIS

Bites are characteristically painful, and a chancre may develop at the bite location. Identification of parasites in specimens of blood, chancre fluid or tissue, lymph node aspirate, or cerebrospinal fluid. Buffy-coat preparations concentrate the parasite, enabling easier visualization for diagnosis. Diagnostic assistance is available through CDC (www.cdc.gov/dpdx; 404-718-4745; parasites@cdc.gov).

TREATMENT

Infection can usually be cured by a course of antitrypanosomal therapy, although long-term sequelae, including permanent damage to the central nervous system, may remain. Treatment drugs (suramin, melarsoprol, eflornithine) are provided by CDC under investigational protocols. Clinicians can consult with CDC for assistance with treatment.

PREVENTION

Avoid tsetse fly bites. Travelers should wear clothing of wrist and ankle length made of medium-weight fabric in neutral colors, as tsetse flies are attracted to bright or dark colors and can bite through lightweight clothing. Permethrin-impregnated clothing and use of DEET repellent may reduce the number of fly bites.

CDC website: www.cdc.gov/parasites/sleepingsickness

BIBLIOGRAPHY

1. Brun R, Blum J, Chappuis F, Burri C. Human African trypanosomiasis. Lancet. 2010 Jan 9;375(9709): 148–59.

2. Simarro PP, Franco JR, Cecchi G, Paone M, Diarra A, Ruiz Postigo JA, et al. Human African trypanosomiasis in non-endemic countries (2000–2010). J Travel Med. 2012 Jan–Feb; 19(1):44–53.

TRYPANOSOMIASIS, AMERICAN (CHAGAS DISEASE)

Susan Montgomery

INFECTIOUS AGENT

The protozoan parasite *Trypanosoma cruzi*.

TRANSMISSION

Typically through feces of an infected triatomine insect (reduviid bug), may occur when a bug bite is scratched or by consuming food or beverages contaminated with infected bug feces; may also be transmitted through blood transfusion or organ transplantation and from mother to infant.

EPIDEMIOLOGY

Endemic in many parts of Mexico and Central and South America. In the United States, Chagas disease is primarily a disease of immigrants from endemic areas of Latin America. The risk to travelers is extremely low, but they could be at risk if staying in poor-quality housing or from consuming contaminated food or beverages in endemic areas.

CLINICAL PRESENTATION

Acute illness typically develops ≥1 week after exposure and lasts up to 60 days. A chagoma may develop at the site of infection; for example, the Romaña sign (edema of the eyelid and ocular tissues). Most infected people never develop symptoms but remain infected throughout their lives. Approximately 30% of patients will develop chronic manifestations of Chagas disease after a prolonged period without any clinical disease. Chronic Chagas disease usually affects the heart; clinical signs include conduction system abnormalities, ventricular arrhythmias, and in late-stage disease, congestive cardiomyopathy. Less common chronic gastrointestinal problems (such as megaesophagus or megacolon) may develop with or without cardiac manifestations. Reactivation disease can occur in immunocompromised patients.

DIAGNOSIS

During the acute phase, parasites may be detectable in fresh preparations of buffy coat or stained peripheral blood specimens; PCR testing may also help detect acute infection. After the acute phase, diagnosis requires 2 or more serologic tests (most commonly, ELISA, immunoblot, and immunofluorescent antibody test) to detect *T. cruzi*–specific antibodies. PCR is not a useful diagnostic test for chronic-phase infections since parasites are not detectable in the peripheral blood during this phase.

TREATMENT

Antitrypanosomal drug treatment is always recommended for acute, early congenital, and reactivated *T. cruzi* infection and for chronic *T. cruzi* infection in children aged <18 years old. In adults, treatment is usually recommended. In the United States, treatment drugs (benznidazole and nifurtimox) are provided by CDC under investigational protocols. Contact CDC (chagas@cdc.gov; 404-718-4745) for assistance with clinical management.

PREVENTION

Insect precautions (see Chapter 2, Protection against Mosquitoes, Ticks, & Other Arthropods) and food and water precautions (see Chapter 2, Food & Water Precautions).

CDC website: www.cdc.gov/parasites/chagas

BIBLIOGRAPHY

1. Bern C. Antitrypanosomal therapy for chronic Chagas' disease. N Engl J Med. 2011 Jun 30;364(26):2527–34.
2. Bern C, Montgomery SP, Herwaldt BL, Rassi A Jr, Marin-Neto JA, Dantas RO, et al. Evaluation and treatment of Chagas disease in the United States: a systematic review. JAMA. 2007 Nov 14;298(18):2171–81.
3. Carter YL, Juliano JJ, Montgomery SP, Qvarnstrom Y. Acute Chagas disease in a returning traveler. Am J Trop Med Hyg. 2012 Dec;87(6):1038–40.
4. Rassi A Jr, Rassi A, Marin-Neto JA. Chagas disease. Lancet. 2010 Apr 17;375(9723):1388–402.

TUBERCULOSIS

Philip LoBue

INFECTIOUS AGENT

Mycobacterium tuberculosis is a rod-shaped, nonmotile, slow-growing, acid-fast bacterium.

TRANSMISSION

Tuberculosis (TB) transmission occurs when a contagious patient coughs, spreading bacilli through the air. Bovine TB (caused by the closely related *M. bovis*) can be transmitted by consuming unpasteurized dairy products from infected cattle.

EPIDEMIOLOGY

Globally, nearly 9 million new TB cases and approximately 1.3 million TB-related deaths occur each year. TB occurs throughout the world, but the incidence varies (see Map 3-13). In the United States, the annual incidence is <4 per 100,000 population, but in some countries in sub-Saharan Africa and Asia, the annual incidence is several hundred per 100,000.

Drug-resistant TB is of increasing concern. Multidrug-resistant (MDR) TB is resistant to the 2 most effective drugs, isoniazid and rifampin. Extensively drug-resistant (XDR) TB is resistant to isoniazid and rifampin, any fluoroquinolone, and ≥1 of 3 injectable second-line drugs (amikacin, kanamycin, or capreomycin). MDR TB is less common than drug-susceptible TB, but approximately 450,000 new cases of MDR TB are diagnosed each year, and some countries have proportions of MDR TB as high as 20% (see Map 3-14). MDR and XDR TB are of particular concern among HIV-infected or other immunocompromised people. As of October 2011, XDR TB had been reported in 92 countries

Before leaving the United States, travelers who anticipate possible prolonged exposure to TB (such as those who would spend time in health care facilities, correctional facilities, or homeless shelters) or those who plan to stay for years in an endemic country should have a 2-step tuberculin skin test (TST) or a single interferon-γ release assay (IGRA), either the QuantiFERON TB test (Gold In-Tube version) or T-SPOT.TB test (see *Perspectives*: Tuberculin Skin Testing of Travelers, later in this chapter). If the predeparture test result is negative, a single TST or IGRA should be repeated 8–10 weeks after returning from travel. Because people with HIV infection or other immunocompromising conditions are more likely to have an impaired response to either a skin or blood test, travelers should inform their clinicians about such conditions.

The risk of TB transmission on an airplane does not appear to be higher than in any other enclosed space. To prevent TB transmission, people who have infectious TB (TB that can be transmitted to other people) should not travel by commercial airplanes or other commercial conveyances. Only TB of the lung is infectious, and health department authorities determine whether a person is infectious based on the person's chest radiograph, sputum tests, symptoms, and treatment received. The World Health Organization (WHO) has issued guidelines for notifying passengers who might have been exposed to TB aboard airplanes. Passengers concerned about possible exposure to TB should see their primary health care provider or visit their local health department clinic for evaluation.

Bovine TB (*M. bovis*) is a risk in travelers who consume unpasteurized dairy products in countries where *M. bovis* in cattle is common. Mexico is a common place of infection for US travelers.

CLINICAL PRESENTATION

TB disease can affect any organ but most commonly occurs in the lungs (70%–80%). Common TB symptoms include prolonged cough, fever, decreased appetite, weight loss, night sweats, and coughing up blood (hemoptysis). The most common sites for TB outside the lungs are the lymph nodes, pleura, bones and joints, brain and spinal cord lining (meningitis), kidneys, bladder, and genitalia.

Infection is manifested by a positive TST or IGRA result 8–10 weeks after exposure. Overall, only 5%–10% of otherwise healthy people have an infection that progresses to disease during their lifetime. Progression to disease can occur weeks to decades after initial infection. People with TB disease have symptoms or other manifestations of illness such as an abnormal chest radiograph. In the remainder, the infection remains in a latent state (latent TB infection or LTBI) in which the infected person has no symptoms and cannot spread TB to others. The risk of progression is much higher in immunosuppressed people (8%–10% per year in HIV-infected people not receiving antiretroviral therapy). People who are receiving tumor necrosis factor inhibitors to treat rheumatoid arthritis and other chronic inflammatory conditions have also been found to be at increased risk for disease progression.

DIAGNOSIS

Diagnosis of TB disease is confirmed by culturing *M. tuberculosis* from sputum or other respiratory specimens for pulmonary

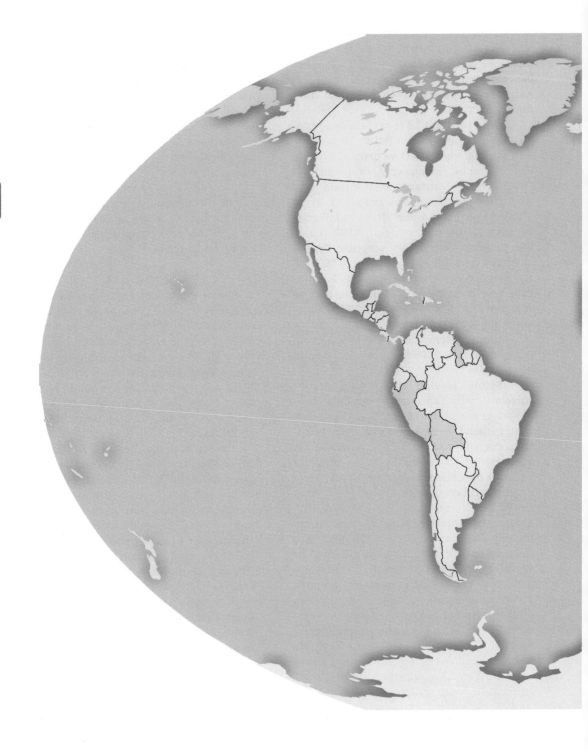

MAP 3-13. ESTIMATED TUBERCULOSIS INCIDENCE RATES, 2012[1]

[1] Data from the World Health Organization's tuberculosis database. Available from: www.who.int/tb/country/data/download/en/index.html. Data accessed July 2014.

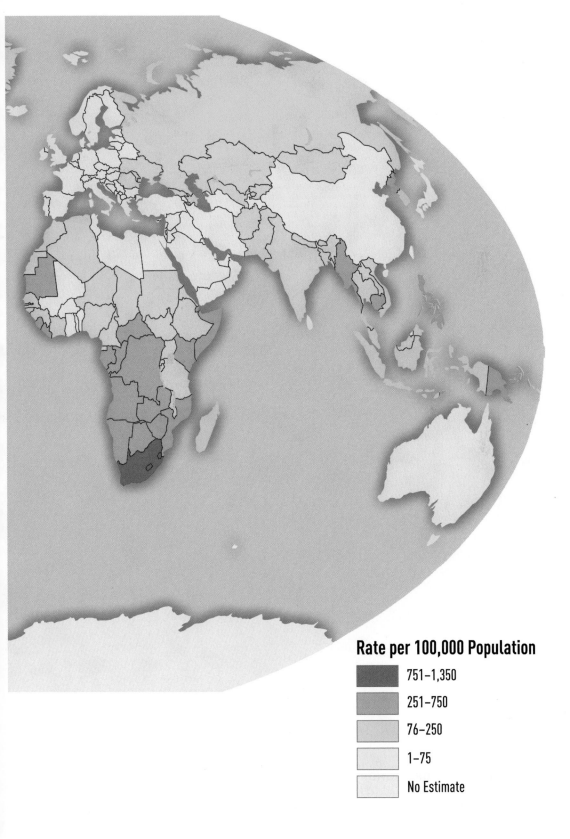

Rate per 100,000 Population

- 751–1,350
- 251–750
- 76–250
- 1–75
- No Estimate

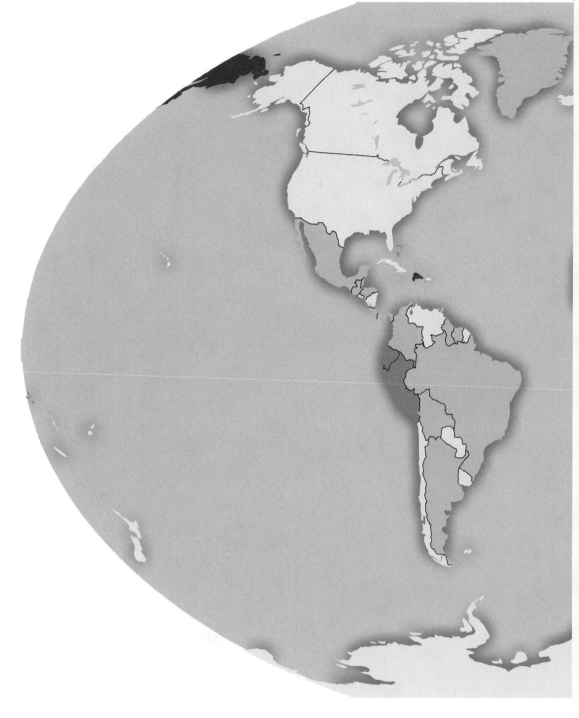

MAP 3-14. PROPORTION OF MULTIDRUG-RESISTANT TUBERCULOSIS (MDR TB) AMONG NEW TUBERCULOSIS CASES, 2012[1]

[1] Data from the World Health Organization's tuberculosis database. Available from: www.who.int/tb/country/data/download/en/index.html. Accessed July 2014.

Proportion of MDR TB

- >6%
- 3%–6%
- <3%
- No Data

3

TB and from other affected body tissues or fluids for extrapulmonary TB. On average, it takes about 2 weeks to culture and identify M. tuberculosis, even with rapid culture techniques. A preliminary diagnosis of TB can be made when acid-fast bacilli are seen by microscope on sputum smear or in other body tissues or fluids. However, microscopy cannot distinguish between M. tuberculosis and nontuberculous mycobacteria. This is particularly problematic in countries such as the United States where TB incidence is low. Nucleic acid amplification tests are more rapid than culture and specific for M. tuberculosis. They are also more sensitive than the acid-fast bacillus smear but less sensitive than culture. A diagnosis of TB disease can be made by using clinical criteria in the absence of microbiologic confirmation. However, laboratory testing should be performed when feasible to confirm the diagnosis. In addition, a culture is necessary to conduct conventional drug susceptibility testing to guide treatment. LTBI is diagnosed by a positive TST or IGRA after further examinations (such as chest radiograph, symptom review) have excluded TB disease.

TREATMENT

People with LTBI can be treated to prevent progression to TB disease. American Thoracic Society (ATS)/CDC guidelines for treatment of LTBI recommend 9 months of isoniazid as the preferred treatment. The combination regimen of isoniazid and rifapentine given as 12 weekly doses using directly observed therapy is recommended as equivalent to 9 months of isoniazid for treating LTBI in otherwise healthy patients aged ≥12 years who are at higher risk of developing active TB, for example after recent exposure to contagious TB. For people who have been exposed to isoniazid-resistant, rifampin-susceptible TB or who cannot tolerate isoniazid, 4 months of rifampin is a reasonable alternative. Travelers who suspect that they have been exposed to TB should inform their health care provider of the possible exposure and receive medical evaluation. CDC and ATS have published guidelines for targeted testing and treatment of LTBI. Because drug resistance is relatively common in some parts of the world, travelers who have TST

or IGRA conversion associated with international travel should consult experts in infectious diseases or pulmonary medicine.

TB disease is treated with a multiple-drug regimen administered by directly observed therapy for 6–9 months (usually isoniazid, rifampin, ethambutol, and pyrazinamide for 2 months, followed by isoniazid and rifampin for an additional 4 months) if the TB is not MDR TB. MDR TB treatment is more difficult, requiring 4–6 drugs for 18–24 months; it should be managed by an expert in MDR TB. ATS/CDC/Infectious Diseases Society of America have published guidelines on TB treatment (www.cdc.gov/mmwr/preview/mmwrhtml/rr5211a1.htm).

PREVENTION

Travelers should avoid exposure to TB patients in crowded and enclosed environments (such as health care facilities, correctional facilities, or homeless shelters). Travelers who will be working in hospitals or health care settings where TB patients are likely to be encountered should be advised to consult infection control or occupational health experts about procedures for obtaining personal respiratory protective devices (such as N-95 respirators), along with respirator selection and training.

Based on WHO recommendations, bacillus Calmette-Guérin (BCG) vaccine is used once at birth in most developing countries to reduce the severe consequences of TB in infants and children. However, BCG vaccine has variable efficacy in preventing the adult forms of TB and interferes with testing for LTBI with the TST. Therefore, BCG is not routinely recommended for use in the United States. Recently, some experts have advocated BCG vaccination for health care providers who are likely to be exposed to MDR or XDR TB patients in settings where the TB infection control measures recommended in the United States are not fully implemented. BCG may offer some protection in this circumstance; however, people who receive BCG vaccination must follow all recommended TB infection control precautions to the extent possible. Additionally, IGRA is preferred over the TST for pre- and post-travel testing in people vaccinated with BCG.

To prevent infections due to *M. bovis*, travelers should also avoid eating or drinking unpasteurized dairy products.

CDC website: www.cdc.gov/tb

BIBLIOGRAPHY

1. American Thoracic Society and CDC. Diagnostic standards and classification of tuberculosis in adults and children. Am J Respir Crit Care Med. 2000 Apr;161(4 Pt 1):1376–95.

2. American Thoracic Society and CDC. Targeted tuberculin testing and treatment of latent tuberculosis infection. Am J Respir Crit Care Med. 2000 Apr;161(4 Pt 2):S221–47.

3. CDC. Recommendations for use of an isoniazid-rifapentine regimen with direct observation to treat latent *Mycobacterium tuberculosis* infection. MMWR Morb Mortal Wkly Rep. 2011 Dec 9;60(48):1650–3.

4. CDC. The role of BCG vaccine in the prevention and control of tuberculosis in the United States. A joint statement by the Advisory Council for the Elimination of Tuberculosis and the Advisory Committee on Immunization Practices. MMWR Recomm Rep. 1996 Apr 26;45(RR-4):1–18.

5. CDC. Treatment of tuberculosis. MMWR Recomm Rep. 2003 Jun 20;52(RR-11):1–77.

6. CDC. Updated guidelines for using interferon gamma release assays to detect *Mycobacterium*

tuberculosis infection, United States. MMWR Recomm Rep. 2010.

7. Jensen PA, Lambert LA, Iademarco MF, Ridzon R. Guidelines for preventing the transmission of *Mycobacterium tuberculosis* in health-care settings, 2005. MMWR Recomm Rep. 2005 Dec 30;54(RR-17):1–141.

8. World Health Organization. Global tuberculosis report 2013. Geneva: World Health Organization; 2013 [cited 2014 Sep 24]. Available from: http://apps.who.int/iris/bitstream/10665/91355/1/9789241564656_eng.pdf.

9. World Health Organization. Multidrug and extensively drug-resistant TB (M/XDR-TB): 2010 global report on surveillance and response. Geneva: World Health Organization; 2010. Available from: http://www.who.int/tb/features_archive/m_xdrtb_facts/en/index.html.

10. World Health Organization. Tuberculosis and air travel: guidelines for prevention and control. Geneva: World Health Organization; 2008 [cited 2014 Sep 24]. Available from: http://www.who.int/tb/publications/2008/WHO_HTM_TB_2008.399_eng.pdf.

Perspectives

TUBERCULIN SKIN TESTING OF TRAVELERS

Philip LoBue

Screening for asymptomatic tuberculosis (TB) infections should only be carried out among travelers who will be at risk of acquiring TB if they are exposed at their destinations (see the preceding section on Tuberculosis). Screening with a tuberculin skin test (TST) in very low-risk travelers may

Perspectives sections are written as editorial discussions aiming to add depth and clinical perspective to the official recommendations contained in the book. The views and opinions expressed in this section are those of the author and do not necessarily represent the official position of CDC.

result in false-positive test results, leading to unnecessary additional screening or unnecessary treatment. Using screening tests in very low-prevalence populations will likely produce more false positives than true positives.

Therefore, the TST should be considered only for travelers who are spending years in a country with a high risk of TB or for those travelers who will spend any length of time in routine contact with health care facilities, prisons, or homeless shelter populations. The general recommendation is that people at low risk for exposure to TB, which includes most travelers, do not need to be screened before or after travel.

For travelers who anticipate a long stay or contact with a high-risk population, careful pre-travel screening should be carried out, with use of 2-step pre-travel TST screening. For 2-step TSTs, people whose baseline TSTs yield a negative result are retested 1–3 weeks after the initial test; if the second test result is negative, they are considered not infected. If the second test result is positive, they are classified as having had previous TB infection. The 2-step TST is recommended in this population for the following reasons:

- The use of 2-step testing can reduce the number of positive TSTs that would otherwise be misclassified as recent skin test conversions during future periodic screenings.
- Certain people who were infected with *Mycobacterium tuberculosis* years earlier exhibit waning delayed-type hypersensitivity to tuberculin. When they are skin tested years after infection, they might have a false-negative TST result (even though they are truly infected). However, the first TST might stimulate the ability to react to subsequent tests, resulting in a "booster" reaction. When the test is repeated, the reaction might be misinterpreted as a new infection (recent conversion) rather than a boosted reaction.

Two-step testing is important for travelers who will have potential prolonged or substantial TB exposure. Two-step testing before travel will detect boosting and potentially prevent "false conversions"—positive TST results that appear to indicate infection acquired during travel, but which are really the result of previous TB infection. This distinction is particularly important if the traveler is going to a country where multidrug-resistant (MDR) and extensively drug-resistant XDR TB are present: it would be critical to know whether the person's skin test had been positive before travel.

If the 2-step pre-travel TST result is negative, the traveler should have a repeat TST 8–10 weeks after returning from the trip. During extended (>6 months) stays in or repeated travel to high-risk settings, a TST should be performed every 6–12 months, depending on the risk of exposure while traveling outside the United States, and 8–10 weeks after final return. Two-step testing should be considered for the baseline testing of people who report no history of a recent TST and who will receive repeated TSTs as part of ongoing monitoring.

People who have repeat TSTs must be tested with the same commercial antigen, since switching antigens can also lead to false TST conversions. Two commercial tuberculin skin test antigens are approved by the Food and Drug Administration (FDA) and are commercially available in the United States: Aplisol (JHP Pharmaceuticals) and Tubersol (Sanofi Pasteur).

An alternative to the 2-step TST is a single FDA-approved interferon-γ release assay (IGRA), either the QuantiFERON TB test (Gold In-Tube versions) or T-SPOT.TB test. IGRAs, which require a blood draw, are approximately as specific as TST in people who have not been vaccinated with bacillus Calmette-Guérin (BCG) and are much more specific in BCG-vaccinated populations. For a traveler whose time before departure is short, a single-step TST would be an acceptable alternative if time is insufficient for the 2-step TST and the IGRAs are not available.

In general, it is best not to mix tests. There is approximately 15% discordance between TST and IGRA, usually with the TST positive and the IGRA negative. There are multiple reasons for the discordance, and in any single person, it is often difficult to be confident about the reason for discordance. However, if the clinician decides to mix tests, it is better to go from TST to IGRA than the other way around, because the likelihood of having a discordant result with the TST negative and the IGRA positive is much lower. Such discordant results may become unavoidable as more medical establishments switch from TSTs to IGRAs.

The use of TSTs among travelers who are visiting friends and relatives in TB-endemic areas should take into account that the rate of TST positivity in people visiting their country of birth is often high. In a study among 53,000 adults in Tennessee, the prevalence of a positive TST among the foreign born was 11 times that among the US born (34% vs 3%). Confirming TST status before travel would prevent the conclusion that a positive TST after travel was due to recent infection.

BIBLIOGRAPHY

1. Al-Jahdali H, Memish ZA, Menzies D. Tuberculosis in association with travel. Int J Antimicrob Agents. 2003 Feb;21(2):125–30.
2. Cobelens FG, van Deutekom H, Draayer-Jansen IW, Schepp-Beelen AC, van Gerven PJ, van Kessel RP, et al. Risk of infection with *Mycobacterium tuberculosis* in travellers to areas of high tuberculosis endemicity. Lancet. 2000 Aug 5;356(9228):461–5.
3. Haley CA, Cain KP, Yu C, Garman KF, Wells CD, Laserson KF. Risk-based screening for latent tuberculosis infection. South Med J. 2008 Feb;101(2):142–9.
4. Johnston VJ, Grant AD. Tuberculosis in travellers. Travel Med Infect Dis. 2003 Nov;1(4):205–12.
5. Jung P, Banks RH. Tuberculosis risk in US Peace Corps volunteers, 1996 to 2005. J Travel Med. 2008 Mar–Apr;15(2):87–94.
6. Leder K, Tong S, Weld L, Kain KC, Wilder-Smith A, von Sonnenburg F, et al. Illness in travelers visiting friends and relatives: a review of the GeoSentinel Surveillance Network. Clin Infect Dis. 2006 Nov 1;43(9):1185–93.
7. Mancuso JD, Tobler SK, Keep LW. Pseudoepidemics of tuberculin skin test conversions in the US Army after recent deployments. Am J Respir Crit Care Med. 2008 Jun 1;177(11):1285–9.
8. Mazurek M, Jereb J, Vernon A, LoBue P, Goldberg S, Castro K. Updated guidelines for using interferon gamma release assays to detect *Mycobacterium tuberculosis* infection—United States, 2010. MMWR Recomm Rep. 2010 Jun 25;59 (RR-5):1–25.
9. Villarino ME, Burman W, Wang YC, Lundergan L, Catanzaro A, Bock N, et al. Comparable specificity of 2 commercial tuberculin reagents in persons at low risk for tuberculous infection. JAMA. 1999 Jan 13;281(2):169–71.

TYPHOID & PARATYPHOID FEVER

Anna E. Newton, Janell A. Routh, Barbara E. Mahon

INFECTIOUS AGENT

Typhoid fever is a potentially severe and occasionally life-threatening febrile illness caused by the bacterium *Salmonella enterica* serotype Typhi. Paratyphoid fever is a similar illness caused by *S. enterica* serotype Paratyphi A, B (tartrate negative), or C.

TRANSMISSION

Humans are the only source of these bacteria; no animal or environmental reservoirs have been identified. Typhoid and paratyphoid fever are most often acquired through consumption of water or food that has been contaminated by feces of an acutely infected or convalescent person or a chronic, asymptomatic carrier. Transmission through sexual contact, especially among men who have sex with men, has been documented rarely.

EPIDEMIOLOGY

An estimated 22 million cases of typhoid fever and 200,000 related deaths occur worldwide each year; an additional 6 million cases of paratyphoid fever are estimated to occur annually. Each year in the United States, approximately 300 culture-confirmed cases of typhoid fever and 100 cases of paratyphoid fever are reported. More than 80% of reports of typhoid fever and >90% of reports of paratyphoid fever caused by *Salmonella* Paratyphi A are of travelers to southern Asia. Other areas of risk include East and Southeast Asia, Africa, the Caribbean, and Central and South America. In certain regions, the risk of typhoid fever has decreased. As a result, CDC removed pre-travel typhoid vaccination recommendations for 26 countries in Eastern Europe and the Middle East; the most recent pre-travel vaccination guidelines can be found at www.cdc.gov/travel.

Travelers who are visiting friends and relatives are at increased risk (see Chapter 8, Immigrants Returning Home to Visit Friends and Relatives [VFRs]). Although the risk of acquiring typhoid or paratyphoid fever increases with the duration of stay, travelers have acquired typhoid fever even during visits of <1 week to countries where the disease is endemic.

CLINICAL PRESENTATION

The incubation period of typhoid and paratyphoid infections is 6–30 days. The onset of illness is insidious, with gradually increasing fatigue and a fever that increases daily from low-grade to as high as 102°F–104°F (38°C–40°C) by the third to fourth day of illness. Headache, malaise, and anorexia are nearly universal and abdominal pain, diarrhea, or constipation are common. Hepatosplenomegaly can often be detected. A transient, macular rash of rose-colored spots can occasionally be seen on the trunk. Fever is commonly lowest in the morning, reaching a peak in late afternoon or evening. This clinical presentation is often confused with malaria, and typhoid fever should be suspected in a person with a history of travel to an endemic area who is not responding to antimalarial medication. Untreated, the disease can last for a month. The serious complications of typhoid fever generally occur after 2–3 weeks of illness and may include intestinal hemorrhage or perforation, which can be life threatening.

DIAGNOSIS

Infection with typhoid or paratyphoid fever results in a low-grade septicemia. Although blood culture is the mainstay of diagnosis in typhoid fever, a single culture is positive in only approximately 50% of cases. Multiple cultures increase the sensitivity and may be required to make the diagnosis. Bone marrow culture increases the diagnostic yield to approximately 80% of cases. Stool culture is not usually positive during the earliest phase of the disease.

The Widal test is unreliable but is widely used in developing countries because of its low cost. It is a serologic assay for IgM and IgG to the O and H antigens of *Salmonella* Typhi, but is not specific and false positives may occur. Acute- and convalescent-phase titers are more sensitive than a single serum sample. Newer serologic assays for *Salmonella* Typhi infection are occasionally used in outbreak situations, and are somewhat more sensitive and specific than the Widal test, but are not an adequate substitute for blood, stool, or bone marrow culture.

Because there is no definitive serologic test for typhoid or paratyphoid fever, the initial diagnosis often has to be made clinically. The combination of a history of risk for infection and a gradual onset of fever that increases in severity over several days should raise suspicion of typhoid or paratyphoid fever.

TREATMENT

Specific antimicrobial therapy shortens the clinical course of typhoid fever and reduces the risk for death. A fluoroquinolone, most often ciprofloxacin, is used for empiric treatment in most parts of the world. However, fluoroquinolone-resistant or multidrug-resistant (resistant to ampicillin, chloramphenicol, and trimethoprim-sulfamethoxazole) strains are common in the Indian subcontinent and increasing in other areas, such as Africa. Injectable third-generation cephalosporins are often the empiric drug of choice when the possibility of fluoroquinolone resistance is high. Azithromycin is increasingly used to treat typhoid fever or paratyphoid fever because of the emergence of multidrug-resistant strains, although increasing resistance to azithromycin in *Salmonella* Typhi strains has already been documented.

Patients treated with an antibiotic may remain febrile for 3–5 days, although the height of the fever generally decreases each day. Patients may actually feel worse during the several days it takes for the fever to end. If fever in a person with culture-confirmed typhoid or paratyphoid fever does not subside within 5 days, alternative antimicrobial agents or other foci of infection should be considered.

PREVENTION
Food and Water

Safe food and water precautions and frequent handwashing are important in preventing typhoid and paratyphoid fever

(see Chapter 2, Food & Water Precautions). Although vaccines are recommended to prevent typhoid fever, they are not 100% effective; therefore, even vaccinated travelers should follow recommended food and water precautions. For paratyphoid fever, these precautions are the only prevention method, as no vaccines are available.

Vaccine
Indications for Use

CDC recommends typhoid vaccine for travelers to areas where there is an increased risk of exposure to *Salmonella* Typhi. Two typhoid vaccines are available in the United States:

- Oral live attenuated vaccine (Vivotif, manufactured from the Ty21a strain of *Salmonella* Typhi by PaxVax)
- Vi capsular polysaccharide vaccine (ViCPS) (Typhim Vi, manufactured by Sanofi Pasteur) for intramuscular use

Both typhoid vaccines protect 50%–80% of recipients; travelers should be reminded that typhoid immunization is not 100% effective, and typhoid fever could still occur. Available typhoid vaccines offer limited or no protection against *Salmonella* Paratyphi infection.

Vaccine Administration

Table 3-20 provides information on vaccine dosage, administration, and revaccination. The time required for primary vaccination differs for the 2 vaccines, as do the lower age limits.

Primary vaccination with oral Ty21a vaccine consists of 4 capsules, 1 taken every other day. The capsules should be kept refrigerated (not frozen), and all 4 doses must be taken to achieve maximum efficacy. Each capsule should be taken with cool liquid no warmer than 98.6°F (37°C), approximately 1 hour before a meal. This regimen should be completed 1 week before potential exposure. The vaccine manufacturer recommends that Ty21a not be administered to infants or children aged <6 years.

Primary vaccination with ViCPS consists of one 0.5-mL (25-mg) dose administered intramuscularly. One dose of this vaccine should be given ≥2 weeks before expected exposure. The manufacturer does

Table 3-20. Vaccines to prevent typhoid fever

VACCINATION	AGE (Y)	DOSE, MODE OF ADMINISTRATION	NUMBER OF DOSES	DOSING INTERVAL	BOOSTING INTERVAL
Oral, Live, Attenuated Ty21a Vaccine (Vivotif)[1]					
Primary series	≥6	1 capsule,[2] oral	4	48 hours	Not applicable
Booster	≥6	1 capsule,[2] oral	4	48 hours	Every 5 years
Vi Capsular Polysaccharide Vaccine (Typhim Vi)					
Primary series	≥2	0.5 mL, intramuscular	1	Not applicable	Not applicable
Booster	≥2	0.5 mL, intramuscular	1	Not applicable	Every 2 years

[1] The vaccine must be kept refrigerated (35.6°F–46.4°F, 2°C–8°C).
[2] Administer with cool liquid no warmer than 98.6°F (37°C).

not recommend the vaccine for infants and children aged <2 years.

Vaccine Safety and Adverse Reactions

Adverse reactions to Ty21a vaccine are rare and mainly consist of abdominal discomfort, nausea, vomiting, and rash. ViCPS vaccine is most often associated with headache (16%–20%) and injection-site reactions (7%).

Precautions and Contraindications

No information is available on the safety of these vaccines in pregnancy; it is prudent on theoretical grounds to avoid vaccinating pregnant women. Live attenuated Ty21a vaccine should not be given to immunocompromised travelers, including those infected with HIV. The intramuscular vaccine presents a theoretically safer alternative for immunocompromised travelers. (The Advisory Committee on Immunization Practices does not recommend against vaccinating household contacts of immunocompromised people with Ty21a; although vaccine organisms can be shed transiently in the stool of vaccine recipients, secondary transmission of vaccine organisms has not

been documented.) The only contraindication to vaccination with ViCPS vaccine is a history of severe local or systemic reactions after a previous dose. Neither vaccine should be given to people with an acute febrile illness.

Theoretical concerns have been raised about the immunogenicity of live, attenuated Ty21a vaccine in people concurrently receiving antimicrobial agents (including antimalarial chemoprophylaxis), viral vaccines, or immune globulin. The growth of the live Ty21a strain is inhibited in vitro by various antibacterial agents, and vaccination with Ty21a should be delayed for >72 hours after the administration of any antibacterial agent. Available data do not suggest that simultaneous administration of oral polio or yellow fever vaccine decreases the immunogenicity of Ty21a. If typhoid vaccination is warranted, it should not be delayed because of administration of viral vaccines. Simultaneous administration of Ty21a and immune globulin does not appear to pose a problem.

CDC website: www.cdc.gov/nczved/divisions/dfbmd/diseases/typhoid_fever

BIBLIOGRAPHY

1. Beeching NJ, Clarke PD, Kitchin NR, Pirmohamed J, Veitch K, Weber F. Comparison of two combined vaccines against typhoid fever and hepatitis A in healthy adults. Vaccine. 2004 Nov 15;23(1):29–35.

2. CDC. Typhoid immunization: recommendations of the Advisory Committee on Immunization Practices (ACIP). MMWR Recomm Rep. 1994 Dec 9;43(RR-14):1–7.

3. Crump JA, Mintz ED. Global trends in typhoid and paratyphoid fever. Clin Infect Dis. 2010 Jan 15;50(2):241–6.

4. Effa EE, Bukirwa H. Azithromycin for treating uncomplicated typhoid and paratyphoid fever (enteric fever). Cochrane Database Syst Rev. 2008(4):CD006083.

5. Gupta SK, Medalla F, Omondi MW, Whichard JM, Fields PI, Gerner-Smidt P, et al. Laboratory-based surveillance of paratyphoid fever in the United States: travel and antimicrobial resistance. Clin Infect Dis. 2008 Jun 1;46(11):1656–63.

6. Johnson KJ, Gallagher NM, Mintz ED, Newton AE, Brunette GW, Kozarsky PE. From the CDC: new country-specific recommendations for pre-travel typhoid vaccination. J Travel Med. 2011 Nov–Dec;18(6):430–3.

7. Kollaritsch H, Que JU, Kunz C, Wiedermann G, Herzog C, Cryz SJ, Jr. Safety and immunogenicity of live oral cholera and typhoid vaccines administered alone or in combination with antimalarial drugs, oral polio vaccine, or yellow fever vaccine. J Infect Dis. 1997 Apr;175(4):871–5.

8. Lynch MF, Blanton EM, Bulens S, Polyak C, Vojdani J, Stevenson J, et al. Typhoid fever in the United States, 1999–2006. JAMA. 2009 Aug 26;302(8):859–65.

9. Parry CM, Hien TT, Dougan G, White NJ, Farrar JJ. Typhoid fever. N Engl J Med. 2002 Nov 28;347(22):1770–82.

10. Steinberg EB, Bishop R, Haber P, Dempsey AF, Hoekstra RM, Nelson JM, et al. Typhoid fever in travelers: who should be targeted for prevention? Clin Infect Dis. 2004 Jul 15;39(2):186–91.

VARICELLA (CHICKENPOX)

Mona Marin, Stephanie R. Bialek

INFECTIOUS AGENT

Varicella-zoster virus, a member of the herpesvirus family. Humans are the only reservoir of the virus, and disease occurs only in humans. After primary infection as varicella (chickenpox), the virus remains dormant in the sensory-nerve ganglia and can reactivate at a later time, causing herpes zoster (shingles).

TRANSMISSION

Varicella-zoster virus is transmitted from person to person, primarily via the respiratory route by inhalation of aerosols from vesicular fluid of skin lesions of varicella or herpes zoster; it can also spread by direct contact with the vesicular fluid of skin lesions and possibly infected respiratory tract secretions. The varicella zoster virus enters the host through the upper respiratory tract or the conjunctiva. Varicella is a highly contagious viral disease with secondary attack ratios of approximately 85% (range, 61%–100%) in susceptible household contacts; contagiousness after community exposure is lower. Herpes zoster is approximately 20% as infectious as varicella; contact with herpes zoster rash causes varicella, not herpes zoster. The period of communicability of varicella patients is estimated to begin 1–2 days before the onset of rash and ends when all lesions are crusted, typically 4–7 days after onset of rash in immunocompetent people, but this period may be longer in immunocompromised people. People with varicella should be isolated until the lesions crust over. Herpes zoster patients are contagious while they have active, vesicular lesions (usually 7–10 days).

In utero infection can also occur as a result of transplacental passage of virus during maternal varicella infection.

EPIDEMIOLOGY

Varicella occurs worldwide. In temperate climates, varicella tends to be a childhood disease, with peak incidence among preschool and school-aged children and during late winter and early spring. In these countries, <5% of adults are susceptible to varicella. In tropical climates, the highest incidence was described in the driest, coolest months; overall, infection tends to be acquired later in childhood, resulting in higher susceptibility among adults than in temperate climates, especially in less densely populated areas.

With the implementation of the childhood varicella vaccination program in the United States, substantial declines have occurred in disease incidence, and, although varicella is still endemic, the risk of exposure to varicella zoster virus is higher in most other parts of the world than it is in the United States. Varicella vaccine is used routinely to vaccinate healthy young children in only a few other countries, including Australia, Canada, Costa Rica, Germany, Greece, Korea, Latvia, Luxembourg, Qatar, Saudi Arabia, United Arab Emirates, Uruguay, and certain regions in Italy and Spain. The risk of exposure is expected to be low in these countries.

Because varicella is endemic worldwide, all susceptible travelers are at risk of contracting varicella during travel. Additionally, exposure to herpes zoster poses a risk for varicella in susceptible travelers, although localized herpes zoster is much less contagious than varicella. Travelers at highest risk for severe varicella are infants, adults, and immunocompromised people without evidence of immunity (see criteria for evidence of immunity in "Prevention," below).

CLINICAL PRESENTATION
Varicella is generally a mild disease in children, and most people recover without serious complications. The average incubation period is 14–16 days (range, 10–21 days). Infection is often characterized by a short (1- or 2-day) prodromal period (fever, malaise), although this may be absent in children, and a pruritic rash consisting of crops of macules, papules, and vesicles (typically 250–500 lesions), which appear in ≥3 successive waves and resolve by crusting. Characteristic for varicella is presence of lesions in different stages of development at the same time. Serious complications can occur, most commonly in infants, adults, and

immunocompromised people. Complications include secondary bacterial infections of skin lesions, pneumonia, cerebellar ataxia, encephalitis, and hemorrhagic conditions; rarely (about 1 case in 40,000), these complications may result in death.

Modified varicella, also known as breakthrough varicella, can occur in vaccinated people. Breakthrough varicella is usually mild, with <50 lesions, low or no fever, and shorter duration of rash. The rash may be atypical in appearance with fewer vesicles and predominance of maculopapular lesions. Breakthrough varicella is contagious, although less so than varicella in unvaccinated people.

DIAGNOSIS
Varicella is often diagnosed clinically on the basis of a generalized maculopapulovesicular rash. The clinical diagnosis of varicella in the United States has become increasingly challenging as a growing proportion of cases occur in vaccinated people in whom disease is mild and rash is atypical. Although not routinely recommended, laboratory diagnosis is likely to become increasingly useful. For laboratory confirmation, skin lesions are the preferred specimen. Vesicular swabs or scrapings and scabs from crusted lesions can be used to identify varicella-zoster virus by PCR or direct fluorescent antibody. In the absence of vesicles or scabs, scrapings of maculopapular lesions can be collected for testing.

Serologic tests may also be used to confirm disease:

- A significant rise in serum varicella IgG from acute- and convalescent-phase samples by any standard serologic assay can confirm a diagnosis retrospectively; these antibody tests may not be reliable in immunocompromised people.
- Testing for varicella-zoster IgM by using commercial kits is not recommended, because available methods lack sensitivity and specificity; false-positive IgM results are common in the presence of high IgG levels.

TREATMENT
Treatment with antivirals is not routinely recommended for otherwise healthy

children with varicella. Treatment with oral acyclovir should be considered for people at increased risk for moderate to severe disease, such as people aged >12 years, people with chronic cutaneous or pulmonary disorders, people who are receiving long-term salicylate therapy, and people who are receiving short, intermittent, or aerosolized courses of corticosteroids. Intravenous acyclovir is recommended for immunocompromised people, including patients being treated with high-dose corticosteroids, and people with serious, virally mediated complications (such as pneumonia). Therapy initiated within 24 hours of onset maximizes efficacy.

PREVENTION
Vaccine
All people, including those traveling or living abroad, should be assessed for varicella immunity, and those who do not have evidence of immunity or contraindications to vaccination should receive age-appropriate vaccination. Vaccination against varicella is not a requirement for entry into any country (including the United States), but people who do not have evidence of immunity should be considered at risk for varicella during international travel. Evidence of immunity to varicella includes any of the following:

- Documentation of age-appropriate vaccination:
  > Preschool-aged children aged ≥12 months: 1 dose
  > School-aged children, adolescents, and adults: 2 doses
- Laboratory evidence of immunity or laboratory confirmation of disease
- Birth in the United States before 1980 (not a criterion for health care personnel, pregnant women, and immunocompromised people)
- A health care provider's diagnosis of varicella or verification of a history of varicella
- A health care provider's diagnosis of herpes zoster or verification of a history of herpes zoster

Varicella vaccine contains live, attenuated varicella-zoster virus. Single-antigen varicella vaccine is licensed for people aged ≥12 months, and the combination measles-mumps-rubella-varicella (MMRV) vaccine is licensed only for children 1–12 years. CDC recommends varicella vaccination for all people aged ≥12 months without evidence of immunity to varicella who do not have contraindications to the vaccine: 1 dose for children aged 1–4 years and 2 doses for people aged ≥4 years. The minimum interval between doses is 3 months for children aged <13 years and 4 weeks for people aged ≥13 years. Contraindications for vaccination include allergy to vaccine components, immune-compromising conditions or treatments, and pregnancy. When evidence of immunity is uncertain, a possible history of varicella is not a contraindication to varicella vaccination. Vaccine effectiveness is approximately 80% after 1 dose and 95% after 2 doses.

Vaccine Safety and Adverse Reactions
The varicella vaccine is generally well tolerated. The most common adverse events after vaccination are self-limited injection-site reactions (pain, soreness, redness, and swelling). Fever or a varicellalike rash, usually consisting of a few lesions at the injection site or generalized rash with a small number of lesions, are reported less frequently.

Compared with use of MMR and varicella vaccines at the same visit, use of MMRV vaccine is associated with a higher risk for fever and febrile seizures 5–12 days after the first dose among children aged 12–23 months and approximately 1 additional febrile seizure for every 2,300–2,600 MMRV vaccine doses administered. Use of separate MMR and varicella vaccines avoids this increased risk for fever and febrile seizures in this age group. For detailed information regarding the varicella vaccine, visit www.cdc.gov/vaccines/vpd-vac/varicella/default.htm.

POSTEXPOSURE PROPHYLAXIS
Vaccine
Varicella vaccine is recommended for postexposure administration for unvaccinated healthy people aged ≥12 months and without other evidence of immunity, to prevent or modify the disease. The vaccine should be administered as soon as possible within 5 days after exposure to rash, if there are no contraindications to use. Among children, protective efficacy was reported as ≥90% when vaccination occurred within 3 days of

exposure. No data are available regarding a potential benefit of administering a second dose to 1-dose vaccine recipients after exposure. However, administration of the second dose is recommended for exposed people to bring them up-to-date on vaccination.

Varicella Zoster Immune Globulin

People without evidence of immunity who have contraindications for vaccination and who are at risk for severe varicella and complications are recommended to receive postexposure prophylaxis with varicella zoster immune globulin. The varicella zoster immune globulin product licensed in the United States is VariZIG (FFF Enterprises, Temecula, California).

People who should receive VariZIG after exposure include immunocompromised people, pregnant women without evidence of immunity, and some infants. VariZIG provides maximum benefit when administered as soon as possible after exposure but may be effective if administered as late as 10 days after exposure. VariZIG can be obtained from FFF Enterprises by calling 800-843-7477 or visiting www.fffenterprises.com.

If VariZIG is not available, intravenous immune globulin (IVIG) can be considered (also within 10 days of exposure). Additionally, in the absence of both VariZIG and IVIG, some experts recommend prophylaxis with acyclovir (80 mg/kg/day, administered 4 times per day for 7 days; maximum dose, 800 mg, 4 times per day), beginning 7–10 days after exposure for people without evidence of immunity and with contraindications for varicella vaccination. Published data on the benefit of acyclovir as postexposure prophylaxis among immunocompromised people are limited.

CDC website: www.cdc.gov/chickenpox

BIBLIOGRAPHY

1. American Academy of Pediatrics. Varicella-zoster infections. In: Pickering LK, editor. Red Book: 2012 Report of the Committee on Infectious Diseases. 29th ed. Elk Grove Village, IL: American Academy of Pediatrics; 2012. p. 774–89.
2. Bialek SR, Perella D, Zhang J, Mascola L, Viner K, Jackson C, et al. Impact of a routine two-dose varicella vaccination program on varicella epidemiology. Pediatrics. 2013 Nov;132(5):e1134–40.
3. CDC. Updated recommendations for use of VariZIG—United States, 2013. MMWR Morb Mortal Wkly Rep. 2013 Jul 19;62(28):574–6.
4. Gershon AA, Takahasi M, Seward JF. Varicella vaccine. In: Plotkin SA, Orenstein WA, Offit PA, editors. Vaccines. 6th ed. Philadelphia: Saunders Elsevier; 2012. p. 837–69.
5. Harpaz R, Ortega-Sanchez IR, Seward JF. Prevention of herpes zoster: recommendations of the Advisory Committee on Immunization Practices (ACIP). MMWR Recomm Rep. 2008 Jun 6;57(RR-5):1–30.
6. Marin M, Broder KR, Temte JL, Snider DE, Seward JF. Use of combination measles, mumps, rubella, and varicella vaccine: recommendations of the Advisory Committee on Immunization Practices (ACIP). MMWR Recomm Rep. 2010 May 7;59(RR-3):1–12.
7. Marin M, Guris D, Chaves SS, Schmid S, Seward JF. Prevention of varicella: recommendations of the Advisory Committee on Immunization Practices (ACIP). MMWR Recomm Rep. 2007 Jun 22;56 (RR-4):1–40.
8. World Health Organization. Immunization summary: the 2014 edition. Geneva: World Health Organization; 2013 [cited 2014 Sep 18]. Available from: http://www.childinfo.org/files/immunization_summary_2012_en.pdf.

VIRAL HEMORRHAGIC FEVERS

Barbara Knust

INFECTIOUS AGENT

Viral hemorrhagic fevers (VHFs) are caused by several families of enveloped RNA viruses: filoviruses (Ebola and Marburg hemorrhagic fever), arenaviruses (Lassa fever, Lujo, Guanarito, Machupo, Junin, Sabia, and

Chapare viruses), bunyaviruses (Rift Valley fever [RVF], Crimean-Congo hemorrhagic fever [CCHF], and hantaviruses), and flaviviruses (dengue, yellow fever, Omsk hemorrhagic fever, Kyasanur Forest disease, and Alkhurma viruses) (also see the Dengue and Yellow Fever sections in this chapter).

TRANSMISSION

Some VHFs are spread person to person through direct contact with symptomatic patients, body fluids, or cadavers or through inadequate infection control in a hospital setting (filoviruses, arenaviruses, CCHF virus). Zoonotic spread may occur from contact with the following:

- Livestock via slaughter or consumption of raw meat from infected animals or unpasteurized milk (CCHF, RVF, Alkhurma viruses)
- Bushmeat, likely via slaughter or consumption of infected animals (Ebola, Marburg viruses)
- Rodent (arenaviruses, hantaviruses) via inhalation of or contact with materials contaminated with rodent excreta
- Other reservoir species, such as bats (Ebola, Marburg viruses)
- Vectorborne transmission also occurs via mosquito (RVF virus) or tick (CCHF, Omsk, Kyasanur Forest disease, Alkhurma viruses) bites or by crushing infected ticks

EPIDEMIOLOGY

The viruses that cause VHF are distributed over much of the globe. Each virus is associated with 1 or more nonhuman host or vector species, restricting the virus and the initial contamination to the areas inhabited by these species. The diseases caused by these viruses are seen in people living in or having visited these areas. Humans are incidental hosts for these enzootic diseases; however, person-to-person transmission of some viruses can result in large human outbreaks. Specific viruses are addressed below.

Ebola and Marburg: Filoviral Diseases

Ebola and Marburg viruses cause hemorrhagic fever in humans and nonhuman primates. Five species within the genus *Ebolavirus* have been identified: *Tai Forest ebolavirus* (Taï Forest virus), *Sudan ebolavirus*

(Sudan virus), *Zaire ebolavirus* (Ebola virus), *Bundibugyo ebolavirus* (Bundibugyo virus), and *Reston ebolavirus* (Reston virus). Countries with confirmed human cases of Ebola hemorrhagic fever include Republic of the Congo, Côte d'Ivoire, Democratic Republic of the Congo, Gabon, Sudan, Uganda, Guinea, Liberia, Sierra Leone, and Nigeria. In March of 2014, an outbreak of Ebola virus was detected in a rural area of Guinea near the border with Liberia and Sierra Leone. By June, cases were reported in all three countries, and across many districts. The outbreak is the largest and most complex Ebola epidemic ever reported. As of February 2015, additional cases have occurred in Nigeria, Senegal, Mali, Spain, the United Kingdom, and the United States after importation of infected individuals from West Africa. CDC confirmed on September 30, 2014, the first laboratory-confirmed case of Ebola to be diagnosed in the United States in a person who had traveled from West Africa; this resulted in limited secondary transmission to two US health care workers who cared for the index patient. Several patients have also been evacuated to Europe and the USA. Genetic analysis of the virus indicated that it was 97% identical to *Zaire ebolavirus* previously identified in the Democratic Republic of Congo and Gabon. For the most current information on this outbreak, visit www.cdc.gov/vhf/ebola/outbreaks/guinea/index.html.

Ebola-Reston virus is believed to be endemic in the Philippines and potentially in neighboring countries, but has not been shown to cause human disease. Countries with confirmed human cases of Marburg hemorrhagic fever include Uganda, Kenya, Democratic Republic of the Congo, Angola, and possibly Zimbabwe.

Fruit bats (*Rousettus aegypticacus*) are the natural reservoirs for Marburg virus, and bats are also the suspected reservoir species for the viruses within the genus *Ebolavirus*. Outbreaks occur when a person becomes infected after exposure to the reservoir species or a secondarily infected nonhuman primate and then transmits the virus to other people in the community. Four cases of Marburg hemorrhagic fever have occurred in travelers visiting caves harboring bats, including Kitum cave in Kenya and Python cave in Maramagambo Forest, Uganda.

Miners have also acquired Marburg infection from working in underground mines harboring bats in the Democratic Republic of the Congo and Uganda.

Lassa Fever and Other Arenaviral Diseases

Arenaviruses are transmitted from rodents to humans, except Tacaribe virus, which was found in bats. Most infections are mild, but some result in hemorrhagic fever with high death rates. Old World (Eastern Hemisphere) and New World (Western Hemisphere) viruses cause the following diseases:

- Old World arenaviruses: Lassa virus (Lassa fever), Lujo virus, and Lymphocytic choriomeningitis virus (meningitis, encephalitis, and congenital fetal infection in normal hosts, hemorrhagic fever in organ transplant recipients). Lassa fever occurs in rural West Africa, with hyperendemic areas in Sierra Leone, Guinea, Liberia, and Nigeria. Lujo virus has been recently described in Zambia and the Republic of South Africa during a health care–associated outbreak.
- New World arenaviruses: Junin (Argentine hemorrhagic fever), Machupo (Bolivian hemorrhagic fever), Guanarito (Venezuelan hemorrhagic fever), Sabia (Brazilian hemorrhagic fever), and the recently discovered Chapare virus (single case in Bolivia).

Reservoir host species are Old World rats and mice (family Muridae, subfamily Murinae) and New World rats and mice (family Muridae, subfamily Sigmodontinae). These rodent types are found worldwide, including Europe, Asia, Africa, and the Americas. Virus is transmitted through inhalation of aerosols from rodent urine, ingestion of rodent-contaminated food, or direct contact of broken skin or mucosa with rodent excreta. Risk of Lassa virus infection is associated with peridomestic rodent exposure. Inappropriate food storage increases the risk for exposure. Health care–associated transmission of Lassa, Lujo, and Machupo viruses has occurred through droplet and contact. One anecdotal report of possible airborne transmission exists. Several cases of Lassa fever have been confirmed in international travelers staying in traditional dwellings in the countryside.

Rift Valley Fever and Other Bunyaviral Diseases

RVF causes fever, hemorrhage, encephalitis, and retinitis in humans, but primarily affects livestock. RVF is endemic to sub-Saharan Africa. Sporadic outbreaks have occurred in humans in Egypt, Madagascar, and Mauritania. Large epidemics occurred in Kenya, Somalia, and Tanzania in 1997–1998 and 2006–2007; Saudi Arabia and Yemen in 2000; Madagascar in 2008; and South Africa, Botswana, Namibia, and Mauritania in 2010. RVF virus is transmitted by mosquito, percutaneous inoculation, and slaughter or consumption of infected animals.

CCHF is endemic where ticks of the genus *Hyalomma* are found in Africa and Eurasia, including South Africa, the Balkans, the Middle East, Russia, and western China, and is highly endemic in Afghanistan, Iran, Pakistan, and Turkey. CCHF virus is transmitted to humans by infected ticks or direct handling and preparation of fresh carcasses of infected animals, usually domestic livestock. Health care–associated transmission can occur through droplet or direct contact.

Hantaviruses cause hantavirus pulmonary syndrome (HPS) and hemorrhagic fever with renal syndrome (HFRS). The viruses that cause HPS are present in the New World; those that cause HFRS occur worldwide. The viruses that cause both HPS and HFRS are transmitted to humans through contact with urine, feces, or saliva of infected rodents. Travelers staying in rodent-infested dwellings are at risk for HPS and HFRS. Human-to-human transmission has been reported only with Andes virus in Chile and Argentina.

CLINICAL PRESENTATION

Signs and symptoms vary by disease, but in general, patients with VHF present with abrupt onset of fever, myalgias, and prostration, followed in severe forms by coagulopathy with a petechial rash or ecchymoses and sometimes overt bleeding. Gastrointestinal symptoms (diarrhea, vomiting, abdominal pain) are commonly observed. Vascular endothelial damage leads to shock and pulmonary edema, and liver injury is common. Signs seen with specific viruses include renal failure (HFRS), ecchymoses and bruises (CCHF), hearing loss, anasarca and shock in newborns (Lassa fever), and spontaneous abortion and birth defects (Lassa and lymphocytic choriomeningitis viruses). Laboratory abnormalities include elevations in liver enzymes, initial drop in white blood cell count, and thrombocytopenia. Because the incubation period may be as long as 21 days, patients may not develop illness until returning from travel; therefore, a thorough travel and exposure history is critical.

DIAGNOSIS

US-based clinicians should notify local health authorities and CDC's Viral Special Pathogens Branch immediately of any suspected cases of VHF occurring in patients residing in or requiring evacuation to the United States: 404-639-1115 or the CDC Emergency Operations Center at 770-488-7100 after hours. CDC also provides consultation for international clinicians and health ministries. Whole blood or serum may be tested for virologic (RT-PCR, antigen detection, virus isolation) and immunologic (IgM, IgG) evidence of infection. Tissue may be tested by immunohistochemistry, RT-PCR, and virus isolation. Postmortem skin biopsies fixed in formalin and blood collected within a few hours after death by cardiac puncture can be used for diagnosis. Samples should be sent for testing to a reference laboratory with biosafety level 3 and 4 capability.

TREATMENT

Ribavirin is effective for treating Lassa fever and other Old World arenaviruses, New World arenaviruses, and potentially CCHF, but it is not approved by the Food and Drug Administration (FDA) for these indications. Convalescent-phase plasma is effective in treating Argentine hemorrhagic fever. Intravenous ribavirin can be obtained for compassionate use through FDA from Valeant Pharmaceuticals (Aliso Viejo, California).

Requests should be initiated by the provider through FDA (301-796-1500 or after hours 866-300-4374), with simultaneous notification to Valeant Pharmaceuticals: 800-548-5100, extension 5 (domestic telephone). The process is explained on FDA's website (www.fda.gov/Drugs/DevelopmentApprovalProcess/HowDrugsareDevelopedandApproved/ApprovalApplications/InvestigationalNewDrugINDApplication/ucm090039.htm).

PREVENTION

The risk of acquiring VHF is very low for international travelers. Travelers at increased risk for exposure include those engaging in animal research, health care workers, and others providing care for patients in the community without adequate personal protection, particularly where outbreaks of VHF are occurring.

Prevention should focus on avoiding unprotected contact with people suspected of having VHF or host or vector species in endemic countries. Travelers should not visit locations where an outbreak is occurring, avoid contact with rodents and bats, and avoid livestock in RVF- and CCHF-endemic areas. To prevent vectorborne disease, travelers should use insecticide-treated bed nets and wear insect repellent.

Standard precautions and contact and droplet precautions for suspected VHF patients are recommended to avoid transmission. Direct contact should be avoided with corpses of patients suspected of having died of Ebola, Marburg, or Old World arenavirus infection. Contact with or consumption of primates, bats, and other bushmeat should be avoided. Bat-inhabited caves or mines should be avoided. Investigational vaccines exist for Argentine hemorrhagic fever and RVF; however, neither is approved by FDA, nor are they commonly available in the United States.

BIBLIOGRAPHY

1. Ergonul O, Holbrook MR. Crimean-Congo hemorrhagic fever. In: Guerrant RL, Walker DH, Weller PF, editors. Tropical Infectious Diseases: Principles, Pathogens and Practice. 3rd ed. Philadelphia: Elsevier; 2011. p. 466–9.

2. Feldmann H, Jones SM, Schnittler HJ, Geisbert T. Therapy and prophylaxis of Ebola virus infections. Curr Opin Investig Drugs. 2005 Aug;6(8):823–30.

3. Gunther S, Lenz O. Lassa virus. Crit Rev Clin Lab Sci. 2004;41(4):339–90.

4. Heyman P, Vaheri A, Lundkvist A, Avsic-Zupanc T. Hantavirus infections in Europe: from virus carriers to a major public-health problem. Expert Rev Anti Infect Ther. 2009 Mar;7(2):205–17.

5. Marty AM, Jahrling PB, Geisbert TW. Viral hemorrhagic fevers. Clin Lab Med. 2006 Jun;26(2):345–86, viii.

6. Ozkurt Z, Kiki I, Erol S, Erdem F, Yilmaz N, Parlak M, et al. Crimean-Congo hemorrhagic fever in eastern Turkey: clinical features, risk factors and efficacy of ribavirin therapy. J Infect. 2006 Mar;52(3):207–15.

7. Paweska JT, Sewlall NH, Ksiazek TG, Blumberg LH, Hale MJ, Lipkin WI, et al. Nosocomial outbreak of novel arenavirus infection, southern Africa. Emerg Infect Dis. 2009 Oct;15(10):1598–602.

8. Peters CJ, Makino S, Morrill JC. Rift valley fever. In: Guerrant RL, Walker DH, Weller PF, editors. Tropical Infectious Diseases: Principles, Pathogens and Practice. 3rd ed. Philadelphia: Saunders Elsevier; 2011. p. 462–5.

9. Peters CJ, Zaki SR. Overview of viral hemorrhagic fevers. In: Guerrant RL, Walker DH, Weller PF, editors. Tropical Infectious Diseases: Principles,
Pathogens & Practice. 3rd ed. Philadelphia: Elsevier; 2011. p. 441–8.

10. Rollin PE, Nichol ST, Zaki S, Ksiazek TG. Arenaviruses and filoviruses. In: Versalovic J, Carroll KC, Funke G, Jorgensen JH, Landry ML, Warnock DW, editors. Manual of Clinical Microbiology. 10th ed. Washington, DC: ASM Press; 2011. p. 1514–29.

11. Rouquet P, Froment JM, Bermejo M, Kilbourn A, Karesh W, Reed P, et al. Wild animal mortality monitoring and human Ebola outbreaks, Gabon and Republic of Congo, 2001–2003. Emerg Infect Dis. 2005 Feb;11(2):283–90.

12. Wahl-Jensen V, Peters CJ, Jahrling PB, Feldman H, Kuhn JH. Filovirus infections. In: Guerrant RL, Walker DH, Weller PF, editors. Tropical Infectious Diseases: Principles, Pathogens & Practice. 3rd ed. Philadelphia: Elsevier; 2011. p. 483–91.

YELLOW FEVER
Mark D. Gershman, J. Erin Staples

INFECTIOUS AGENT
Yellow fever virus (YFV) is a single-stranded RNA virus that belongs to the genus *Flavivirus*.

TRANSMISSION
Vectorborne transmission occurs via the bite of an infected mosquito, primarily *Aedes* or *Haemagogus* spp. Nonhuman and human primates are the main reservoirs of the virus, with anthroponotic (human-to-vector-to-human) transmission occurring. There are 3 transmission cycles for yellow fever: sylvatic (jungle), intermediate (savannah), and urban.

- The sylvatic (jungle) cycle involves transmission of the virus between nonhuman primates and mosquito species found in the forest canopy. The virus is transmitted via mosquitoes from monkeys to humans when the humans encroach into the jungle during occupational or recreational activities.
- In Africa, an intermediate (savannah) cycle involves transmission of YFV from tree hole-breeding *Aedes* spp. to humans living or working in jungle border areas. In this cycle, the virus may be transmitted from monkeys to humans or from human to human via these mosquitoes.
- The urban cycle involves transmission of the virus between humans and peridomestic mosquitoes, primarily A. *aegypti*.

Humans infected with YFV experience the highest levels of viremia and can transmit the virus to mosquitoes shortly before onset of fever and for the first 3–5 days of illness. Given the high level of viremia, bloodborne transmission theoretically can occur via transfusion or needlesticks.

EPIDEMIOLOGY
Yellow fever occurs in sub-Saharan Africa and tropical South America, where it is endemic and intermittently epidemic (see Tables 3-21 and 3-22 for a list of countries with risk of YFV transmission). Most yellow fever disease in humans is due to sylvatic or intermediate transmission cycles. However, urban yellow fever occurs periodically in Africa and sporadically in the Americas. In Africa, natural immunity accumulates with age, and thus, infants and children are at highest risk for disease. In South America, yellow fever occurs most frequently in unimmunized young men who are exposed to mosquito vectors through their work in forested areas.

Table 3-21. Countries with risk of yellow fever virus (YFV) transmission[1]

AFRICA			CENTRAL AND SOUTH AMERICA
Angola	Ethiopia[2]	Nigeria	Argentina[2]
Benin	Gabon	Rwanda	Bolivia[2]
Burkina Faso	The Gambia	Senegal	Brazil[2]
Burundi	Ghana	Sierra Leone	Colombia[2]
Cameroon	Guinea	South Sudan	Ecuador[2]
Central African Republic	Guinea-Bissau	Sudan[2]	French Guiana
Chad[2]	Kenya[2]	Togo	Guyana
Congo, Republic of the	Liberia	Uganda	Panama[2]
Côte d'Ivoire	Mali[2]		Paraguay
Democratic Republic of the Congo[2]	Mauritania[2]		Peru[2]
	Niger[2]		Suriname
Equatorial Guinea			Trinidad and Tobago[2]
			Venezuela[2]

[1] Countries or areas where "a risk of YFV transmission is present," as defined by the World Health Organization, are countries or areas where "yellow fever has been reported currently or in the past, plus vectors and animal reservoirs currently exist" (see the current country list within the *International Travel and Health* publication (Annex 1) at www.who.int/ith/en/index.html).
[2] These countries are not holoendemic (only a portion of the country has risk of yellow fever transmission). See Maps 3-15 and 3-16 and yellow fever vaccine recommendations (Yellow Fever & Malaria Information, by Country) for details.

Table 3-22. Countries with low potential for exposure to yellow fever virus (YFV)[1]

AFRICA
Eritrea[2]
São Tomé and Príncipe[3]
Somalia[2]
Tanzania[3]
Zambia[2]

[1] Countries listed in this table are not contained on the official World Health Organization list of countries with risk of YFV transmission (Table 3-21). Therefore, proof of yellow fever vaccination should not be required if traveling from any of these countries to another country with a vaccination entry requirement (unless that country requires proof of yellow fever vaccination from all arriving travelers; see Table 3-25).
[2] These countries are classified as "low potential for exposure to YFV" in only some areas; the remaining areas of these countries are classified as having no risk of exposure to YFV.
[3] The entire area of these countries is classified as "low potential for exposure to YFV."

RISK FOR TRAVELERS

A traveler's risk for acquiring yellow fever is determined by various factors, including immunization status, location of travel, season, duration of exposure, occupational and recreational activities while traveling, and local rate of virus transmission at the time of travel. Although reported cases of human disease are the principal indicator of disease risk, case reports may be absent because of a low level of transmission, a high level of immunity in the population (because of vaccination, for example), or failure of local surveillance systems to detect cases. This "epidemiologic silence" does not equate to absence of risk and should not lead to travel without taking protective measures.

YFV transmission in rural West Africa is seasonal, with an elevated risk during the end of the rainy season and the beginning of the dry season (usually July–October). However, YFV may be episodically transmitted by *Ae. aegypti* even during the dry season in both rural and densely settled urban areas.

The risk for infection in South America is highest during the rainy season (January–May, with a peak incidence in February and March). Given the high level of viremia that may occur in infected humans and the widespread distribution of *Ae. aegypti* in many towns and cities, South America is at risk for a large-scale urban epidemic.

From 1970 through 2013, a total of 10 cases of yellow fever were reported in unvaccinated travelers from the United States and Europe who traveled to West Africa (5 cases) or South America (5 cases). Eight (80%) of these 10 travelers died. There has been only 1 documented case of yellow fever in a vaccinated traveler. This nonfatal case occurred in a traveler from Spain who visited several West African countries in 1988.

The risk of acquiring yellow fever is difficult to predict because of variations in ecologic determinants of virus transmission. For a 2-week stay, the estimated risks for illness and death due to yellow fever for an unvaccinated traveler visiting an endemic area in

- West Africa are 50 per 100,000 and 10 per 100,000, respectively

- South America are 5 per 100,000 and 1 per 100,000, respectively

These estimates are a rough guideline based on the risk to indigenous populations, often during peak transmission season. Thus, these risk estimates may not accurately reflect the true risk to travelers, who may have a different immunity profile, take precautions against getting bitten by mosquitoes, and have less outdoor exposure.

The risk of acquiring yellow fever in South America is lower than that in Africa, because the mosquitoes that transmit the virus between monkeys in the forest canopy in South America do not often come in contact with humans. Additionally, there is a relatively high level of immunity in local residents because of vaccine use, which might reduce the risk of transmission.

CLINICAL PRESENTATION

Asymptomatic or clinically inapparent infection is believed to occur in most people infected with YFV. For people who develop symptomatic illness, the incubation period is typically 3–6 days. The initial illness presents as a nonspecific influenzalike syndrome with sudden onset of fever, chills, headache, backache, myalgias, prostration, nausea, and vomiting. Most patients improve after the initial presentation. After a brief remission of hours to a day, approximately 15% of patients progress to a more serious or toxic form of the disease, characterized by jaundice, hemorrhagic symptoms, and eventually shock and multisystem organ failure. The case-fatality ratio for severe cases with hepatorenal dysfunction is 20%–50%.

DIAGNOSIS

The preliminary diagnosis is based on the patient's clinical features, places and dates of travel, and activities. Laboratory diagnosis is best performed by

- Serologic assays to detect virus-specific IgM and IgG antibodies. Because of cross-reactivity between antibodies raised against other flaviviruses, more specific antibody testing, such as a plaque reduction neutralization test, should be done to confirm the infection.

3

- Virus isolation or nucleic acid amplification tests performed early in the illness for YFV or yellow fever viral RNA. However, by the time more overt symptoms are recognized, the virus or viral RNA might be undetectable. Therefore, virus isolation and nucleic acid amplification should not be used to rule out a diagnosis of yellow fever.

Clinicians should contact their state or local health department or call the CDC Arboviral Diseases Branch at 970-221-6400 for assistance with diagnostic testing for yellow fever infections and for questions about antibody response to vaccination.

TREATMENT

There are no specific medications to treat YFV infections; treatment is directed at symptomatic relief or life-saving interventions. Rest, fluids, and use of analgesics and antipyretics may relieve symptoms of fever and aching. Care should be taken to avoid certain medications, such as aspirin or nonsteroidal anti-inflammatory drugs, which may increase the risk for bleeding. Infected people should be protected from further mosquito exposure (staying indoors or under a mosquito net) during the first few days of illness, so they do not contribute to the transmission cycle.

PREVENTION

Personal Protection Measures

The best way to prevent mosquitoborne diseases, including yellow fever, is to avoid mosquito bites (see Chapter 2, Protection against Mosquitoes, Ticks, & Other Arthropods).

Vaccine

Yellow fever is preventable by a relatively safe, effective vaccine. All yellow fever vaccines currently manufactured are live-attenuated viral vaccines. Only 1 yellow fever vaccine is licensed for use in the United States (Table 3-23). Studies comparing the reactogenicity and immunogenicity of various yellow fever vaccines, including those manufactured outside the United States, suggest that there is no substantial difference in the reactogenicity or immune response generated by the various vaccines. Thus, people who receive yellow fever vaccines in other countries should be considered protected against yellow fever.

Indications for Use

Yellow fever vaccine is recommended for people aged ≥9 months who are traveling to or living in areas with risk for YFV transmission in South America and Africa. In addition, some countries require proof of yellow fever vaccination for entry. See the Yellow Fever & Malaria Information, by Country section at the end of this chapter for more detailed information on the requirements and recommendations for yellow fever vaccination for specific countries.

Because of the risk of serious adverse events that can occur after yellow fever vaccination, clinicians should only vaccinate people who 1) are at risk of exposure to YFV or 2) require proof of vaccination to enter

Table 3-23. Vaccine to prevent yellow fever

VACCINE	TRADE NAME (MANUFACTURER)	AGE	DOSE	ROUTE	SCHEDULE	BOOSTER
17D yellow fever vaccine	YF-Vax (Sanofi Pasteur)	≥9 months[1]	0.5 mL[2]	SC	1 dose	Not recommended for most[3]

Abbreviation: SC, subcutaneous.
[1] Ages 6–8 months and ≥60 years are precautions and age <6 months is a contraindication to the use of yellow fever vaccine.
[2] YF-Vax is available in single-dose and multiple-dose (5-dose) vials.
[3] For further details about recent changes to ACIP recommendations and WHO policy regarding revaccination, see "Vaccine Administration" in this section.

a country. To further minimize the risk of serious adverse events, clinicians should carefully observe the contraindications and consider the precautions to vaccination before administering yellow fever vaccine (Table 3-24). For additional information, refer to the yellow fever vaccine recommendations of the Advisory Committee on Immunization Practices (ACIP) at www.cdc.gov/vaccines/hcp/acip-recs/vacc-specific/yf.html.

Vaccine Administration

For all eligible people, a single injection of reconstituted vaccine should be administered subcutaneously. Revaccination has been required by certain countries at 10-year intervals to comply with International Health Regulations (IHR) of the World Health Organization (WHO).

Note: In 2014, the World Health Assembly (of the WHO) adopted the recommendation to remove the 10-year booster dose requirement from the IHR as of June 2016. Once this change is instituted, a completed International Certificate of Vaccination or Prophylaxis will be valid for the lifetime of the vaccinee. It is uncertain when and if all countries with yellow fever vaccination entry requirements will adopt this change.

In February 2015, ACIP approved a new recommendation that one dose of yellow fever vaccine provides long-lasting protection and is adequate for most travelers. The recommendations also identify specific groups of travelers who should receive additional doses and others for whom additional doses may be considered. The official recommendations were published after this edition went to press. For current booster information, consult the ACIP website (www.cdc.gov/vaccines/hcp/acip-recs/).

Vaccine Safety and Adverse Reactions
Common adverse reactions

Reactions to yellow fever vaccine are generally mild; 10%–30% of vaccinees report mild systemic adverse events. Reported events typically include low-grade fever, headache, and myalgias that begin within days after vaccination and last 5–10 days. Approximately 1% of vaccinees temporarily curtail their regular activities because of these reactions.

Severe adverse reactions
Hypersensitivity

Immediate hypersensitivity reactions, characterized by rash, urticaria, or bronchospasm

Table 3-24. Contraindications and precautions to yellow fever vaccine administration

CONTRAINDICATIONS	PRECAUTIONS
<ul><li>Allergy to vaccine component</li><li>Age <6 months</li><li>Symptomatic HIV infection or CD4 T-lymphocytes <200/mm³ (or <15% of total lymphocytes in children aged <6 years)[1]</li><li>Thymus disorder associated with abnormal immune-cell function</li><li>Primary immunodeficiencies</li><li>Malignant neoplasms</li><li>Transplantation</li><li>Immunosuppressive and immunomodulatory therapies</li></ul>	<ul><li>Age 6–8 months</li><li>Age ≥60 years</li><li>Asymptomatic HIV infection and CD4 T-lymphocytes 200–499/mm³ (or 15%–24% of total lymphocytes in children aged <6 years)[1]</li><li>Pregnancy</li><li>Breastfeeding</li></ul>

[1] Symptoms of HIV are classified in 1) Adults and Adolescents, Table 1. CDC. 1993 Revised classification system for HIV infection and expanded surveillance case definition for AIDS among adolescents and adults. MMWR Recomm Rep 1992 Dec 18: 41(RR-17). Available from: www.cdc.gov/mmwr/preview/mmwrhtml/00018871.htm and 2) Panel on Antiretroviral Therapy and Medical Management of HIV-Infected Children. Guidelines for the use of antiretroviral agents in pediatric HIV infection. 2010. Available from: http://aidsinfo.nih.gov/ContentFiles/PediatricGuidelines.pdf. p. 20–2.

are uncommon. Anaphylaxis after yellow fever vaccine is reported to occur at a rate of 1.8 cases per 100,000 doses administered.

Yellow fever vaccine–associated neurologic disease (YEL-AND)

YEL-AND represents a conglomerate of clinical syndromes, including meningoencephalitis, Guillain-Barré syndrome, acute disseminated encephalomyelitis, and rarely, cranial nerve palsies. Historically, YEL-AND was seen primarily among infants as encephalitis, but more recent reports have been among people of all ages.

The onset of illness for documented cases is 3–28 days after vaccination, and almost all cases were in first-time vaccine recipients. YEL-AND is rarely fatal. The incidence of YEL-AND in the United States is 0.8 per 100,000 doses administered. The rate is higher in people aged ≥60 years, with a rate of 1.6 per 100,000 doses in people aged 60–69 years and 2.3 per 100,000 doses in people aged ≥70 years.

Yellow fever vaccine–associated viscerotropic disease (YEL-AVD)

YEL-AVD is a severe illness similar to wild-type disease, with vaccine virus proliferating in multiple organs and often leading to multiple organ dysfunction syndrome or multiorgan failure and death. Since the initial cases of YEL-AVD were published in 2001, >65 confirmed and suspected cases have been reported throughout the world.

YEL-AVD has been reported to occur only after the first dose of yellow fever vaccine; there have been no reports of YEL-AVD following booster doses. The median time from yellow fever vaccination until symptom onset for YEL-AVD cases was 4 days (range, 0–8 days). The case-fatality ratio for all reported YEL-AVD cases worldwide is approximately 60%. The incidence of YEL-AVD in the United States is 0.4 cases per 100,000 doses of vaccine administered. The rate is higher for people aged ≥60 years, with a rate of 1.0 per 100,000 doses in people aged 60–69 years and 2.3 per 100,000 doses in people aged ≥70 years.

Contraindications

Infants younger than 6 months

Yellow fever vaccine is contraindicated for infants aged <6 months. This contraindication was instituted in the late 1960s in response to a high rate of YEL-AND documented in vaccinated young infants (50–400 per 100,000). The mechanism of increased neurovirulence in infants is unknown but may be due to the immaturity of the blood-brain barrier, higher or more prolonged viremia, or immune system immaturity.

Hypersensitivity

Yellow fever vaccine is contraindicated for people with a history of acute hypersensitivity reaction to a previous dose of the vaccine, as well as those who have a history of an allergic reaction to any of the vaccine components, including eggs, egg products, chicken proteins, or gelatin. The stopper used in vials of vaccine also contains dry natural latex rubber, which may cause an allergic reaction.

If vaccination of a person with a questionable history of hypersensitivity to any of the vaccine components is considered essential because of a high risk for acquiring yellow fever, skin testing, as described in the vaccine package insert, should be performed under close medical supervision. If a person has a positive skin test to the vaccine or has severe egg sensitivity and the vaccination is recommended, desensitization, as described in the package insert, can be performed under direct supervision of a physician experienced in the management of anaphylaxis.

Altered immune status

Thymus disorder

Yellow fever vaccine is contraindicated for people with a thymus disorder that is associated with abnormal immune cell function, such as thymoma or myasthenia gravis. If travel to a yellow fever–endemic area cannot be avoided in a person with such a thymus disorder, a medical waiver should be provided and counseling on protective measures against mosquito bites should be emphasized. Because there is no evidence of immune dysfunction or increased risk of yellow fever vaccine–associated serious adverse events in people who have undergone incidental surgical removal of their thymus or have had indirect radiation therapy in the distant past, these people can be given yellow fever vaccine if recommended or required.

HIV infection

Yellow fever vaccine is contraindicated for people with AIDS or other clinical manifestations of HIV, including people with CD4 T-lymphocyte values <200/mm^3 or <15% of total lymphocytes for children aged <6 years. This recommendation is based on a theoretical increased risk of encephalitis in this population (see HIV infection under the following section, Precautions).

If travel to a yellow fever–endemic area cannot be avoided by a person with severe immune suppression based on CD4 counts (<200/mm^3 or <15% total lymphocytes for children aged <6 years) or symptomatic HIV, a medical waiver should be provided, and counseling on protective measures against mosquito bites should be emphasized. See the following section, Precautions, for other HIV-infected people not meeting the above criteria.

Immunodeficiencies (other than thymus disorder or HIV infection)

Yellow fever vaccine is contraindicated for people with primary immunodeficiencies, malignant neoplasms, or transplantation. While there are no data on the use of yellow fever vaccine in these people, they presumably are at increased risk for yellow fever vaccine–associated serious adverse events (see Chapter 8, Immunocompromised Travelers). If someone with an immunodeficiency cannot avoid travel to a yellow fever–endemic area, a medical waiver should be provided, and counseling on protective measures against mosquito bites should be emphasized.

Immunosuppressive and immunomodulatory therapies

Yellow fever vaccine is contraindicated for people whose immunologic response is either suppressed or modulated by current or recent radiation therapies or drugs. Drugs with known immunosuppressive or immunomodulatory properties include, but are not limited to, high-dose systemic corticosteroids, alkylating drugs, antimetabolites, tumor necrosis factor-α inhibitors (such as etanercept), interleukin-1 and interleukin-6 blocking agents (such as anakinra and tocilizumab), or other monoclonal antibodies targeting immune cells (such as rituximab or alemtuzumab. There are no specific data on the use of yellow fever vaccine in people receiving these therapies. However, these people are presumed to be at increased risk for yellow fever vaccine–associated serious adverse events, and the use of live attenuated vaccines is contraindicated in the package insert for most of these therapies (see Chapter 8, Immunocompromised Travelers).

Live viral vaccines should be deferred in people who have discontinued these therapies until immune function has improved. If travel to a yellow fever–endemic area cannot be avoided for someone receiving immunosuppressive or immunomodulatory therapies, a medical waiver should be provided and counseling on protective measures against mosquito bites should be emphasized.

Family members of people with altered immune status, who themselves have no contraindications, can receive yellow fever vaccine.

Precautions
Infants aged 6–8 months

Age 6–8 months is a precaution for yellow fever vaccination. Two cases of YEL-AND have been reported among infants aged 6–8 months. In infants <6 months of age, the rates of YEL-AND are elevated (50–400 per 100,000). By 9 months of age, risk for YEL-AND is believed to be substantially lower. ACIP generally recommends that, whenever possible, travel to yellow fever–endemic countries should be postponed or avoided for children aged 6–8 months. If travel is unavoidable, the decision of whether to vaccinate these infants needs to balance the risks of YFV exposure with the risk for adverse events after vaccination.

Adults 60 years of age or older

Age ≥60 years is a precaution for yellow fever vaccination, particularly if this is the first dose of the yellow fever vaccine given. An analysis of adverse events passively reported to the Vaccine Adverse Events Reporting System from 2000 through 2006 indicates that people aged ≥60 years are at increased risk for any serious adverse event after vaccination, compared with younger people. The rate of serious adverse events in people aged

≥60 years was 8.3 per 100,000 doses distributed, compared with 4.7 per 100,000 for all vaccine recipients. The risk of YEL-AND and YEL-AVD is also increased in this age group, at 1.8 and 1.4 per 100,000 doses, respectively, compared with 0.8 and 0.4 per 100,000 for all vaccine recipients. Given that YEL-AVD has been reported exclusively, and YEL-AND almost exclusively, in primary vaccine recipients, more caution should be exercised with older travelers who may be receiving yellow fever vaccine for the first time. If travel is unavoidable, the decision to vaccinate travelers aged ≥60 years needs to weigh the risks and benefits of the vaccination in the context of their destination-specific risk for exposure to YFV.

HIV infection

Asymptomatic HIV infection with CD4 T-lymphocyte values 200–499/mm³ or 15%–24% of total lymphocytes for children aged <6 years is a precaution for yellow fever vaccination (see also the discussion of HIV infection in the Contraindications section above). Large prospective, randomized trials have not been performed to adequately address the safety and efficacy of yellow fever vaccine among this group. Retrospective and prospective studies that combined included >500 HIV-infected people reported no serious adverse events among patients considered moderately immunosuppressed based on their CD4 counts. However, HIV infection has been associated with a reduced immunologic response to a number of inactivated and live attenuated vaccines, including yellow fever vaccine. The mechanisms for the diminished immune response in HIV-infected people are uncertain but appear to be correlated with HIV RNA levels and CD4 T-cell counts.

If an asymptomatic HIV-infected person with moderate immune suppression (CD4 T-lymphocyte values 200–499/mm³ or 15%–24% of total lymphocytes for children aged <6 years) is traveling to a yellow fever–endemic area, vaccination may be considered. Vaccinated people should be monitored closely after vaccination for evidence of adverse events, and the state health department or CDC should be notified if an adverse event occurs. However, if international travel requirements—not risk of yellow fever—are the only reason to vaccinate an HIV-infected person, the person should be excused from immunization and issued a medical waiver to fulfill health regulations.

If an asymptomatic HIV-infected person has no evidence of immune suppression based on CD4 counts (CD4 T-lymphocyte values ≥500/mm³ or ≥25% of total lymphocytes for children aged <6 years), yellow fever vaccine can be administered if recommended.

Because vaccinating asymptomatic HIV-infected people might be less effective than vaccinating people not infected with HIV, measuring their neutralizing antibody response to vaccination should be considered before travel. Contact the state health department or the CDC Arboviral Diseases Branch (970-221-6400) to discuss serologic testing.

Pregnancy

Pregnancy is a precaution for yellow fever vaccine administration. The safety of yellow fever vaccination during pregnancy has not been studied in a large prospective trial. However, a recent study of women who were vaccinated with yellow fever vaccine early in their pregnancies found no major malformations in their infants. A slight increased risk was noted for minor, mostly skin, malformations in infants. A higher rate of spontaneous abortions in pregnant women receiving the vaccine was reported but not substantiated. The proportion of women vaccinated during pregnancy who develop YFV-specific IgG antibodies is variable depending on the study (39% or 98%) and may be correlated with the trimester in which they received the vaccine. Because pregnancy may affect immunologic function, serologic testing can be considered to document a protective immune response to the vaccine.

If travel is unavoidable and the vaccination risks are felt to outweigh the risks of YFV exposure, pregnant women should be excused from immunization and issued a medical waiver to fulfill health regulations. Pregnant women who must travel to areas where YFV exposure is likely should be vaccinated. Although there are no specific data, ACIP recommends that a woman wait 4 weeks after receiving the yellow fever vaccine before conceiving.

Breastfeeding

Breastfeeding is a precaution for yellow fever vaccine administration. Three YEL-AND cases have been reported in exclusively breastfed infants whose mothers were vaccinated with yellow fever vaccine. All 3 infants were diagnosed with encephalitis and aged <1 month at the time of exposure. Further research is needed to document the risk of potential vaccine exposure through breastfeeding. Until more information is available, yellow fever vaccine should be avoided in breastfeeding women. However, when travel of nursing mothers to a yellow fever–endemic area cannot be avoided or postponed, these women should be vaccinated.

Other Considerations

There are no data regarding possible increased adverse events or decreased vaccine efficacy after administration of yellow fever vaccine to patients with other chronic medical conditions (such as renal disease, hepatitis C virus infection, other liver disease, or diabetes mellitus). Caution should be used if considering vaccination of such patients. Factors to consider in assessing patients' general level of immune competence include disease severity, duration, clinical stability, complications, and comorbidities.

Simultaneous Administration of Other Vaccines and Drugs

Determination of whether to administer yellow fever vaccine and other immunobiologics simultaneously (administration on the same day but at a different injection site) should be made on the basis of convenience to the traveler in completing the desired vaccinations before travel and on information regarding potential immune interference. No evidence exists that inactivated vaccines interfere with the immune response to yellow fever vaccine. Therefore, inactivated vaccines can be administered either simultaneously or at any time before or after yellow fever vaccination. ACIP recommends that yellow fever vaccine be given at the same time as other live viral vaccines. Otherwise, the clinician should wait 30 days between vaccinations, as the immune response to a live viral vaccine might be impaired if administered within 30 days of another live viral vaccine. A recent study involving the simultaneous administration of yellow fever and measles-mumps-rubella (MMR) vaccines in children found a decrease in the immune response against yellow fever, mumps, and rubella when the vaccines were given on the same day versus 30 days apart. Additional studies are needed to confirm these findings, but they suggest that if possible, yellow fever and MMR should be given 30 days apart. Because of the different routes of administration, oral Ty21a typhoid vaccine, a live bacterial vaccine, can be administered simultaneously or at any interval before or after yellow fever vaccine.

INTERNATIONAL CERTIFICATE OF VACCINATION OR PROPHYLAXIS (ICVP)

The IHR allow countries to require proof of yellow fever vaccination documented on an ICVP as a condition of entry for travelers arriving from certain countries, even if only in transit, to prevent importation and indigenous transmission of YFV. Some countries require evidence of vaccination from all entering travelers, which includes direct travel from the United States (Table 3-25). Travelers who arrive in a country with a yellow fever vaccination entry requirement without proof of yellow fever vaccination may be quarantined for up to 6 days, refused entry, or vaccinated on site. A traveler who has a specific contraindication to yellow fever vaccine and who cannot avoid travel to a country requiring vaccination should request a waiver from a physician before embarking on travel (see the Medical Waivers [Exemptions] section below).

Authorization to Provide Vaccinations and to Validate the ICVP

Under the revised IHR (2005), effective December 15, 2007, all countries are required to issue a new ICVP. This is intended to replace the former International Certificate of Vaccination against Yellow Fever (ICV). People who received a yellow fever vaccination after December 15, 2007, must provide proof of vaccination on the new ICVP. If the person received the vaccine before December 15, 2007, the original ICV card is still valid, provided that the vaccination was given <10 years previously. Vaccinees should receive a completed ICVP (Figure 3-2),

Table 3-25. Countries that require proof of yellow fever vaccination from all arriving travelers[1]

Angola	Guinea-Bissau
Benin	Liberia
Burkina Faso	Mali
Burundi	Niger
Cameroon	Rwanda
Central African Republic	Sierra Leone
Congo, Republic of the	Togo
Côte d'Ivoire	
Democratic Republic of the Congo	
French Guiana	
Gabon	

[1] Country requirements for yellow fever vaccination are subject to change at any time; therefore, CDC encourages travelers to check with the destination country's embassy or consulate before departure.

validated (stamped and signed) with the stamp of the center where the vaccine was given (see below). An incomplete or inaccurate ICVP is not valid. Failure to secure validations can cause a traveler to be quarantined, denied entry, or possibly revaccinated at the point of entry to a country. Revaccination at the point of entry is not a recommended option for the traveler.

Clinics may purchase ICVPs, CDC 731 (formerly PHS 731), from the US Government Printing Office (http://bookstore.gpo.gov/, 866-512-1800). This certificate of vaccination is valid for a period of 10 years, beginning 10 days after the date of vaccination. When a booster dose of the vaccine is given within this 10-year period, the certificate is considered valid from the date of revaccination.

People Authorized to Sign the ICVP and Designated Yellow Fever Vaccination Centers

The ICVP must be signed by a medical provider, who may be a licensed physician or a health care worker designated by the physician, supervising the administration of the vaccine (Figure 3-2). A signature stamp is not acceptable. Yellow fever vaccination must be given at a certified center in possession of an official "uniform stamp," which can be used to validate the ICVP.

State health departments are responsible for designating nonfederal yellow fever vaccination centers and issuing uniform stamps to clinicians. Information about the location and hours of yellow fever vaccination centers may be obtained by visiting CDC's website at wwwnc.cdc.gov/travel/yellow-fever-vaccination-clinics-search.aspx.

Medical Waivers (Exemptions)

Some countries do not require an ICVP for infants younger than a certain age (<6 months, <9 months, or <1 year of age, depending on the country). Age requirements for vaccination for individual countries can be found in the Yellow Fever & Malaria Information, by Country section at the end of this chapter. For medical contraindications, a clinician who has decided to issue a waiver should fill out and sign the Medical Contraindications to Vaccination section of the ICVP (Figure 3-3). The clinician should also do the following:

- Give the traveler a signed and dated exemption letter on letterhead stationery, clearly stating the contraindications to vaccination and bearing the stamp used by the yellow fever vaccination center to validate the ICVP.
- Inform the traveler of any increased risk for yellow fever infection associated with lack of vaccination and how to minimize this risk by avoiding mosquito bites.

 YELLOW FEVER | 355

INTERNATIONAL CERTIFICATE OF VACCINATION OR PROPHYLAXIS
Certificat international de vaccination ou de prophylaxie

This is to certify that ① _Jane Mary Doe_ ② _22 March 1960_ _F_ _United States_
Nous certifions que (name – nom) (date of birth – né(e) le) (sex – de sexe) (nationality – et de nationalité)

[passport number] whose signature follows ③ _Jane Mary Doe_
(national identification document, if applicable – document d'identification nationale, le cas échéant) dont la signature suit

has on the date indicated been vaccinated or received prophylaxis against ④ _Yellow Fever_ in accordance with the International Health Regulations.
a été vacciné(e) ou a reçu une prophylaxie à la date indiquée (name of disease or condition – nom de la maladie ou de l'affection) conformément au Règlement sanitaire international.

Vaccine or prophylaxis Vaccin ou agent prophylactique	Date	Signature and professional status of supervising clinician Signature et titre du professional de santé responsable	Manufacturer and batch no. of vaccine or prophylaxis Fabricant du vaccin ou de l'agent prophylactique et numéro du lot	Certificate valid from: until: Certificat valable à partir du : jusqu'au :	Official stamp of the administering center Cachet officiel du centre habilité
④ Yellow Fever	⑤ 15 June 2016	⑥ John M. Smith, MD	[Batch (or lot) #]	⑦ 25 June 2016 24 June 2022	[⑧]

FIGURE 3-2. EXAMPLE INTERNATIONAL CERTIFICATE OF VACCINATION OR PROPHYLAXIS (ICVP)

(1) Name should appear exactly as on the patient's passport.
(2, 5, 7) All dates should be entered with the day in numerals, followed by the month in letters, then the year. For example: in the above example, the patient's date of birth is 22 March 1960.
(3) This space is for the patient's signature.
(4) For a yellow fever vaccination, 'Yellow Fever' should be written in both spaces. Should the ICVP be used for a required vaccination or prophylaxis against another disease or condition (following an amendment to the International Health Regulations or by recommendation of the World Health Organization), that disease or condition should be written in this space. Other vaccinations may be listed on the other side.
(5) The date on which the vaccination is given should be entered as shown above.
(6) A handwritten signature of the clinician—either the stamp holder or another health care provider authorized by the stamp holder—administering or supervising the administration of the vaccine (or prophylaxis) should appear in this box. A signature stamp is not acceptable.
(7) The certificate of yellow fever vaccination is valid for 10 years, beginning 10 days after the date of primary vaccination. The ending date for a valid vaccination recorded on the ICVP is 1 calendar day prior to the calendar day on which the vaccine became valid. For example, a vaccination given on 15 June 2012 will be valid on 25 June 2012 and will expire on 24 June 2022. In the case of revaccination, the certificate of yellow fever vaccination is valid immediately if documentation exists on an ICVP demonstrating that the previous yellow fever vaccination was given within the last 10 years.
(8) The Uniform Stamp of the vaccinating center should appear in this box.

Reasons other than medical contraindications are not acceptable for exemption from vaccination. The traveler should be advised that issuance of a waiver does not guarantee its acceptance by the destination country. On arrival at the destination, the traveler may be faced with quarantine, refusal of entry, or vaccination on site. To improve the likelihood that the waiver will be accepted at the destination country, clinicians can suggest that the traveler take the following additional measures before beginning travel:

- Obtain specific and authoritative advice from the embassy or consulate of the destination country or countries.
- Request documentation of requirements for waivers from embassies or consulates and retain these, along with the completed Medical Contraindication to Vaccination section of the ICVP.

MEDICAL CONTRAINDICATION TO VACCINATION
Contre-indication médicale à la vaccination

This is to certify that immunization against
Je soussigné(e) certifie que la vaccination contre

_____ for
(Name of disease – Nom de la maladie)   pour

_____ is medically
(Name of traveler – Nom du voyageur)   est médicalement

contraindicated because of the following conditions:
contre-indiquée pour les raisons suivantes :

_____

_____

_____

_____
(Signature and address of physician)
(Signature et adresse du médecin)

FIGURE 3-3. MEDICAL CONTRAINDICATION TO VACCINATION SECTION OF THE INTERNATIONAL CERTIFICATE OF VACCINATION OR PROPHYLAXIS (ICVP)

REQUIREMENTS VERSUS RECOMMENDATIONS

Country entry *requirements* for proof of yellow fever vaccination under the IHR differ from CDC's *recommendations*. Yellow fever vaccine entry requirements are established by countries to prevent the importation and transmission of YFV and are allowed under the IHR. Travelers must comply with these to enter the country, unless they have been issued a medical waiver. Certain countries require vaccination from travelers arriving from all countries (Table 3-25), while some countries require vaccination only for travelers coming from a country with risk of YFV transmission (see Yellow Fever & Malaria Information, by Country at the end of this chapter). WHO defines those areas with risk of YFV transmission as countries or areas where yellow fever has been reported currently or in the past, plus where vectors and animal reservoirs exist. Country requirements are subject to change at any time; therefore, CDC encourages travelers to check with the relevant embassy or consulate before departure.

The information in the section on yellow fever vaccine recommendations is advice given by CDC to prevent yellow fever infections among travelers. Recommendations are subject to change at any time because of changes in YFV circulation; therefore, CDC encourages travelers to check the destination pages for up-to-date vaccine information and to check for relevant travel notices on the CDC website before departure (www.cdc.gov/travel).

Yellow fever vaccine recommendations for travelers going to specific destinations are based on the risk classification for YFV transmission: endemic, transitional, low potential for exposure, and no risk. Yellow fever vaccination is recommended for travel to endemic and transitional areas (Maps 3-15 and 3-16). Although vaccination is generally not recommended for travel to areas with low potential for exposure, it might be considered for a small subset of travelers whose itinerary could place them at increased risk for exposure to YFV (such as prolonged travel, heavy exposure to mosquitoes, or inability to avoid mosquito bites). Yellow fever vaccination is not recommended in areas with no risk.

Countries that only contain areas with low potential for exposure to YFV (Table 3-22) are not included on the official WHO list of

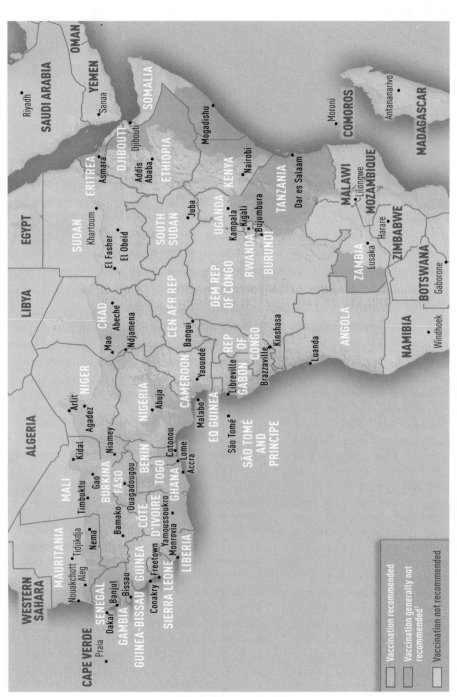

MAP 3-15. YELLOW FEVER VACCINE RECOMMENDATIONS IN AFRICA [2]

[1] Yellow fever (YF) vaccination is generally not recommended in areas where there is low potential for YF virus exposure. However, vaccination might be considered for a small subset of travelers to these areas who are at increased risk for exposure to YF virus because of prolonged travel, heavy exposure to mosquitoes, or inability to avoid mosquito bites. Consideration for vaccination of any traveler must take into account the traveler's risk of being infected with YF virus, country entry requirements, and individual risk factors for serious vaccine-associated adverse events (e.g., age, immune status).

[2] Current as of March 2014. This map is an updated version of the 2010 map created by the Informal WHO Working Group on the Geographic Risk of Yellow Fever.

Vaccination recommended

Vaccination generally not recommended[1]

Vaccination not recommended

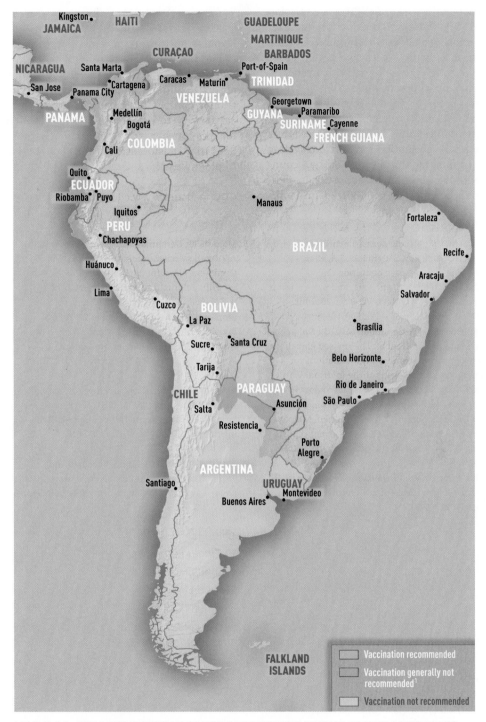

Vaccination recommended

Vaccination generally not recommended[1]

Vaccination not recommended

MAP 3-16. YELLOW FEVER VACCINE RECOMMENDATIONS IN THE AMERICAS[2]

[1] Yellow fever (YF) vaccination is generally not recommended in areas where there is low potential for YF virus exposure. However, vaccination might be considered for a small subset of travelers to these areas who are at increased risk for exposure to YF virus because of prolonged travel, heavy exposure to mosquitoes, or inability to avoid mosquito bites. Consideration for vaccination of any traveler must take into account the traveler's risk of being infected with YF virus, country entry requirements, and individual risk factors for serious vaccine-associated adverse events (e.g., age, immune status).

[2] Current as of March 2014. This map is an updated version of the 2010 map created by the Informal WHO Working Group on the Geographic Risk of Yellow Fever.

countries with risk of YFV transmission (Table 3-21). Therefore, proof of yellow fever vaccination should not be required if traveling from a country with low potential for exposure to YFV to a country with a vaccination entry requirement (unless that country requires proof of yellow fever vaccination from all arriving travelers; see Table 3-25). An exception is South Africa, which requires yellow fever vaccination for people traveling from or transiting through any of the 5 countries with low potential for exposure, in addition to those with risk of YFV transmission.

VACCINATION FOR TRAVEL ON MILITARY ORDERS

Because military requirements may exceed those indicated in this publication, any person who plans to travel on military orders (civilians and military personnel) should contact the nearest military medical facility to determine the requirements for his or her trip (see also Chapter 8, Special Considerations for US Military Deployments).

CDC website: www.cdc.gov/yellowfever

BIBLIOGRAPHY

1. Gershman MD, Staples JE, Bentsi-Enchill AD, Breugelmans JG, Brito GS, Camacho LA, et al. Viscerotropic disease: case definition and guidelines for collection, analysis, and presentation of immunization safety data. Vaccine. 2012 Jul 13;30(33):5038–58.

2. Jentes ES, Poumerol G, Gershman MD, Hill DR, Lemarchand J, Lewis RF, et al. The revised global yellow fever risk map and recommendations for vaccination, 2010: consensus of the Informal WHO Working Group on Geographic Risk for Yellow Fever. Lancet Infect Dis. 2011 Aug;11(8):622–32.

3. Lindsey NP, Schroeder BA, Miller ER, Braun MM, Hinckley AF, Marano N, et al. Adverse event reports following yellow fever vaccination. Vaccine. 2008 Nov 11;26(48):6077–82.

4. Monath TP, Cetron MS. Prevention of yellow fever in people traveling to the tropics. Clin Infect Dis. 2002 May 15;34(10):1369–78.

5. Monath TP, Gershman M, Staples JE, Barrett ADT. Yellow fever vaccine. In: Plotkin SA, Orenstein WA, Offit PA, editors. Vaccines. 6th ed. Philadelphia: Saunders Elsevier; 2012. p. 870–968.

6. Staples JE, Gershman M, Fischer M. Yellow fever vaccine: recommendations of the Advisory Committee on Immunization Practices (ACIP). MMWR Recomm Rep. 2010 Jul 30;59(RR-7):1–27.

7. World Health Organization. International Health Regulations, 2005. 2008 [cited 2014 Sep 24]. Available from: http://whqlibdoc.who. int/publications/2008/9789241580410_ eng. pdf.

8. World Health Organization. Vaccines and vaccination against yellow fever. WHO position paper—June 2013. Wkly Epidemiol Rec. 2013 Jul 5;88(27):269–83.

For the Record

A HISTORY OF YELLOW FEVER VACCINATION REQUIREMENTS
Mark D. Gershman

The history of yellow fever vaccination requirements is best understood in the larger context of the history of international measures to prevent the spread of infectious diseases. The first international disease control measures were instituted in Europe in the 14th century in an attempt to prevent the spread of bubonic plague. Subsequently, cholera became the next major target of international disease control efforts. The lack of agreement between countries on the most effective means of disease prevention and lack of consistency in quarantine regulations eventually led to a series of International Sanitary Conferences.

The first International Sanitary Conference was held in Paris in 1851, and others were held periodically until 1944. Several international health organizations, including the Health Organization of the League of Nations, were established to oversee the various international regulations on disease control. The onset of World War II in 1939 severely disrupted the international public health functions of these agencies. The United Nations Relief and Rehabilitation Administration (UNRRA) was created by the Allies in 1943 to provide economic assistance to war-ravaged European nations, assist refugees, and conduct public health functions. (The UNRRA is unrelated to the more familiar United Nations organization, founded in 1945.) The public health responsibilities included the oversight of international quarantine activities, particularly those delineated in the updated International Sanitary Conventions of 1944, which contained yellow fever control measures. Specific provisions for national governments included quarantining a traveler from an endemic area who did not possess a valid vaccination certificate. This provision, which directed countries how to deal with unvaccinated travelers who may have been exposed to yellow fever virus, was the precursor to formal yellow fever vaccination requirements.

In order for the provisions of the Sanitary Conventions of 1944 to be carried out, areas where yellow fever was endemic had to be delineated. The conventions delegated this responsibility to the UNRRA, which appointed the Expert Commission on Quarantine. This commission created the first official map of yellow fever–endemic areas in 1945. Soon after the end of World War II, the responsibilities of the UNRRA were assumed by the newly formed World Health Organization (WHO), which appointed the Yellow Fever Panel. In 1949, the Yellow Fever Panel modified the original UNRRA map and issued its first report, which recommended that "measures may be applied permanently against arrivals from endemic areas."

The International Sanitary Regulations (ISR), drafted by WHO to replace the previous International Sanitary Conventions, were adopted by the World Health Assembly in 1951. The ISR stipulated that "vaccination against yellow fever shall be required of any person leaving an infected local area on an international voyage and proceeding to a yellow fever receptive area." Although only alluded to in previous International Sanitary Conventions, this was the first regulatory language that overtly mandated yellow fever vaccination requirements for country entry. The ISR were modified and renamed the International Health Regulations (IHR) in 1969; the IHR were completely revised in 2005, the most current iteration. The text regarding yellow fever vaccination requirements has been gradually modified. The IHR (2005) stipulate, "Vaccination against yellow fever may be required of any traveler leaving an area where the Organization has determined that a risk of yellow fever transmission is present."

In 1960, WHO started to publish annually a listing of all the national yellow fever vaccination requirements in the booklet *Vaccination Certificate Requirements for International Travel*. This booklet gradually evolved into the current book *International Travel and Health*, which is also published annually and lists country-specific vaccination requirements. To keep its list current, WHO sends a questionnaire to all member countries yearly requesting any updates to their vaccination requirements. CDC publishes these same country requirements.

BIBLIOGRAPHY

1. Strode GK, editor. Yellow Fever. 1st ed. New York: McGraw Hill; 1951.
2. Wilder-Smith A, Martinez L, Rietveld A, Duclos P, Hardiman M, Gollogly L. World Health Organization and *International Travel and Health*. Travel Med Infect Dis. 2007 May;5(3):147–9.
3. World Health Organization. International Health Regulations (1969): 1st annotated edition. Geneva: World Health Organization; 1971.
4. World Health Organization. International Health Regulations, 2005. Geneva: World Health Organization; 2008 [cited 2014 Sep 24]. Available from: http://whqlibdoc.who.int/publications/2008/9789241580410_eng.pdf.
5. World Health Organization. International Sanitary Regulations: 2nd annotated edition. Geneva: World Health Organization; 1961.

YERSINIOSIS

L. Hannah Gould

INFECTIOUS AGENT

Facultative anaerobic gram-negative coccobacilli in the genus *Yersinia* (most commonly *Yersinia enterocolitica* serogroups O:3; O:5,27; O:8; and O:9).

TRANSMISSION

Consuming or handling contaminated food, most commonly raw or undercooked pork products; milk that was not pasteurized, inadequately pasteurized, or contaminated after pasteurization; or untreated water. Also transmitted by direct or indirect contact with animals.

EPIDEMIOLOGY

Most common in northern Europe (particularly Scandinavia), Japan, and Canada. In temperate climates, risk is higher in cooler months. The incidence among travelers to developing countries is generally low. A recent study in the United States found that approximately 6% of *Y. enterocolitica* infections were travel associated. People with high iron levels are at higher risk of infection and severe disease.

CLINICAL PRESENTATION
Incubation period is 4–6 days (range, 1–14 days). Symptoms include fever, abdominal pain (may mimic appendicitis), and diarrhea (may be bloody and can persist for several weeks). Necrotizing enterocolitis has been described in young infants. Reactive arthritis affecting the wrists, knees, and ankles can occur, usually 1 month after the initial diarrhea episode, resolving after 1–6 months. Erythema nodosum can also occur, manifesting as painful, raised red or purple lesions along the trunk and legs, usually resolving spontaneously within 1 month.

DIAGNOSIS
Isolation of the organism from stool, blood, bile, wound, throat swab, mesenteric lymph node, cerebrospinal fluid, or peritoneal fluid.

BIBLIOGRAPHY
1. Cover TL, Aber RC. *Yersinia enterocolitica*. N Engl J Med. 1989 Jul 6;321(1):16–24.
2. Dennis DT, Mead PS. *Yersinia* species, including plague. In: Mandell GL, Bennett JE, Dolin R, editors. Principles and Practices of Infectious Diseases. 7th ed. Philadelphia: Elsevier Churchill Livingstone 2009. p. 2943–54.
3. Kendall ME, Crim S, Fullerton K, Han PV, Cronquist AB, Shiferaw B, et al. Travel-associated enteric infections diagnosed after return to the United States, Foodborne Diseases Active Surveillance Network (FoodNet), 2004–2009. Clin Infect Dis. 2012 Jun;54 Suppl 5:S480–7.
4. Perdikogianni C, Galanakis E, Michalakis M, Giannoussi E, Maraki S, Tselentis Y, et al. *Yersinia enterocolitica* infection mimicking surgical conditions. Pediatr Surg Int. 2006 Jul;22(7):589–92.

If yersiniosis is suspected, the clinical laboratory should be notified and instructed to culture on CIN agar.

TREATMENT
Most infections are self-limited. Antibiotics should be given for severe cases. *Y. enterocolitica* isolates are usually susceptible to trimethoprim-sulfamethoxazole, aminoglycosides, third-generation cephalosporins, fluoroquinolones, and tetracyclines; they are typically resistant to first-generation cephalosporins and most penicillins. Antimicrobial therapy has no effect on postinfectious sequelae.

PREVENTION
Avoid eating raw or undercooked pork products, unpasteurized milk products, and untreated water (see Chapter 2, Food & Water Precautions). Wash hands with soap and water before eating and preparing food, after contact with animals, and after handling raw meat.

CDC website: www.cdc.gov/nczved/divisions/dfbmd/diseases/yersinia

ZIKA
Tai-Ho Chen, Ronnie Henry, Marc Fischer

INFECTIOUS AGENT
Zika virus (ZIKV) is a single-stranded RNA virus of the Flaviviridae family, genus *Flavivirus*.

TRANSMISSION
Transmission occurs through the bite of an infected *Aedes* mosquito. Perinatal transmission and possible person-to-person transmission have also been reported.

EPIDEMIOLOGY
Serologic evidence and case reports of human ZIKV infection have been documented in Africa (including Central African Republic, Egypt, Gabon, Nigeria, Senegal, Sierra

Leone, and Tanzania) and Asia (including India, Indonesia, Malaysia, the Philippines, Thailand, and Vietnam). In addition, larger sporadic outbreaks caused by ZIKV have been documented in the Pacific Islands in Yap State (Micronesia), French Polynesia, New Caledonia, the Cook Islands, and Easter Island. Cases have been detected in travelers returning from countries with suspected ZIKV activity.

CLINICAL PRESENTATION

Commonly reported signs and symptoms include fever, maculopapular rash, arthralgia, arthritis, myalgia, headache, retroorbital pain, and conjunctivitis. Other symptoms may include fatigue, edema, sore throat, cough, vomiting, and loose stools. Unlike in dengue infection, hemorrhagic manifestations have rarely been reported among people infected with ZIKV. The proportion of asymptomatic cases among people infected with ZIKV has not been established.

DIAGNOSIS

Because of the typical clinical features of fever, rash, and arthralgia, the differential diagnosis of ZIKV infection is broad. Preliminary diagnosis should be based on clinical findings and epidemiologic characteristics, including travel history and

activities, although ZIKV infection may share these with other arboviral infections, including dengue and chikungunya.

Diagnostic testing can include nucleic acid testing (RT-PCR), virus isolation, or antibody detection; cross-reactivity with antibodies for other flaviviruses has been noted. Clinicians are encouraged to report suspected ZIKV infections to state or local health departments to determine if confirmatory testing is indicated and to reduce the risk of local transmission.

TREATMENT

No specific antiviral treatment is available for ZIKV infection. Treatment of symptoms may include rest, fluids, antipyretics, and analgesics. As in other arboviral diseases, infected people should avoid mosquitoes while they are sick to reduce the risk of ongoing transmission.

PREVENTION

Avoiding mosquito bites can protect against ZIKV infection (see Chapter 2, Protection against Mosquitoes, Ticks, & Other Arthropods). Avoiding exposure to bodily fluids (including unprotected sexual contact) of people with suspected ZIKV infection may also reduce transmission risk.

BIBLIOGRAPHY

1. Besnard M, Lastere S, Teissier A, Cao-Lormeau V, Musso D. Evidence of perinatal transmission of Zika virus, French Polynesia, December 2013 and February 2014. Euro Surveill. 2014;19(13).

2. Duffy MR, Chen TH, Hancock WT, Powers AM, Kool JL, Lanciotti RS, et al. Zika virus outbreak on Yap Island, Federated States of Micronesia. N Engl J Med. 2009 Jun 11;360(24):2536–43.

3. Foy BD, Kobylinski KC, Chilson Foy JL, Blitvich BJ, Travassos da Rosa A, Haddow AD, et al.

Probable non-vector-borne transmission of Zika virus, Colorado, USA. Emerg Infect Dis. 2011 May;17(5):880–2.

4. Hayes EB. Zika virus outside Africa. Emerg Infect Dis. 2009 Sep;15(9):1347–50.

5. Tappe D, Rissland J, Gabriel M, Emmerich P, Gunther S, Held G, et al. First case of laboratory-confirmed Zika virus infection imported into Europe, November 2013. Euro Surveill. 2014;19(4).

Yellow Fever & Malaria Information, by Country

Mark D. Gershman, Emily S. Jentes, Rhett J. Stoney (YELLOW FEVER)

Kathrine R. Tan, Paul M. Arguin, Stefanie F. Steele (MALARIA)

The following pages present country-specific information on yellow fever vaccine requirements and recommendations (see Table 3–26) and malaria transmission information and prophylaxis recommendations. Fifteen country-specific maps of malaria transmission areas, 10 country-specific maps depicting yellow fever vaccine recommendations, and reference maps of 2 countries are included to aid in interpreting the recommendations. The information was accurate at the time of publication; however, this information is subject to change at any time as a result of changes in disease transmission or, in the case of yellow fever, changing country entry requirements. Updated information, reflecting changes since publication, can be found in the online version of this book (www.cdc.gov/yellowbook) and on the CDC Travelers' Health website (www.cdc.gov/travel). General recommendations for other vaccines to consider during the pre-travel consultation can be found on the CDC Travelers' Health website (www.cdc.gov/travel).

Yellow Fever

Since publication of the 2014 edition of *CDC Health Information for International Travel*, additional country-specific data on the geographic risk of yellow fever virus (YFV) transmission was provided by certain countries and the Pan American Health Organization (PAHO). Based on a review of these data by CDC, the World Health Organization (WHO), PAHO, and other yellow fever and travel medicine experts, updated yellow fever vaccination recommendations were made for Argentina, Colombia, Peru, and Venezuela. Furthermore, an updated recommendation for the Democratic Republic of the Congo was made after an outbreak of yellow fever was confirmed in Katanga Province in early 2014.

Revaccination for yellow fever has been required by certain countries at 10-year intervals to comply with International Health Regulations (IHR). In 2014, the World Health Assembly (of WHO) adopted the recommendation to remove the 10-year booster dose requirement from the IHR as of June 2016. Once this change is instituted, a completed International Certificate of Vaccination or Prophylaxis will be valid for the lifetime of the vaccinee. **It is uncertain when and if all countries with current yellow fever vaccination entry requirements will adopt this change.**

In the United States, the Advisory Committee on Immunization Practices (ACIP) is considering the issue of the continued need for yellow fever vaccine boosters. **In February 2015, ACIP approved a new recommendation that one dose of yellow fever vaccine provides long-lasting protection and is adequate for most travelers. The recommendations also identify specific groups of travelers who should receive additional doses and others for whom additional doses may be considered. The official recommendations were published after this edition went to press.** For the most up-to-date information about yellow fever vaccine boosters, consult the CDC Travelers' Health website or the ACIP website (www.cdc.gov/vaccines/hcp/acip-recs/).

Ultimately, the clinician's decision whether or not to vaccinate any traveler must take into account the traveler's risk of being infected with YFV, country entry requirements, and individual risk factors for serious adverse events after yellow fever vaccination (such as age and immune status). For a thorough discussion of yellow fever and guidance for vaccination, see the Yellow Fever section earlier in this chapter.

Malaria

The recommendations for malaria prevention include estimates of malaria risk to US travelers. These estimates are based on numbers of malaria cases reported in US travelers and the estimated volume of travel to these countries. In some instances, the risk may be low because the actual intensity of transmission is low in that country. In other instances, malaria transmission may occur only in small focal areas of the country where US travelers seldom

Table 3-26. Categories of recommendations for yellow fever vaccination

YELLOW FEVER VACCINATION CATEGORY	RATIONALE FOR RECOMMENDATION
Recommended	Vaccination recommended for all travelers ≥9 months of age to areas with endemic or transitional yellow fever risk, as determined by persistent or periodic YFV transmission.
Generally not recommended	Vaccination generally not recommended in areas where the potential for YFV exposure is low, as determined by absence of reports of human yellow fever and past evidence suggestive of only low levels of YFV transmission. However, vaccination might be considered for a small subset of travelers who are at increased risk for exposure to YFV because of prolonged travel, heavy exposure to mosquitoes, or inability to avoid mosquito bites.
Not recommended	Vaccination not recommended in areas where there is no risk of YFV transmission, as determined by absence of past or present evidence of YFV circulation in the area or environmental conditions not conducive to YFV transmission.

Abbreviation: YFV, yellow fever virus.

go. Thus, even though the risk for the average traveler to that country may be low, the risk for the rare traveler going to the areas with higher transmission intensity will be higher. For some countries rarely visited by US travelers, insufficient information exists to make a risk estimate. Information about malaria species present in each country is based on the best available data from multiple sources.

Several medications are available for malaria chemoprophylaxis. When deciding on which drug to use, clinicians should consider the specific itinerary, length of trip, cost of the drugs, previous adverse reactions to antimalarials, drug allergies, and medical history.

For a thorough discussion of malaria and guidance for prophylaxis, see the Malaria section earlier in this chapter.

Country-Specific Information

AFGHANISTAN
Yellow Fever
Requirements: Required if traveling from a country with risk of YFV transmission.[1]
Recommendations: None.

Malaria
Areas with malaria: April–December in all areas <2,500 m (8,202 ft).
Estimated relative risk of malaria for US travelers: High.[3]
Drug resistance[4]: Chloroquine.
Malaria species: *P. vivax* 80%–90%, *P. falciparum* 10%–20%.
Recommended chemoprophylaxis: Atovaquone-proguanil, doxycycline, or mefloquine.

ALBANIA
Yellow Fever
Requirements: Required if traveling from a country with risk of YFV transmission and ≥1 year of age.[1]
Recommendations: None.

Malaria
No malaria transmission.

ALGERIA
Yellow Fever
Requirements: Required if traveling from a country with risk of YFV transmission and ≥1 year of age, including transit >12 hours in an airport located in a country with risk of YFV transmission.[1]
Recommendations: None.

Malaria
Areas with malaria: Rare indigenous cases.
Estimated relative risk of malaria for US travelers: No information.
Drug resistance: Chloroquine.
Malaria species: *P. falciparum, P. vivax.*
Recommended chemoprophylaxis: Mosquito avoidance only.

AMERICAN SAMOA (US)
Yellow Fever
No requirements or recommendations.

Malaria
No malaria transmission.

ANDORRA
Yellow Fever
No requirements or recommendations.

Malaria
No malaria transmission.

ANGOLA
Yellow Fever
Requirements: Required for arriving travelers from all countries if traveler is ≥1 year of age.
Recommendations: *Recommended* for all travelers ≥9 months of age.

Malaria
Areas with malaria: All.
Estimated relative risk of malaria for US travelers: High.
Drug resistance[4]: Chloroquine.
Malaria species: *P. falciparum* 90%, *P. ovale* 5%, *P. vivax* 5%.
Recommended chemoprophylaxis: Atovaquone-proguanil, doxycycline, or mefloquine.

ANGUILLA (UK)
Yellow Fever
Requirements: Required if traveling from a country with risk of YFV transmission and ≥1 year of age, including transit in an airport located in a country with risk of YFV transmission.[1]
Recommendations: None.

Malaria
No malaria transmission.

ANTARCTICA
Yellow Fever
No requirements or recommendations.

Malaria
No malaria transmission.

ANTIGUA AND BARBUDA
Yellow Fever
Requirements: Required if traveling from a country with risk of YFV transmission and ≥1 year of age.[1]
Recommendations: None.

ARGENTINA (See Map 3-17.)
Yellow Fever
Requirements: None.
Recommendations:
Recommended for travelers ≥ 9 months of age going to Corrientes and Misiones Provinces.
Generally not recommended for travelers going to Formosa Province and designated areas of Chaco, Jujuy, and Salta Provinces (see Map 3-17).
Not recommended for all travelers whose itineraries are limited to areas and provinces not listed above.

Malaria
No malaria transmission.

ARMENIA
Yellow Fever
No requirements or recommendations.

Malaria
No malaria transmission.

ARUBA
Yellow Fever
Requirements: This country has not stated its yellow fever vaccination certificate requirements.
Recommendations: None.

Malaria
No malaria transmission.

AUSTRALIA
Yellow Fever
Requirements: Required if traveling from a country with risk of YFV transmission and ≥1 year of age, including transit >12 hours in an airport located in a country with risk of YFV transmission. This requirement excludes Galapagos Islands in Ecuador and the island of Tobago and is limited to Misiones Province in Argentina.
Recommendations: None.

Malaria
No malaria transmission.

AUSTRIA
Yellow Fever
No requirements or recommendations.

Malaria
No malaria transmission.

AZERBAIJAN
Yellow Fever
No requirements or recommendations.

Malaria
Areas with malaria: May–October in rural areas <1,500 m (4,921 ft). None in Baku.
Estimated relative risk of malaria for US travelers: Very low.
Drug resistance[4]: None.
Malaria species: *P. vivax* 100%.
Recommended chemoprophylaxis: Mosquito avoidance only.

AZORES (PORTUGAL)
Yellow Fever
No requirements or recommendations.

Malaria
No malaria transmission.

BAHAMAS, THE
Yellow Fever
Requirements: Required if traveling from a country with risk of YFV transmission and ≥1 year of age, including transit >12 hours in an airport located in a country with risk of YFV transmission.[1] This requirement excludes Guyana, Suriname, and Trinidad and Tobago but includes São Tomé and Príncipe, Somalia, and the United Republic of Tanzania.
Recommendations: None.

Malaria
No malaria transmission.

BAHRAIN
Yellow Fever
Requirements: Required if traveling from a country with risk of YFV transmission and ≥9 months of age, including transit >12 hours in an airport located in a country with risk of YFV transmission.[1]
Recommendations: None.

Malaria
No malaria transmission.

BANGLADESH
Yellow Fever
Requirements: Required if traveling from a country with risk of YFV transmission and ≥1 year of age.[1]
Recommendations: None.

Malaria
Areas with malaria: All areas, except in the city of Dhaka.
Estimated relative risk of malaria for US travelers: Low.

---

*All footnotes are located on page 420.

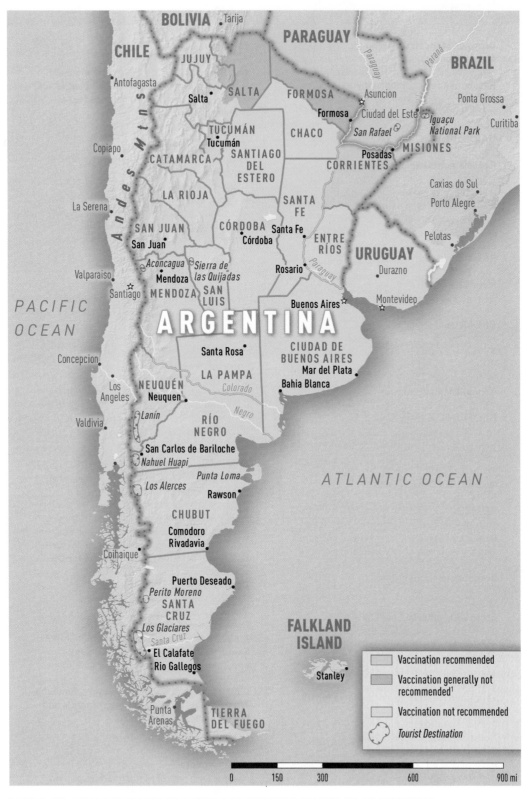

MAP 3-17. YELLOW FEVER VACCINE RECOMMENDATIONS IN ARGENTINA[2]

[1,2] See footnotes on page 420 for an explanation of "Vaccination generally not recommended."

Legend:
- Vaccination recommended
- Vaccination generally not recommended[1]
- Vaccination not recommended
- Tourist Destination

Drug resistance[4]: Chloroquine.
Malaria species: More than half *P. falciparum*, remainder *P. vivax* and *P. malariae*.
Recommended chemoprophylaxis: Atovaquone-proguanil, doxycycline, or mefloquine.

BARBADOS
Yellow Fever
Requirements: Required if traveling from a country with risk of YFV transmission and ≥1 year of age, including transit >12 hours in an airport located in a country with risk of YFV transmission.[1] This requirement excludes Guyana and Trinidad and Tobago.
Recommendations: None.

Malaria
No malaria transmission.

BELARUS
Yellow Fever
No requirements or recommendations.

Malaria
No malaria transmission.

BELGIUM
Yellow Fever
No requirements or recommendations.

Malaria
No malaria transmission.

BELIZE
Yellow Fever
Requirements: Required if traveling from a country with risk of YFV transmission and ≥1 year of age.[1]
Recommendations: None.

Malaria
Areas with malaria: Small foci of transmission, primarily in Stann Creek and Toledo. Rare locally transmitted cases in other districts. None in Belize City and islands frequented by tourists, such as Ambergris Caye.
Estimated relative risk of malaria for US travelers: Very low.
Drug resistance[4]: None.
Malaria species: *P. vivax* 95%, *P. falciparum* 5%.
Recommended chemoprophylaxis: Mosquito avoidance only.

BENIN
Yellow Fever
Requirements: Required for arriving travelers from all countries if traveler is ≥1 year of age.
Recommendations: *Recommended* for all travelers ≥9 months of age.

Malaria
Areas with malaria: All.
Estimated relative risk of malaria for US travelers: High.
Drug resistance[4]: Chloroquine.
Malaria species: *P. falciparum* 85%, *P. ovale* 5%–10%, *P. vivax* rare.
Recommended chemoprophylaxis: Atovaquone-proguanil, doxycycline, or mefloquine.

BERMUDA (UK)
Yellow Fever
No requirements or recommendations.

Malaria
No malaria transmission.

BHUTAN
Yellow Fever
Requirements: Required if traveling from a country with risk of YFV transmission, including transit in an airport located in a country with risk of YFV transmission.[1]
Recommendations: None.

Malaria
Areas with malaria: All rural areas <1,700 m (5,577 ft) in districts of Chukha, Dagana, Pemagatshel, Samdrug Jongkhar, Samtse, Sarpang, and Zhemgang. Rare seasonal cases May–September in Ha, Lhuentse, Monggar, Punakha, Trashigang, Trongsa, Tsirang, Yangtse, and Wangdue. None in districts of Bumthang, Gaza, Paro, and Thimphu.
Estimated relative risk of malaria for US travelers: Very low.
Drug resistance[4]: Chloroquine.
Malaria species: *P. falciparum* 50%, *P. vivax* 50%.
Recommended chemoprophylaxis: **Districts of Chukha, Dagana, Pemagatshel, Samdrug Jongkhar, Samtse, Sarpang, and Zhemgang:** Atovaquone-proguanil, doxycycline, or mefloquine.
Districts of Ha, Lhuentse, Monggar, Punakha, Trashigang, Trongsa, Tsirang, Yangtse, and Wangdue: Mosquito avoidance only.

BOLIVIA (See Maps 3-18 and 3-19.)
Yellow Fever
Requirements: Required if traveling from a country with risk of YFV transmission and

---

*All footnotes are located on page 420.

≥1 year of age, including transit >12 hours in an airport located in a country with risk of YFV transmission.[1]

Recommendations:

Recommended for all travelers ≥9 months of age traveling to the following areas <2,300 m in elevation[2] and east of the Andes Mountains: the entire departments of Beni, Pando, Santa Cruz, and designated areas (see Map 3-18) of Chuquisaca, Cochabamba, La Paz, and Tarija departments.

Not recommended for travelers whose itineraries are limited to areas >2,300 m in elevation[2] and all areas not listed above, including the cities of La Paz and Sucre.

Malaria

Areas with malaria: All areas <2,500 m (8,202 ft). None in the city of La Paz (see Map 3-19).

Estimated relative risk of malaria for US travelers: Low.

Drug resistance[4]: Chloroquine.

Malaria species: *P. vivax* 93%, *P. falciparum* 7%.

Recommended chemoprophylaxis: Atovaquone-proguanil, doxycycline, mefloquine, or primaquine.[5]

MAP 3-18. YELLOW FEVER VACCINE RECOMMENDATIONS IN BOLIVIA[2]

[1,2] See footnotes on page 420 for an explanation of "Vaccination generally not recommended."

BONAIRE
Yellow Fever
Requirements: Required if traveling from a country with risk of YFV transmission and ≥6 months of age.[1]
Recommendations: None.

Malaria
No malaria transmission.

BOSNIA AND HERZEGOVINA
Yellow Fever
No requirements or recommendations.

Malaria
No malaria transmission.

BOTSWANA (See Map 3-20.)
Yellow Fever
Requirements: Required if traveling from a country with risk of YFV transmission and ≥1 year of age, including transit >12 hours in an airport located in a country with risk of YFV transmission.[1]
Recommendations: None.

Malaria
Areas with malaria: Present in the following districts: Central and North West (including Chobe National Park). None in the cities of Francistown and Gaborone.
Estimated relative risk of malaria for US travelers: Very low.
Drug resistance[4]: Chloroquine.

MAP 3-19. MALARIA TRANSMISSION AREAS IN BOLIVIA

*All footnotes are located on page 420.

Malaria species: *P. falciparum* 90%, *P. vivax* 5%, *P. ovale* 5%.

Recommended chemoprophylaxis: Atovaquone-proguanil, doxycycline, or mefloquine.

BRAZIL (See Maps 3-21 and 3-22.)

Yellow Fever

Requirements: None.

Recommendations:

Recommended for all travelers ≥9 months of age going to the following areas: the entire states of Acre, Amapá, Amazonas, Distrito Federal (including the capital city of Brasília), Goiás, Maranhão, Mato Grosso, Mato Grosso do Sul, Minas Gerais, Pará, Rondônia, Roraima, Tocantins, and designated areas (see Map 3-21) of the following states: Bahia, Paraná, Piauí, Rio Grande do Sul, Santa Catarina, and São Paulo (state). Vaccination is also recommended for travelers visiting Iguaçu Falls.

Not recommended for travelers whose itineraries are limited to areas not listed above, including the cities of Fortaleza, Recife, Rio de Janeiro, Salvador, and São Paulo (see Map 3-21).

Malaria

Areas with malaria: States of Acre, Amapá, Amazonas, Maranhão, Mato Grosso, Para,

MAP 3-20. MALARIA TRANSMISSION AREAS IN BOTSWANA

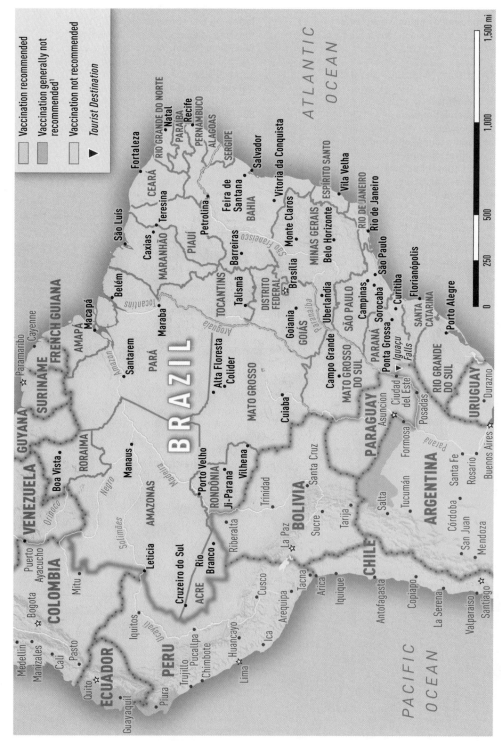

MAP 3-21. YELLOW FEVER VACCINE RECOMMENDATIONS IN BRAZIL. [2]

[1,2] See footnotes on page 420 for an explanation of "Vaccination generally not recommended."

Legend:
- Vaccination recommended
- Vaccination generally not recommended [1]
- Vaccination not recommended
- ▶ *Tourist Destination*

Scale: 0 — 250 — 500 — 1,000 — 1,500 mi

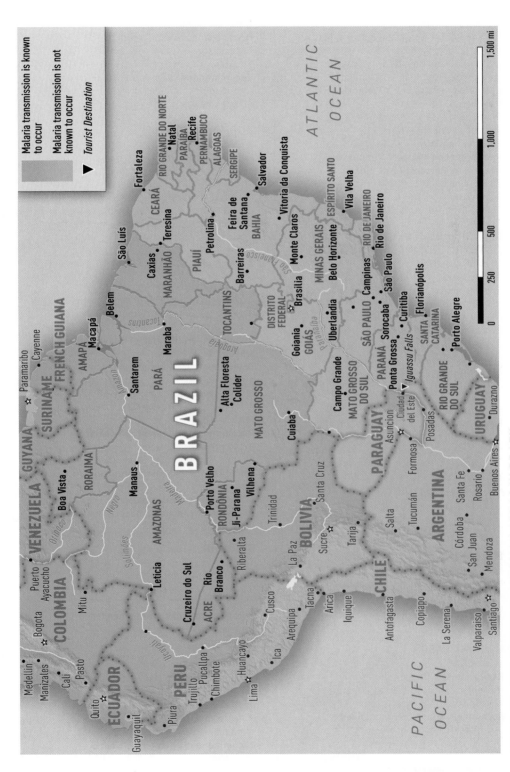

MAP 3-22. MALARIA TRANSMISSION AREAS IN BRAZIL

Malaria transmission is known to occur

Malaria transmission is not known to occur

▶ *Tourist Destination*

0   250   500   1,000   1,500 mi

Rondonia, Roraima, and Tocantins. Also present in urban areas, including cities such as Belem, Boa Vista, Macapa, Manaus, Maraba, Porto Velho, and Santarem. Rare cases in Cuiaba City. No transmission at Iguaçu Falls (see Map 3-22).
Estimated relative risk of malaria for US travelers: Low.
Drug resistance[4]: Chloroquine.
Malaria species: *P. vivax* 85%, *P. falciparum* 15%.
Recommended chemoprophylaxis:
Areas with malaria except Cuiaba City: Atovaquone-proguanil, doxycycline, or mefloquine.
Cuiaba City: Mosquito avoidance only.

BRITISH INDIAN OCEAN TERRITORY, INCLUDES DIEGO GARCIA (UK)
Yellow Fever
Requirements: This territory has not stated its yellow fever vaccination certificate requirements.
Recommendations: None.

Malaria
No malaria transmission.

BRUNEI
Yellow Fever
Requirements: Required if traveling from a country with risk of YFV transmission and ≥1 year of age, including transit >12 hours in an airport located in a country with risk of YFV transmission.
Recommendations: None.

Malaria
No malaria transmission.

BULGARIA
Yellow Fever
No requirements or recommendations.

Malaria
No malaria transmission.

BURKINA FASO
Yellow Fever
Requirements: Required for arriving travelers from all countries if traveler is ≥1 year of age.
Recommendations: *Recommended* for all travelers ≥9 months of age.

Malaria
Areas with malaria: All.

Estimated relative risk of malaria for US travelers: High.
Drug resistance[4]: Chloroquine.
Malaria species: *P. falciparum* 80%, *P. ovale* 5%–10%, *P. vivax* rare.
Recommended chemoprophylaxis:
Atovaquone-proguanil, doxycycline, or mefloquine.

BURMA (MYANMAR)
Yellow Fever
Requirements: Required if traveling from a country with risk of YFV transmission and ≥1 year of age, including transit >12 hours in an airport located in a country with risk of YFV transmission. Required also for nationals and residents of Burma (Myanmar) departing for a country with risk of YFV transmission.
Recommendations: None.

Malaria
Areas with malaria: Present at altitudes <1,000 m (3,281 ft), including Bagan. Rare transmission above 1,000 m.
Estimated relative risk of malaria for US travelers: Moderate.
Drug resistance[4]: Chloroquine and mefloquine.
Malaria species: *P. falciparum* 60%, *P. vivax* 35%, remainder *P. malariae*, *P. ovale*, and *P. knowlesi*.
Recommended chemoprophylaxis:
In the provinces of Bago, Kachin, Kayah, Kayin, Shan, and Tanintharyi: Atovaquone-proguanil or doxycycline.
All other areas with malaria: Atovaquone-proguanil, doxycycline, or mefloquine.

BURUNDI
Yellow Fever
Requirements: Required for arriving travelers from all countries if traveler is ≥1 year of age.
Recommendations: *Recommended* for all travelers ≥9 months of age.

Malaria
Areas with malaria: All.
Estimated relative risk of malaria for US travelers: Moderate.
Drug resistance[4]: Chloroquine.
Malaria species: *P. falciparum* 86%, remainder *P. malariae*, *P. ovale*, and *P. vivax*.
Recommended chemoprophylaxis:
Atovaquone-proguanil, doxycycline, or mefloquine.

*All footnotes are located on page 420.

CAMBODIA
Yellow Fever
Requirements: Required if traveling from a country with risk of YFV transmission and ≥1 year of age, including transit >12 hours in an airport located in a country with risk of YFV transmission.
Recommendations: None.

Malaria
Areas with malaria: Present throughout the country, including Siem Reap city. None in the city of Phnom Penh and at the temple complex at Angkor Wat.
Estimated relative risk of malaria for US travelers: Low.
Drug resistance[4]: Chloroquine and mefloquine.
Malaria species: *P. falciparum* 86%, *P. vivax* 12%, *P. malariae* 2%.
Recommended chemoprophylaxis: In the provinces of Banteay Meanchey, Battambang, Kampot, Koh Kong, Odder Meanchey, Pailin, Preah Vihear, Pursat, and Siem Reap bordering Thailand: Atovaquone-proguanil or doxycycline. All other areas with malaria: Atovaquone-proguanil, doxycycline, or mefloquine.

CAMEROON
Yellow Fever
Requirements: Required for arriving travelers from all countries if traveler is ≥1 year of age.
Recommendations: *Recommended* for all travelers ≥9 months of age.

Malaria
Areas with malaria: All.
Estimated relative risk of malaria for US travelers: High.
Drug resistance[4]: Chloroquine.
Malaria species: *P. falciparum* 85%, *P. ovale* 5%–10%, *P. vivax* rare.
Recommended chemoprophylaxis: Atovaquone-proguanil, doxycycline, or mefloquine.

CANADA
Yellow Fever
No requirements or recommendations.

Malaria
No malaria transmission.

CANARY ISLANDS (SPAIN)
Yellow Fever
No requirements or recommendations.

Malaria
No malaria transmission.

CAPE VERDE
Yellow Fever
Requirements: Required if traveling from a country with risk of YFV transmission and ≥1 year of age, including transit >12 hours in an airport located in a country with risk of YFV transmission.[1]
Recommendations: None.

Malaria
Areas with malaria: Limited cases in São Tiago Island.
Estimated relative risk of malaria for US travelers: Very low.
Drug resistance[4]: Chloroquine.
Malaria species: Primarily *P. falciparum*.
Recommended chemoprophylaxis: Mosquito avoidance only.

CAYMAN ISLANDS (UK)
Yellow Fever
No requirements or recommendations.

Malaria
No malaria transmission.

CENTRAL AFRICAN REPUBLIC
Yellow Fever
Requirements: Required for arriving travelers from all countries if traveler is ≥9 months of age.
Recommendations: *Recommended* for all travelers ≥9 months of age.

Malaria
Areas with malaria: All.
Estimated relative risk of malaria for US travelers: High.
Drug resistance[4]: Chloroquine.
Malaria species: *P. falciparum* 85%; *P. malariae*, *P. ovale*, and *P. vivax* 15% combined.
Recommended chemoprophylaxis: Atovaquone-proguanil, doxycycline, or mefloquine.

CHAD
Yellow Fever
Requirements: Required if traveling from a country with risk of YFV transmission.[1]
Recommendations:

Recommended for all travelers ≥9 months of age traveling to areas south of the Sahara Desert (see Map 3-15).
Not recommended for travelers whose itineraries are limited to areas in the Sahara Desert (see Map 3-15).

Malaria
Areas with malaria: All.
Estimated relative risk of malaria for US travelers: High.
Drug resistance[4]: Chloroquine.
Malaria species: *P. falciparum* 85%; *P. malariae, P. ovale,* and *P. vivax* 15% combined.
Recommended chemoprophylaxis: Atovaquone-proguanil, doxycycline, or mefloquine.

CHILE
Yellow Fever
No requirements or recommendations.

Malaria
No malaria transmission.

CHINA (See Map 3-23.)
Yellow Fever
Requirements: Required if traveling from a country with risk of YFV transmission and ≥9 months of age, including transit in an airport located in a country with risk of YFV transmission.[1]
Recommendations: None.

Malaria
Areas with malaria: Present year round in rural parts of Yunnan Province, primarily in the counties along the China–Burma (Myanmar) border. Limited transmission in rural areas of Anhui, Hubei, Guangxi, and Motuo County in Tibet. Some major river cruises may go through malaria-endemic areas in Anhui and Hubei Provinces.
Estimated relative risk of malaria for US travelers: Very low.
Drug resistance[4]: Chloroquine and mefloquine.
Malaria species: Primarily *P. vivax*; *P. falciparum* in Yunnan Province only.
Recommended chemoprophylaxis: Along China–Burma (Myanmar) border in the western part of Yunnan Province: Atovaquone-proguanil or doxycycline.

Other parts of Yunnan Province: Atovaquone-proguanil, doxycycline, or mefloquine.
All other areas with malaria, including river cruises that pass through malaria-endemic provinces: Mosquito avoidance only.

CHRISTMAS ISLAND (AUSTRALIA)
Yellow Fever
Requirements: Required if traveling from a country with risk of YFV transmission and ≥1 year of age, including transit >12 hours in an airport located in a country with risk of YFV transmission.[1] This requirement excludes Galapagos Islands in Ecuador and the island of Tobago and is limited to Misiones Province in Argentina.
Recommendations: None.

Malaria
No malaria transmission.

COCOS (KEELING) ISLANDS (AUSTRALIA)
Yellow Fever
Requirements: Required if traveling from a country with risk of YFV transmission and ≥1 year of age, including transit >12 hours in an airport located in a country with risk of YFV transmission.[1] This requirement excludes Galapagos Islands in Ecuador and the island of Tobago and is limited to Misiones Province in Argentina.
Recommendations: None.

Malaria
No malaria transmission.

COLOMBIA (See Maps 3-24 and 3-25.)
Yellow Fever
Requirements: None.
Recommendations:
Recommended for all travelers ≥9 months of age except as mentioned below.
Generally not recommended for travelers to the cities of Barranquilla, Cali, Cartagena, and Medellín (See Map 3-24).
Not recommended for travelers whose itineraries are limited to all areas >2,300 m in elevation,[2] the department of San Andrés y Providencia, and the capital city of Bogotá.

Malaria
Areas with malaria: All areas <1,700 m (5,577 ft). None in Bogotá and Cartagena (See Map 3-25).

---

*All footnotes are located on page 420.

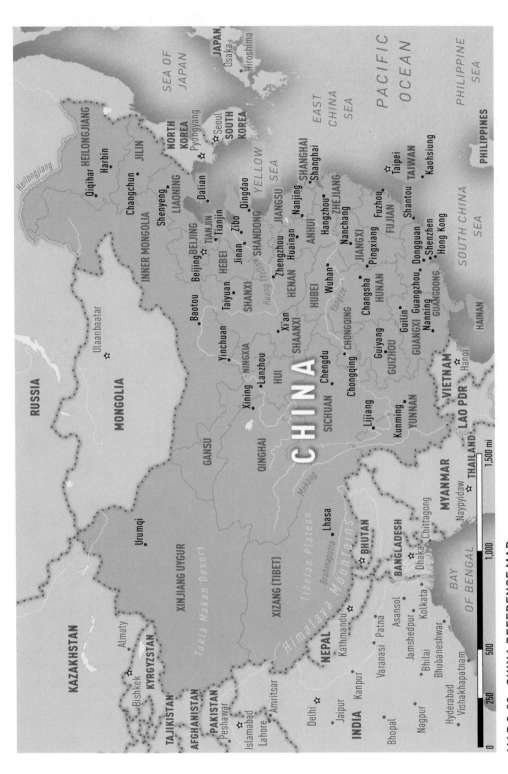

MAP 3-23. CHINA REFERENCE MAP

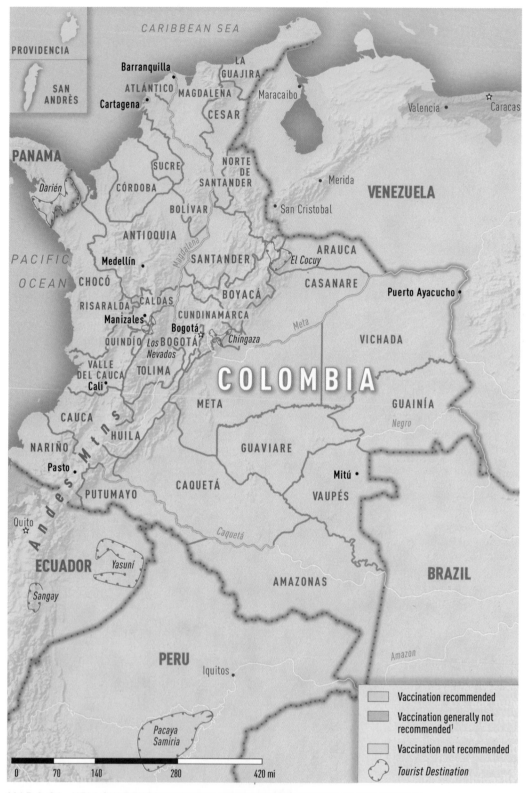

MAP 3-24. YELLOW FEVER VACCINE RECOMMENDATIONS IN COLOMBIA[2]

[1,2] See footnotes on page 420 for an explanation of "Vaccination generally not recommended."

Legend:
- Vaccination recommended
- Vaccination generally not recommended[1]
- Vaccination not recommended
- Tourist Destination

Scale: 0 — 70 — 140 — 280 — 420 mi

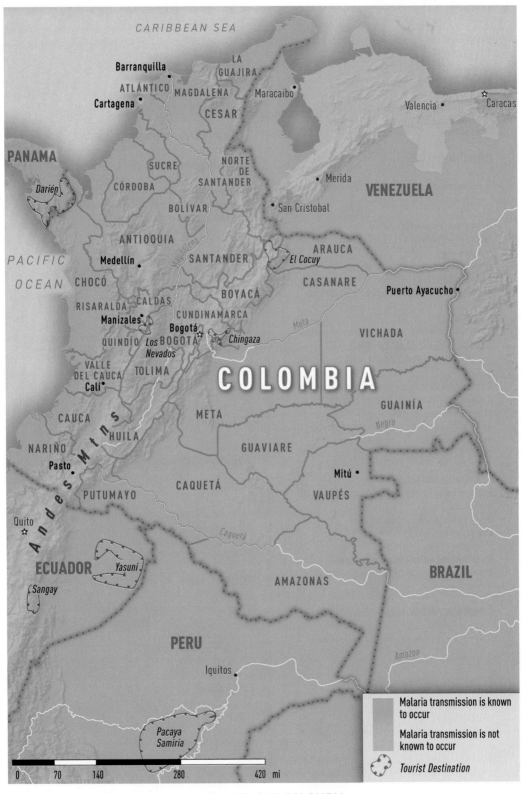

MAP 3-25. MALARIA TRANSMISSION AREAS IN COLOMBIA

Legend:

- Malaria transmission is known to occur
- Malaria transmission is not known to occur
- Tourist Destination

Scale: 0 — 70 — 140 — 280 — 420 mi

Estimated relative risk of malaria for US travelers: Low.
Drug resistance[4]: Chloroquine.
Malaria species: *P. falciparum* 30%, *P. vivax* 70%.
Recommended chemoprophylaxis: Atovaquone-proguanil, doxycycline, or mefloquine.

COMOROS
Yellow Fever
No requirements or recommendations.

Malaria
Areas with malaria: All.
Estimated relative risk of malaria for US travelers: No data.
Drug resistance[4]: Chloroquine.
Malaria species: Primarily *P. falciparum*.
Recommended chemoprophylaxis: Atovaquone-proguanil, doxycycline, or mefloquine.

CONGO, REPUBLIC OF THE (CONGO-BRAZZAVILLE)
Yellow Fever
Requirements: Required for arriving travelers from all countries if traveler is ≥1 year of age.
Recommendations: *Recommended* for all travelers ≥9 months of age.

Malaria
Areas with malaria: All.
Estimated relative risk of malaria for US travelers: High.
Drug resistance[4]: Chloroquine.
Malaria species: *P. falciparum* 90%, *P. ovale* 5%–10%, *P. vivax* rare.
Recommended chemoprophylaxis: Atovaquone-proguanil, doxycycline, or mefloquine.

COOK ISLANDS (NEW ZEALAND)
Yellow Fever
No requirements or recommendations.

Malaria
No malaria transmission.

COSTA RICA
Yellow Fever
Requirements: Required if traveling from a country with risk of YFV transmission and ≥9 months of age, including transit >12 hours in an airport located in a country with risk of YFV transmission.[1] This requirement

excludes Argentina, Panama, and Trinidad and Tobago.
Recommendations: None.

Malaria
No malaria transmission.

CÔTE D'IVOIRE (IVORY COAST)
Yellow Fever
Requirements: Required for arriving travelers from all countries if traveler is ≥9 months of age.
Recommendations: *Recommended* for all travelers ≥9 months of age.

Malaria
Areas with malaria: All.
Estimated relative risk of malaria for US travelers: High.
Drug resistance[4]: Chloroquine.
Malaria species: *P. falciparum* 85%, *P. ovale* 5%–10%, *P. vivax* rare.
Recommended chemoprophylaxis: Atovaquone-proguanil, doxycycline, or mefloquine.

CROATIA
Yellow Fever
No requirements or recommendations.

Malaria
No malaria transmission.

CUBA
Yellow Fever
No requirements or recommendations.

Malaria
No malaria transmission.

CURAÇAO
Yellow Fever
Requirements: Required if traveling from a country with risk of YFV transmission and ≥6 months of age.[1]
Recommendations: None.

Malaria
No malaria transmission.

CYPRUS
Yellow Fever
No requirements or recommendations.

Malaria
No malaria transmission.

*All footnotes are located on page 420.

CZECH REPUBLIC
Yellow Fever
No requirements or recommendations.

Malaria
No malaria transmission.

DEMOCRATIC REPUBLIC OF THE CONGO (CONGO-KINSHASA)
Yellow Fever
Requirements: Required for arriving travelers from all countries if traveler is ≥1 year of age.
Recommendations: *Recommended* for all travelers ≥9 months of age.

Malaria
Areas with malaria: All.
Estimated relative risk of malaria for US travelers: Moderate.
Drug resistance[4]: Chloroquine.
Malaria species: *P. falciparum* 90%, *P. ovale* 5%, *P. vivax* rare.
Recommended chemoprophylaxis: Atovaquone-proguanil, doxycycline, or mefloquine.

DENMARK
Yellow Fever
No requirements or recommendations.

Malaria
No malaria transmission.

DJIBOUTI
Yellow Fever
Requirements: Required if traveling from a country with risk of YFV transmission and ≥1 year of age.[1]
Recommendations: None.

Malaria
Areas with malaria: All.
Estimated relative risk of malaria for US travelers: No data.
Drug resistance[4]: Chloroquine.
Malaria species: *P. falciparum* 90%, *P. vivax* 5%–10%.
Recommended chemoprophylaxis: Atovaquone-proguanil, doxycycline, or mefloquine.

DOMINICA
Yellow Fever
Requirements: Required if traveling from a country with risk of YFV transmission and ≥1 year of age, including transit >12 hours in an airport located in a country with risk of YFV transmission.[1]
Recommendations: None.

Malaria
No malaria transmission.

DOMINICAN REPUBLIC
Yellow Fever
No requirements or recommendations.

Malaria
Areas with malaria: All areas (including resort areas), except none in the cities of Santiago and Santo Domingo.
Estimated relative risk of malaria for US travelers: Low.
Drug resistance[4]: None.
Malaria species: *P. falciparum* 100%.
Recommended chemoprophylaxis: Atovaquone-proguanil, chloroquine, doxycycline, or mefloquine.

EASTER ISLAND (CHILE)
Yellow Fever
Requirements: This country has not stated its yellow fever vaccination certificate requirements.
Recommendations: None.

Malaria
No malaria transmission.

ECUADOR, INCLUDING THE GALÁPAGOS ISLANDS (See Maps 3-26 and 3-27.)
Yellow Fever
Requirements: Required if traveling from a country with risk of YFV transmission and ≥1 year of age.[1]
Recommendations:
Recommended for all travelers ≥9 months of age traveling to areas <2,300 m in elevation[2] in the following provinces east of the Andes Mountains: Morona-Santiago, Napo, Orellana, Pastaza, Sucumbios, and Zamora-Chinchipe (see Map 3-26).
Generally not recommended for travelers whose itinerary is limited to areas <2,300 m in elevation[2] in the following provinces west of the Andes mountains: Esmeraldas, Guayas, Los Rios, Manabi, Santa Elena, Santo Domingo de los Tsachilas, and designated areas of Azuay, Bolivar, Canar, Carchi, Chimborazo, Cotopaxi, El Oro, Imbabura, Loja, Pichincha, and Tungurahua (see Map 3-26).

Not recommended for travelers whose itineraries are limited to all areas >2,300 m in elevation,[2] the cities of Guayaquil and Quito, or the Galápagos Islands (see Map 3-26).

Malaria

Areas with malaria: All areas <1,500 m (4,921 ft). Not present in the cities of Guayaquil and Quito or the Galápagos Islands (see Map 3-27).

Estimated relative risk of malaria for US travelers: Low.

Drug resistance[4]: Chloroquine.

Malaria species: *P. vivax* 90%, *P. falciparum* 10%.

Recommended chemoprophylaxis: Guayas, Esmeraldes, and Canar Provinces: Atovaquone-proguanil, doxycycline, or mefloquine.

All other areas with malaria: Atovaquone-proguanil, doxycycline, mefloquine, or primaquine.[5]

EGYPT

Yellow Fever

Requirements: Required if traveling from a country with risk of YFV transmission and ≥9 months of age, including transit >12 hours in an airport located in a country with risk of YFV transmission.[1] All travelers arriving from Sudan are required to have a vaccination certificate or a location certificate issued by a Sudanese official center that states that they have not been in Sudan south of 15°N within the previous 6 days.

Recommendations: None.

Malaria

No malaria transmission.

EL SALVADOR

Yellow Fever

Requirements: Required if traveling from a country with risk of YFV transmission and

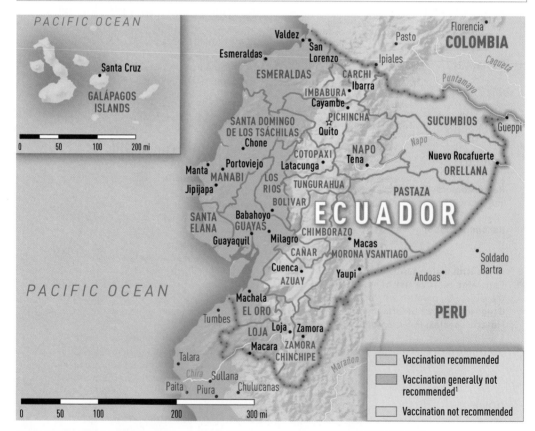

MAP 3-26. YELLOW FEVER VACCINE RECOMMENDATIONS IN ECUADOR[2]

[1,2] See footnotes on page 420 for an explanation of "Vaccination generally not recommended."

*All footnotes are located on page 420.

≥1 year of age, including transit >12 hours in an airport located in a country with risk of YFV transmission.[1]
Recommendations: None.

Malaria
Areas with malaria: Rare cases along Guatemalan border.
Estimated relative risk of malaria for US travelers: Very low.
Drug resistance[4]: None.
Malaria species: *P. vivax* 99%, *P. falciparum* <1%.
Recommended chemoprophylaxis: Mosquito avoidance only.

EQUATORIAL GUINEA
Yellow Fever
Requirements: Required if traveling from a country with risk of YFV transmission and ≥6 months of age.[1]
Recommendations: *Recommended* for all travelers ≥9 months of age.

Malaria
Areas with malaria: All.

Estimated relative risk of malaria for US travelers: Moderate.
Drug resistance[4]: Chloroquine.
Malaria species: *P. falciparum* 85%; *P. malariae*, *P. ovale*, and *P. vivax* 15% combined.
Recommended chemoprophylaxis: Atovaquone-proguanil, doxycycline, or mefloquine.

ERITREA
Yellow Fever
Requirements: Required if traveling from a country with risk of YFV transmission.[1]
Recommendations:
Generally not recommended for travelers going to the following states: Anseba, Debub, Gash Barka, Mae Kel, and Semenawi Keih Bahri.
Not recommended for all areas not listed above, including the Dahlak Archipelago (see Map 3-15).

Malaria
Areas with malaria: All areas <2,200 m (7,218 ft). None in Asmara.
Estimated relative risk of malaria for US travelers: Moderate.

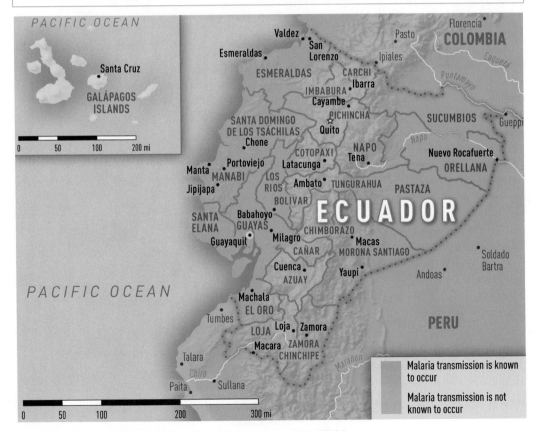

MAP 3-27. MALARIA TRANSMISSION AREAS IN ECUADOR

Drug resistance[4]: Chloroquine.
Malaria species: *P. falciparum* 85%, *P. vivax* 10%–15%, *P. ovale* rare.
Recommended chemoprophylaxis: Atovaquone-proguanil, doxycycline, or mefloquine.

ESTONIA
Yellow Fever
No requirements or recommendations.

Malaria
No malaria transmission.

ETHIOPIA (See Maps 3-28 and 3-29.)
Yellow Fever
Requirements: Required if traveling from a country with risk of YFV transmission and ≥1 year of age, including transit >12 hours in an airport located in a country with risk of YFV transmission.[1]
Recommendations:
Recommended for all travelers ≥9 months of age, except as mentioned below.

Generally not recommended for travelers whose itinerary is limited to the Afar and Somali Provinces (see Map 3-28).

Malaria
Areas with malaria: All areas <2,500 m (8,202 ft), except none in the highly urbanized, central part of the city of Addis Ababa (see Map 3-29).
Estimated relative risk of malaria for US travelers: Moderate.
Drug resistance[4]: Chloroquine.
Malaria species: *P. falciparum* 60%–70%, *P. vivax* 30%–40%, *P. malariae* and *P. ovale* rare.
Recommended chemoprophylaxis: Atovaquone-proguanil, doxycycline, or mefloquine.

FALKLAND ISLANDS (ISLAS MALVINAS)
Yellow Fever
No requirements or recommendations.

MAP 3-28. YELLOW FEVER VACCINE RECOMMENDATIONS IN ETHIOPIA[2]

[1, 2] See footnotes on page 420 for an explanation of "Vaccination generally not recommended."
   *All footnotes are located on page 420.

Malaria
No malaria transmission.

FAROE ISLANDS (DENMARK)
Yellow Fever
No requirements or recommendations.

Malaria
No malaria transmission.

FIJI
Yellow Fever
Requirements: Required if traveling from a country with risk of YFV transmission and ≥1 year of age, including transit >12 hours in an airport located in a country with risk of YFV transmission.[1]
Recommendations: None.

Malaria
No malaria transmission.

FINLAND
Yellow Fever
No requirements or recommendations.

Malaria
No malaria transmission.

FRANCE
Yellow Fever
No requirements or recommendations.

Malaria
No malaria transmission.

FRENCH GUIANA
Yellow Fever
Requirements: Required for arriving travelers from all countries if traveler is ≥1 year of age.
Recommendations: *Recommended* for all travelers ≥9 months of age.

Malaria
Areas with malaria: All areas, including Matoury, Macouria, and Kourou, except none in coastal areas west of Kourou and Cayenne City.
Estimated relative risk of malaria for US travelers: Moderate.

MAP 3-29. MALARIA TRANSMISSION AREAS IN ETHIOPIA

Drug resistance⁴: Chloroquine.
Malaria species: *P. falciparum* <50%, remainder *P. vivax, P. malariae* rare.
Recommended chemoprophylaxis: Atovaquone-proguanil, doxycycline, or mefloquine.

FRENCH POLYNESIA, INCLUDING THE ISLAND GROUPS OF SOCIETY ISLANDS (TAHITI, MOOREA, AND BORA-BORA), MARQUESAS ISLANDS (HIVA OA AND UA HUKA), AND AUSTRAL ISLANDS (TUBUAI AND RURUTU)

Yellow Fever
Requirements: Required if traveling from a country with risk of YFV transmission and ≥1 year of age, including transit >12 hours in an airport located in a country with risk of YFV transmission.[1]
Recommendations: None.

Malaria
No malaria transmission.

GABON
Yellow Fever
Requirements: Required for arriving travelers from all countries if traveler is ≥1 year of age.
Recommendations: *Recommended* for all travelers ≥9 months of age.

Malaria
Areas with malaria: All.
Estimated relative risk of malaria for US travelers: Moderate.
Drug resistance⁴: Chloroquine.
Malaria species: *P. falciparum* 90%; remainder *P. malariae, P. ovale,* and *P. vivax.*
Recommended chemoprophylaxis: Atovaquone-proguanil, doxycycline, or mefloquine.

GAMBIA, THE
Yellow Fever
Requirements: Required if traveling from a country with risk of YFV transmission and ≥9 months of age.[1]
Recommendations: *Recommended* for all travelers ≥9 months of age.

Malaria
Areas with malaria: All.
Estimated relative risk of malaria for US travelers: High.

Drug resistance⁴: Chloroquine.
Malaria species: *P. falciparum* ≥85%, *P. ovale* 5%–10%, *P. malariae* and *P. vivax* rare.
Recommended chemoprophylaxis: Atovaquone-proguanil, doxycycline, or mefloquine.

GEORGIA
Yellow Fever
No requirements or recommendations.

Malaria
No malaria transmission.

GERMANY
Yellow Fever
No requirements or recommendations.

Malaria
No malaria transmission.

GHANA
Yellow Fever
Requirements: Required if traveling from a country with risk of YFV transmission and ≥9 months of age, including transit >12 hours in an airport located in a country with risk of YFV transmission.[1]
Recommendations: *Recommended* for all travelers ≥9 months of age.

Malaria
Areas with malaria: All.
Estimated relative risk of malaria for US travelers: High.
Drug resistance⁴: Chloroquine.
Malaria species: *P. falciparum* 90%, *P. ovale* 5%–10%, *P. vivax* rare.
Recommended chemoprophylaxis: Atovaquone-proguanil, doxycycline, or mefloquine.

GIBRALTAR (UK)
Yellow Fever
No requirements or recommendations.

Malaria
No malaria transmission.

GREECE
Yellow Fever
No requirements or recommendations.

Malaria
Areas with malaria: Sporadic cases and outbreaks last occurring May–November

*All footnotes are located on page 420.

2013 in the agricultural areas of the municipalities of Alexandroupolis (Evros), Avdira (Xanthi), Evrotas (Lakonia), Evia, Lake Paralimni (Viotia), Larisa, Marathon (East Attiki), Markopoulo (East Attiki), Tanagra (Viotia), and Sofades (Karditsa).
Estimated relative risk of malaria for US travelers: None.
Drug resistance: Not applicable.
Malaria species: *P. vivax* in past outbreaks.
Recommended chemoprophylaxis: Not applicable.

GREENLAND (DENMARK)
Yellow Fever
No requirements or recommendations.

Malaria
No malaria transmission.

GRENADA
Yellow Fever
Requirements: Required if traveling from a country with risk of YFV transmission and ≥1 year of age, including transit >12 hours in an airport located in a country with risk of YFV transmission.[1]
Recommendations: None.

Malaria
No malaria transmission.

GUADELOUPE, INCLUDING SAINT-BARTHÉLEMY AND SAINT MARTIN (FRANCE)
Yellow Fever
Requirements: Required if traveling from a country with risk of YFV transmission and ≥1 year of age, including transit >12 hours in an airport located in a country with risk of YFV transmission.[1]
Recommendations: None.

Malaria
No malaria transmission.

GUAM (US)
Yellow Fever
No requirements or recommendations.

Malaria
No malaria transmission.

GUATEMALA
Yellow Fever
Requirements: Required if traveling from a country with risk of YFV transmission and ≥1 year of age.[1]
Recommendations: None.

Malaria
Areas with malaria: Rural areas only at altitudes <1,500 m (4,921 ft). None in Antigua, Guatemala City, or Lake Atitlán.
Estimated relative risk of malaria for US travelers: Low.
Drug resistance[4]: None.
Malaria species: *P. vivax* 97%, *P. falciparum* 3%.
Recommended chemoprophylaxis: Escuintla Province: Atovaquone-proguanil, chloroquine, doxycycline, or mefloquine. All other areas with malaria: Atovaquone-proguanil, chloroquine, doxycycline, mefloquine, or primaquine.[5]

GUINEA
Yellow Fever
Requirements: Required if traveling from a country with risk of YFV transmission and ≥1 year of age.[1]
Recommendations: *Recommended* for all travelers ≥9 months of age.

Malaria
Areas with malaria: All.
Estimated relative risk of malaria for US travelers: High.
Drug resistance[4]: Chloroquine.
Malaria species: *P. falciparum* 85%, *P. ovale* 5%–10%, *P. vivax* rare.
Recommended chemoprophylaxis: Atovaquone-proguanil, doxycycline, or mefloquine.

GUINEA-BISSAU
Yellow Fever
Requirements: Required for arriving travelers from all countries if traveler is ≥1 year of age.
Recommendations: *Recommended* for all travelers ≥9 months of age.

Malaria
Areas with malaria: All.
Estimated relative risk of malaria for US travelers: Moderate.
Drug resistance[4]: Chloroquine.
Malaria species: *P. falciparum* 85%, *P. ovale* 5%–10%, *P. vivax* rare.
Recommended chemoprophylaxis: Atovaquone-proguanil, doxycycline, or mefloquine.

GUYANA
Yellow Fever
Requirements: Required if traveling from a country with risk of YFV transmission and

≥1 year of age.[1] This requirement excludes Argentina, Paraguay, Suriname, and Trinidad and Tobago.

Recommendations: *Recommended* for all travelers ≥9 months of age.

Malaria

Areas with malaria: All areas <900 m (2,953 ft). Rare cases in the cities of Amsterdam and Georgetown.

Estimated relative risk of malaria for US travelers: Moderate.

Drug resistance[4]: Chloroquine.

Malaria species: *P. falciparum* 50%, *P. vivax* 50%.

Recommended chemoprophylaxis: Areas with malaria except cities of Amsterdam and Georgetown: Atovaquone-proguanil, doxycycline, or mefloquine. Cities of Georgetown and Amsterdam: Mosquito avoidance only.

HAITI

Yellow Fever

No requirements or recommendations.

Malaria

Areas with malaria: All (including Port Labadee).

Estimated relative risk of malaria for US travelers: Moderate.

Drug resistance[4]: None.

Malaria species: *P. falciparum* 99%, *P. malariae* rare.

Recommended chemoprophylaxis: Atovaquone-proguanil, chloroquine, doxycycline, or mefloquine.

HONDURAS

Yellow Fever

Requirements: Required if traveling from a country with risk of YFV transmission and ≥1 year of age, including transit >12 hours in an airport located in a country with risk of YFV transmission.[1] This requirement excludes Panama.

Recommendations: None.

Malaria

Areas with malaria: Present throughout the country and in Roatán and other Bay Islands. None in San Pedro Sula and Tegucigalpa.

Estimated relative risk of malaria for US travelers: Moderate.

Drug resistance[4]: None.

Malaria species: *P. vivax* 93%, *P. falciparum* 7%.

Recommended chemoprophylaxis: Atovaquone-proguanil, chloroquine, doxycycline, mefloquine, or primaquine.[5]

HONG KONG SAR (CHINA)

Yellow Fever

No requirements or recommendations.

Malaria

No malaria transmission.

HUNGARY

Yellow Fever

No requirements or recommendations.

Malaria

No malaria transmission.

ICELAND

Yellow Fever

No requirements or recommendations.

Malaria

No malaria transmission.

INDIA (See Map 3-30.)

Yellow Fever

Requirements: Any traveler (except infants <6 months old) arriving by air or sea without a yellow fever vaccination certificate is detained in isolation for up to 6 days if that person—

1) arrives within 6 days of departure from an area with risk of YFV transmission,
2) has been in such an area in transit (except those passengers and members of flight crews who, while in transit through an airport in an area with risk of YFV transmission, remained in the airport during their entire stay and the health officer agrees to such an exemption),
3) arrives on a ship that started from or touched at any port in an area with risk of YFV transmission up to 30 days before its arrival in India, unless such a ship has been disinsected in accordance with the procedure recommended by WHO, or
4) arrives on an aircraft that has been in an area with risk of YFV transmission and has not been disinsected in accordance with the Indian Aircraft Public Health Rules, 1954, or as recommended by WHO.

The following are regarded as countries and areas with risk of YFV transmission:

*All footnotes are located on page 420.

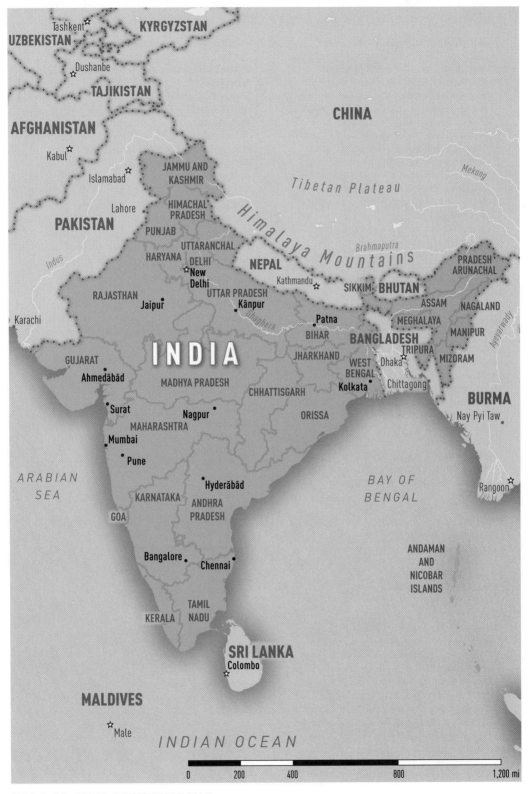

MAP 3-30. INDIA REFERENCE MAP

Africa: Angola, Benin, Burkina Faso, Burundi, Cameroon, Central African Republic, Chad, Congo, Côte d'Ivoire, Democratic Republic of the Congo, Equatorial Guinea, Ethiopia, Gabon, The Gambia, Ghana, Guinea, Guinea-Bissau, Kenya, Liberia, Mali, Mauritania, Niger, Nigeria, Rwanda, Senegal, Sierra Leone, Sudan, South Sudan, Togo, and Uganda.
Americas: Argentina, Bolivia, Brazil, Colombia, Ecuador, French Guiana, Guyana, Panama, Paraguay, Peru, Suriname, Trinidad (Trinidad only), and Venezuela.
Note: When a case of yellow fever is reported from any country, that country is regarded by the government of India as a country with risk of YFV transmission and is added to the above list.
Recommendations: None.

Malaria
Areas with malaria: All areas throughout the country, including cities of Bombay (Mumbai) and Delhi, except none in areas >2,000 m (6,561 ft) in Himachal Pradesh, Jammu and Kashmir, and Sikkim.
Estimated relative risk of malaria for US travelers: Moderate.
Drug resistance[4]: Chloroquine.
Malaria species: *P. vivax* 50%, *P. falciparum* >40%, *P. malariae* and *P. ovale* rare.
Recommended chemoprophylaxis: Atovaquone-proguanil, doxycycline, or mefloquine.

INDONESIA
Yellow Fever
Requirements: Required if traveling from a country with risk of YFV transmission and ≥9 months of age.[1]
Recommendations: None.

Malaria
Areas with malaria: All areas of eastern Indonesia (provinces of Maluku, Maluku Utara, Nusa Tenggara Timur, Papua, and Papua Barat), including the town of Labuan Bajo and Komodo Islands in the Nusa Tenggara region. Rural areas of Kalimantan (Borneo), Nusa Tenggara Barat (includes the island of Lombok), Sulawesi, and Sumatra. Low transmission in rural areas of Java, including Pangandaran, Sukalumi, and Ujung Kulong. None in cities of Jakarta and Ubud, resort areas of Bali and Java, and Gili Islands and the Thousand Islands (Pulau Seribu).
Estimated relative risk of malaria for US travelers: Moderate.
Drug resistance[4]: Chloroquine (*P. falciparum* and *P. vivax*).
Malaria species: *P. falciparum* 66%, remainder primarily *P. vivax*.
Recommended chemoprophylaxis: Atovaquone-proguanil, doxycycline, or mefloquine.

IRAN
Yellow Fever
Requirements: Required if traveling from a country with risk of YFV transmission.[1]
Recommendations: None.

Malaria
Areas with malaria: Rural areas of Fars Province, Sistan-Baluchestan Province, and southern, tropical parts of Hormozgan and Kerman Provinces.
Estimated relative risk of malaria for US travelers: Very low.
Drug resistance[4]: Chloroquine.
Malaria species: *P. vivax* 88%, *P. falciparum* 12%.
Recommended chemoprophylaxis: Atovaquone-proguanil, doxycycline, or mefloquine.

IRAQ
Yellow Fever
Requirements: Required if traveling from a country with risk of YFV transmission and ≥6 months of age.[1]
Recommendations: None.

Malaria
No malaria transmission.

IRELAND
Yellow Fever
No requirements or recommendations.

Malaria
No malaria transmission.

ISRAEL
Yellow Fever
No requirements or recommendations.

Malaria
No malaria transmission.

*All footnotes are located on page 420.

ITALY, INCLUDING HOLY SEE (VATICAN CITY)
Yellow Fever
No requirements or recommendations.

Malaria
No malaria transmission.

JAMAICA
Yellow Fever
Requirements: Required if traveling from a country with risk of YFV transmission and ≥1 year of age, including transit in an airport located in a country with risk of YFV transmission.
Recommendations: None.

Malaria
No malaria transmission.

JAPAN
Yellow Fever
No requirements or recommendations.

Malaria
No malaria transmission.

JORDAN
Yellow Fever
Requirements: Required if traveling from a country with risk of YFV transmission and ≥1 year of age.[1]
Recommendations: None.

Malaria
No malaria transmission.

KAZAKHSTAN
Yellow Fever
Requirements: Required if traveling from a country with risk of YFV transmission.[1]
Recommendations: None.

Malaria
No malaria transmission.

KENYA (See Maps 3-31 and 3-32.)
Yellow Fever
Requirements: Required if traveling from a country with risk of YFV transmission and ≥1 year of age.[1]
Recommendations:
Recommended for all travelers ≥9 months of age, except as mentioned below.
Generally not recommended for travelers whose itinerary is limited to the following areas: the entire North Eastern Province; the states of Kilifi, Kwale, Lamu, Malindi, and Tanariver in the Coast Province; and the cities of Mombasa and Nairobi (see Map 3-31).

Malaria
Areas with malaria: Present in all areas (including game parks) <2,500 m (8,202 ft). None in the highly urbanized, central part of the city of Nairobi (see Map 3-32).
Estimated relative risk of malaria for US travelers: Moderate.
Drug resistance[4]: Chloroquine.
Malaria species: *P. falciparum* 85%, *P. vivax* 5%–10%, *P. ovale* up to 5%.
Recommended chemoprophylaxis: Atovaquone-proguanil, doxycycline, or mefloquine.

KIRIBATI (FORMERLY GILBERT ISLANDS), INCLUDES TARAWA, TABUAERAN (FANNING ISLAND), AND BANABA (OCEAN ISLAND)
Yellow Fever
Requirements: Required if traveling from a country with risk of YFV transmission and ≥1 year of age.[1]
Recommendations: None.

Malaria
No malaria transmission.

KOSOVO
Yellow Fever
Requirements: This country has not stated its yellow fever vaccination certificate requirements.
Recommendations: None.

Malaria
No malaria transmission.

KUWAIT
Yellow Fever
No requirements or recommendations.

Malaria
No malaria transmission.

KYRGYZSTAN
Yellow Fever
Requirements: Required if traveling from a country with risk of YFV transmission and ≥1 year of age, including transit >12 hours in an airport located in a country with risk of YFV transmission.[1]
Recommendations: None.

Malaria
No malaria transmission.

LAOS
Yellow Fever
Requirements: Required if traveling from a country with risk of YFV transmission.[1]
Recommendations: None.

Malaria

Areas with malaria: All, except rare cases in Luang Prabong City, the provinces of Bokeo, Huaphan, and Oudomxay. None in the city of Vientiane.

Estimated relative risk of malaria for US travelers: Very low.

Drug resistance⁴: Chloroquine and mefloquine.

Malaria species: *P. falciparum* 65%, *P. vivax* 34%, *P. malariae* and *P. ovale* 1% combined.

Recommended chemoprophylaxis:
Along the Laos-Burma (Myanmar) border in the provinces of Bokeo and Louang Namtha, along the Laos-Thailand border in the province of Champasak and Saravan, along the Laos-Cambodia border, and along the Laos-Vietnam border: Atovaquone-proguanil or doxycycline.

All other areas with malaria except Luang Prabang City: Atovaquone-proguanil, doxycycline, or mefloquine.

Luang Prabang City: Mosquito avoidance only.

LATVIA

Yellow Fever

No requirements or recommendations.

Malaria

No malaria transmission.

LEBANON

Yellow Fever

Requirements: Required if traveling from a country with risk of YFV transmission and ≥9 months of age, including transit >12 hours in an airport located in a country with risk of YFV transmission.[1]

Recommendations: None.

Malaria

No malaria transmission.

MAP 3-31. YELLOW FEVER VACCINE RECOMMENDATIONS IN KENYA²

[1,2] See footnotes on page 420 for an explanation of "Vaccination generally not recommended."

*All footnotes are located on page 420.

3

LESOTHO
Yellow Fever
Requirements: Required if traveling from a country with risk of YFV transmission and ≥9 months of age, including transit >12 hours in an airport located in a country with risk of YFV transmission.[1]
Recommendations: None.

Malaria
No malaria transmission.

LIBERIA
Yellow Fever
Requirements: Required for arriving travelers from all countries if traveler is ≥1 year of age.
Recommendations: *Recommended* for all travelers ≥9 months of age.

Malaria
Areas with malaria: All.
Estimated relative risk of malaria for US travelers: High.
Drug resistance[4]**:** Chloroquine.

Malaria species: *P. falciparum* 85%, *P. ovale* 5%–10%, *P. vivax* rare.
Recommended chemoprophylaxis: Atovaquone-proguanil, doxycycline, or mefloquine.

LIBYA
Yellow Fever
Requirements: Required if traveling from a country with risk of YFV transmission.[1]
Recommendations: None.

Malaria
No malaria transmission.

LIECHTENSTEIN
Yellow Fever
No requirements or recommendations.

Malaria
No malaria transmission.

LITHUANIA
Yellow Fever
No requirements or recommendations.

MAP 3-32. MALARIA TRANSMISSION AREAS IN KENYA

Malaria
No malaria transmission.

LUXEMBOURG
Yellow Fever
No requirements or recommendations.

Malaria
No malaria transmission.

MACAU SAR (CHINA)
Yellow Fever
No requirements or recommendations.

Malaria
No malaria transmission.

MACEDONIA
Yellow Fever
No requirements or recommendations.

Malaria
No malaria transmission.

MADAGASCAR
Yellow Fever
Requirements: Required if traveling from a country with risk of YFV transmission.[1]
Recommendations: None.

Malaria
Areas with malaria: All areas, except rare cases in the city of Antananarivo.
Estimated relative risk of malaria for US travelers: Moderate.
Drug resistance[4]: Chloroquine.
Malaria species: *P. falciparum* 85%, *P. vivax* 5%–10%, *P. ovale* 5%.
Recommended chemoprophylaxis:
All areas except the city of Antananarivo: Atovaquone-proguanil, doxycycline, or mefloquine.
Antananarivo: Mosquito avoidance only.

MADEIRA ISLANDS (PORTUGAL)
Yellow Fever
No requirements or recommendations.

Malaria
No malaria transmission.

MALAWI
Yellow Fever
Requirements: Required if traveling from a country with risk of YFV transmission and ≥1 year of age, including transit >12 hours in an airport located in a country with risk of YFV transmission.[1]
Recommendations: None.

Malaria
Areas with malaria: All.
Estimated relative risk of malaria for US travelers: Moderate.
Drug resistance[4]: Chloroquine.
Malaria species: *P. falciparum* 90%; *P. malariae, P. ovale,* and *P. vivax* 10% combined.
Recommended chemoprophylaxis:
Atovaquone-proguanil, doxycycline, or mefloquine.

MALAYSIA
Yellow Fever
Requirements: Required if traveling from a country with risk of YFV transmission and ≥1 year of age, including transit >12 hours in an airport located in a country with risk of YFV transmission.[1]
Recommendations: None.

Malaria
Areas with malaria: Present in rural areas.
Estimated relative risk of malaria for US travelers: Low.
Drug resistance[4]: Chloroquine.
Malaria species: *P. falciparum, P. vivax, P. knowlesi, P. malariae,* and *P. ovale.*
Recommended chemoprophylaxis:
Atovaquone-proguanil, doxycycline, or mefloquine.

MALDIVES
Yellow Fever
Requirements: Required if traveling from a country with risk of YFV transmission and ≥1 year of age, including transit >12 hours in an airport located in a country with risk of YFV transmission.[1]
Recommendations: None.

Malaria
No malaria transmission.

MALI
Yellow Fever
Requirements: Required for arriving travelers from all countries if traveler is ≥1 year of age.
Recommendations: *Recommended* for all travelers ≥9 months of age going to areas south of the Sahara Desert (see Map 3-15).

*All footnotes are located on page 420.

Not recommended for travelers whose itineraries are limited to areas in the Sahara Desert (see Map 3-15).

Malaria
Areas with malaria: All.
Estimated relative risk of malaria for US travelers: High.
Drug resistance[4]: Chloroquine.
Malaria species: *P. falciparum* 85%, *P. ovale* 5%–10%, *P. vivax* rare.
Recommended chemoprophylaxis: Atovaquone-proguanil, doxycycline, or mefloquine.

MALTA
Yellow Fever
Requirements: Required if traveling from a country with risk of YFV transmission and ≥9 months of age.[1] If indicated on epidemiologic grounds, infants <9 months of age are subject to isolation or surveillance if coming from an area with risk of YFV transmission. No certificate of yellow fever vaccination is required for travelers having transited through an airport located in a country with risk of YFV transmission.[1]
Recommendations: None.

Malaria
No malaria transmission.

MARSHALL ISLANDS
Yellow Fever
No requirements or recommendations.

Malaria
No malaria transmission.

MARTINIQUE (FRANCE)
Yellow Fever
Requirements: Required if traveling from a country with risk of YFV transmission and ≥1 year of age, including transit >12 hours in an airport located in a country with risk of YFV transmission.[1]
Recommendations: None.

Malaria
No malaria transmission.

MAURITANIA
Yellow Fever
Requirements: Required if traveling from a country with risk of YFV transmission and ≥1 year of age.[1]
Recommendations:

Recommended for all travelers ≥9 months of age traveling to areas south of the Sahara Desert (see Map 3-15).
Not recommended for travelers whose itineraries are limited to areas in the Sahara Desert (see Map 3-15).

Malaria
Areas with malaria: All areas, including the city of Nouakchott.
Estimated relative risk of malaria for US travelers: High.
Drug resistance[4]: Chloroquine.
Malaria species: *P. falciparum* 85%, *P. ovale* 5%–10%, *P. vivax* rare.
Recommended chemoprophylaxis: Atovaquone-proguanil, doxycycline, or mefloquine.

MAURITIUS
Yellow Fever
Requirements: Required if traveling from a country with risk of YFV transmission and ≥1 year of age, including transit >12 hours in an airport located in a country with risk of YFV transmission.[1]
Recommendations: None.

Malaria
No malaria transmission.

MAYOTTE (FRANCE)
Yellow Fever
Requirements: Required if traveling from a country with risk of YFV transmission and ≥1 year of age, including transit >12 hours in an airport located in a country with risk of YFV transmission.[1]
Recommendations: None.

Malaria
Areas with malaria: All.
Estimated relative risk of malaria for US travelers: No data.
Drug resistance[4]: Chloroquine.
Malaria species: *P. falciparum* 40%–50%, *P. vivax* 35%–40%, *P. ovale* <1%.
Recommended chemoprophylaxis: Atovaquone-proguanil, doxycycline, or mefloquine.

MEXICO (See Map 3-33.)
Yellow Fever
Requirements: Required if traveling from a country with risk of YFV transmission and ≥1 year of age, including transit >12 hours in

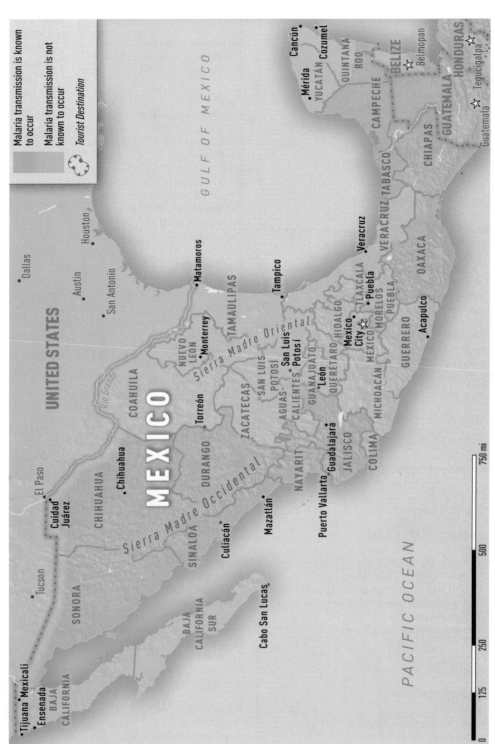

MAP 3-33. MALARIA TRANSMISSION AREAS IN MEXICO

Legend:
- Malaria transmission is known to occur
- Malaria transmission is not known to occur
- ☆ Tourist Destination

an airport located in a country with risk of YFV transmission.[1]
Recommendations: None.

Malaria
Areas with malaria: Present in Chihuahua, Chiapas, Durango, Nayarit, and Sinaloa. Rare cases in Campeche, Jalisco, Oaxaca, Sonora, and Tabasco. Rare cases in the municipality of Othon P. Blanco in the southern part of Quintana Roo bordering Belize. No malaria along the United States–Mexico border (see Map 3-33).
Estimated relative risk of malaria for US travelers: Very low.
Drug resistance[4]: None.
Malaria species: *P. vivax* 100%.
Recommended chemoprophylaxis:
States of Chiapas, Chihuahua, Durango, Nayarit, and Sinaloa: Atovaquone-proguanil, chloroquine, doxycycline, mefloquine, or primaquine.[5]
States of Campeche, Jalisco, Oaxaca, Sonora, Tabasco, and Orthón P. Blanco municipality of Quintana Roo: Mosquito avoidance only.

MICRONESIA, FEDERATED STATES OF; INCLUDES YAP ISLANDS, POHNPEI, CHUUK, AND KOSRAE
Yellow Fever
No requirements or recommendations.

Malaria
No malaria transmission.

MOLDOVA
Yellow Fever
No requirements or recommendations.

Malaria
No malaria transmission.

MONACO
Yellow Fever
No requirements or recommendations.

Malaria
No malaria transmission.

MONGOLIA
Yellow Fever
No requirements or recommendations.

Malaria
No malaria transmission.

MONTENEGRO
Yellow Fever
No requirements or recommendations.

Malaria
No malaria transmission.

MONTSERRAT (UK)
Yellow Fever
Requirements: Required if traveling from a country with risk of YFV transmission and ⩾1 year of age.[1]
Recommendations: None.

Malaria
No malaria transmission.

MOROCCO
Yellow Fever
No requirements or recommendations.

Malaria
No malaria transmission.

MOZAMBIQUE
Yellow Fever
Requirements: Required if traveling from a country with risk of YFV transmission and ⩾1 year of age.[1]
Recommendations: None.

Malaria
Areas with malaria: All.
Estimated relative risk of malaria for US travelers: Moderate.
Drug resistance[4]: Chloroquine.
Malaria species: *P. falciparum* 90%, *P. malariae*, *P. ovale*, and *P. vivax* rare.
Recommended chemoprophylaxis: Atovaquone-proguanil, doxycycline, or mefloquine.

NAMIBIA (See Map 3-34.)
Yellow Fever
Requirements: Required if traveling from a country with risk of YFV transmission. The countries or parts of countries included in the endemic zones in Africa and South America are regarded as areas with risk of YFV transmission.[1] Travelers on scheduled flights that originated outside the countries with risk of YFV transmission, but who have been in transit through these areas, are not required to possess a certificate provided that they remained at the airport or in the adjacent town during transit. All travelers whose flights originated in countries with

*All footnotes are located on page 420.

risk of YFV transmission or who have been in transit through these countries on unscheduled flights are required to possess a certificate. The certificate is not required for children <1 year of age, but such infants may be subject to surveillance.

Recommendations: None.

Malaria

Areas with malaria: Present in the provinces of Kavango (East and West), Kunene, Ohangwena, Omaheke, Omusati, Oshana, Oshikoto, and Otjozondjupa and in the Caprivi Strip. Rare cases in the Gobabis constituency of Omaheke Province and in the constituencies of Grootfontein, Okahandja,

Okakarara, and Otjiwarongo in Otjozundjupa Province.

Estimated relative risk of malaria for US travelers: Low.

Drug resistance[4]: Chloroquine.

Malaria species: *P. falciparum* 90%; *P. malariae*, *P. ovale*, and *P. vivax* 10% combined.

Recommended chemoprophylaxis: Areas with malaria except Omaheke and Otjozundjupa Provinces: Atovaquone-proguanil, doxycycline, or mefloquine. Constituencies of Omaheke and Otjozundjupa Provinces with rare cases: Mosquito avoidance only.

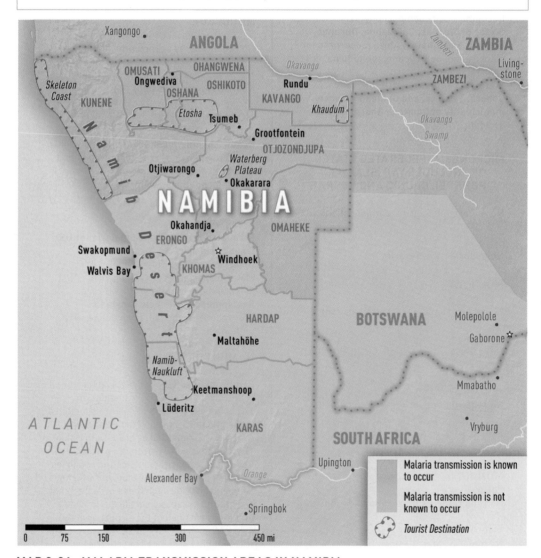

MAP 3-34. MALARIA TRANSMISSION AREAS IN NAMIBIA

*All footnotes are located on page 420.

NAURU
Yellow Fever
Requirements: Required if traveling from a country with risk of YFV transmission and ≥1 year of age.[1]
Recommendations: None.

Malaria
No malaria transmission.

NEPAL
Yellow Fever
Requirements: Required if traveling from a country with risk of YFV transmission.[1]
Recommendations: None.

Malaria
Areas with malaria: Present throughout the country at altitudes <2,000 m (6,561 ft). None in Kathmandu and on typical Himalayan treks.
Estimated relative risk of malaria for US travelers: Low.
Drug resistance[4]: Chloroquine.
Malaria species: *P. vivax* 85%, *P. falciparum* 15%.
Recommended chemoprophylaxis: Atovaquone-proguanil, doxycycline, or mefloquine.

NETHERLANDS, THE
Yellow Fever
No requirements or recommendations.

Malaria
No malaria transmission.

NEW CALEDONIA (FRANCE)
Yellow Fever
Requirements: Required if traveling from a country with risk of YFV transmission and ≥1 year of age, including transit >12 hours in an airport located in a country with risk of YFV transmission.[1] *Note:* In the event of an epidemic threat to the territory, a specific vaccination certificate may be required.
Recommendations: None.

Malaria
No malaria transmission.

NEW ZEALAND
Yellow Fever
No requirements or recommendations.

Malaria
No malaria transmission.

NICARAGUA (See Map 3-35.)
Yellow Fever
No requirements or recommendations.

Malaria
Areas with malaria: Present in districts of Chinandega, Jinotega, Leon, Managua, Matagalpa, Región Autónoma Atlántico Norte (RAAN), and Región Autónoma Atlántico Sur (RAAS). Rare cases in Boaco, Carazo, Masaya, and Rio San Juan.
Estimated relative risk of malaria for US travelers: Low.
Drug resistance[4]: None.
Malaria species: *P. vivax* 90%, *P. falciparum* 10%.
Recommended chemoprophylaxis: Districts with malaria except Boaco, Masaya, Carazo, and Rio San Juan: Atovaquone-proguanil, chloroquine, doxycycline, mefloquine, or primaquine.[5] For Boaco, Masaya, Carazo, and Rio San Juan: Mosquito avoidance only.

NIGER
Yellow Fever
Requirements: Required for arriving travelers from all countries if traveler is ≥1 year of age. The government of Niger recommends vaccine for travelers departing Niger.
Recommendations:
Recommended for all travelers ≥9 months of age traveling to areas south of the Sahara Desert (see Map 3-15).
Not recommended for travelers whose itineraries are limited to areas in the Sahara Desert (see Map 3-15).

Malaria
Areas with malaria: All.
Estimated relative risk of malaria for US travelers: High.
Drug resistance[4]: Chloroquine.
Malaria species: *P. falciparum* 85%, *P. ovale* 5%–10%, *P. vivax* rare.
Recommended chemoprophylaxis: Atovaquone-proguanil, doxycycline, or mefloquine.

NIGERIA
Yellow Fever
Requirements: Required if traveling from a country with risk of YFV transmission and ≥1 year of age.[1]
Recommendations: *Recommended* for all travelers ≥9 months of age.

Malaria
Areas with malaria: All.
Estimated relative risk of malaria for US travelers: High.
Drug resistance⁴: Chloroquine.
Malaria species: *P. falciparum* 85%, *P. ovale* 5%–10%, *P. vivax* rare.
Recommended chemoprophylaxis: Atovaquone-proguanil, doxycycline, or mefloquine.

NIUE (NEW ZEALAND)
Yellow Fever
Requirements: Required if traveling from a country with risk of YFV transmission and ≥9 months of age.¹
Recommendations: None.

Malaria
No malaria transmission.

NORFOLK ISLAND (AUSTRALIA)
Yellow Fever
Requirements: Required if traveling from a country with risk of YFV transmission and ≥1 year of age, including transit >12 hours in an airport located in a country with risk of YFV transmission. This requirement excludes Galapagos Islands in Ecuador and the island of Tobago and is limited to Misiones Province in Argentina.
Recommendations: None.

Malaria
No malaria transmission.

NORTH KOREA
Yellow Fever
Requirements: Required if traveling from a country with risk of YFV transmission and ≥1 year of age.¹
Recommendations: None.

Malaria
Areas with malaria: Present in southern provinces.
Estimated relative risk of malaria for US travelers: No data.
Drug resistance⁴: None.
Malaria species: Presumed to be 100% *P. vivax*.

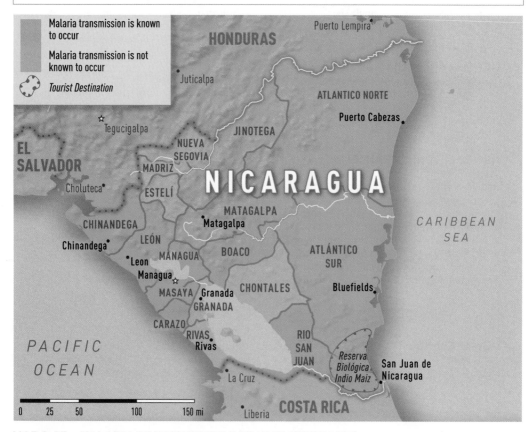

MAP 3-35 . MALARIA TRANSMISSION AREAS IN NICARAGUA

*All footnotes are located on page 420.

Recommended chemoprophylaxis:
Atovaquone-proguanil, chloroquine,
doxycycline, mefloquine, or primaquine.[5]

NORTHERN MARIANA ISLANDS (US), INCLUDES SAIPAN, TINIAN, AND ROTA ISLAND
Yellow Fever
No requirements or recommendations.

Malaria
No malaria transmission.

NORWAY
Yellow Fever
No requirements or recommendations.

Malaria
No malaria transmission.

OMAN
Yellow Fever
Requirements: Required if traveling from a
country with risk of YFV transmission and
≥9 months of age, including transit >12 hours
in an airport located in a country with risk of
YFV transmission.[1]
Recommendations: None.

Malaria
Areas with malaria: Sporadic transmission
in Dakhliyah, North Batinah, and North and
South Sharqiyah.
**Estimated relative risk of malaria for US
travelers:** Very low.
Drug resistance[4]: Chloroquine.
Malaria species: *P. falciparum* and *P. vivax*.
Recommended chemoprophylaxis: Mosquito
avoidance only.

PAKISTAN
Yellow Fever
Requirements: Required if traveling from
any part of a country where there is risk
of YFV transmission and ≥9 months of age,
including transit >12 hours in an airport
located in a country with risk of YFV
transmission.[1]
Recommendations: None.

Malaria
Areas with malaria: All areas (including all
cities) <2,500 m (8,202 ft).
**Estimated relative risk of malaria for US
travelers:** Moderate.
Drug resistance[4]: Chloroquine.

Malaria species: *P. falciparum* 30%,
P. vivax 70%.
Recommended chemoprophylaxis:
Atovaquone-proguanil, doxycycline, or
mefloquine.

PALAU
Yellow Fever
No requirements or recommendations.

Malaria
No malaria transmission.

PANAMA (See Maps 3-36 and 3-37.)
Yellow Fever
Requirements: None.
Recommendations:
Recommended for all travelers ≥9 months
of age traveling to all mainland areas
east of the area surrounding the canal
(the entire *comarcas* of Emberá and Kuna
Yala, the entire province of Darién, and areas
of the provinces of Colón and Panamá that
are east of the Canal) (see Map 3-36).
Not recommended for travelers whose
itineraries are limited to areas west
of the canal, the city of Panama, the
canal area itself, and the Balboa Islands
(Pearl Islands) and San Blas Islands (see
Map 3-36).

Malaria
Areas with malaria: Transmission occurs
primarily in the provinces east of the Panama
Canal and Ngäbe-Buglé Comarca. Rare cases
in the provinces of Bocas del Toro, Colón, and
Veraguas. None in the provinces of Coclé,
Chiriquí, Herrera, Los Santos, San Miguelito,
and the part of Panamá Province west of
the canal. None in the city of Panama (see
Map 3-37).
**Estimated relative risk of malaria for US
travelers:** Low.
Drug resistance[4]: Chloroquine (east of the
Panama Canal).
Malaria species: *P. vivax* 99%,
P. falciparum 1%.
Recommended chemoprophylaxis:
Provinces east of the Panama
Canal: Atovaquone-proguanil, doxycycline,
mefloquine, or primaquine.[5]
Ngäbe-Buglé Comarca:
Atovaquone-proguanil, chloroquine,
doxycycline, mefloquine, or primaquine[7].
Other areas with malaria: Mosquito
avoidance only.

PAPUA NEW GUINEA

Yellow Fever

Requirements: Required if traveling from a country with risk of YFV transmission and ≥1 year of age.[1]
Recommendations: None.

Malaria

Areas with malaria: Present throughout the country at altitudes <2,000 m (6,561 ft).
Estimated relative risk of malaria for US travelers: High.
Drug resistance[4]: Chloroquine (both *P. falciparum* and *P. vivax*).
Malaria species: *P. falciparum* 65%–80%, *P. vivax* 10%–30%, remainder *P. malariae* and *P. ovale*.
Recommended chemoprophylaxis: Atovaquone-proguanil, doxycycline, or mefloquine.

PARAGUAY (See Map 3-38.)

Yellow Fever

Requirements: Required if traveling from a country with risk of YFV transmission and ≥1 year of age.[1]
Recommendations:
Recommended for all travelers ≥9 months of age, except as mentioned below.
Generally not recommended for travelers whose itinerary is limited to the city of Asunción.

Malaria

Areas with malaria: Rare cases in the departments of Alto Paraná, Caaguazú, and Canendiyú.
Estimated relative risk of malaria for US travelers: Very low.
Drug resistance[4]: None.
Malaria species: *P. vivax* 95%, *P. falciparum* 5%.

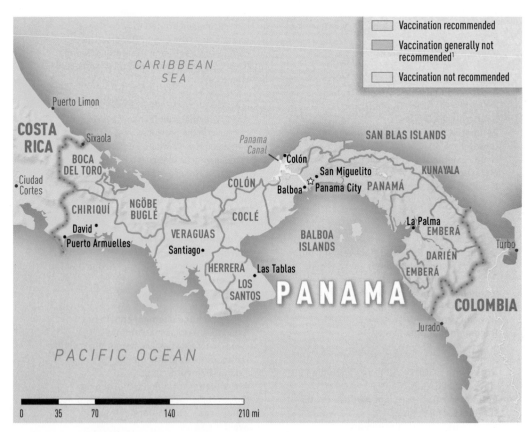

MAP 3-36. YELLOW FEVER VACCINE RECOMMENDATIONS IN PANAMA[2]

[1,2] See footnotes on page 420 for an explanation of "Vaccination generally not recommended."

*All footnotes are located on page 420.

3

Recommended chemoprophylaxis: Mosquito avoidance only.

PERU (See Maps 3-39 and 3-40.)
Yellow Fever
Requirements: None.
Recommendations:
Recommended for all travelers ≥9 months of age going to the following areas at elevations below 2,300 m: the Regions of Amazonas, Loreto, Madre de Dios, San Martin, Ucayali, Puno, Cusco, Junín, Pasco, and Huánuco, and designated areas (see Map 3-39) of the following Regions: far north of Apurimac, far northern Huancavelica, far northeastern Ancash, eastern La Libertad, northern and eastern Cajamarca, northern and northeastern Ayacucho, and eastern Piura.
Generally not recommended for travelers whose itineraries are limited to the following areas west of the Andes: Regions of Lambayeque and Tumbes and the designated areas (see Map 3-39) of western Piura and south, west, and central Cajamarca.

Not recommended for travelers whose itineraries are limited to the following areas: all areas above 2,300 m elevation, areas west of the Andes not listed above, the city of Cusco, the capital city of Lima, Machu Picchu, and the Inca Trail (see Map 3-39).

Malaria
Areas with malaria: All departments <2,000 m (6,561 ft), including the cities of Iquitos and Puerto Maldonado and only the remote eastern regions of La Libertad and Lambayeque. None in the following areas: Lima Province; the cities of Arequipa, Ica, Moquegua, Nazca, Puno, and Tacna; the highland tourist areas (Cusco, Machu Picchu, and Lake Titicaca); and along the Pacific Coast (see Map 3-40).
Estimated relative risk of malaria for US travelers: Low.
Drug resistance[4]: Chloroquine.
Malaria species: *P. vivax* 85%, *P. falciparum* 15%.

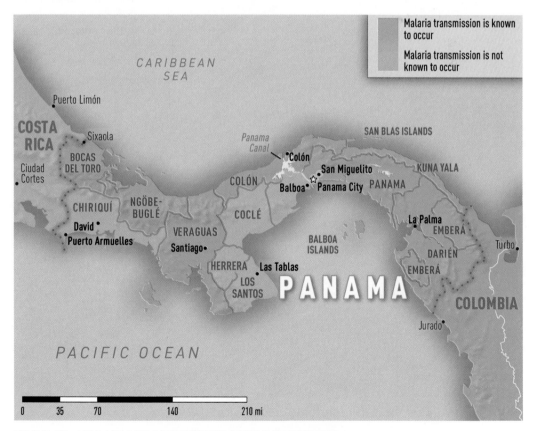

MAP 3-37. MALARIA TRANSMISSION AREAS IN PANAMA

Recommended chemoprophylaxis:
Atovaquone-proguanil, doxycycline, or mefloquine.

PHILIPPINES

Yellow Fever

Requirements: Required if traveling from a country with risk of YFV transmission and ≥1 year of age, including transit in an airport located in a country with risk of YFV transmission.[1]
Recommendations: None.

Malaria

Areas with malaria: Present in rural areas <600 m (1,969 ft) on the islands of Basilu, Luzon, Mindanao, Mindoro, Palawan, Sulu (Jolo), and Tawi-Tawi. None in Manila and other urban areas.
Estimated relative risk of malaria for US travelers: Low.
Drug resistance[4]: Chloroquine.
Malaria species: *P. falciparum* 70%–80%, *P. vivax* 20%–30%.

Recommended chemoprophylaxis:
Atovaquone-proguanil, doxycycline, or mefloquine.

PITCAIRN ISLANDS (UK)

Yellow Fever

Requirements: Required if traveling from a country with risk of YFV transmission and ≥1 year of age.[1]
Recommendations: None.

Malaria
No malaria transmission.

POLAND

Yellow Fever
No requirements or recommendations.

Malaria
No malaria transmission.

PORTUGAL

Yellow Fever
No requirements or recommendations.

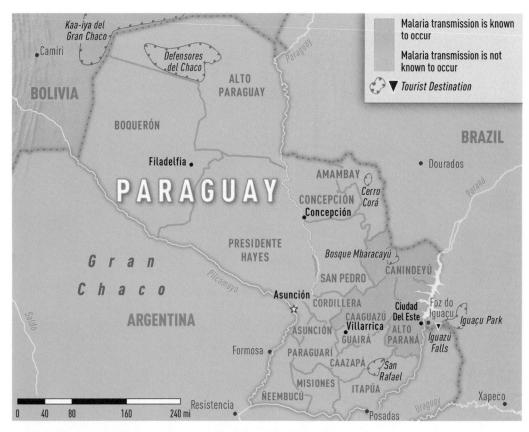

MAP 3-38. MALARIA TRANSMISSION AREAS IN PARAGUAY

*All footnotes are located on page 420.

MAP 3-39. YELLOW FEVER VACCINE RECOMMENDATIONS IN PERU[2]

[1,2] See footnotes on page 420 for an explanation of "Vaccination generally not recommended."

MAP 3-40. MALARIA TRANSMISSION AREAS IN PERU

Malaria
No malaria transmission.

PUERTO RICO (US)
Yellow Fever
No requirements or recommendations.

Malaria
No malaria transmission.

QATAR
Yellow Fever
No requirements or recommendations.

Malaria
No malaria transmission.

RÉUNION (FRANCE)
Yellow Fever
Requirements: Required if traveling from a country with risk of YFV transmission and ⩾1 year of age, including transit >12 hours in an airport located in a country with risk of YFV transmission.[1]
Recommendations: None.

Malaria
No malaria transmission.

ROMANIA
Yellow Fever
No requirements or recommendations.

Malaria
No malaria transmission.

RUSSIA
Yellow Fever
No requirements or recommendations.

Malaria
No malaria transmission.

RWANDA
Yellow Fever
Requirements: Required for arriving travelers from all countries if traveler is ⩾1 year of age.
Recommendations: *Recommended* for all travelers ⩾9 months of age.

Malaria
Areas with malaria: All.
Estimated relative risk of malaria for US travelers: Moderate.

Drug resistance[4]: Chloroquine.
Malaria species: *P. falciparum* 90%, *P. vivax* 5%, *P. ovale* 5%.
Recommended chemoprophylaxis: Atovaquone-proguanil, doxycycline, or mefloquine.

SABA
Yellow Fever
Requirements: Required if traveling from a country with risk of YFV transmission and ⩾6 months of age.[1]
Recommendations: None.

Malaria
No malaria transmission.

SAINT HELENA (UK)
Yellow Fever
Requirements: Required if traveling from a country with risk of YFV transmission and ⩾1 year of age.[1]
Recommendations: None.

Malaria
No malaria transmission.

SAINT KITTS (SAINT CHRISTOPHER) AND NEVIS (UK)
Yellow Fever
Requirements: Required if traveling from a country with risk of YFV transmission and ⩾1 year of age.[1]
Recommendations: None.

Malaria
No malaria transmission.

SAINT LUCIA
Yellow Fever
Requirements: Required if traveling from a country with risk of YFV transmission and ⩾1 year of age.[1]
Recommendations: None.

Malaria
No malaria transmission.

SAINT PIERRE AND MIQUELON (FRANCE)
Yellow Fever
No requirements or recommendations.

Malaria
No malaria transmission.

*All footnotes are located on page 420.

SAINT VINCENT AND THE GRENADINES
Yellow Fever
Requirements: Required if traveling from a country with risk of YFV transmission and ≥1 year of age.[1]
Recommendations: None.

Malaria
No malaria transmission.

SAMOA (FORMERLY WESTERN SAMOA)
Yellow Fever
Requirements: Required if traveling from a country with risk of YFV transmission and ≥1 year of age, including transit >12 hours in an airport located in a country with risk of YFV transmission.[1]
Recommendations: None.

Malaria
No malaria transmission.

SAN MARINO
Yellow Fever
No requirements or recommendations.

Malaria
No malaria transmission.

SÃO TOMÉ AND PRÍNCIPE
Yellow Fever
Requirements: Required if traveling from a country with risk of YFV transmission and ≥1 year of age, including transit >12 hours in an airport located in a country with risk of YFV transmission.[1]
Recommendations: *Generally not recommended* for travelers to São Tomé and Príncipe.

Malaria
Areas with malaria: All.
Estimated relative risk of malaria for US travelers: Very low.
Drug resistance[4]**:** Chloroquine.
Malaria species: *P. falciparum* 85%; remainder *P. malariae*, *P. ovale*, and *P. vivax*.
Recommended chemoprophylaxis: Atovaquone-proguanil, doxycycline, or mefloquine.

SAUDI ARABIA
Yellow Fever
Requirements: Required if traveling from a country with risk of YFV transmission and ≥1 year of age, including transit in an airport located in a country with risk of YFV transmission.[1]
Recommendations: None.

Malaria
Areas with malaria: Present in emirates by border with Yemen, specifically Asir and Jizan. None in the cities of Jeddah, Mecca, Medina, Riyadh, and Ta'if.
Estimated relative risk of malaria for US travelers: Very low.
Drug resistance[4]**:** Chloroquine.
Malaria species: *P. falciparum* predominantly, remainder *P. vivax*.
Recommended chemoprophylaxis: Atovaquone-proguanil, doxycycline, or mefloquine.

SENEGAL
Yellow Fever
Requirements: Required if traveling from a country with risk of YFV transmission and ≥9 months of age, including transit in an airport located in a country with risk of YFV transmission.[1]
Recommendations: *Recommended* for all travelers ≥9 months of age.

Malaria
Areas with malaria: All.
Estimated relative risk of malaria for US travelers: High.
Drug resistance[4]**:** Chloroquine.
Malaria species: *P. falciparum* >85%, *P. ovale* 5%–10%, *P. vivax* rare.
Recommended chemoprophylaxis: Atovaquone-proguanil, doxycycline, or mefloquine.

SERBIA
Yellow Fever
No requirements or recommendations.

Malaria
No malaria transmission.

SEYCHELLES
Yellow Fever
Requirements: Required if traveling from a country with risk of YFV transmission and ≥1 year of age, including transit in an airport located in a country with risk of YFV transmission.[1]
Recommendations: None.

Malaria
No malaria transmission.

*All footnotes are located on page 420.

SIERRA LEONE
Yellow Fever
Requirements: Required for arriving travelers from all countries.
Recommendations: *Recommended* for all travelers ≥9 months of age.

Malaria
Areas with malaria: All.
Estimated relative risk of malaria for US travelers: High.
Drug resistance[4]: Chloroquine.
Malaria species: *P. falciparum* 85%, *P. ovale potentially* 5%–10%, *P. malariae* and *P. vivax* rare.
Recommended chemoprophylaxis: Atovaquone-proguanil, doxycycline, or mefloquine.

SINGAPORE
Yellow Fever
Requirements: Required for travelers who are ≥1 year of age who, within the preceding 6 days, have been in or have been in transit >12 hours in an airport located in a country with risk of YFV transmission.[1]
Recommendations: None.

Malaria
No malaria transmission.

SINT EUSTATIUS
Yellow Fever
Requirements: Required if traveling from a country with risk of YFV transmission and ≥6 months of age.[1]
Recommendations: None.

Malaria
No malaria transmission.

SINT MAARTEN
Yellow Fever
Requirements: Required if traveling from a country with risk of YFV transmission and ≥6 months of age.[1]
Recommendations: None.

Malaria
No malaria transmission.

SLOVAKIA
Yellow Fever
No requirements or recommendations.

Malaria
No malaria transmission.

SLOVENIA
Yellow Fever
No requirements or recommendations.

Malaria
No malaria transmission.

SOLOMON ISLANDS
Yellow Fever
Requirements: Required if traveling from a country with risk of YFV transmission.[1]
Recommendations: None.

Malaria
Areas with malaria: All.
Estimated relative risk of malaria for US travelers: High.
Drug resistance[4]: Chloroquine.
Malaria species: *P. falciparum* 60%, *P. vivax* 35%–40%, *P. ovale* <1%.
Recommended chemoprophylaxis: Atovaquone-proguanil, doxycycline, or mefloquine.

SOMALIA
Yellow Fever
Requirements: Required if traveling from a country with risk of YFV transmission.[1]
Recommendations:
Generally not recommended for travelers going to the following regions: Bakool, Banaadir, Bay, Galguduud, Gedo, Hiiraan, Lower Jubabada, Lower Shabelle, Middle Jubabada, and Middle Shabelle (see Map 3-15).
Not recommended for all other areas not listed above.

Malaria
Areas with malaria: All.
Estimated relative risk of malaria for US travelers: High.
Drug resistance[4]: Chloroquine.
Malaria species: *P. falciparum* 90%, *P. vivax* 5%–10%, *P. malariae* and *P. ovale* rare.
Recommended chemoprophylaxis: Atovaquone-proguanil, doxycycline, or mefloquine.

SOUTH AFRICA (See Map 3-41.)
Yellow Fever
Requirements: Required if traveling from a country with risk of YFV transmission and ≥1 year of age, including transit >12 hours in an airport located in a country with risk of YFV transmission.[1]
Recommendations: None.

Malaria

Areas with malaria: Present in northeastern KwaZulu-Natal Province as far south as the Tugela River, Limpopo (Northern) Province, and Mpumalanga Province. Present in Kruger National Park.

Estimated relative risk of malaria for US travelers: Low.

Drug resistance[4]: Chloroquine.

Malaria species: *P. falciparum* 90%, *P. vivax* 5%, *P. ovale* 5%.

Recommended chemoprophylaxis: Atovaquone-proguanil, doxycycline, or mefloquine.

SOUTH GEORGIA AND SOUTH SANDWICH ISLANDS (UK)

Yellow Fever

Requirements: This country has not stated its yellow fever vaccination certificate requirements.

Recommendations: None.

Malaria

No malaria transmission.

SOUTH KOREA

Yellow Fever

No requirements or recommendations.

Malaria

Areas with malaria: Limited to the months of March–December in rural areas in the northern parts of Incheon, Kangwon-do, and Kyônggi-do Provinces, including the demilitarized zone (DMZ).

Estimated relative risk of malaria for US travelers: Low.

Drug resistance[4]: None.

Malaria species: *P. vivax* 100%.

MAP 3-41. MALARIA TRANSMISSION AREAS IN SOUTH AFRICA

*All footnotes are located on page 420.

Recommended chemoprophylaxis:
Atovaquone-proguanil, chloroquine,
doxycycline, mefloquine, or primaquine.[5]

SOUTH SUDAN, REPUBLIC OF
Yellow Fever
Requirements: None.
Recommendations: *Recommended* for all
travelers ≥9 months of age.

Malaria
Areas with malaria: All.
**Estimated relative risk of malaria for US
travelers:** High.
Drug resistance[4]: Chloroquine.
Malaria species: *P. falciparum* 90%, *P. vivax*
5%–10%, *P. malariae* and *P. ovale* rare.
Recommended chemoprophylaxis:
Atovaquone-proguanil, doxycycline, or
mefloquine.

SPAIN
Yellow Fever
No requirements or recommendations.

Malaria
No malaria transmission.

SRI LANKA
Yellow Fever
Requirements: Required if traveling
from a country with risk of YFV
transmission and ≥9 months of age,
including transit >12 hours in an airport
located in a country with risk of YFV
transmission.[1]
Recommendations: None.

Malaria
Areas with malaria: Last locally transmitted
cases in October 2012.
**Estimated relative risk of malaria for US
travelers:** None.
Drug resistance[4]: Not applicable.
Malaria species: Not applicable.
Recommended chemoprophylaxis: Not
applicable.

SUDAN
Yellow Fever
Requirements: Required if traveling
from a country with risk of YFV
transmission and ≥9 months of age.[1]
A certificate may be required for travelers
departing Sudan.
Recommendations:
Recommended for all travelers ≥9 months of
age traveling to areas south of the Sahara
Desert (see Map 3-15).

Not recommended for travelers whose
itineraries are limited to areas in the Sahara
Desert and the city of Khartoum (see
Map 3-15).

Malaria
Areas with malaria: All.
**Estimated relative risk of malaria for US
travelers:** High.
Drug resistance[4]: Chloroquine.
Malaria species: *P. falciparum* 90%, *P. vivax*
5%–10%, *P. malariae* and *P. ovale* rare.
Recommended chemoprophylaxis:
Atovaquone-proguanil, doxycycline, or
mefloquine.

SURINAME
Yellow Fever
Requirements: Required if traveling from a
country with risk of YFV transmission and
≥1 year of age.[1]
Recommendations: *Recommended* for all
travelers ≥9 months of age.

Malaria
Areas with malaria: Present in provinces of
Brokopondo and Sipaliwini. Rare cases in
Paramaribo.
**Estimated relative risk of malaria for US
travelers:** Moderate.
Drug resistance[4]: Chloroquine.
Malaria species: *P. falciparum* 70%, *P. vivax*
15%–20%.
Recommended chemoprophylaxis:
Brokopondo and Sipaliwini:
Atovaquone-proguanil, doxycycline, or
mefloquine.
Paramaribo: Mosquito avoidance only.

SWAZILAND
Yellow Fever
Requirements: Required if traveling from a
country with risk of YFV transmission.[1]
Recommendations: None.

Malaria
Areas with malaria: Present in eastern
areas bordering Mozambique and South
Africa, including all of Lubombo district and
the eastern half of Hhohho, Manzini, and
Shiselweni districts.
**Estimated relative risk of malaria for US
travelers:** Very low.
Drug resistance[4]: Chloroquine.
Malaria species: *P. falciparum* 90%, *P. vivax*
5%, *P. ovale* 5%.
Recommended chemoprophylaxis:
Atovaquone-proguanil, doxycycline, or
mefloquine.

SWEDEN
Yellow Fever
No requirements or recommendations.

Malaria
No malaria transmission.

SWITZERLAND
Yellow Fever
No requirements or recommendations.

Malaria
No malaria transmission.

SYRIA
Yellow Fever
No requirements or recommendations.

Malaria
No malaria transmission.

TAIWAN
Yellow Fever
No requirements or recommendations.

Malaria
No malaria transmission.

TAJIKISTAN
Yellow Fever
No requirements or recommendations.

Malaria
Areas with malaria: Rare indigenous cases.
Estimated relative risk of malaria for US travelers: Very low.
Drug resistance[4]: Chloroquine.
Malaria species: *P. vivax* 90%, *P. falciparum* 10%.
Recommended chemoprophylaxis: Mosquito avoidance only.

TANZANIA
Yellow Fever
Requirements: Required if traveling from a country with risk of YFV transmission and ≥1 year of age, including transit >12 hours in an airport located in a country with risk of YFV transmission.[1]
Recommendations: *Generally not recommended* for travelers to Tanzania.

Malaria
Areas with malaria: All areas <1,800 m (5,906 ft).
Estimated relative risk of malaria for US travelers: Moderate.

Drug resistance[4]: Chloroquine.
Malaria species: *P. falciparum* >85%, *P. ovale* >10%, *P. malariae* and *P. vivax* rare.
Recommended chemoprophylaxis: Atovaquone-proguanil, doxycycline, or mefloquine.

THAILAND
Yellow Fever
Requirements: Required if traveling from a country with risk of YFV transmission and ≥1 year of age, including transit in an airport located in a country with risk of YFV transmission.[1]
Recommendations: None.

Malaria
Areas with malaria: Primarily in provinces that border Burma (Myanmar), Cambodia, and Laos and the provinces of Kalasin, Krabi (Plai Phraya district), Nakhon Si Thammarat, Narathiwat, Pattani, Phang Nga (including Phang Nga City), Rayong, Sakon Nakhon, Songkhla, Surat Thani, and Yala, especially the forest and forest fringe areas of these provinces. Rare to few cases in other parts of Thailand, including other parts of Krabi Province and the cities of Bangkok, Chang Mai, Chang Rai, Koh Phangan, Koh Samui, and Phuket. None in the islands of Krabi Province (Koh Phi Phi, Koh Yao Noi, Koh Yao Yai, and Ko Lanta) and Pattaya City.
Estimated relative risk of malaria for US travelers: Low.
Drug resistance[4]: Chloroquine and mefloquine.
Malaria species: *P. falciparum* 50% (up to 75% in some areas), *P. vivax* 50% (up to 60% in some areas), remainder *P. ovale*.
Recommended chemoprophylaxis: Provinces that border Burma (Myanmar), Cambodia, and Laos, the provinces of Kalasin, Plai Phraya district of Krabi, Nakhon Si Thammarat, Narathiwat, Pattani, Phang Nga (including Phang Nga City), Rayong, Sakon Nakhon, Songkhla, Surat Thani, and Yala: Atovaquone-proguanil or doxycycline. All other areas of Thailand with malaria including the cities of Bangkok, Chang Mai, Chang Rai, Koh Phangan, Koh Samui, and Phuket: Mosquito avoidance only.

TIMOR-LESTE
Yellow Fever
Requirements: Required if traveling from a country with risk of YFV transmission and ≥1 year of age.[1]

*All footnotes are located on page 420.

Recommendations: None.

Malaria
Areas with malaria: All.
Estimated relative risk of malaria for US travelers: No data.
Drug resistance⁴: Chloroquine.
Malaria Species: *P. falciparum* 50%, *P. vivax* 50%, *P. ovale* <1%, *P. malariae* <1%.
Recommended chemoprophylaxis: Atovaquone-proguanil, doxycycline, or mefloquine.

TOGO
Yellow Fever
Requirements: Required for arriving travelers from all countries if traveler is ≥1 year of age.
Recommendations: *Recommended* for all travelers ≥9 months of age.

Malaria
Areas with malaria: All.
Estimated relative risk of malaria for US travelers: High.
Drug resistance⁴: Chloroquine.
Malaria species: *P. falciparum* 85%, *P. ovale* 5%–10%, remainder *P. vivax*.
Recommended chemoprophylaxis: Atovaquone-proguanil, doxycycline, or mefloquine.

TOKELAU (NEW ZEALAND)
Yellow Fever
No requirements or recommendations.

Malaria
No malaria transmission.

TONGA
Yellow Fever
No requirements or recommendations.

Malaria
No malaria transmission.

TRINIDAD AND TOBAGO
Yellow Fever
Requirements: Required if traveling from a country with risk of YFV transmission and ≥1 year of age, including transit in an airport located in a country with risk of YFV transmission.¹
Recommendations:
Recommended for all travelers ≥9 months of age traveling to the island of Trinidad, except as mentioned below.
Generally not recommended for travelers whose itinerary is limited to the urban

areas of the capital city of Port of Spain, cruise ship passengers who do not disembark from the ship, and airplane passengers in transit.
Not recommended for travelers whose itineraries are limited to the island of Tobago.

Malaria
No malaria transmission.

TUNISIA
Yellow Fever
Requirements: Required if traveling from a country with risk of YFV transmission and ≥1 year of age.¹
Recommendations: None.

Malaria
No malaria transmission.

TURKEY
Yellow Fever
No requirements or recommendations.

Malaria
Areas with malaria: Rare indigenous cases in Mardin. None on the Incerlik US Air Force Base or on typical cruise itineraries.
Estimated relative risk of malaria for US travelers: Very low.
Drug resistance⁴: None.
Malaria species: *P. vivax* predominantly, *P. falciparum* sporadically.
Recommended chemoprophylaxis: Mosquito avoidance only.

TURKMENISTAN
Yellow Fever
No requirements or recommendations.

Malaria
No malaria transmission.

TURKS AND CAICOS ISLANDS (UK)
Yellow Fever
Requirements: This country has not stated its yellow fever vaccination certificate requirements.
Recommendations: None.

Malaria
No malaria transmission.

TUVALU
Yellow Fever
No requirements or recommendations.

Malaria
No malaria transmission.

UGANDA

Yellow Fever

Requirements: Required if traveling from a country with risk of YFV transmission and ≥1 year of age.[1]
Recommendations: *Recommended* for all travelers ≥9 months of age.

Malaria
Areas with malaria: All.
Estimated relative risk of malaria for US travelers: High.
Drug resistance[4]: Chloroquine.
Malaria species: *P. falciparum* >85%; remainder *P. malariae, P. ovale,* and *P. vivax.*
Recommended chemoprophylaxis: Atovaquone-proguanil, doxycycline, or mefloquine.

UKRAINE

Yellow Fever
No requirements or recommendations.

Malaria
No malaria transmission.

UNITED ARAB EMIRATES

Yellow Fever
No requirements or recommendations.

Malaria
No malaria transmission.

UNITED KINGDOM, WITH CHANNEL ISLANDS AND ISLE OF MAN

Yellow Fever
No requirements or recommendations.

Malaria
No malaria transmission.

UNITED STATES

Yellow Fever
No requirements or recommendations.

Malaria
No malaria transmission.

URUGUAY

Yellow Fever
No requirements or recommendations.

Malaria
No malaria transmission.

UZBEKISTAN

Yellow Fever
No requirements or recommendations.

Malaria
No malaria transmission.

VANUATU

Yellow Fever
No requirements or recommendations.

Malaria
Areas with malaria: All.
Estimated relative risk of malaria for US travelers: Moderate.
Drug resistance[4]: Chloroquine.
Malaria species: *P. falciparum* 60%, *P. vivax* 35%–40%, *P. ovale* <1%.
Recommended chemoprophylaxis: Atovaquone-proguanil, doxycycline, or mefloquine.

VENEZUELA (See Maps 3-42 and 3-43.)

Yellow Fever
Requirements: None.
Recommendations:
Recommended for all travelers ≥9 months of age, except as mentioned below.
Generally not recommended for travelers whose itinerary is limited to the following areas: the states of Aragua, Carabobo, Miranda, Vargas, and Yaracuy, and the Distrito Federal (see Map 3-42).
Not recommended for travelers whose itineraries are limited to the following areas: all areas > 2,300m in elevation in the states of Trujillo, Merida, and Tachira; the states of Falcón and Lara; Margarita Island; the capital city of Caracas; and the city of Valencia (see Map 3-42).

Malaria
Areas with malaria: Present in the following states: Amazonas, 1 municipality in Apure (Pedro Camejo), Bolivar, Delta Amacuro, Monagas, Sucre, and 2 municipalities in Zulia (Jesus M. Semprum, Machiques de Perija). Few cases in the following states: Anzoategui, other parts of Apure, Barinas, Guarico, Miranda, Monagas, Marcano municipality in Margarita Island of Nueva Esparta, Portuguesa, Tachira, and other parts of Zulia. Present in Angel Falls. None in the cities of Caracas, La Asuncion, Maracaibo, and other parts of Margarita Island (see Map 3-43).

*All footnotes are located on page 420.

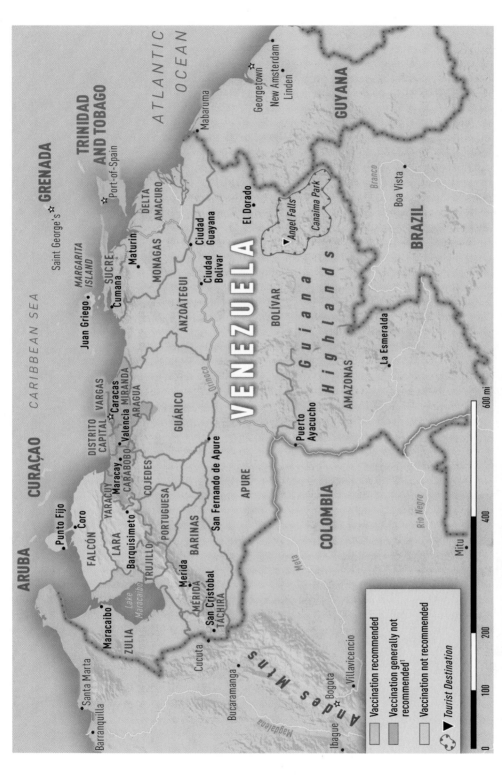

MAP 3-42. YELLOW FEVER VACCINE RECOMMENDATIONS IN VENEZUELA[2]

[1],[2] See footnotes on page 420 for an explanation of "Vaccination generally not recommended."

Legend:
- Vaccination recommended
- Vaccination generally not recommended[1]
- Vaccination not recommended
- ▼ Tourist Destination

Scale: 0 — 100 — 200 — 400 — 600 mi

3

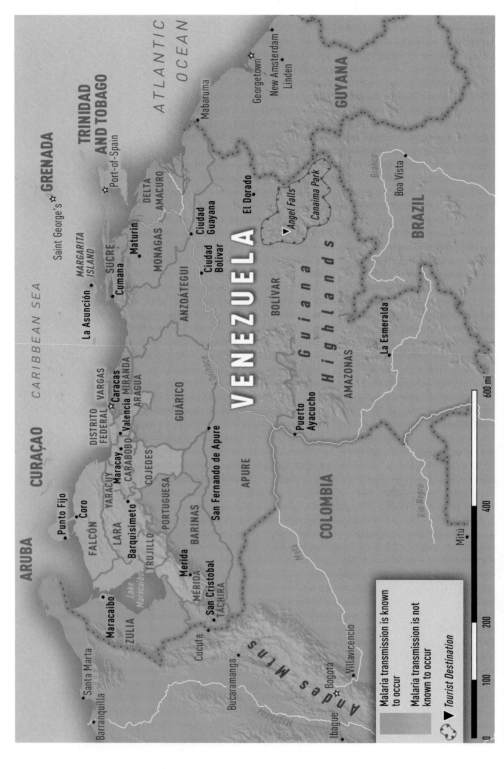

MAP 3-43. MALARIA TRANSMISSION AREAS IN VENEZUELA

Malaria transmission is known to occur

Malaria transmission is not known to occur

▼ *Tourist Destination*

Estimated relative risk of malaria for US travelers: Low.
Drug resistance[4]: Chloroquine.
Malaria species: *P. vivax* 75%,
P. falciparum 25%.
Recommended chemoprophylaxis:
For the states of Amazonas, 1 municipality in Apure (Pedro Camejo), Bolivar, Delta Amacuro, Monagas, Sucre, and 2 municipalities in Zulia (Jesus M. Semprum, Machiques de Perija): Atovaquone-proguanil, doxycycline, or mefloquine.
All other areas with malaria: Mosquito avoidance only.

VIETNAM
Yellow Fever
Requirements: Required if traveling from a country with risk of YFV transmission and ⩾1 year of age.[1]
Recommendations: None.

Malaria
Areas with malaria: Rural areas only. Rare cases in the Mekong Delta. None in Da Nang, Haiphong, Hanoi, Ho Chi Minh City (Saigon), Nha Trang, Qui Nhon, and the Red River Delta.
Estimated relative risk of malaria for US travelers: Low.
Drug resistance[4]: Chloroquine and mefloquine.
Malaria species: *P. falciparum* 50%–90%, remainder *P. vivax*.
Recommended chemoprophylaxis:
Southern part of the country in the provinces of Dac Lac, Gia Lai, Khanh Hoa, Kon Tum, Lam Dong, Ninh Thuan, Song Be, Tay Ninh: Atovaquone-proguanil or doxycycline.
Other areas with malaria except Mekong Delta: Atovaquone-proguanil, doxycycline, or mefloquine.
Mekong Delta: Mosquito avoidance only.

VIRGIN ISLANDS, BRITISH
Yellow Fever
No requirements or recommendations.

Malaria
No malaria transmission.

VIRGIN ISLANDS, US
Yellow Fever
No requirements or recommendations.

Malaria
No malaria transmission.

WAKE ISLAND, US
Yellow Fever
No requirements or recommendations.

Malaria
No malaria transmission.

WALLIS AND FUTUNA ISLANDS (FRANCE)
Yellow Fever
Requirements: Required if traveling from a country with risk of YFV transmission and ⩾1 year of age, including transit >12 hours in an airport located in a country with risk of YFV transmission.[1]
Recommendations: None.

Malaria
No malaria transmission.

WESTERN SAHARA
Yellow Fever
Requirements: This territory has not stated its yellow fever vaccination certificate requirements.
Recommendations: None.

Malaria
Areas with malaria: Rare cases.
Estimated relative risk of malaria for US travelers: No data.
Drug resistance[4]: Chloroquine.
Malaria species: Unknown.
Recommended chemoprophylaxis: Mosquito avoidance only.

YEMEN
Yellow Fever
Requirements: Required if traveling from a country with risk of YFV transmission and ⩾1 year of age.[1]
Recommendations: None.

Malaria
Areas with malaria: All areas <2,000 m (6,561 ft). None in Sana'a.
Estimated relative risk of malaria for US travelers: Low.
Drug resistance[4]: Chloroquine.
Malaria species: *P. falciparum* 95%; *P. malariae*, *P. vivax*, and *P. ovale* 5% combined.
Recommended chemoprophylaxis:
Atovaquone-proguanil, doxycycline, or mefloquine.

*All footnotes are located on page 420.

ZAMBIA

Yellow Fever

Requirements: Required if traveling from a country with risk of YFV transmission and ≥9 months of age, including transit >12 hours in an airport located in a country with risk of YFV transmission.[1]

Recommendations:

Generally not recommended for travelers going to the North West and Western Provinces.

Not recommended in all other areas not listed above.

Malaria

Areas with malaria: All.

Estimated relative risk of malaria for US travelers: Moderate.

Drug resistance[4]: Chloroquine.

Malaria species: *P. falciparum* >90%, *P. vivax* up to 5%, *P. ovale* up to 5%.

Recommended chemoprophylaxis: Atovaquone-proguanil, doxycycline, or mefloquine.

ZIMBABWE

Yellow Fever

Requirements: Required if traveling from a country with risk of YFV transmission and ≥9 months of age, including transit >12 hours in an airport located in a country with risk of YFV transmission.[1]

Recommendations: None.

Malaria

Areas with malaria: All.

Estimated relative risk of malaria for US travelers: Moderate.

Drug resistance[4]: Chloroquine.

Malaria species: *P. falciparum* >90%, *P. vivax* up to 5%, *P. ovale* up to 5%.

Recommended chemoprophylaxis: Atovaquone-proguanil, doxycycline, or mefloquine.

FOOTNOTES

Yellow Fever

[1] The official WHO list of countries with risk of YFV transmission can be found in Table 3-21. Proof of yellow fever vaccination should be required only if traveling from a country on the WHO list, unless otherwise specified. The following countries, containing only areas with low potential for exposure to YFV, are not on the WHO list: Eritrea, São Tomé and Príncipe, Somalia, Tanzania, Zambia.

[2] An elevation of 2,300 m is equivalent to 7,546 ft.

Malaria

[3] This risk estimate is based largely on cases occurring in US military personnel who travel for extended periods of time with unique itineraries that likely do not reflect the risk for the average US traveler.

[4] Refers to *P. falciparum* malaria unless otherwise noted.

[5] Primaquine can cause hemolytic anemia in people with glucose-6-phosphate dehydrogenase (G6PD) deficiency. Patients must be screened for G6PD deficiency before starting primaquine.

Yellow Fever Maps

[1] Yellow fever (YF) vaccination is generally not recommended in areas where there is low potential for YF virus exposure. However, vaccination might be considered for a small subset of travelers to these areas who are at increased risk for exposure to YF virus because of prolonged travel, heavy exposure to mosquitoes, or inability to avoid mosquito bites. Consideration for vaccination of any traveler must take into account the traveler's risk of being infected with YF virus, country entry requirements, and individual risk factors for serious vaccine-associated adverse events (e.g., age, immune status).

[2] Current as of September 2014. This map, which aligns with recommendations also published by the World Health Organization (WHO), is an updated version of the 2010 map created by the Informal WHO Working Group on the Geographic Risk of Yellow Fever.

Select Destinations

RATIONALE FOR SELECT DESTINATIONS
David R. Shlim

The quality of travel health advice is based on trying to reduce risks for the traveler in a particular destination. Our ability to counsel travelers is improved when we have visited a particular destination ourselves, or at least are familiar with typical itineraries and the specifics of health risks. However, our own travel experiences rarely encompass all the destinations that our clients plan to visit. Thus, this chapter of the Yellow Book was created to allow experts who have lived in or have frequently visited particular destinations to share their insider's knowledge of these places.

Each of these sections should be considered a personal perspective on the area discussed. They are editorial in nature, containing the author's expressed opinions, and aim to present topics for consideration; they should not necessarily be taken as a prescription for pre-travel care. Preventive recommendations that are covered elsewhere in the book are usually not repeated in these chapters, other than to address controversies or to emphasize important points.

The destination sections have proved to be one of the most popular features of the Yellow Book. The goals of these sections are to help a travel health provider feel more comfortable giving advice about specific destinations that he or she may have never visited, and to provide a level of detail about the attractions and health risks at select destinations that has not been provided elsewhere in this book.

AFRICA

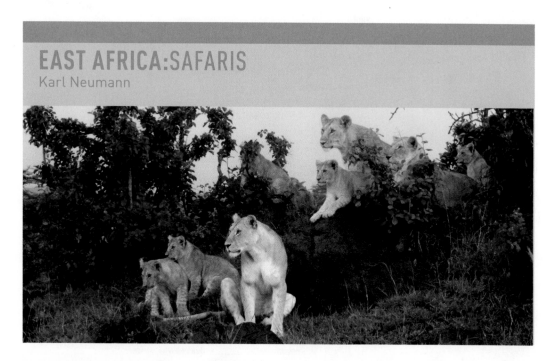

DESTINATION OVERVIEW

Arguably the ultimate in adventure travel, an African safari is also an easily doable family vacation, an experience of a lifetime for people of all ages, and, with a little research, not much more difficult to arrange than a week at a Caribbean resort. While the centerpiece of safari-going remains viewing majestic animals in their natural habitats, many tour operators now include programs on local culture, history, geology, and ecosystems and encourage travelers to get to know the people not merely as subjects of photos. Safaris can also be differentiated by the topography, vegetation, and bird life of the region. There are safaris for families, honeymooners, and people with similar interests (serious photography, for example). Many safaris accept children as young as 6 years and have special age-appropriate programs for children and adolescents aged 6–16 years.

Animals can be viewed from open trucks, air-conditioned vans, private aircraft, hot air balloons, or while hiking (where animals are friendly). Trips need not be strenuous. Accommodations range from crawl-in tents to air-conditioned, walk-in tents with full bathrooms. There are even luxurious 5-star lodges with floodlit water holes to view animals at night. Lunch in the wilderness varies from prepackaged sandwiches eaten sitting on a tree stump to 3-course meals served on tables covered with linen cloths and matching napkins. Some safaris include side trips to exotic places—to see or climb Mount Kilimanjaro, or visit Zanzibar or Lake Victoria, for example.

Travelers on their first safari often choose game parks in Kenya and Tanzania, in East Africa. The most famous game park in Kenya is the Masai Mara National Reserve, which, in effect, is the northern continuation of the Serengeti National Park game reserve in Tanzania, together forming the home of perhaps the grandest and most complete collection of the large wild animals for which Africa is famous. The Serengeti is the starting point of the annual migration of about 2 million wildebeest and several hundred thousand zebras as they search

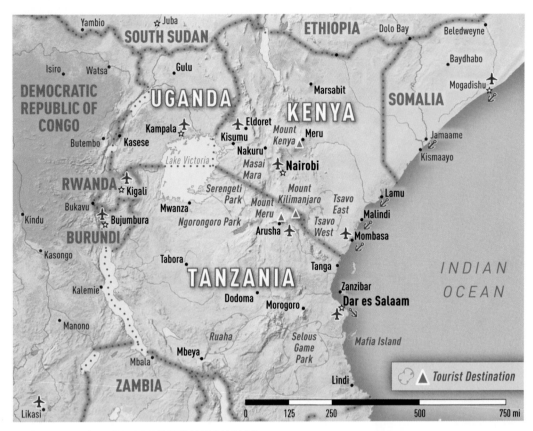

MAP 4-1. EAST AFRICA DESTINATION MAP

for pasture and water. Tanzania also has the Ngorongoro Crater, a 100-square mile depression (caldera) formed when a giant volcano, perhaps the size of Mount Kilimanjaro, exploded and collapsed on itself millions of years ago. The crater has most of the same animals as the Masai Mara reserve. The major East African game parks are shown on Map 4-1.

Travelers should research the optimum time of the year for their safari. The wildebeest migration in the Serengeti is a seasonal event, for example, although the precise time of the migration may vary from year to year. Some parks have a dry season, offering better views of the animals, as the vegetation is sparser and animals gather where water is present, but roads are dustier. And many areas of Africa have times of the year that are more comfortable for visitors, with cooler weather, less humidity, and less chance of rain.

HEALTH ISSUES

Health and safety issues that safari-goers are likely to encounter are mostly predictable and largely avoidable. The best insurance for carefree trips is a pre-travel consultation with a travel health provider, choosing an experienced and sophisticated tour operator, and taking along a small, personalized medical kit (see Chapter 2, Travel Health Kits).

Experienced tour operators generally require that clients buy medical evacuation insurance, supply clients with ample literature relating to local conditions, and employ knowledgeable guides who carry first aid kits and communication equipment to summon help, if necessary (see Chapter 2, Travel Insurance, Travel Health Insurance, & Medical Evacuation Insurance).

Much of East Africa is in the "meningitis belt," and polio recently reemerged in Kenya. In addition, health advice must be itinerary- and game park–specific. Immunizations and preventive medications necessary for one park may not be necessary for others. Parks may be long distances apart and located in countries with different health standards and dissimilar climates. Some parks are located at higher elevations and close to the equator, making proper sun precautions imperative. Significant sunburns can occur in less than an hour. Sunglasses are also essential.

Generally, proper preparations, common-sense precautions, the short duration of most trips (usually <2 weeks), experienced guides, and leaving the driving to others make safaris relatively low-risk undertakings for travelers of all ages.

Food and Water
Travelers' diarrhea appears to be the most common ailment, and most cases are mild. Sensible food and water selections may reduce the incidence (see Chapter 2, Food & Water Precautions). Illness may occur even on deluxe trips. Carrying medication for self-treatment is generally recommended (see Chapter 2, Travelers' Diarrhea).

Animals
Wild animals are unpredictable. Travelers should follow oral and written instructions provided by safari operators. Animal-related injuries are extremely rare and are usually the result of disregarding rules, for example approaching animals too closely to feed or photograph them.

Rabies exists throughout Africa. While most cases result from bites from dogs, all mammals are susceptible and could transmit the virus. Wounds from mammals should be considered a risk for rabies exposure unless proven otherwise. Licks can also result in rabies; the virus can enter through minor breaks in the skin. The incidence of rabies from bats seems to be increasing. In addition to rabies, bats may also transmit other diseases to humans, such as viral hemorrhagic fevers. Travelers should be encouraged to avoid entering caves where bats are known to be present. Cases of Marburg fever have occurred in travelers who visited a python cave in western Uganda.

Malaria
Malaria transmission occurs in most game parks. Most infections are caused by *Plasmodium falciparum*, and all *P. falciparum* in sub-Saharan Africa should be considered to be chloroquine-resistant. Safari activities often include sleeping in tents and observing animals at dusk or after dark, sometimes near water holes, all increasing the risk of being bitten by malaria-carrying mosquitoes. Taking preventive medication and using personal protection techniques—wearing long-sleeved shirts and pants, using insect repellents, and sleeping under permethrin-impregnated mosquito netting—are essential.

Yellow Fever
Travelers to East Africa must consult a travel medicine professional for the very latest information regarding yellow fever in that area. Yellow fever activity and vaccination recommendations can change frequently. Currently, yellow fever vaccination is recommended for much of East Africa (see Chapter 3, Yellow Fever & Malaria Information, by Country). In 2010, the World Health Organization and CDC reclassified a portion of East Africa to "low potential for exposure" to yellow fever virus and consequently downgraded the vaccination recommendation for these areas to "generally not recommended." This recommendation limits the need for vaccination to a small subset of travelers who are at increased risk for exposure to yellow fever virus (such as prolonged travel, heavy exposure to mosquitoes, or inability to avoid mosquito bites). These areas of East Africa where vaccine is generally not recommended include, but are not limited to, eastern Kenya, the cities of Nairobi and Mombasa, and all of Tanzania (see Chapter 3, Yellow Fever & Malaria Information, by Country).

However, some countries require proof of yellow fever vaccination in the form of a valid International Certificate of Vaccination or Prophylaxis (ICVP) as a condition of entry. Moreover, some safaris include more than one country. Travelers must check the requirements of each country on their itinerary, including countries they only transit through on the way to their destination. Some countries may require a valid ICVP even if there is no yellow fever in the country travelers are leaving or entering.

Other Health Risks

African trypanosomiasis (sleeping sickness), a disease only rarely seen among travelers, is transmitted by day-biting tsetse flies (*Glossina*). Wearing light-colored clothing (and avoiding wearing blue) seems to deter the flies. Insect repellents are only partially effective. Symptoms include fever, eschar at the site of the bite, headache, and signs of central nervous system involvement. Several cases of trypanosomiasis (*rhodesiense*) have recently been reported in European tourists visiting the Masai Mara National Reserve in Kenya and wildlife reserves in Tanzania.

Dengue, filariasis, leishmaniasis, and onchocerciasis (river blindness) are other diseases carried by insects that occur in East Africa. Swimming in freshwater ponds, lakes, and rivers can result in schistosomiasis (bilharzia), a parasite found in freshwater snails and transmitted by exposure to water. All freshwater sources should be considered contaminated. Swimming in the ocean or well-chlorinated pools is safe.

Myiasis and tungiasis are rare skin diseases among travelers. Myiasis is caused by fly larvae penetrating the skin and causing a boil-like lesion with a central aperture. Eggs are usually laid on clothing left to dry outdoors, and the larvae enter the skin when the clothing is worn. Clothing should be dried indoors or ironed before wearing. Tungiasis is caused by direct penetration of skin by sand fleas, causing small, painful nodules, often on the foot adjacent to toenails. Prevention includes wearing closed-toed footwear and not walking barefoot.

Symptoms of many diseases acquired in Africa may surface weeks and occasionally months after exposure, sometimes long after the traveler has returned home. Patients should mention all travel to their health care provider if they become ill after a trip.

Other Safety Risks

Although being a crime victim is an unusual occurrence for those on safari, robbery, muggings, and carjacking may occur in major urban centers, notably Nairobi and Mombasa. Street muggings during the day and night are common. The rates of fatal motor vehicle crashes in sub-Saharan Africa are among the highest in the world. Within game parks, serious motor vehicle crashes are rare, as the poor roads discourage speeding. However, travel in rural areas between parks is high risk, especially after dark. If at all possible, nighttime driving in sub-Saharan Africa should be avoided, and pedestrians should take extra care for speeding vehicles. Boarding an overcrowded bus should be avoided.

BIBLIOGRAPHY

1. Gautret P, Schlagenhauf P, Gaudart J, Castelli F, Brouqui P, von Sonnenburg F, et al. Multicenter EuroTravNet/GeoSentinel study of travel-related infectious diseases in Europe. Emerg Infect Dis. 2009 Nov;15(11):1783–90.

2. Meltzer E, Artom G, Marva E, Assous MV, Rahav G, Schwartz E. Schistosomiasis among travelers: new aspects of an old disease. Emerg Infect Dis. 2006 Nov;12(11):1696–700.

3. Sinha A, Grace C, Alston WK, Westenfeld F, Maguire JH. African trypanosomiasis in two travelers from the United States. Clin Infect Dis. 1999 Oct;29(4):840–4.

4. Thrower Y, Goodyer LI. Application of insect repellents by travelers to malaria endemic areas. J Travel Med. 2006 Jul–Aug;13(4):198–202.

5. Trypanosomiasis (sleeping sickness and Chagas disease). In: Field VK, Ford L, Hill DR, editors. Health Information for Overseas Travel. London: National Travel Health Network and Centre; 2010. p. 329–30.

6. United Nations office at Nairobi. Security in Kenya. Nairobi: United Nations office at Nairobi [cited 2014 Sep 17]. Available from: http://dcs.unon.org/index.php?option=com_content&view=article&id=127&Itemid=177&lang=en.

7. World Health Organization. Global status report on road safety: time for action. Geneva: World Health Organization; 2009 [cited 2014 Sep 21]. Available from: http://www.who.int/violence_injury_prevention/road_safety_status/2009/en.

SOUTH AFRICA
Gary W. Brunette

DESTINATION OVERVIEW

South Africa has been called "a world in one country." This refers, in part, to the diversity in the geography, which includes lush subtropical regions, old hardwood forests, sweeping Highveld vistas, and the deep desert of the Kalahari; the splendor of the animal species found throughout the country and protected in expansive game reserves; the diverse origins of the locals (from Africa, Europe, India, and Southeast Asia); the cultural, artistic, and culinary variety; and access to the conveniences of a developed infrastructure amid the challenges of Africa.

South Africa has experienced a surge in tourism in the last 2 decades, with visitors from within the African continent, as well as those from Europe and North America. Business travelers typically head to the commercial centers of Johannesburg, Cape Town, and Durban. Tourists may be attracted by the game reserves, the largest of which is Kruger National Park, located along the Mozambique border in the northeast (see Map 4-2). Kwa-Zulu Natal has a number of game parks (Hluhluwe-Umfolozi and Saint Lucia) set inland from Durban, and the Eastern Cape has parks (Addo Elephant Park and Shamwari) easily accessed from Port Elizabeth on the southern coast. Many smaller luxury reserves have emerged to cater to the high-end traveler. Visitors may be attracted to itineraries that include a trip from Cape Town along the south coast through the small scenic towns of Knysna and Plettenberg Bay; a tour of the old gold-mining towns in Mpumalanga, many of which are in near-original condition; spectacular drives and fascinating tours of the old wineries along the wine routes in the Western Cape; or visits to the southernmost point of Africa at Cape Agulhas or Cape Point, where the Indian and Atlantic Oceans meet in a roar of foam.

South Africa is also a common destination of humanitarian workers, missionaries, and students. A sizable number of South Africans live outside the country and would be considered visiting friends and relatives when returning to the country for a visit.

While there is a wide range of living standards in South Africa, most visitors experience standards comparable to those in developed countries. A smaller number of visitors may go to less developed areas, either the lower-income townships outside most towns and cities or to rural areas. Hikers, adventure-seekers, and missionaries will experience a wider range of living standards. Similarly, the quality and availability of health care are variable. Middle- and upper-income South Africans live in low-risk environments, have a standard of health comparable to that of North Americans, and have access to world-class medical facilities. Poorer South Africans live in areas with few amenities, are exposed to a wide range of diseases, and have limited access to adequate health care.

HEALTH ISSUES

Vaccine-Preventable Diseases

All travelers to South Africa should be up-to-date with their routine vaccinations. Infectious diseases such as measles and mumps are endemic in the region. In addition, travelers should obtain vaccinations for hepatitis A and B. Travelers should also consider typhoid vaccine, especially those who are more adventuresome or staying in less sanitary surroundings.

Yellow Fever Vaccine Requirements

South Africa requires a valid International Certificate of Vaccination or Prophylaxis documenting yellow fever vaccination ≥10 days before arrival in South Africa for all travelers aged ≥1 year who are traveling from or transiting for >12 hours through the airport of a country with risk of yellow fever virus transmission. Travelers not meeting this requirement can be refused entry to South Africa or be quarantined for up to 6 days. Unvaccinated travelers with a valid medical waiver should be allowed entry.

Travelers going to or transiting through South Africa are advised to seek the most current information by consulting the CDC Travelers' Health website (www.cdc.gov/travel), and also the website of the US embassy in South Africa (Pretoria) and the embassy of South Africa in Washington, DC.

HIV and Sexually Transmitted Diseases

South Africa has the largest estimated number of people living with HIV of any other country in the world. The prevalence of HIV infection is approximately 18% among people aged 15–49 years, and the prevalence among sex workers is even higher. Other sexually transmitted diseases (STDs) are also present at high rates in this population. Travelers should be aware of STD risks and use condoms if they have sex with someone whose HIV or STD status is unknown.

Vectorborne Diseases

Malaria transmission only occurs in the northeast of the country in the Mpumalanga and Limpopo Provinces (including Kruger National Park) and in Kwa-Zulu Natal north of the Tugela River (see Map 3-41). *Plasmodium falciparum* is the predominant species and is universally resistant to chloroquine. Visitors to these areas should be on a malaria chemoprophylaxis regimen and should be advised about mosquito precautions. Malaria in the northeastern game reserves occurs throughout the year but is seasonal; the highest transmission occurs from October through May, peaking from February to early May. The risk to visiting travelers is low. A study conducted in 1999 estimated a case rate of 4.5 cases per 10,000 visitors in April, a high-transmission month. The South African Department of Health recommends malaria chemoprophylaxis for all travelers visiting from September through May and mosquito-avoidance measures for the rest of the year. CDC recommends chemoprophylaxis at all times of the year (see Chapter 3, Yellow Fever & Malaria Information, by Country).

Tick-bite fever caused by rickettsial species is common in South Africa. The disease is characterized by an eschar at the bite site, regional adenopathy, and a maculopapular to petechial rash. Hikers and campers in rural areas who are exposed to ticks are especially at risk. Measures should be taken to prevent tick bites (see Chapter 2, Protection against

MAP 4-2. SOUTH AFRICA DESTINATION MAP

Mosquitoes, Ticks, & Other Arthropods). Travelers who are taking doxycycline for malaria chemoprophylaxis may have some protection against tick-bite fever, but no studies exist to support or refute this viewpoint. Taking doxycycline only as prophylaxis for tick-bite fever (as opposed to taking it for malaria chemoprophylaxis) is not recommended.

Travelers' Diarrhea
As with most destinations, the risk of travelers' diarrhea depends on style of traveling and food choices. A fluoroquinolone, such as ciprofloxacin, can be prescribed to self-treat diarrhea.

Waterborne Diseases
Schistosomiasis, a common parasite throughout Africa, may be present in any body of freshwater, such as lakes, streams, and ponds. Travelers should avoid swimming in fresh, unchlorinated water.

Animal Avoidance
Although most travelers avoid wild animals in game reserves, rabies is common in dogs and other mammals throughout the country. The KwaZulu-Natal Province has the highest incidence of rabies. Travelers have no way of telling if a given animal is rabid and should avoid all contact with animals. Any bite or scratch from an animal should be washed with soap and water immediately and be evaluated as soon as possible by a clinician. Postexposure prophylaxis and medical care for rabies exposures can be obtained in South Africa. Rabies vaccine is available throughout South Africa, and human rabies immune globulin is available in major urban medical centers.

Safety and Security

South Africa has struggled with a rise in violent crime, which includes armed robberies, carjackings, home invasions, and rape. Most of these incidents occur in poor areas and, as such, most visitors will not be affected. However, awareness of personal safety and security should be stressed to all visitors. Travelers should rely on local guidance about the security precautions to take in specific areas.

Although South Africa has a modern road system, drivers should be alert for dangerous driving practices, stray animals, and poor roads in remote rural areas.

BIBLIOGRAPHY

1. Blumberg LH, de Frey A, Frean J, Mendelson M. The 2010 FIFA World Cup: communicable disease risks and advice for visitors to South Africa. J Travel Med. 2010 May–Jun;17(3):150–2.
2. Durrheim DN, Braack LE, Waner S, Gammon S. Risk of malaria in visitors to the Kruger National Park, South Africa. J Travel Med. 1998 Dec;5(4):173–7.
3. Maharaj R, Raman J, Morris N, Moonasar D, Durrheim DN, Seocharan I, et al. Epidemiology of malaria in South Africa: from control to elimination. S Afr Med J. 2013 Oct;103(10 Pt2):779–83.
4. South African National Travel Health Network. SaNTHNet [homepage on the Internet]. Dunvegan (South Africa): South African National Travel Health Network; c2013 [cited 2014 Jun 30]. Available from: http://www.santhnet.co.za/.

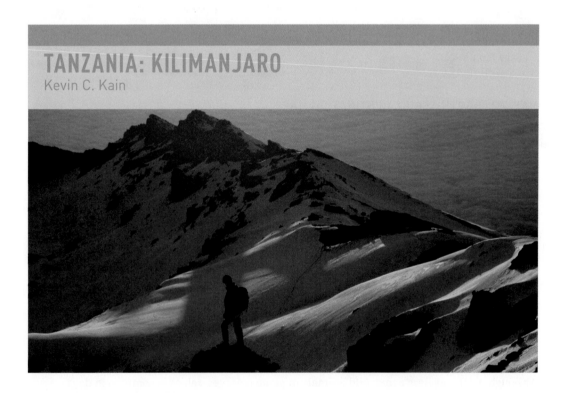

TANZANIA: KILIMANJARO
Kevin C. Kain

DESTINATION OVERVIEW

As the highest mountain in Africa and one of the largest freestanding volcanoes in the world, Kilimanjaro remains a revered and classic image of East Africa. Its snow-capped peak rising 19,341 ft (5,895 m) above the tropical African savanna is an irresistible draw for trekkers, particularly since no technical climbing is required to reach the summit. Kilimanjaro is one of the "seven summits" representing the highest peaks on each continent. However, because it does not involve technical climbing, the difficulties are often misjudged. Climbing Kilimanjaro is a serious undertaking, requiring serious preparation. Despite being higher than classic trekking destinations in Nepal, such as Kala Pattar (18,450 ft; 5,625 m) or Everest base camp (17,598 ft; 5,364 m), typical ascent rates on Kilimanjaro are considerably faster (4–6 days vs 8–12 days).

The classic route up Kilimanjaro is the Marangu route (64 km), usually sold as a "5 day, 4 night" trip. Marangu is frequently nicknamed the "Coca-Cola" route, since accommodation and food are provided in bunkhouses and the trail is wide and relatively easy compared with other routes. There are at least 9 alternative routes (Map 4-3), including the stunningly beautiful Machame route (the so-called "whiskey" route, since the days are generally longer, with tougher climbs). Machame and other routes involve camping but are usually sold as

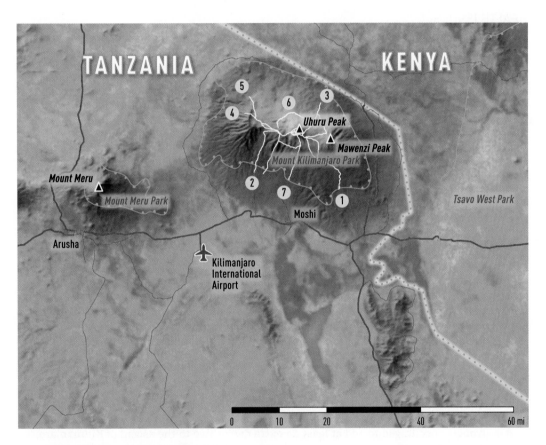

Sleeping altitude (feet) per night

	Route	Night 1	Night 2	Night 3	Night 4	Night 5	Night 6	Night 7	Night 8	Night 9
1	Marangu	8,858	12,205	14,160	15,430	12,205	6,046	n/a	n/a	n/a
2	Machame	9,350	12,500	13,044	13,106	15,331	10,065	5,380	n/a	n/a
3	Rongai	9,300	11,811	14,160	14,160	15,430	12,205	6,046	n/a	n/a
4	Lemosho	9,498	11,500	13,800	13,044	13,106	15,331	10,065	5,380	n/a
5	Shira	11,800	12,500	13,044	13,106	15,331	10,065	5,380	n/a	n/a
6	Northern	9,498	11,500	12,500	13,580	13,200	12,700	15,600	10,065	5,380
7	Umbwe	9,514	13,044	13,106	15,331	10,065	5,380	n/a	n/a	n/a

MAP 4-3. KILIMANJARO DESTINATION MAP

6- to 9-day packages, providing more opportunity to acclimatize and greater chances to successfully summit. Kilimanjaro can be climbed throughout the year (March–April are often the wettest months), but the weather is unpredictable, and the climber must be prepared for extreme weather and rain at any time of the year. A 2011 review of UK companies arranging high-altitude trekking reported that only 16 of 93 (17%) companies offering Kilimanjaro treks complied with Wilderness Medical Society guidelines on ascending to altitude, compared with 92% of treks to Everest base camp.

Climbing Kilimanjaro is a dream for many who visit Africa. However, a large number of travelers are ill-prepared, ascend too quickly, and consequently fail to summit. With due preparation and more reasonable ascent rates, climbing "Kili" is an aspiration that can be successfully and safely accomplished by many.

HEALTH ISSUES

The main medical issues for those attempting Kilimanjaro include the prevention and treatment of altitude illness and the potential for drug interactions between medications used for altitude illness and antimalarial or antidiarrheal agents commonly used by travelers to Tanzania.

Altitude and Acute Mountain Sickness (AMS)

Altitude illness is a problem on Kilimanjaro and a major contributor to the reason that only 50% of those attempting the standard 4- to 5-day Marangu route reach the crater rim, known as Gilman's Point (18,652 ft; 5,685 m), and as few as 10% reach the summit, known as Uhuru (Freedom) Peak (19,341 ft; 5,895 m). Prevalence rates of AMS were 75%–77% in recent studies of 4- and 5-day ascents on the Marangu route. Those using acetazolamide were significantly less likely to develop AMS on the 5-day ascents, but 40%–50% of those taking acetazolamide may still report AMS symptoms.

Every hiker on Kilimanjaro should receive pre-travel advice on AMS, be able to recognize symptoms, and know how to prevent and treat it. People with certain underlying medical conditions, including pregnancy, significant underlying lung or cardiac disease, and ocular and neurologic conditions, may be more susceptible to altitude-associated problems or may be taking medications that may interact with altitude medications, and should consult a travel health provider with knowledge of altitude illness before travel.

Enjoying the experience and successfully reaching the summit can be enhanced by allowing more time to acclimatize:

> If Ngorongoro crater is part of the planned combined itinerary, try to spend the last few nights of the safari here, because its elevation (7,500 ft; 2,286 m) will aid acclimatization for the Kilimanjaro trek.
> It is strongly encouraged to add at least an extra day or two to the ascent of Kilimanjaro, regardless of the route, but especially on routes normally promoted as 4- to 6-day trips.
> If possible before attempting Kilimanjaro, acclimatize by hiking nearby Mount Meru (14,978 ft; 4,565 m) or Mount Kenya (to Point Lenana, 16,355 ft; 4,895 m). A number of combined climbing trips for Mount Kenya and Kilimanjaro are now offered commercially.

For those with a past history of susceptibility to AMS and for those in whom adequate acclimatization is not possible (most "Kili" clients), the use of medications such as acetazolamide to prevent altitude illness is recommended. Acetazolamide accelerates acclimatization, is effective in preventing (beginning the day before ascent) and treating AMS, and is safe in children.

For those who are intolerant or allergic to acetazolamide, dexamethasone is an alternative for prevention of AMS, but there are cautions involved in using dexamethasone for ascent. Consideration should be given to carrying a treatment course of dexamethasone for high-altitude cerebral edema (HACE). Travelers with symptoms of altitude illness must not continue to ascend and need to descend if symptoms are worsening at the same altitude. A flexible itinerary and having an extra guide who can accompany any member of the group down the mountain if he or she becomes ill are considerations. See Chapter 2, Altitude Illness for more information about prevention and treatment of altitude illness.

Malaria

Kilimanjaro is unique in that its tropical malaria-endemic location means that many trekkers will be on antimalarial drugs and may need to continue them after their climb, particularly if they are also visiting game parks and staying overnight at altitudes <1,800 m (5,906 ft). Malaria chemoprophylaxis is recommended for Tanzania (even if only for a short trip). If a traveler flew directly into Kilimanjaro International Airport (2,932 ft; 894 m) and went the same day to an altitude above 1,800 m, there would be no risk of malaria. However, most people will be on safari or traveling before or after their Kilimanjaro trip, and therefore will be on prophylaxis.

Kilimanjaro is also a unique destination in that high altitude will affect everyone, and possible interactions should be considered between drugs commonly used for chemoprophylaxis or treatment of AMS, high-altitude pulmonary edema, or HACE, such as acetazolamide, dexamethasone, and nifedipine. Fortunately, there are few reported clinically significant drug interactions between common malaria chemoprophylaxis agents (atovaquone-proguanil, doxycycline, or mefloquine) and acetazolamide or dexamethasone used to prevent or treat AMS. Nifedipine is metabolized by the CYP3A4 enzyme and concurrent use of CYP3A4 inhibitors, such as doxycycline, could lead to elevated plasma levels of nifedipine and potentially lower blood pressure. Therefore, it would not be advised to take nifedipine for altitude illness prophylaxis concurrently with doxycycline.

Treatment of Travelers' Diarrhea

There are no reported drug interactions between acetazolamide and the fluoroquinolones (ciprofloxacin, levofloxacin) or macrolides (azithromycin) commonly used to treat travelers' diarrhea. There is a potential increased risk of tendon rupture when dexamethasone is used with fluoroquinolones. Avoid concurrent use of macrolides and nifedipine.

Remote Travel

Treks on Kilimanjaro are physically demanding and require a good level of fitness and preparation for the elements. Kilimanjaro weather is characterized by extremes: be prepared for tropical heat, heavy rains, and bitter cold. Keep gear, especially one's sleeping bag, in waterproof bags. Travelers should have adequate health insurance, including medical evacuation insurance. Travelers are advised to make sure their medical care and medical evacuation policy will cover any potential costs for a rescue or evacuation from the top of the mountain.

Carry a first aid kit that includes bandages, tape, blister kit, antibacterial and antifungal cream, antibiotics for travelers' diarrhea, antimalarials, antiemetics, antihistamines, analgesics, cold and flu medications, throat lozenges, and altitude medications.

BIBLIOGRAPHY

1. Bartsch P, Gibbs JS. Effect of altitude on the heart and the lungs. Circulation. 2007 Nov 6;116(19):2191–202.
2. Baumgartner RW, Siegel AM, Hackett PH. Going high with preexisting neurological conditions. High Alt Med Biol. 2007 Summer;8(2):108–16.
3. Davies AJ, Kalson NS, Stokes S, Earl MD, Whitehead AG, Frost H, et al. Determinants of summiting success and acute mountain sickness on Mt Kilimanjaro (5895 m). Wilderness Environ Med. 2009 Winter;20(4):311–7.
4. Jackson SJ, Varley J, Sellers C, Josephs K, Codrington L, Duke G, et al. Incidence and predictors of acute mountain sickness among trekkers on Mount Kilimanjaro. High Alt Med Biol. 2010 Fall;11(3):217–22.
5. Low EV, Avery AJ, Gupta V, Schedlbauer A, Grocott MP. Identifying the lowest effective dose of acetazolamide for the prophylaxis of acute mountain sickness: systematic review and meta-analysis. BMJ. 2012 Oct;345:e6779.

6. Luks AM, Swenson ER. Medication and dosage considerations in the prophylaxis and treatment of high-altitude illness. Chest. 2008 Mar;133(3):744–55.

7. Luks AM, Swenson ER. Travel to high altitude with pre-existing lung disease. Eur Respir J. 2007 Apr;29(4):770–92.

8. Rimoldi SF, Sartori C, Seiler C, Delacretaz E, Mattle HP, Scherrer U, et al. High-altitude exposure in patients with cardiovascular disease: risk assessment and practical recommendations. Prog Cardiovasc Dis. 2010 May–Jun;52(6):512–24.

9. Ritchie ND, Baggott AV, Andrew Todd WT. Acetazolamide for the prevention of acute mountain sickness—a systematic review and meta-analysis. J Travel Med. 2012 Sep–Oct;19(5):298–307.

10. Shah NM, Windsor JS, Meijer H, Hillebrandt D. Are UK commercial expeditions complying with wilderness medical society guidelines on ascent rates to altitude? J Travel Med. 2011 May–Jun;18(3):214–6.

THE AMERICAS & THE CARIBBEAN

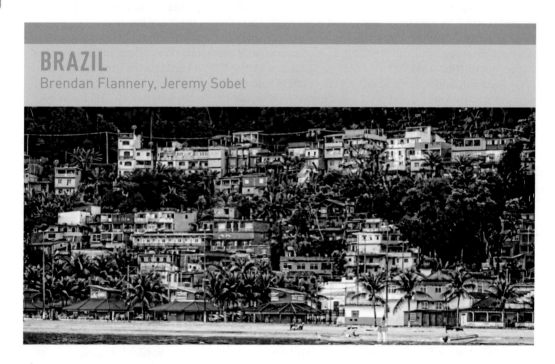

BRAZIL
Brendan Flannery, Jeremy Sobel

DESTINATION OVERVIEW

Brazil is the fifth largest country in the world and the largest country in South America, occupying nearly half of the land area of the continent. With a population of >200 million, Brazil has the world's largest Portuguese-speaking population. Brazil has the world's seventh largest economy and is classified as an upper-middle-income country. The population is highly urbanized; 84% live in urban areas.

Tourism is an important part of the Brazilian economy. In 2011, Brazil received over 5 million international visitors. As host of the World Cup in 2014 and the Summer Olympic Games in 2016, Brazil is receiving an increasing number of international visitors. Brazil's beaches and natural areas are popular tourist destinations. Rio de Janeiro is Brazil's second largest city (with a population of >6 million) and most frequently visited tourist destination for its beaches, landmarks, and annual Carnival Parade. Many of Brazil's major cities,

MAP 4-4. BRAZIL DESTINATION MAP

including Salvador, Recife, Florianópolis, Fortaleza, and Natal, are tourist destinations for beaches as well as regional culture. Brazil has a number of UNESCO World Heritage sites, including Iguaçu National Park in Paraná (the largest waterfalls in the Americas), historic towns of Olinda (Pernambuco), Ouro Preto (Minas Gerais), Salvador (Bahia) and San Luis (Maranhão), the modern capital of Brasília, and natural areas of the Amazon forest, Pantanal Conservation Area (Mato Grosso and Mato Grosso do Sul), Atlantic forests (Rio de Janeiro and São Paulo), and the archipelago of Fernando de Noronha in the Atlantic Ocean (see Map 4-4). São Paulo, one of the world's largest cities (>20 million people in the metropolitan area), is the economic center of Brazil and the most visited destination for business travel.

HEALTH ISSUES

Immunizations

Travelers to Brazil should be up-to-date on routine vaccines. Hepatitis A vaccination is recommended for most travelers ≥1 year of age; immunoglobulin injection may be used for infants. Hepatitis B vaccination should be considered for most travelers and is recommended for those who might be exposed to blood or other body fluids, including through sexual contact. Typhoid vaccine is recommended for most travelers, especially those more likely to be exposed to potentially contaminated food or water, such as those staying with friends or relatives; visiting smaller cities, villages, or rural areas; or prone to "adventurous eating." Yellow fever vaccine is recommended for travelers to certain areas.

Travelers' Diarrhea and Foodborne Infections

Travelers should take food and water precautions throughout Brazil (see Chapter 2, Food & Water Precautions). Travelers' diarrhea is the most common travel-related ailment, but travelers who consume foods or beverages from street vendors, raw fruits or vegetables, or unpasteurized dairy products are at risk for more serious foodborne infections. Oral rehydration salts are available from public health clinics and in almost all pharmacies in Brazil. Clinicians may wish to prescribe an antibiotic for empiric self-treatment of diarrhea (see Chapter 2, Travelers' Diarrhea).

Dengue

Dengue is the leading cause of febrile illness among travelers returning from South America. Risk of dengue is considered high in many Brazilian states because of high indices of *Aedes* infestation. From 2000 through 2010, cases of dengue increased throughout Brazil, and epidemics were reported from large Brazilian cities, including Rio de Janeiro and Salvador; >1 million cases were reported in 2010. Travelers to Brazil should take measures to protect themselves from mosquito bites (see Chapter 2, Protection against Mosquitoes, Ticks, & Other Arthropods).

Malaria

Almost all malaria in Brazil occurs in the Amazon Basin, although the mosquito vector is present in much of Brazil. *Plasmodium vivax* is the main species of malaria parasite, although approximately 15% of cases are caused by *P. falciparum*. Prophylactic treatment with antimalarial medication is recommended for travelers to malaria-endemic areas in Brazil (See Chapter 3, Yellow Fever & Malaria Information, by Country, and Map 3-22).

Yellow Fever

Yellow fever virus circulates in monkeys and is transmitted by mosquitoes throughout the Amazon Basin and in forested regions along all major river basins in Brazil, including Iguaçu Falls and as far south as Rio Grande do Sul. Vaccination against yellow fever is recommended for all travelers aged >9 months going to areas at risk of yellow fever. In 2011, the Brazilian

Ministry of Health expanded the list of municipalities for which yellow fever vaccination is recommended in the states of São Paulo, Paraná, Santa Catarina, and Rio Grande do Sul. (See Chapter 3, Yellow Fever & Malaria Information, by Country, and Map 3-21.)

Other Infections

Sexually Transmitted Diseases (STDs)

In Brazil, condoms are distributed free of charge by the government and are available in health clinics, tourist service centers, and other distribution points in many cities. Male condoms are available throughout Brazil in pharmacies, convenience stores, and large supermarkets; female condoms are also available in some locations. Vaccination against hepatitis A and B is recommended, as these infections can be sexually transmissible. Travelers, particularly those at high risk for acquiring HIV infection (such as men who have sex with men), may consider discussing preexposure prophylaxis with their health care provider (www.cdc.gov/hiv/prep).

Respiratory Diseases

Peak influenza circulation occurs from April through September in most of Brazil but may occur throughout the year in tropical areas. Seasonal influenza vaccination is recommended at least 2 weeks before travel. A number of fungal diseases endemic to parts of Brazil, including coccidioidomycosis, histoplasmosis, paracoccidioidomycosis, and cryptococcosis, are caused by inhalation of fungal spores typically present in soil, resulting in respiratory illness and occasionally more severe disease such as meningitis or bone infection. Travelers should exercise caution before disturbing soil, particularly if it is contaminated by bird or bat feces, and should beware of bat guano in caves.

Leptospirosis

Outbreaks of leptospirosis have occurred in urban areas in Brazil following heavy flooding. Travelers participating in recreational water activities are at increased risk, particularly after heavy rainfall or flooding.

Parasitic Infections

Chagas disease has been eliminated in most Brazilian states through insecticide spraying. Although risk to travelers is extremely low, outbreaks associated with contaminated food or drink have been reported, including locally prepared juice containing açaí, an Amazonian fruit eaten throughout Brazil. Travelers and ecotourists staying in poor-quality housing may be at higher risk.

Schistosomiasis is found in freshwater lakes and rivers in many states of Brazil, especially in the northeast. Swimming, bathing, and wading in fresh, unchlorinated water can result in infection. Schistosomiasis is not acquired by contact with saltwater (oceans or seas).

Both cutaneous and visceral leishmaniasis occur in Brazil and are most common in the Amazon and northeast regions. The risk is highest from dusk to dawn because sand flies typically feed (bite) at night and during twilight hours. Ecotourists and adventure travelers might have an increased risk, but even short-term travelers in endemic areas have developed leishmaniasis.

Rabies

Preexposure rabies vaccination is recommended for prolonged stays, particularly for children and those planning rural travel. For shorter stays, rabies vaccination is recommended for adventure travelers, those who may be occupationally exposed to animals, and those staying in locations >24 hours from access to rabies immune globulin.

Rickettsial Disease

Several tickborne rickettsial diseases have been identified in Brazil, including febre maculosa and Brazilian spotted fever, caused by the etiologic agent of Rocky Mountain spotted fever, *Rickettsia rickettsii*. Travelers should take precautions to avoid flea and tick bites both indoors and outdoors. For more detailed information, see Chapter 2, Protection against Mosquitoes, Ticks, & Other Arthropods.

Tuberculosis (TB)

Tuberculosis is prevalent in Brazil, but short-term travelers are not considered at high risk for infection unless they will be spending time in specific crowded environments. Travelers who anticipate possible prolonged exposure to people with TB because they will routinely come into contact with clinic, hospital, prison, or homeless shelter populations should have a tuberculin skin test or TB blood test before leaving the United States. If the test is negative, the traveler should have a repeat test 8–10 weeks after returning from Brazil.

Other Health and Safety Risks

Good health care is available in most sizable Brazilian cities. Brazilian public health services are free. Foreign visitors who have health problems can seek treatment in the emergency care network of Brazil's public health system, known as the Unified Health System or by its acronym, SUS, or through private facilities. The toll-free emergency number for ambulance services throughout Brazil is 192. The website of the Brazilian Ministry of Health provides information for international visitors in English (http://portalsaude.saude.gov.br/index. php?option=com_content&view=article&id=9652&Itemid=509), including a list of reference hospitals for mass events in Brazil.

Brazil has a growing number of private clinics that offer medical procedures using advanced technologies and cater to international clientele. Travel to Brazil for cosmetic surgery, assisted reproductive technology, or other elective medical procedures has increased in recent years (see Chapter 2, Medical Tourism) and is a major medical industry in Brazil. Although Brazil has many cosmetic surgery facilities that are on par with those found in the United States, the quality of care varies widely. Patients seeking to undergo cosmetic surgery or other elective procedures in Brazil should be advised to make sure that emergency medical facilities are available.

As in many foreign countries, motor vehicle crashes are among the leading causes of injury and death of US citizens in Brazil. Road conditions in Brazil differ significantly from those in the United States, and driving at night can be dangerous. The national toll-free number for emergency road-side assistance is 193 (in Portuguese only). It is illegal to drive after drinking alcohol, even in small quantities. Seat belt use is mandatory in vehicles, and children aged ≤10 years must be seated in the back seat. Brazilian federal law requires car seats for all children under the age of 7.5 years. Travelers with small children (weighing <40 lb) should travel with car or booster seats, since safety seats may be limited or unavailable. Helmets are required for motorcycles.

Travelers to Brazil should familiarize themselves with climatic conditions at their destinations before travel. Temperatures >40°C (104°F) are common from October through January in some Brazilian cities (see Chapter 2, Problems with Heat & Cold).

Poisonous snakes are hazards in many locations in Brazil, although deaths from snakebites are rare. Travelers should be advised to seek immediate medical attention any time a bite wound breaks the skin or when snake venom is ejected into their eyes. Specific antivenoms are available for some snakes in some areas of Brazil, so trying to ascertain the species of snake that bit the victim may be critical.

Although travel in Brazil is generally safe, crime remains a problem in urban areas and has increased in rural areas. The incidence of crime against tourists is higher in areas surrounding beaches, hotels, nightclubs, and other tourist destinations. Drug-related violence has resulted in violent clashes with police in tourist areas. Demonstrations may disrupt public and private transportation. Department of State advisories should be monitored for alerts in areas where travelers plan to visit. Several Brazilian cities have established specialized tourist police units to patrol areas frequented by tourists.

BIBLIOGRAPHY

1. Jentes ES, Poumerol G, Gershman MD, Hill DR, Lemarchand J, Lewis RF, et al. The revised global yellow fever risk map and recommendations for vaccination, 2010: consensus of the Informal WHO Working Group on Geographic Risk for Yellow Fever. Lancet Infect Dis. 2011 Aug;11(8):622–32.

2. Nobrega AA, Garcia MH, Tatto E, Obara MT, Costa E, Sobel J, et al. Oral transmission of Chagas disease by consumption of acai palm fruit, Brazil. Emerg Infect Dis. 2009 Apr;15(4):653–5.

3. Oliveira-Ferreira J, Lacerda MV, Brasil P, Ladislau JL, Tauil PL, Daniel-Ribeiro CT. Malaria in Brazil: an overview. Malar J. 2010;9:115.

4. Malaria Atlas Project. The spatial limits of *Plasmodium vivax* malaria transmission map in 2010 in Brazil. [cited 2014 Jun 30]. Available from: http://www.map.ox.ac.uk/explore/countries/BRA/.

5. Teixeira MG, Siqueira JB Jr, Ferreira GL, Bricks L, Joint G. Epidemiological trends of dengue disease in Brazil (2000–2010): a systematic literature search and analysis. PLoS Negl Trop Dis. 2013;7(12):e2520.

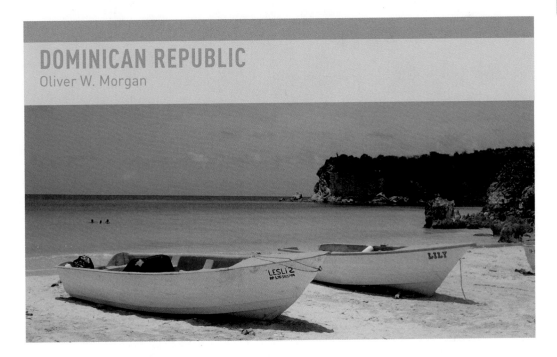

DOMINICAN REPUBLIC
Oliver W. Morgan

DESTINATION OVERVIEW

The Dominican Republic covers the eastern two-thirds of the Caribbean island of Hispaniola; the other third is covered by Haiti. The capital city, Santo Domingo, is located on the south coast of the island (see Map 4-5). Spanish is the official language, although English is spoken in most tourist areas. In 2013, >5 million foreign tourists visited the Dominican Republic, of which approximately 1.6 million were from the United States.

The Dominican Republic has a diverse geography of beaches, mountain ranges (including the highest point in the Caribbean, Pico Duarte, at 3,098 m [10,164 ft]), sugar cane plantations, and farming areas. The average temperature ranges from 73.5°F in January to 80°F in August. The island receives more rain from May through November, and tropical storms or hurricanes are a possibility. Most of the tourism is concentrated in the east of the country around Punta Cana, which offers all-inclusive beach resorts. Kite- and wind-surfing attract visitors to the northern areas of Puerto Plata, Sosua, and Cabarete. A small number of travelers visit other

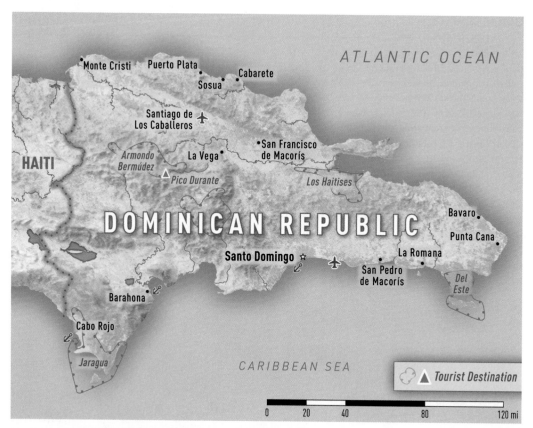

MAP 4-5. DOMINICAN REPUBLIC DESTINATION MAP

parts of the country, where tourist infrastructure is limited or nonexistent. The capital city, Santo Domingo, has an attractive colonial district that contains many historical sites dating back to Christopher Columbus's arrival in the New World. A highway completed in 2014 connects Punta Cana to Santo Domingo and is expected to increase tourism in the capital.

HEALTH ISSUES

Vaccine-Preventable Diseases

All travelers should be up-to-date on routine vaccinations, including measles-mumps-rubella (MMR), diphtheria-tetanus-pertussis, varicella (chickenpox), polio, and seasonal influenza. Cases of vaccine-preventable diseases have been reported among the local population and unvaccinated tourists from Europe and other parts of the world.

Most travelers should also be vaccinated against hepatitis A and, depending upon the traveler's itinerary and activities, typhoid—especially those who are staying with friends or family. Hepatitis B vaccine is recommended for people who might be exposed to blood through needles or medical procedures or bodily fluids during sexual intercourse with a new partner.

Cases of rabies among animals continue to be reported in the Dominican Republic, and several human cases of rabies have been reported over the last few years. In 2013, there were 34,473 reports of people bitten by animals, 112 cases of animal rabies, and 1 human rabies case. Travelers potentially at risk for animal bites (such as those undertaking outdoor pursuits, working with or around animals, taking long trips or moving to the Dominican Republic, or children who may play with animals) should be vaccinated against rabies before travel.

HIV and Sexually Transmitted Infections
Commercial sex work occurs throughout the Dominican Republic, and some locations, such as Sosua and Puerto Plata, are known as sex tourism destinations. HIV prevalence among female commercial sex workers is as high as 6% in some areas, syphilis 12%, hepatitis B virus 2.4%, and hepatitis C virus 0.9%. Data about sexually transmitted infections among male commercial sex workers are not available. Among men who have sex with men, HIV prevalence is as high as 6.9% and active syphilis as high as 13.9%. Travelers should avoid sexual intercourse with commercial sex workers and always use condoms with any partner whose HIV or sexually transmitted disease status is unknown.

Vectorborne Diseases
Dengue and malaria are potential concerns for travelers to the Dominican Republic. All travelers should take precautions to prevent mosquito bites by wearing long-sleeved shirts and long pants and using mosquito repellent. See Chapter 2, Protection against Mosquitoes, Ticks, & Other Arthropods for more information.

The malaria in the Dominican Republic is not drug resistant. CDC recommends that travelers to the Dominican Republic take malaria chemoprophylaxis unless they are only visiting in the urban areas of Santiago or Santo Domingo. Dengue is widespread throughout the Dominican Republic. In 2013, 16,658 cases were reported, of which 78% had laboratory confirmation, and 111 were fatal. Although cases of dengue are reported year round, transmission frequently increases during the rainy season from May through November. The mosquito vector for dengue is found in urban as well as rural areas.

Chikungunya virus has recently been introduced into the Caribbean, and cases have been detected in the Dominican Republic. The virus is transmitted by the same mosquito as dengue, and prevention is the same as for other mosquitoborne diseases.

Food and Water Safety
Travelers should only drink water that is purified or bottled. Ice served in well-established tourist locations is usually made from purified water and is safe to consume. However, when traveling to remote or nontourist areas, ice may not be safe. Food hygiene at large, all-inclusive, and popular tourist locations has improved over the last few years. However, travelers' diarrhea continues to be the most common problem for visitors to the Dominican Republic. Food purchased on the street or sold on beaches by informal sellers presents a higher risk of illness. Although cholera was introduced to the Dominican Republic in 2010, disease transmission is mostly limited to poor, urban areas or certain rural communities; cholera is not an ongoing concern in major tourist locations. Nevertheless, tourists are advised not to eat raw or undercooked seafood in the Dominican Republic.

Sun and Heat Safety
Visitors to the Dominican Republic often underestimate the strength of the sun and the dehydrating effect of the humid environment. Visitors should take precautions to avoid sunburn by wearing hats, suitable clothing, and proper application of sunblock against UVA and UVB. Travelers should also drink plenty of fluids throughout the day.

Safety and Security
Driving in the Dominican Republic is hazardous. Traffic laws are rarely enforced, and drivers commonly drink and drive, exceed speed limits, do not respect red lights or stop signs, and drive without seatbelts or helmets. The Dominican Republic has among the highest number of traffic deaths per capita in the world (41.7 per 100,000 population). Many fatal or serious traffic

crashes involve motorcycles and pedestrians. Motorcycle taxis, which are used throughout the country, including in tourist areas, frequently carry 2 or more passengers without helmets. Visitors should avoid motorcycle taxis, use only licensed taxis, and always wear a seatbelt.

Foreign tourists may become victims of crime in the Dominican Republic. The risks are similar to most major US cities. Although much crime involving tourists involves robbery or pickpocketing, more serious assaults occasionally occur, and criminals may react violently if resisted. Visitors to the Dominican Republic should follow normal precautions such as going out in groups, especially at night; using only licensed taxi drivers; drinking alcohol in moderation; and being cautious of strangers. Criminal activity is often higher in the Christmas and New Year season, and additional caution is advised during those months.

MEDICAL TOURISM

The market for medical tourism, including plastic surgery and dental care, is growing in the Dominican Republic. Several companies offer package deals that include postsurgical recovery at a tourist resort. As of March 2014, no public or private health care facilities have standards accredited by bodies such as the Joint Commission International. Outbreaks of health care–associated infections, medical malpractice, and even deaths have been reported among foreign visitors traveling to the Dominican Republic for medical tourism. People considering traveling to the Dominican Republic for medical procedures, including plastic surgery or dental care, should consult with a health care provider before travel and consider whether foreign health care providers meet quality standards of care.

BIBLIOGRAPHY

1. Banco Central de la República Dominicana [Internet]. Estadísticas económicas: sector turismo. Santo Domingo, Dominican Republic: Banco Central de la República Dominicana; c2012 [cited 2014 Sep 22]. Available from: http://www.bancentral.gov.do/estadisticas_economicas/turismo/. Spanish.
2. CDC. Dengue fever among US travelers returning from the Dominican Republic—Minnesota and Iowa, 2008. MMWR Morb Mortal Wkly Rep. 2010 Jun 4;59(21):654–6.
3. CDC. Notes from the field: rapidly growing nontuberculous *Mycobacterium* wound infections among medical tourists undergoing cosmetic surgeries in the Dominican Republic—multiple states, March 2013–February 2014. MMWR Morb Mortal Wkly Rep. 2014 Mar 7;63(9):201–2.
4. CONAVIHSIDA (Consejo Nacional para el VIH y sida). Segunda encuesta de vigilancia de comportamiento con vinculación serológica en poblaciones claves. Gais, trans y hombres que tienen sexo con hombres (GTH) trabajadoras sexuales (TRSX) usuarios de drogas (UD), 2012. Santo Domingo, Dominican Republic: CONAVIHSIDA; 2014 [cited 2014 Sep 22]. Available from: http://countryoffice.unfpa.org/dominicanrepublic/drive/CONAVIHSIDASegundaEncuestaVigiliancia.pdf. Spanish.
5. Dirección General de Epidemiología [Internet]. Sistema nacional de vigilancia epidemiológica, boletín semanal 2013. Santo Domingo, Dominican Republic: Minsterio de Salud Colectiva República Dominicana; 2014 [cited 2014 Sep 22]. Available from: http://digepisalud.gob.do/boletines/boletines-semanales/cat_view/34-boletines-semanales/108-2013.html. Spanish.
6. World Health Organization. Global status report on road safety 2013: supporting a decade of action. Geneva: World Health Organization; 2013 [cited 2014 Sep 22]. Available from: http://www.who.int/violence_injury_prevention/road_safety_status/2013/en/.

HAITI

J. Nadine Gracia, Clive M. Brown, Lacreisha Ejike-King

4

DESTINATION OVERVIEW

Nestled between the Caribbean Sea and the Atlantic Ocean, the Republic of Haiti occupies the western third of the island of Hispaniola, with the Dominican Republic on the eastern two-thirds of the island (Map 4-6). Originally inhabited by the native Taíno, *Ayiti* ("land of high mountains") was introduced to European influence through periods of Spanish and French colonization from the 15th through 18th centuries. After a successful slave rebellion, on January 1, 1804, Haiti became the first independent black republic in the Western Hemisphere, the first independent state in the Caribbean, and the second independent state in the Western Hemisphere after the United States.

Although it was once the wealthiest French colony in the Caribbean because of its rich soil with gold and bountiful land and crops, such as sugar, rum, coffee, cotton, wood, and lumber, Haiti has experienced considerable environmental degradation due to deforestation, poor agricultural practices, and soil erosion. It is reported to be the poorest country in the Western Hemisphere, having suffered from political and economic instability for most of its history.

French and Creole are the official languages of the country. French is the principal written and administratively authorized language. It is the medium of instruction in most schools. The majority (approximately 90%) of Haitians, however, use Creole as their primary language. Because of the mix of indigenous, African, and European influences, Haiti possesses a "mosaic culture" that is reflected in local art, music, and cuisine.

Once called the Pearl of the Antilles because of its natural beauty, Haiti is home to a vibrant and diverse landscape that includes beaches, waterfalls, caves, and the most mountains of any nation in the Caribbean. The people of Haiti are known for their resilience, strength, and warm and kind spirit, leaving travelers to often say after a visit to Haiti that they have fallen in love with the country and its people.

Haiti has suffered significant environmental degradation, contributing to poor sanitation and water quality. As a result, various public health risks exist for Haitians and for people traveling to Haiti.

Immunizations

All people traveling to Haiti should be up-to-date on routine vaccinations. Additionally, hepatitis A vaccine is strongly recommended and typhoid as well, especially if travelers are staying with friends or relatives or visiting smaller cities or rural areas. Providers should also consider administering hepatitis B vaccine. Rabies affects Haiti more than any other nation in the Americas. Prevention efforts have decreased the number of human cases of rabies transmitted by dogs, but deaths continue to be reported in Haiti. Rabies vaccination is recommended for travelers anticipating contact with animals. Yellow fever vaccination is required for people traveling from countries where the disease is endemic.

Vectorborne Diseases

Vectorborne diseases are common in Haiti and include *Plasmodium falciparum* malaria, dengue, and chikungunya.

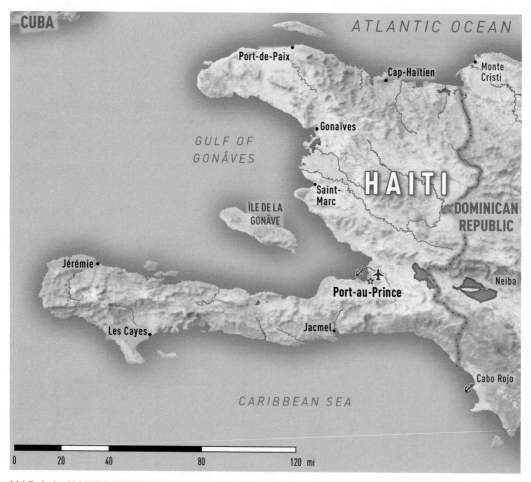

MAP 4-6. HAITI DESTINATION MAP

Malaria

The *P. falciparum* species of malaria is endemic in Haiti. The prevalence of malaria in Haiti is approximately 2%–3%. Highest transmission rates are reported to occur after the rainy seasons from March through May and October through November. Travelers are advised to begin malaria prophylaxis before travel. Suggested prophylactic medications for people traveling to Haiti include atovaquone-proguanil, chloroquine, doxycycline, or mefloquine. Travelers to Haiti should also take measures to protect themselves from mosquito bites to prevent malaria (see Chapter 2, Protection against Mosquitoes, Ticks, & Other Arthropods).

Dengue and Chikungunya

Dengue is endemic in the Caribbean, including Haiti. Cases of dengue have been reported before and after the 2010 earthquake among military personnel and US missionaries. Travelers to Haiti should take measures to protect themselves from mosquito bites to prevent dengue (see Chapter 2, Protection against Mosquitoes, Ticks, & Other Arthropods). Chikungunya virus transmission was first reported in Haiti in May 2014. Chikungunya is transmitted by the same mosquito that transmits dengue, so travelers are urged to adhere to the same mosquito precautions.

Travelers' Diarrhea and Food- or Water-Related Diseases

Travelers to Haiti will want to experience the local, flavorful cuisine, such as rice with red beans, plantains, *griot* (seasoned, fried pork), and a variety of fish and shellfish, including conch. While enjoying the incredible Haitian cuisine, travelers should select food and beverages carefully (see Chapter 2, Food & Water Precautions). People traveling to Haiti are at an intermediate risk (8%–20% attack rate) of developing travelers' diarrhea. Travelers to Haiti are at additional risk of contracting hepatitis A and typhoid fever.

Cholera

A cholera outbreak that began in Haiti in October 2010, 10 months after the January 2010 earthquake, has caused more than 8,500 deaths and 700,000 cases of illness. After the outbreak, cases of cholera were reported in people returning to the United States from Haiti. The incidence of the disease has lessened over the years because of improved access to clean water and sanitation, as well as the operations of cholera treatment centers and training of health care workers in the prevention, diagnosis, and treatment of cholera. Use of oral cholera vaccine as part of a complementary set of ongoing treatment and control measures was eventually implemented in a region of the Artibonite Department of Haiti. Although the use of oral cholera vaccine is accepted as an option for cholera control, there are as yet no guidelines for use in epidemic and emergency settings, including its appropriateness for use by travelers to an epidemic or endemic area. Travelers are urged to adhere to food and water precautions.

Leptospirosis

Leptospirosis is endemic in the Caribbean. Haiti may pose a higher risk than other areas because of natural disasters such as tropical storms or flooding. Many cases have been reported in Haiti since the 2010 earthquake. The incidence of leptospirosis is highest during the rainy season. The disease can be transmitted from contact with the urine or tissues of an infected animal or with water or soil tainted by the urine of an infected animal. Travelers are advised to avoid freshwater (such as streams or lakes) that may be contaminated by animal urine.

Physical Concerns for the Traveler

Motor Vehicle Safety

Motor vehicle crashes are the most common cause of death for healthy Americans traveling abroad. Road conditions in Haiti are significantly different from those in the United States: roads and lanes are generally unmarked, speed limits are seldom posted or adhered to, right of way is not widely observed, a variety of people and objects may appear on roads (such as carts, animals, and vendors), and roads may be unpaved or have large potholes. The main roads have been cleared of rubble from the 2010 earthquake, although some rubble remains in certain areas. Traffic is usually chaotic and congested in urban areas. *Tap taps* (vibrantly painted buses or pick-up trucks that serve as share taxis in Haiti but are open-air vehicles that are often overloaded with passengers and not mechanically sound) are a common form of public transportation for Haitians but are not recommended for visitors to the country because of safety concerns (such as accidents, robbery, or kidnapping). Travelers can exercise safety while traveling in Haiti by keeping alert when traveling on foot, choosing safe vehicles, and observing safety practices when operating vehicles.

Crime

The crime rate in Haiti is high, particularly in the capital of Port-au-Prince, which presents persistent safety concerns for travelers. Although much of the violent crime is perpetuated by Haitians on other Haitians, American citizens have also been victims of crime. Travelers arriving from US flights have been targeted for attack and robbery. Crime, disorderly conduct, and general congestion of local areas increase during Carnival. Travelers are advised to exercise caution throughout their trip including keeping valuables well hidden, ensuring possessions are not left in parked vehicles, keeping doors and window in homes and vehicles closed and locked, avoiding nighttime travel, and remaining alert.

Natural Disasters

Natural disasters common to Haiti include tropical storms, flooding, hurricanes, and earthquakes. Haiti experiences 2 rainy seasons, from April through June and from October through November. Hurricane season lasts from June through November. In 2008, Haiti experienced a series of 4 hurricanes and tropical storms within 2 months.

On January 12, 2010, Haiti experienced a 7.0 magnitude earthquake. More than 200,000 people died, and 1.5 million people were displaced from their homes. Multiple powerful aftershocks added to the widespread devastation and destruction. As a result, the health, emergency response, and safety infrastructure in the nation was significantly weakened.

BIBLIOGRAPHY

1. Brown C, Ripp J, Kazura J. Perspectives on Haiti two years after the earthquake. Am J Trop Med Hyg. 2012 Jan;86(1):5–6.
2. CDC. Dengue virus infections among travelers returning from Haiti—Georgia and Nebraska, October 2010. MMWR Morb Mortal Wkly Rep. 2011 Jul 15;60(27):914–7.
3. CDC. Malaria in post-earthquake Haiti: CDC's recommendations for prevention and treatment. Atlanta: CDC; 2010 [cited 2014 Sep 17]. Available from: http://www.cdc.gov/malaria/resources/pdf/new_info/2010/malaria-1-pager_dec3v1_508.pdf.
4. Dowell SF, Tappero JW, Frieden TR. Public health in Haiti—challenges and progress. N Engl J Med. 2011 Jan 27;364(4):300–1.
5. FRONTLINE/World. Haiti's history. Berkeley, CA: Public Broadcasting Service; c2002–2011 [cited 2014 Sep 22]. Available from: http://www.pbs.org/frontlineworld/rough/2007/12/haiti_belos_sonlinks.html.
6. Ivers LC, Teng JE, Lascher J, Raymond M, Weigel J, Victor N, et al. Use of oral cholera vaccine in Haiti: a rural demonstration project. Am J Trop Med Hyg. 2013 Oct;89(4):617–24.
7. Pan American Health Organization/World Health Organization (PAHO/WHO), Health Information and Analysis Project (HSD/HA). Health situation in the Americas: basic indicators, 2012. Washington, DC: PAHO; 2012 [cited 2014 Sep 22]. Available from: http://ais.paho.org/chi/brochures/2012/BI_2012_ENG.pdf?ua=1.
8. United Nations Development Programme (UNDP) Human Development Report Office. Human development report 2013. The rise of the South: human progress in a diverse world. New York: UNDP; 2013 [cited 2014 Sep 22]. Available from: http://hdr.undp.org/sites/default/files/reports/14/hdr2013_en_complete.pdf.
9. World Food Programme [Internet]. Haiti overview. Port au Prince (Haiti): World Food Programme; c2014 [cited 2014 Sep 22]. Available from: http://www.wfp.org/countries/haiti/overview.

MEXICO

Margarita E. Villarino, Sonia H. Montiel, Stephen H. Waterman

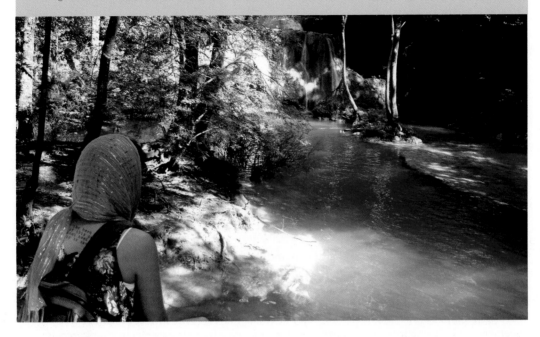

DESTINATION OVERVIEW

Mexico, the second most populous country in Latin America, has a population of >120 million, with 78% living in urban areas. The United States' third-largest trading partner overall and second-largest agricultural trading partner, Mexico is now considered a middle-income country with the world's 14th-largest economy. Mexico has a rich history and proud culture that reflect its pre-Columbian civilizations and Hispanic heritage. With one-fifth the area of the United States (about 3 times the size of Texas), Mexico has diverse geographic features within the 31 states and 1 federal district. The Sonoran desert is in the northwest, beautiful beaches are available on both coasts, and forested mountain ranges traverse the western and eastern mainland. Impressive volcanic peaks rise up to 18,000 feet above the high central plateau. The Yucatán Peninsula and southern regions are tropical. The Copper Canyon in the northwestern state of Chihuahua is larger than the US Grand Canyon.

Mexico City is one of the world's largest cities, with a population >20 million. Despite increasing national prosperity, Mexico's large cities contain much poverty. Extensive migration has taken place from the poor rural south to the northern border for jobs in bustling border cities, such as Ciudad Juárez and Tijuana.

Mexico has the most foreign visitors of any Latin American country and is the country most frequently visited by US tourists. Travel to beach resorts such as Acapulco, Ixtapa, Cancún, Cozumel, Puerto Vallarta, Nuevo Vallarta, and Cabo San Lucas, along with cruise ship tours, makes up a large portion of tourist travel to Mexico. Also common are day trips to northern border cities and longer cultural trips to historical and World Heritage sites. Popular pre-Columbian anthropologic destinations include Teotihuacan outside Mexico City, Great Pyramid of Cholula in Puebla, El Tajin in Veracruz, Chichen Itzá in Yucatán, Monte Alban in Oaxaca, and Palenque in Chiapas. Baja California offers whale watching on the Pacific Coast and sports fishing in the Gulf of California.

Mexico ranks second only to Thailand as the destination for American patients to receive health services outside the United States (medical tourism). The main services sought are dental services, eye care, and cosmetic surgery in the border cities. Increasingly, a complete range of services and specialized procedures are offered in cities with large medical services infrastructure, such as Mexico City, Monterrey, Merida, Cancún, and Guadalajara (see Chapter 2, Medical Tourism).

HEALTH ISSUES

Immunizations

All travelers should be up-to-date with their routine immunizations. Hepatitis A is endemic in Mexico, and all travelers should be immunized with at least the first dose of hepatitis A vaccine before travel to Mexico. Hepatitis B vaccine should be considered for all travelers and is also recommended especially for those with expected long-term stays (≥6 months), those who plan to use medical services, or who are planning activities in Mexico that may expose them to blood or blood products. Other vaccines, such as typhoid and rabies, may be considered, especially for those visitors (such as field biologists, nature adventure tourists) who will be traveling to less-developed, remote areas of the country.

Travelers' Diarrhea and Other Foodborne and Waterborne Infections

Travelers' diarrhea is common among visitors to Mexico. In addition to practicing food and water precautions, travelers should consider bringing an antibiotic for self-treatment of diarrhea (see the Food & Water Precautions and Travelers' Diarrhea sections in Chapter 2). Travelers should avoid consuming raw dairy products, undercooked meat or fish, and raw vegetables. Foodborne infections that are a risk in Mexico include amebiasis, cysticercosis, brucellosis, listeriosis, and infections with *Mycobacterium bovis*.

An outbreak of 181 cholera cases was reported from the Huasteca Region of the state of Hidalgo, Mexico, in 2013. The outbreak was quickly controlled, and the infecting strain was serogroup O1, serotype Ogawa, toxigenic, biotype El Tor, the same strain that caused outbreaks in Haiti, the Dominican Republic, and Cuba. Although cholera is considered a low risk in Mexico, travelers should adhere to food and water precautions.

Dengue

Dengue is endemic throughout Mexico, except for the state of Baja California Norte and at higher elevations (for example, it is not present in Mexico City at 7,350 ft [2,240 m]). Large outbreaks of dengue have been reported in recent years, and dengue virus transmission should be considered a risk year-round. To prevent dengue, travelers to Mexico should take measures against mosquito bites (see Chapter 2, Protection against Mosquitoes, Ticks, & Other Arthropods).

Chikungunya

Aedes aegypti and A. *albopictus* mosquitoes that can transmit chikungunya and dengue viruses are found in Mexico. Introduction into Mexico is a possibility given the outbreaks in the Caribbean Islands. Travelers to Mexico should be advised to reduce the possibility of mosquito bites (see Chapter 2, Protection against Mosquitoes, Ticks, & Other Arthropods).

Malaria

Malaria incidence has decreased dramatically in recent decades in Mexico, and only a few cases of infection with *Plasmodium vivax* are reported among US travelers each year. Major resorts are free of malaria, as is the US–Mexico border region. Malaria prophylaxis is recommended for travelers to Chihuahua, Chiapas, Durango, Nayarit, and Sinaloa. Mosquito

MAP 4-7. MEXICO DESTINATION MAP

avoidance but not chemoprophylaxis is recommended for travelers to Campeche, Jalisco, Oaxaca, Sonora, Tabasco, and the Othón P. Blanco municipality of Quintana Roo.

Other Infections
Respiratory Diseases
Influenza virus strains similar to those in the United States circulate in Mexico, as was demonstrated by the emergence of pandemic influenza A (H1N1) in North America in the spring of 2009. Coccidioidomycosis, a fungal respiratory disease caused by inhaling spores in the soil, is endemic in northwestern Mexico. Several outbreaks of coccidioidomycosis have been reported among missionary groups from the United States doing construction projects in this region. Histoplasmosis, another fungal respiratory disease agent found in soil, is endemic in other regions of Mexico, mainly the central and southeast regions. Occasional clusters of legionellosis have been reported in association with hotel stays in Mexico. Legionellosis should be considered in elderly and immunocompromised travelers who develop pneumonia, within 14 days of travel.

Parasitic Infections
Cutaneous leishmaniasis, transmitted by sand flies, is found in focal areas of coastal and southern Mexico. The risk is higher for ecotourists, field biologists, and long-term travelers. Travelers should practice preventive measures against fly bites, including avoiding outdoor activities at night. Travelers to beach areas may be at risk for cutaneous larva migrans (CLM), a creeping skin eruption most commonly associated with dog hookworm infection. CLM is preventable by wearing shoes and avoiding direct skin contact with sand. Chagas disease is endemic throughout Mexico (see Chapter 3, Trypanosomiasis, American [Chagas Disease]).

Rabies
Travelers should be educated on how to prevent animal bites to reduce the risk of rabies. In Mexico, the most common animal species that carry rabies are unvaccinated dogs or cats and wild animals such as raccoons, skunks, coyotes, bats, and foxes. Preexposure rabies vaccination should be considered for travelers who are likely to come into contact with these animals or those who will be traveling to areas with limited access to medical care.

Rickettsial Disease
In Mexico, rickettsial diseases, febrile rash illnesses transmitted by ticks or fleas, include Rocky Mountain spotted fever, which is potentially fatal unless treated promptly with antibiotics, and fleaborne typhus, which usually causes symptoms that are similar to dengue. Travelers should take precautions to avoid flea and tick bites both indoors and outside. Rocky Mountain spotted fever associated with *Rhipicephalus sanguineus*, the brown dog tick, has been identified recently in northern Mexico in urban and rural areas with large stray dog populations.

Tuberculosis (TB)
Mexico's TB incidence is lower than rates in Asia, Africa, and Eastern Europe but is 5 times that of the United States. The potential risk of exposure and infection with tuberculosis should be discussed with travelers planning long-term stays (≥6 months), or those who may be exposed to patients with untreated TB (such as those working in health care settings, homeless shelters, or prisons).

Other Health and Safety Risks
Good health care is available in most Mexican cities, and hotels in tourist resorts usually have well-trained physicians available. Injuries, rather than infectious diseases, appear to pose the largest risk of death among healthy travelers to Mexico. In one review, the leading cause of death to all US travelers to Mexico was injuries (51%), and 18% of deaths resulted from motor vehicle crashes.

Mexico's highway system and roads have become increasingly modernized over the years. Toll highways are often of high quality. Nevertheless, driving in traffic in cities and at night through the countryside can be dangerous. Although travel in Mexico is generally safe, drug-related violence has continued to increase in parts of the country. Department of State advisories should be monitored for alerts in areas where tourists are planning to visit.

Air pollution in Mexico City, while decreased in recent years, can be particularly severe during the dry winter months and can exacerbate asthma and chronic lung and heart conditions. Both healthy travelers from lower elevations and people with lung and heart conditions should cautiously acclimate to Mexico City's altitude.

Most injuries and deaths caused by poisonous scorpions are reported from states in the Pacific Coast (from Sonora to Oaxaca) and in the center states of Morelos, State of Mexico, Guanajuato, and Durango. Travelers should exercise caution when visiting Mexico's rural areas and when participating in outdoor activities, especially during spring and summer.

BIBLIOGRAPHY

1. Brathwaite Dick O, San Martin JL, Montoya RH, del Diego J, Zambrano B, Dayan GH. The history of dengue outbreaks in the Americas. Am J Trop Med Hyg. 2012 Oct;87(4):584–93.
2. CDC. Human rabies from exposure to a vampire bat in Mexico—Louisiana, 2010. MMWR Morb Mortal Wkly Rep. 2011 Aug 12;60(31):1050–2.
3. CDC. Notes from the field: outbreak of *Vibrio cholerae* serogroup O1, serotype Ogawa, biotype El Tor strain—La Huasteca Region, Mexico, 2013. MMWR Morb Mortal Wkly Rep. 2013;63(25):552–3.
4. CDC. Update: novel influenza A (H1N1) virus infection—Mexico, March–May, 2009. MMWR Morb Mortal Wkly Rep. 2009 Jun 5;58(21):585–9.
5. Fitchett JR, Vallecillo AJ, Espitia C. Tuberculosis transmission across the United States–Mexico border. Rev Panam Salud Publica. 2011 Jan;29(1):57–60.
6. Flores-Figueroa J, Okhuysen PC, von Sonnenburg F, DuPont HL, Libman MD, Keystone JS, et al. Patterns of illness in travelers visiting Mexico and Central America: the GeoSentinel experience. Clin Infect Dis. 2011 Sep;53(6):523–31.
7. Laniado-Laborin R. Coccidioidomycosis and other endemic mycoses in Mexico. Rev Iberoam Micol. 2007 Dec 31;24(4):249–58.
8. Leparc-Goffart I, Nougairede A, Cassadou S, Prat C, de Lamballerie X. Chikungunya in the Americas. Lancet. 2014 Feb 8;383(9916):514.
9. Spradling PR, Xing J, Phippard A, Fonseca-Ford M, Montiel S, Guzman NL, et al. Acute viral hepatitis in the United States–Mexico border region: data from the Border Infectious Disease Surveillance (BIDS) project, 2000–2009. J Immigr Minor Health. 2013 Apr;15(2):390–7.

PERU: CUSCO–MACHU PICCHU
Alan J. Magill

DESTINATION OVERVIEW

Peru is almost twice the size of the state of Texas, with a population of 30 million people. Thousands of tourists are drawn to Peru every year to enjoy the country's magnificent geographic, biologic, and cultural diversity. A primary destination for most travelers is the remarkable Incan ruins of Machu Picchu, named a UNESCO World Heritage site in 1983 and voted one of the New Seven Wonders of the World in 2007. Machu Picchu stands in the middle of a tropical mountain forest, in an extraordinarily beautiful setting. It was probably the most amazing urban creation of the Inca Empire at its height; its giant walls, terraces, and ramps seem as if they have been cut naturally in the continuous rock escarpments. The natural setting, on the eastern slopes of the Andes, is in the upper Amazon Basin, with its rich diversity of flora and fauna.

A typical visit to Peru includes arrival at the capital city of Lima, a megacity the size of the state of Rhode Island, with approximately one-third of Peru's population. Interestingly, many people think Lima is a high-altitude Incan city, but it is actually located on the Pacific coast at sea level (Map 4-8). After spending a few days in Lima, one takes an hour-long flight to Cusco, the gateway to Machu Picchu and a worthwhile destination of its own. Tourists can visit multiple Inca-era ruins and Peruvian mountain villages and markets in the Valle Sagrado (Sacred Valley) before taking the train to Machu Picchu. One of the world's most popular and best-known treks, the Inca Trail, begins classically at Piscacucho (82 km) (8,438 ft; 2572 m) on the Cusco–Machu Picchu railway. This moderate 26-mile (43-km) trek is usually done in 4 days and 3 nights, and most fit people should be able to complete the hike. Nevertheless it is quite challenging, with 3 high mountain passes; the highest is Warmiwañusca at 13,796 ft (4,205 m), before ending in the ruins of Machu Picchu (7,970 ft; 2,430 m).

Many people also wish to add a tropical rainforest experience to their Cusco trip and take the 30-minute flight from Cusco to Puerto Maldonado, 34 miles (55 km) west of the Bolivian border, on the confluence of the Rio Tambopata with the Madre de Dios River, a major tributary of the Amazon River. Most travelers take a boat up the Rio Tambopata to one of several rustic lodges. Visitors wanting to see the Amazon rainforest may also go to the more remote Manu National Park in the south, also reached via Cusco.

MAP 4-8. PERU DESTINATION MAP

Other popular tourist destinations in Peru include the northern Amazon rainforest in Loreto that can be visited by traveling to the lodges around Iquitos or by journeying on the increasingly popular Amazon River cruises that go both upstream and downstream from Iquitos. As elsewhere, ecotourism is a growing activity in Peru. Also, Peru is home to the Cordillera Blanca, a hundred-mile range of spectacular snow-covered peaks that form the backbone of the Andes Mountains in Peru. The Cordillera Blanca boasts 33 peaks >18,040 feet (5,500 meters) and has an international reputation for its spectacular trekking and world-class mountaineering.

HEALTH ISSUES

Important pre-travel information for Peru includes advice on preventing high-altitude illness, the risk for cutaneous leishmaniasis in certain jungle areas, use of yellow fever vaccine in some areas, and the risk of malaria for travelers visiting popular jungle lodges.

Altitude and Acute Mountain Sickness

All travelers to Machu Picchu will arrive and transit through Cusco, 11,200 ft (3,400 m) above sea level. Most will quickly note shortness of breath on gathering luggage and making their way to local hotels on the hilly streets. Many arriving travelers will find the elevation leads to some degree of acute mountain sickness (AMS), with the initial symptoms of headache, nausea, and loss of appetite beginning 4–8 hours after arrival. The hypoxemia of high altitude can also affect the quality of sleep in the first few nights in Cusco, causing restless sleep, frequent awakening, and periodic breathing (irregular breathing patterns, often alternating periods of deep breathing and shallow breathing), even in those who appear to be doing well during the day. A few travelers may progress to severe forms of altitude illness, including high-altitude pulmonary edema and high-altitude cerebral edema. The symptoms of AMS can markedly impair the traveler and prevent enjoyment of the sights of Cusco. People with underlying lung disease may not be the best candidates for travel to this destination. Expert medical consultation is advised.

Surveys have shown that most travelers arrive in Cusco with limited or no knowledge of AMS or the fact that AMS can be prevented to a large degree by prophylactic use of acetazolamide. Every traveler to Cusco should be counseled about AMS pre-travel and be prepared to prevent or self-treat AMS with acetazolamide. (More information about prevention and treatment of altitude illness can be found in Chapter 2, Altitude Illness.) Locals refer to AMS as *soroche* and will almost always offer the new arrival a cup of hot coca tea (*mate de coca*) when checking in to the hotel. Although many believe *mate de coca* can prevent and treat *soroche*, no data support its use in the prevention or treatment of AMS. Perhaps of concern to some who may experience random drug screening as a condition of employment, people who drink a single cup of coca tea will test positive for cocaine metabolites in standard drug toxicology screens for several days. However, sitting quietly and resting while enjoying a cup of tea is a most civilized activity and a pleasant memory.

New arrivals may also find it helpful to transit directly from Cusco to the Valle Sagrado of the Rio Urubamba to spend the first few days and nights at a somewhat lower altitude. This spectacular river valley begins 15 miles (24 km) northeast of Cusco in the town of Pisac (9,751 ft; 2,972 m), known for its colorful Sunday markets, and continues downstream toward the northwest for another 37 miles (60 km) to reach the town of Ollantaytambo (9,160 ft; 2,792 m). One can board the train to Machu Picchu in Ollantaytambo, at the northwest end of the Valle Sagrado, and the not-to-be-missed visit to Cusco can be made on return from Machu Picchu, when people are better acclimatized. The train follows the Rio Urubamba north and northwest (downstream) to Aguas Calientes (6,693 ft; 2,040 m). Machu Picchu (7,972 ft; 2,430 m) is located on a ridge above the town.

Cutaneous Leishmaniasis

Many areas in the Pacific valleys of the Andes and the Amazon tropical rainforest are endemic for cutaneous leishmaniasis (CL), a parasitic infection transmitted by bites of sand flies (see

Chapter 3, Leishmaniasis, Cutaneous). While this disease is widespread in southeastern Peru, the highest risk for travelers seems to be in the Manu Park area in Madre de Dios. In Manu, CL is most often caused by *Leishmania braziliensis*, and there is a risk of both localized ulcerative CL and mucosal leishmaniasis. There is no visceral leishmaniasis in Peru. Travelers should be counseled to be meticulous about vector precautions, as there is no vaccine or chemoprophylaxis to prevent leishmaniasis. Any person with a skin lesion persisting more than a few weeks after return from Peru should be evaluated for CL.

Yellow Fever

Proof of yellow fever vaccination is not required for entry into Peru. Travelers who are limiting travel to the cities of Lima, Cusco, and Machu Picchu, and the Inca Trail do not need yellow fever vaccination. Peru recommends vaccination for those who intend to visit any jungle areas of the country <2,300 m (7,546 ft). For complete CDC yellow fever vaccination recommendations for Peru, see Chapter 3, Yellow Fever & Malaria Information, by Country.

Malaria

In general, the risk of malaria in travelers visiting Peru is low. There are, on average, <5 cases reported in the United States each year that were acquired in Peru. Both *Plasmodium vivax* malaria and *P. falciparum* malaria are found in the Peruvian Amazon.

There is no malaria risk for travelers visiting only Lima and vicinity, coastal areas south of Lima, or the popular highland tourist areas (Cusco, Machu Picchu, and Lake Titicaca). The malaria-endemic areas for most tourists are the neotropical rainforests of the Amazon, with 2 major destinations (see Map 3-40). The city of Iquitos in the northern rainforest is a frequent arrival destination for those traveling to jungle lodges around the city or for boarding river cruise boats for rainforest travel. Malaria transmission occurs in the areas in and around Iquitos. Malaria transmission occurs throughout the year but is seasonal, with peak activity between January and May that correlates with the rainy season and the height of the Amazon River. Chemoprophylaxis is recommended for most travelers.

The city of Puerto Maldonado is a 30-minute flight from Cusco and a popular arrival destination for those visiting the rainforest lodges on the Rio Tambopata. Newly arrived travelers usually transit directly from the airport to the boats that take them up the river to numerous lodges. Peruvian Ministry of Health data document that malaria transmission occurs in Puerto Maldonado. Most cases reported in the region occur in local loggers and gold miners in the forests. Travelers transiting Puerto Maldonado for a short 2- to 3-day visit to lodges on the Rio Tambopata may not need chemoprophylaxis, but the decision should be individualized for those who are staying longer or who are engaging in higher-risk activities.

Risk for the traveler varies with itinerary, style of travel, and location of accommodations. Malaria in the Peruvian Amazon is unpredictable from season to season; *P. falciparum* epidemics occasionally occur in the Loreto region. When making a decision on whether to recommend chemoprophylaxis or simply mosquito precautions, all these factors and data need to be taken into consideration.

Other Infectious Diseases

Typical travelers' diarrhea is relatively common. Fluoroquinolone-resistant *Campylobacter* gastrointestinal infections are common and should be suspected in anyone with a gastrointestinal illness with fever and systemic symptoms and failure to clinically improve in 12–24 hours after initial empiric fluoroquinolone treatment. Azithromycin is recommended in this setting. Cyclosporiasis, an intestinal illness caused by the parasite *Cyclospora cayetanensis*, is also common in Peru. This diagnosis should be considered in people with watery diarrhea, loss of appetite, weight loss, cramping, and bloating that persist for days to weeks. Treatment is with trimethoprim-sulfamethoxazole.

Dengue is common in the neotropical areas of Peru and the northern coast. Mayaro virus, an alphavirus found in the Amazon Basin and transmitted by mosquitoes, causes a denguelike illness. As with other alphaviruses, Mayaro can result in lengthy and debilitating arthralgias. Physicians treating patients with signs and symptoms of a denguelike illness and a recent history of travel to the Amazon should consider Mayaro infection in the differential diagnosis, especially if arthralgia is prominent and prolonged and dominates the clinical picture. Travelers to Peru should take measures to protect themselves from daytime mosquito bites to prevent dengue (see Chapter 2, Protection against Mosquitoes, Ticks, & Other Arthropods).

BIBLIOGRAPHY

1. Cabada MM, Maldonado F, Quispe W, Serrano E, Mozo K, Gonzales E, et al. Pretravel health advice among international travelers visiting Cusco, Peru. J Travel Med. 2005 Mar–Apr;12(2):61–5.
2. Mazor SS, Mycyk MB, Wills BK, Brace LD, Gussow L, Erickson T. Coca tea consumption causes positive urine cocaine assay. Eur J Emerg Med. 2006 Dec;13(6):340–1.
3. Merritt AL, Camerlengo A, Meyer C, Mull JD. Mountain sickness knowledge among foreign travelers in Cusco, Peru. Wilderness Environ Med. 2007 Spring;18(1):26–9.
4. Neumayr A, Gabriel M, Fritz J, Gunther S, Hatz C, Schmidt-Chanasit J, et al. Mayaro virus infection in traveler returning from Amazon Basin, northern Peru. Emerg Infect Dis. 2012 Apr;18(4):695–6.
5. Steinhardt LC, Magill AJ, Arguin PM. Review: Malaria chemoprophylaxis for travelers to Latin America. Am J Trop Med Hyg. 2011 Dec;85(6):1015–24.

ASIA

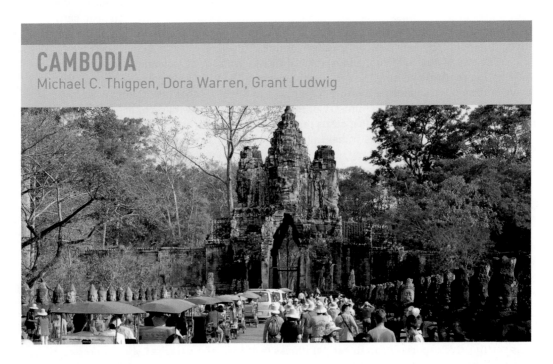

CAMBODIA
Michael C. Thigpen, Dora Warren, Grant Ludwig

DESTINATION OVERVIEW

Every year, >4 million tourists travel to Cambodia, many to visit Angkor Wat, a collection of approximately 100 ancient temples and other structures covering 400 km² (150 square miles) in the northwestern Cambodia jungle (Map 4-9). The Angkor Temple Complex is considered one of the architectural wonders of the world and, in 1992, was designated a World Heritage site. The temples were built between the 9th and 14th centuries AD, at the height of the Khmer Empire. These historical structures are decorated with intricately carved Khmer artwork depicting Hindu and Buddhist themes, providing an archaeological portrayal of the empire that ruled much of Southeast Asia for 5 centuries. After the decline of the Khmer Empire, the site was largely abandoned to the surrounding jungle and remained virtually untouched until descriptions of the "lost temples of Cambodia" were published late in the 19th century. Restorations began as international visitors arrived, but the emergence of the Khmer Rouge and the ensuing decades of civil war halted most tourist travel to the site until the late 1990s. As Cambodia has emerged from >20 years of political and economic turmoil, the Angkor temples have become one of the most popular tourist destinations in Southeast Asia. Increasingly, tourists are also visiting other areas of Cambodia, including beaches along the coast and islands in the Gulf of Thailand. Adventure tourism through the rural and forested areas bordering Vietnam and Laos has also become popular.

Cambodia is one of the poorest countries in Southeast Asia but is rapidly developing. As a result, business-related travel is increasing. Visitors can fly directly to Phnom Penh or Siem Reap from a number of Asian cities, including Bangkok, Singapore, Kuala Lumpur, Seoul, Hong Kong, Vientiane, and Ho Chi Minh City. Overland travel is also possible via direct bus service from Bangkok and Ho Chi Minh City.

HEALTH ISSUES

Immunizations

All travelers to Cambodia should be up-to-date with their routine immunizations, including seasonal influenza, and should be protected against hepatitis A and B and typhoid fever.

Japanese encephalitis (JE) is considered endemic throughout Cambodia; transmission occurs year-round but peaks during the May to October rainy season. The vaccine is recommended for travelers who plan to spend ≥1 month in rural areas and should be considered for short-term travelers who may be at increased risk for JE virus exposure, such as those who will spend substantial time outdoors in rural or agricultural areas, especially during the rainy season. Travelers on a typical 2- to 4-day visit to the close-in Angkor temples, staying in air-conditioned hotels in Siem Reap, are at minimal risk, but mosquito prevention measures should be employed.

Rabies is endemic throughout Cambodia. For most travelers on a short tour of the Angkor Wat temples, the risk is minimal. However, travelers planning more extensive travel in Cambodia should consider rabies immunization before arrival. The chief risk is from dog bites. The Pasteur Institute in Phnom Penh and some private clinics can provide rabies vaccine and consultation; rabies immunoglobulin is available to the public at the Pasteur Institute.

Although yellow fever is not a disease risk in Cambodia, the government requires travelers arriving from countries with a risk of yellow fever virus transmission to present proof of yellow fever vaccination.

Other Health and Safety Risks
Travelers' Diarrhea

Diarrhea and foodborne infections in travelers are common in Cambodia. Avoid water that is not bottled, ice, and food from street vendors. Safe, bottled water is readily available. Travelers should practice safe food and water precautions (see Chapter 2, Food & Water Precautions) and carry an antibiotic for self-treatment. Because fluoroquinolone resistance is widespread in Cambodia and other areas of Southeast Asia, azithromycin may be preferred (see Chapter 2, Travelers' Diarrhea for self-treatment recommendations).

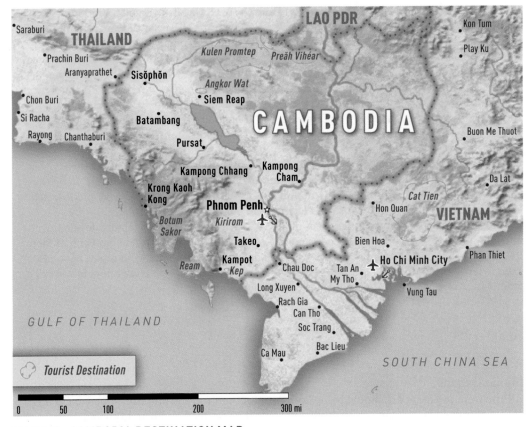

MAP 4-9. CAMBODIA DESTINATION MAP

Dengue

Dengue is endemic throughout Cambodia, and large epidemics occur every several years. Peak transmission occurs during the rainy season, although cases occur year-round even in nonepidemic years. Travelers to Cambodia should take measures to protect themselves from daytime mosquito bites to prevent dengue (see Chapter 2, Protection against Mosquitoes, Ticks, & Other Arthropods).

Malaria

The highest risk of malaria infection for the traveler in Cambodia is in forested areas. There is little transmission of malaria around Angkor Wat, Tonle Sap Lake, Siem Reap city, and Phnom Penh. On a typical 2- to 4-day visit that involves exploring the close-in temples of Angkor Wat during the day and staying in an air-conditioned hotel in Siem Reap at night, malaria risk is minimal. However, mosquito protection measures should still be employed. Travelers planning to visit the more remote Angkor temples deeper in the forest, or who travel outside the main tourist sites in Phnom Penh, especially to forested areas, should consider malaria chemoprophylaxis. The recommended chemoprophylaxis regimen for Banteay Meanchey, Battambang, Kampot, Koh Kong, Odder Meanchey, Pailin, Preah Vihear, Pursat, and Siem Reap is atovaquone-proguanil or doxycycline. Mefloquine is an additional option in all other areas (see Chapter 3, Malaria, for more information).

Chikungunya

Chikungunya was reintroduced into Cambodia in 2011, and a large outbreak occurred in southeastern Cambodia in March 2012. Risk of chikungunya infection exists throughout the day, as the primary vector, *Aedes aegypti*, aggressively bites during the daytime. Travelers can protect themselves by preventing mosquito bites (see Chapter 3, Chikungunya for additional details).

Schistosomiasis
Liver flukes such as *Schistosoma mekongi* are found in the Mekong Basin from the border of Laos to Kratie Province in Cambodia, where the freshwater dolphins attract tourists. Swimming in natural freshwater settings such as lakes, rivers, and ponds should be avoided. (see Chapter 3, Schistosomiasis).

Snakebites
At least 17 known venomous snake species are found in Cambodia; therefore travelers should use precautions to avoid snakebites. Effective antivenom is available in some international hospitals, including the Royal Angkor International Hospital in Siem Reap and the Calmette Hospital in Phnom Penh (see Chapter 2, Animal-Associated Hazards).

Transportation
Motor vehicle crashes are a rapidly rising cause of injury and death to passengers and pedestrians. Most road users are on motorcycles and are required to wear helmets as drivers but not as passengers. Avoid riding on motorcycle taxis. In addition to the ever-growing number of cars and motorcycles, there is lax enforcement of traffic laws and scant understanding of rules of the road. Travelers should carefully look in every direction before crossing the street. In cities and at Angkor Wat, most travelers use *tuk-tuks* (usually 3-wheeled), which are readily available, or hire cars with a driver guide. The fare should be negotiated at the outset. For those who, in spite of the risk, end up riding on the back of a motorcycle, wearing a helmet is essential. Five national highways link Cambodia's capital city, Phnom Penh, to other cities and beach resorts. During the rainy season road conditions deteriorate rapidly, and travel after dark on the highways is discouraged.

Safety
Travelers should be alert at all times and use common-sense measures such as not walking or traveling alone at night. Travelers are also advised to only carry what they are willing to lose. The most common type of theft is "snatch and grab" robbery. Travelers should keep belongings out of sight if traveling via *tuk-tuk* and carry items and bags away from the street side while walking.

Land Mines
Although the areas around the Angkor Wat temples and major towns have been cleared, land mines and unexploded ordnance from the decades of conflict are still found in rural areas in Cambodia, including Battambang, Banteay Meanchey, Pursat, Siem Reap, and Kampong Thom Provinces. Travelers to those areas should exercise caution, especially when venturing out to the more remote temples and forest, by staying on roads and paths and using a guide with knowledge of local hazards. Travelers should not touch anything resembling a mine or unexploded ordnance. If these items are observed, the Cambodia Mine Action Center should be notified.

Counterfeit Drugs
Local pharmacies provide a limited number of prescription and over-the-counter medications, but because the quality of locally obtained medications can vary greatly, travelers should bring an adequate supply of medications. Counterfeit drugs are commonly found and are often indiscernible from authentic medication (see Chapter 2, *Perspectives*: Pharmaceutical Quality & Counterfeit Drugs). If needed, medications should only be purchased from licensed pharmacies, which can easily be recognized by a green cup and snake sign.

Climate
Cambodia has a tropical climate and is generally hot throughout the year. The hottest months are March through May, and heat precautions should be taken when exploring the temples

or visiting other tourist areas. Many travelers explore the temples in the early mornings and late afternoon, taking a midday break in the comfort of an air-conditioned restaurant. Rainy season is from late April or early May through October or November. During this time, risk of vectorborne disease transmission increases.

Medical Care

Medical facilities and services in Cambodia do not generally meet international standards. A few internationally run clinics and hospitals in Siem Reap and Phnom Penh can provide basic medical care and stabilization. Some information on health facilities and pharmacies in Cambodia can be found on the website for the US embassy in Phnom Penh. For anything other than basic care and stabilization, most travelers should seek medical care in Bangkok or Singapore. For this reason, travel health insurance that includes medical evacuation insurance should be strongly considered.

BIBLIOGRAPHY

1. CDC. Chikungunya outbreak—Cambodia, February–March 2012. MMWR Morb Mortal Wkly Rep. 2012 Sep 21;61:737–40.
2. Embassy of the United States, Phnom Penh, Cambodia [Internet]. Medical services in Cambodia. Phnom Penh: US Department of State; 2014 [cited 2014 Jun 25]. Available from: http://cambodia.usembassy.gov/medical_information.html.
3. Ledgerwood J. Landmines in Cambodia. DeKalb, IL: Northern Illinois University [cited 2014 Jun 25]. Available from: http://www.seasite.niu.edu/khmer/Ledgerwood/Landmines.htm.
4. Ly S, Buchy P, Heng NY, Ong S, Chhor N, Bourhy H, et al. Rabies situation in Cambodia. PLoS Negl Trop Dis. 2009;3(9):e511.
5. Muth S, Sayasone S, Odermatt-Biays S, Phompida S, Duong S, Odermatt P. *Schistosoma mekongi* in Cambodia and Lao People's Democratic Republic. Adv Parasitol. 2010;72:179–203.
6. Rogers WO, Sem R, Tero T, Chim P, Lim P, Muth S, et al. Failure of artesunate-mefloquine combination therapy for uncomplicated *Plasmodium falciparum* malaria in southern Cambodia. Malar J. 2009;8:10.
7. Touch S, Hills S, Sokhal B, Samnang C, Sovann L, Khieu V, et al. Epidemiology and burden of disease from Japanese encephalitis in Cambodia: results from two years of sentinel surveillance. Trop Med Int Health. 2009 Nov;14(11):1365–73.
8. US Department of State. Cambodia country specific information. Washington, DC: US Department of State; 2013 [cited 2014 Sep 22]. Available from: http://travel.state.gov/content/passports/english/country/cambodia.html.
9. Vong S, Goyet S, Ly S, Ngan C, Huy R, Duong V, et al. Under-recognition and reporting of dengue in Cambodia: a capture-recapture analysis of the National Dengue Surveillance System. Epidemiol Infect. 2012 Mar;140(3):491–9.
10. World Health Organization. Cambodia. In: World Malaria Report, 2013. Geneva: World Health Organization; 2013 [cited 2014 Sep 22]. Available from: http://www.who.int/malaria/publications/country-profiles/profile_khm_en.pdf.

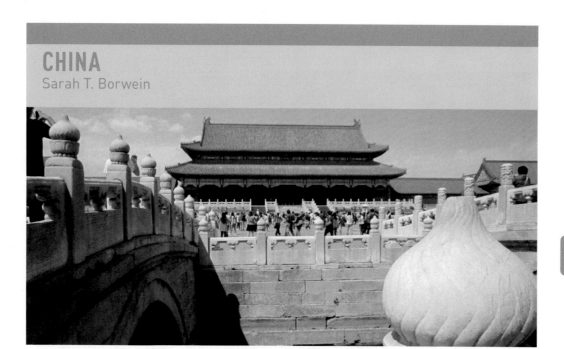

CHINA
Sarah T. Borwein

DESTINATION OVERVIEW

China, with >1.3 billion people, is the world's most populous country and the fourth largest geographically, behind Russia, Canada, and the United States. It shares a border with 14 other countries and has approximately 18,000 km of coastline. China is divided into 23 provinces, 5 autonomous regions, and 4 municipalities (Map 4-10). This large landmass is home to diverse topography, languages, and customs. The climate varies from tropical in the south to subarctic in the north, with wide variations between regions and seasons. Natural hazards include typhoons along the southern and eastern seaboards, dust storms in the north, floods, earthquakes, and landslides. Six of the 10 deadliest natural disasters in history occurred in China, including the 1556 Shaanxi earthquake, which is thought to have killed >800,000 people, making it the most lethal earthquake in history. Chinese superstition holds that natural disasters foretell the death of a ruler or the end of a dynasty, and indeed Mao Tse-tung died only 6 weeks after the 1976 Tangshan earthquake, the death toll of which was also in the hundreds of thousands. More recently, devastating earthquakes have struck the western provinces of Sichuan in 2008 and Qinghai in 2010. Torrential rain, floods, and landslides plagued large areas of China in the summer of 2010, as well as drought and dust storms in the north.

China has one of the world's oldest continuous civilizations, dating back >5,000 years. It has the world's longest continuously used written language system and is the source of many major inventions, including the "four great inventions of Ancient China": paper, the compass, gunpowder, and printing. Today, China is considerably more advanced (with the ability to put men in space, for example) and wealthier than many other developing countries, yet rural poverty and underdevelopment are still problems, particularly in the western part of the country.

Approximately 700 million Chinese live in rural areas. Urban areas are growing rapidly, however, and China is now home to many of the world's largest megacities. Shanghai and Beijing each have close to 20 million inhabitants, and Chongqing, with a metropolitan population >30 million, is among the fastest-growing urban centers in the world. Rivers play a central role in China's economy, history, and culture. The Yangtze River Basin, stretching 4,000 miles from the Tibetan plateau to the East China Sea near Shanghai, is home to >5% of the world's population.

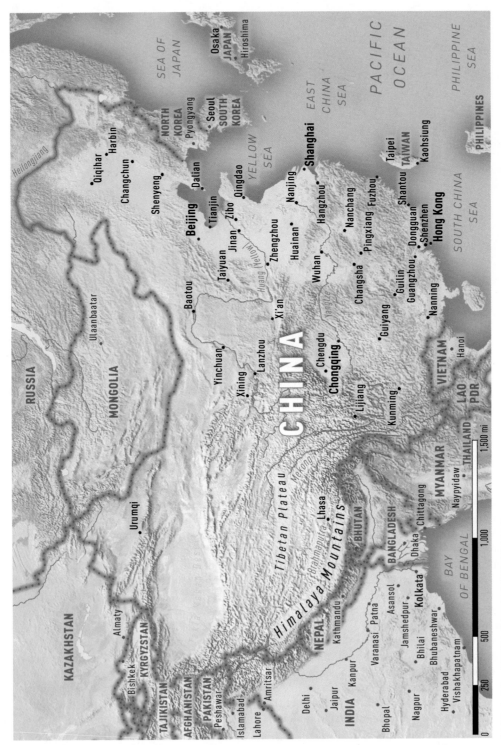

MAP 4-10. CHINA DESTINATION MAP

In 2012, >100 million tourists visited China. There has been extraordinary growth in tourism to China over the past decade, although numbers have leveled off slightly in the past 2 years. What is even more striking is the rapid growth in Chinese outbound tourism, from 29 million in 2004 to nearly 100 million in 2013. Chinese have also become the world's biggest spenders of tourism dollars, spending >$100 billion overseas in 2012, ahead of both US and German tourists.

China's long history and varied natural beauty can be traced in its 41 UNESCO World Heritage sites, from the imperial grandeur of the Forbidden City and the Temple of Heaven to the marvel of the Great Wall, the Terracotta Warriors in Xi'an, and the spectacular mountainous sanctuaries of the west. Popular itineraries often include Beijing and the Great Wall, Xi'an, and the Yangtze River (see Box 4.1 for information specifically about Yangtze River cruises). Other tourist destinations include the following:

> Shanghai and Hong Kong, with their futuristic architecture and East-meets-West mystique
> Lijiang in the province of Yunnan, where many ethnic minorities are concentrated
> Sichuan Province, home to China's iconic symbol, the panda
> Guilin, famous for its uniquely shaped limestone karst mountains that are often featured in Chinese paintings
> Tibet, accessible now by the world's highest railroad directly to Lhasa, with a maximum altitude of 16,640 ft (5,072 m)

Specialized itineraries are increasingly being offered, including hiking, mountain climbing, village tours, the Silk Road, and other more remote regions. Aside from tourism, increasing numbers of people travel to China to visit friends and relatives, to study, or to adopt children. These groups may be at particularly high risk of illness, because they underestimate their risks, are less likely to seek pre-travel advice, and stay in more local or rural accommodations. People traveling to China to adopt children often worry about the health of the child but neglect their own health.

BOX 4.1 CRUISING DOWN THE YANGTZE: WHAT TO CONSIDER

The Yangtze River is the third longest river in the world and one of the world's busiest (and most polluted) waterways. Yangtze River cruises are popular with tourists, and there are several heath considerations for this trip:

- At least 1 case of Japanese encephalitis has been documented in a tourist whose 3-week trip to rural and urban China included a Yangtze River cruise, and documented cases are likely to be an underestimate.
- Malaria is not a substantial risk on this itinerary; only insect bite precautions are recommended.
- Schistosomiasis—*Schistosoma japonicum*—exists in the Yangtze River Basin. Swimming is ill-advised.
- Motion sickness is rare on Yangtze cruises, since much of it takes place on a calm reservoir. However, susceptible travelers should carry antiemetic medication.
- Excursions off the boat often involve steep climbs, many stairs, and long walking distances and may not be appropriate for physically infirm tourists.
- Air pollution can be a problem on Yangtze River cruises and can cause eye and throat irritation, as well as respiratory problems in susceptible travelers. September and October are said to be the clearest months.
- Most non-Chinese-speaking tourists will prefer a 4- or 5-star "luxury" cruise. First class on a Chinese tourist boat may not meet expectations for cleanliness, and English may not be spoken.
- Food and water precautions apply, even on a luxury boat.

Although China is now the world's second-largest economy, in per capita terms income is still below the world average, with wide disparity in wealth and development between rural and urban as well as east and west. Health risks vary accordingly.

Air Pollution

China's rapid economic expansion has resulted in tremendous increases in emissions of air pollutants, particularly in the megacities. Although aggressive efforts are underway to control pollution, 16 of the 20 most polluted cities in the world are in China, and Beijing regularly tops the list. On peak pollution days, sometimes dubbed "airpocalypse" days by expatriate residents, the levels of particulate matter in the air can exceed 40 times the limit considered safe by the World Health Organization. The long-term health risks of this level of pollution are not the concern for most travelers, whose exposure will be relatively brief. However, they may suffer from irritation of the eyes and throat, and those with underlying cardiorespiratory illness, including asthma, chronic obstructive pulmonary disease, or congestive heart failure, may find their condition exacerbated. In addition, exposure to high levels of air pollution significantly increases the risk of respiratory tract infections, including sinusitis, otitis, bronchitis, and pneumonia. Children and the elderly are the most vulnerable to these effects.

Travelers should be sure to carry a good supply of any regular medications such as inhalers. All travelers should have a current influenza vaccine, and pneumococcal vaccine should be considered for anyone who is at higher risk from respiratory infection. Although surgical-style face masks have become increasingly fashionable in the big cities of China, especially Beijing and Shanghai, they provide no protection from air pollution and are not recommended. Properly fitted N95 masks can filter out particulates but not gaseous pollutants and can sometimes actually compound breathing problems, so are not routinely recommended.

Immunizations

Routine vaccinations should be up-to-date, including tetanus, diphtheria, measles, mumps, rubella, varicella, influenza, and pneumococcal vaccines, as indicated. In addition, hepatitis A and B and typhoid vaccinations are usually recommended. Since the Xinjiang Uygur Autonomous Region borders Pakistan, a polio-endemic country, adults traveling to this region who will be working in health care settings, refugee camps, or humanitarian aid settings should be vaccinated against polio, including a single lifetime booster dose of polio vaccine (IPV). Measles and rubella immunity is particularly important, although a massive vaccination campaign begun in September 2010 has decreased the number of reported measles cases in China, from 131,000 in 2008 to 10,000 in 2011. Nonetheless, a few travelers have made news headlines by triggering outbreaks in their home countries after returning from China. Although limited data exist on rubella in China, it was not part of the national immunization program until 2008, and incidence is believed to be high.

Rabies Vaccine

Rabies is a serious problem in China, as in much of Asia, with >3,000 human deaths per year reported in recent years. Mammal bites in any area of China, including urban areas, must be considered high risk for rabies. As international standard rabies immune globulin is generally unavailable, animal bites are often trip-enders, requiring evacuation to Hong Kong, Bangkok, or home for postexposure prophylaxis. Bites are surprisingly common in tourists. For example, dog bites were the most common dermatologic problem seen after China travel in a recent analysis of data from the GeoSentinel Surveillance Network. Rabies risk and prevention should be discussed in pre-travel consultations, and a strategy for dealing with a possible exposure should be developed. Long-term travelers and expatriates living in China should consider the preexposure vaccination series. Travel health insurance, including medical evacuation insurance, should be encouraged (see Chapter 2, Travel Insurance, Travel Health Insurance, & Medical Evacuation Insurance).

Japanese Encephalitis Vaccine

Japanese encephalitis (JE) occurs in all regions except Qinghai, Xinjiang, and Xizang (Tibet) (see Map 3-8 and Table 3-6). China has greatly reduced the incidence of JE through vaccination, and as of 2008, included JE in its expanded national immunization program; however, the disease remains a threat to unimmunized travelers. Although the JE season varies by region, most cases in local residents are reported from June through October. The risk of JE for most travelers to China is low but varies based on season, destination, duration, and activities. Risk is highest among travelers to rural areas during the transmission season. JE vaccine is recommended for travelers who plan to spend ≥1 month in endemic areas during June through October. It should be considered for shorter-term travelers if they plan to travel to rural areas and will have an increased risk for JE virus exposure based on their activities or itineraries, such as spending substantial time outdoors or staying in accommodations without air conditioning, screens, or bed nets. However, rare sporadic cases have occurred on an unpredictable basis in short-term travelers, including in periurban Beijing and Shanghai.

Malaria

Malaria risk is low for travelers to China, with the exception of those visiting rural parts of southern Yunnan Province or Hainan Island. For these areas, chemoprophylaxis should be considered. Mefloquine resistance in southern Yunnan means that travelers should be given doxycycline or atovaquone-proguanil for travel in this area. For travelers to other regions, the risk is too low to warrant chemoprophylaxis. Rare cases occur in other rural parts of the country at <1,500 m (4,921 ft) from May through December, usually *Plasmodium vivax* infections, and only insect precautions are recommended.

Other Health Risks
Foodborne Illnesses

The risk for travelers' diarrhea appears to be low in deluxe accommodations in China but moderate elsewhere. Usual food and water precautions should apply, and travelers should carry an antibiotic for self-treatment. Since highly quinolone-resistant *Campylobacter* is a problem in China, azithromycin may be a good choice. Tap water is not safe to drink even in major cities. Most hotels provide bottled or boiled water, and bottled water is easily available. In addition, there have been several well-publicized episodes of contamination of food with pesticides and other substances. Travelers should strictly avoid undercooked fish and shellfish and unpasteurized milk.

Sexually Transmitted Diseases

Sexually transmitted diseases, including syphilis, HIV, gonorrhea, and chlamydia, are a growing problem in China, particularly along the booming eastern seaboard. Travel is associated with loosened inhibitions and increased casual sexual liaisons. Travelers should be aware of STD risks and use condoms if they have sex with someone whose HIV or STD status is unknown. Hepatitis B vaccination before travel should be considered.

Road Traffic Injuries

Traffic in China is often chaotic, and the rate of traffic crashes, including fatal ones, is among the highest in the world. Driving is on the right side of the road in mainland China but on the left in Hong Kong and Macau. In practice, many people drive down the middle of the road. Child safety seats, rear seat belts, and bicycle or motorcycle helmets are rarely seen and not widely available, even in taxis. Electronic bicycles (E-bikes) are popular and do not have to be registered. They often travel in pedestrian and bicycle lanes as well as with traffic. Because E-bikes are quiet (no engine noise), they can be hard to avoid. Motor vehicles and E-bikes often drive with no lights, making night travel dangerous. Traffic crashes, even minor ones, can create major traffic jams and sometimes turn into violent altercations, particularly when foreigners are involved. China has not signed the convention that created the International Driving Permit, and travelers require a Chinese license to drive in China. For all of these reasons, it is often simpler and safer to hire a local driver than to drive oneself. It is also advisable to avoid driving at night or when weather conditions are bad and not to assume that traffic rules or right-of-way will be respected.

Medical Care in China

Western-style medical facilities that meet international standards are available in Beijing, Shanghai, and Hong Kong. Some hospitals in other cities have "VIP wards" (*gaogan bingfang*), which may have English-speaking staff. The standard of care in such facilities is somewhat unpredictable, and cultural and regulatory differences can cause difficulties for travelers. In rural areas, only rudimentary medical care may be available. Hepatitis B transmission from poorly sterilized medical equipment remains a risk outside major centers.

Ambulances are not staffed with trained paramedics and often have little or no medical equipment. Therefore, injured travelers may need to take taxis or other immediately available vehicles to the nearest major hospital rather than waiting for ambulances to arrive.

Pharmacies often sell prescription medications over the counter. Such medications have sometimes been counterfeit, substandard, or even contaminated. Travelers should carry all their regular medications in sufficient quantity; if more or other medications are required, it is advisable to visit a reputable clinic or hospital.

Some travelers wish to try traditional Chinese medicine and acupuncture. Although most do so uneventfully, there is a risk of bloodborne and skin infections from acupuncture needles, and traditional medicine products may be contaminated with heavy metals or pharmaceutical agents. Acupressure may be preferable to acupuncture.

Travelers are strongly advised to purchase travel health and medical evacuation insurance before travel. Most hospitals will not directly accept foreign medical insurance, however, and patients will often be expected to pay a deposit before care to cover the expected cost of the treatment.

BIBLIOGRAPHY

1. CDC. Measles among adults associated with adoption of children in China—California, Missouri, and Washington, July–August 2006. MMWR Morb Mortal Wkly Rep. 2007 Feb 23;56(7):144–6.
2. Chen XS, Gong XD, Liang GJ, Zhang GC. Epidemiologic trends of sexually transmitted diseases in China. Sex Transm Dis. 2000 Mar;27(3):138–42.
3. Cutfield NJ, Anderson NE, Brickell K, Hueston L, Pikholz C, Roxburgh RH. Japanese encephalitis acquired during travel in China. Intern Med J. 2005 Aug;35(8):497–8.
4. Davis XM, MacDonald S, Borwein S, Freedman DO, Kozarsky PE, von Sonnenburg F, et al. Health risks in travelers to China: the GeoSentinel experience and implications for the 2008 Beijing Olympics. Am J Trop Med Hyg. 2008 Jul;79(1):4–8.
5. Hills SL, Griggs AC, Fischer M. Japanese encephalitis in travelers from non-endemic countries, 1973–2008. Am J Trop Med Hyg. 2010 May;82(5):930–6.
6. Shaw MT, Leggat PA, Borwein S. Travelling to China for the Beijing 2008 Olympic and Paralympic Games. Travel Med Infect Dis. 2007 Nov;5(6):365–73.
7. Shlim DR, Solomon T. Japanese encephalitis vaccine for travelers: exploring the limits of risk. Clin Infect Dis. 2002 Jul 15;35(2):183–8.
8. Tang X, Luo M, Zhang S, Fooks AR, Hu R, Tu C. Pivotal role of dogs in rabies transmission, China. Emerg Infect Dis. 2005 Dec;11(12):1970–2.
9. United Nations World Tourism Organization. UNWTO tourism highlights. Madrid: United Nations World Tourism Organization; 2012 [cited 2014 Sep 18]. Available from: http://mkt.unwto.org/en/publication/unwto-tourism-highlights-2012-edition.
10. World Health Organization. Measles bulletin: Western Pacific region. Geneva: World Health Organization; 2010 [cited 2014 Sep 18]. Available from: http://www.wpro.who.int/entity/immunization/documents/docs/MeasBulletinVol4Issue1_F840.pdf.
11. Zhang J, Jin Z, Sun GQ, Zhou T, Ruan S. Analysis of rabies in China: transmission dynamics and control. PloS One. 2011;6(7):e20891.
12. Zhang YZ, Xiong CL, Xiao DL, Jiang RJ, Wang ZX, Zhang LZ, et al. Human rabies in China. Emerg Infect Dis. 2005 Dec;11(12):1983–4.

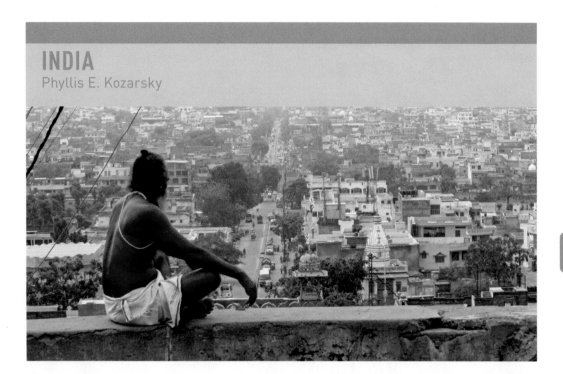

INDIA
Phyllis E. Kozarsky

DESTINATION OVERVIEW

India is approximately one-third the size of the United States and has 4 times the population (almost 1.3 billion people). This makes it the second most populous country in the world, behind China. Rich in history, vibrant culture, and diversity, India is the birthplace of 4 world religions: Hinduism, Buddhism, Jainism, and Sikhism. Despite the growth of megacities such as Mumbai and Delhi (both >15 million people), 70% of the population still resides in rural areas, and 65%–70% work in agriculture. Although India is one of the fastest-growing economies in the world, the literacy rate varies by state (64%–94%), and the level of poverty is high. The topography is varied, ranging from tropical beaches to foothills, deserts, and the Himalayan mountains. The north has a more temperate climate, while the south is more tropical year round. Many travelers prefer India during the winter—November through March, when the temperatures are more agreeable—although some, particularly families with children, must travel during the summer vacation time.

India is becoming more popular for US travelers, and rates of travel from the United States are increasing. International businesses are flourishing in India; tourists are flocking to the temples, beaches, and the Taj Mahal. For some new US residents, India remains their homeland, and they make frequent visits to family and friends.

Because tourists could not possibly visit all the sites in India during a 2-week holiday, they usually select a part of India for any given trip. A typical itinerary in the north of India includes Delhi, Agra, Varanasi, and cities in Rajasthan, such as Jaipur (the Pink City) and Udaipur. Agra is the home of the Taj Mahal, a breathtaking monument to lost love. Along the northern travel circle, one can stop to enjoy the magnificent bird sanctuary at Keoladeo Ghana and the tiger reserve at Ran Thambore (see Map 4-11). Varanasi, sacred to Hindus, Buddhists, and Jains, welcomes Hindu pilgrimages and boasts extraordinary experiences along the Ganges. A more southern route might swing through Goa and its beaches along the western coast, where swaying coconut palms form the backdrop for great parties and old-time hippies. Mumbai, a common entry point to India, hosts Bollywood, the largest film industry in the world. Kolkata is considered the cultural capital of the country. Bengaluru (Bangalore) in the

MAP 4-11. INDIA DESTINATION MAP

south-central region is both the garden city and India's Silicon Valley. The old seaside town of Kochi (Cochin) shows evidence of its Portuguese heritage, and Hyderabad shows off its old granite fort, many mosques, and bazaars. Despite the many and varied itineraries, most health recommendations for travelers to India are similar. The incidences of some illnesses, such as those transmitted by mosquitoes, increase during the monsoon season (May–October) with the high temperatures, heavy rains, and the risk of flooding.

Some of the most important health considerations of travel to India are those for travelers who are visiting friends and relatives (VFRs). These travelers often do not seek pre-travel health advice, since they are returning to their land of origin. Such travelers may stay in rural areas often not visited by tourists or business people, live in homes, and eat and drink with their families and thus are at higher risk of many travel-related illnesses (see Chapter 8, Immigrants Returning Home to Visit Friends and Relatives [VFRs]).

HEALTH ISSUES

Immunizations
All travelers to India should be up-to-date with their routine immunizations and are advised to consider hepatitis B vaccine. Particularly important is making sure that the traveler is immune to measles. As India has not had a case of wild poliovirus since early 2011 and obtained its polio-free certification from the World Health Organization in March 2014, polio vaccine is no longer recommended for US travelers. However, all travelers (residents and nationals) from polio-endemic countries are required to have a recent oral polio vaccination as of March 2014 (http://mohfw.nic.in/showfile.php?lid=2634).

Hepatitis A Vaccine
All travelers to India should be protected against hepatitis A. Although some assume that those born in India would have been exposed to hepatitis A in childhood and thus be immune, this may no longer be true, particularly for younger people. Providers should consider serologic testing for hepatitis A IgG in VFR travelers, or they should be immunized.

Typhoid Vaccine
More than 80% of typhoid fever cases in the United States are in people who traveled to India or other countries in south Asia. Thus, even for short-term travel, a typhoid vaccine should be recommended. Patients who are hesitant to be vaccinated may find it even more compelling that typhoid fever acquired in south Asia is becoming increasingly resistant to quinolone antibiotics, sometimes requiring parenteral therapy.

Paratyphoid fever, a similar disease caused by *Salmonella enterica* serovar Paratyphi A, B, and C, has become increasingly prevalent in south Asia, but typhoid vaccines are not protective against this infection.

Japanese Encephalitis Vaccine
Although there has never been a published case of a traveler acquiring Japanese encephalitis (JE) in India, the disease is present in many parts of the country. Risk is highest during the monsoon season from May through October; however, the season may be extended or year-round in some areas, especially in the south. Vaccination is not recommended for the typical 2-week trip most travelers take to see the major tourist sites in urban areas. However, vaccination is recommended for travelers who plan to spend ≥1 month in endemic areas during the JE virus transmission season and should be considered for short-term travelers if they plan to travel outside an urban area and have an increased risk for JE virus exposures (see Chapter 3, Japanese Encephalitis). Publicized outbreaks in recent years have not been in typical tourist destinations.

Rabies Vaccine

India has the highest burden of rabies in the world, with estimates of 15,000–20,000 human cases per year. Dogs roam in packs in many areas of the country. Unfortunately, human rabies immune globulin is not readily available, except in some clinics in major cities. Information about such clinics can be obtained from the website of the International Society of Travel Medicine (www.istm.org). Otherwise, if a traveler has not received preexposure rabies vaccination, a bite may result in having to leave the country for postexposure prophylaxis. Even so, a preexposure series is not recommended for all travelers to India. Cost is a consideration for many. Long-term travelers, expatriates, missionaries, and volunteers may want to obtain preexposure immunization for themselves and their children. Travelers may want to purchase a medical evacuation insurance policy that will cover travel for recommended rabies postexposure prophylaxis.

Malaria

Although the intensity of malaria transmission may be related to the season, unlike other countries in Asia, malaria is holoendemic in India (except at altitudes >2,000 m [6,561 ft]) and occurs in both rural and urban areas. Rates of *Plasmodium falciparum* have increased in the last few decades, and thus chemoprophylaxis is recommended for all destinations. However, for short-term travelers spending 1–2 days in northern areas in winter, insect precautions alone may be sufficient to prevent malaria. Travelers should be reminded that malaria-transmitting mosquitoes primarily bite between dusk and dawn.

Other Infections
General

More recently in India, new strains of bacteria that are resistant to most antibiotics have been carried by travelers to many other countries, including the United States. For example, resistance to carbapenem antibiotics is conferred by enzymes such as NDM-1, which makes it more difficult to treat problems such as skin and bloodstream infections.

Dengue

Dengue is endemic in all of India, although it is poorly reported at the local and national levels, and large outbreaks have occurred. The incidence is highest during the wet summer season, which includes the monsoon season (September–October). Travelers to India should take measures to protect themselves from daytime mosquito bites to prevent dengue (see Chapter 2, Protection against Mosquitoes, Ticks, & Other Arthropods).

Chikungunya

During the last several years there have been outbreaks of chikungunya, which is transmitted by day- and night-biting mosquitoes. Symptoms are similar to those of dengue and malaria, although often with severe and persistent arthralgia.

Hepatitis E

Hepatitis E is being recognized more frequently in travelers to India. A traveler who develops symptomatic hepatitis, despite being immunized against hepatitis A, will likely have hepatitis E.

Animal Bites and Wounds

In addition to rabies, other diseases can be transmitted by animal bites and wounds. Cellulitis, fasciitis, and wound infections may result from scratches or bites of any animal. B virus is carried by Old World monkeys and may be transmitted by active macaques that are kept as pets, inhabit many of the temples, and scatter themselves in many tourist gathering places (see Chapter 3, B virus). Monkeys can be aggressive and often seek food from travelers. When visiting temple areas that have monkeys, travelers should not carry any food in their hands, pockets, or bags. It is important to stress to travelers that monkeys and other animals should not be approached or handled at all. If travelers are bitten, they should seek medical care.

Travelers' Diarrhea

The risk for travelers' diarrhea is moderate to high in India, with an estimated 30%–50% chance of developing diarrhea during a 2-week journey. Travelers should practice safe food and water precautions (see Chapter 2, Food & Water Precautions) and carry an antibiotic for empiric self-treatment of diarrhea (see Chapter 2, Travelers' Diarrhea).

Tuberculosis (TB)

India has among the highest prevalences of TB; approximately one-fourth of all TB cases worldwide occur there. Roughly 2%–3% of cases are estimated to be multidrug resistant, and a smaller percentage are extensively drug resistant. Travelers who anticipate possible prolonged exposure to people with TB because they will routinely come in contact with clinic, hospital, prison, or homeless shelter populations should have a tuberculin skin test or TB blood test before leaving the United States. If the test is negative, they should have a repeat test 8–10 weeks after returning from India. Travelers who plan to work in high-risk settings or in crowded institutions (such as medical clinics, hospitals, prisons, or homeless shelters) should consult their health care providers about measures for prevention and testing before and after travel.

Miscellaneous

Arrival in India for the first time may be shocking to travelers who have never ventured into the developing world. The crowds, the intense colors, heat, and smells are striking and invade all the senses at once. It is difficult to enjoy the beauty without being touched by the enormity of the poverty. The close juxtaposition of the old and new is noteworthy. At times this can be overwhelming for travelers.

Transportation in India remains problematic. While traveling through India, travelers should be advised to carry food and beverages with them in the event of delays, which are almost inevitable no matter the mode of transport. Traveling by train can be harrowing, particularly having to force one's way through the crowd and onto the train. Travelers should make sure to keep passports and valuables safe while in a crowd. Roadways are some of the most hazardous in the world, and India has a poor record in traffic-related deaths. Animals, rickshaws, motor scooters, people, bicycles, trucks, and overcrowded buses compete for space in an unregulated free-for-all. Avoid overcrowded buses, travel by bus into the interior or on curving, mountainous roads, and long-distance travel at night. Rural, nighttime driving should be discouraged, even when a paid driver has been hired. Air pollution is a problem in the major cities, so those with chronic lung disease or asthma may consider spending time outdoors when there is less traffic or staying in facilities outside major cities.

Medical tourism is a growing industry in India. Many newer medical facilities have recently opened for travelers desiring cardiac, orthopedic, dental, or plastic surgery or transplantations at a substantially lower cost than in the United States. The benefits and hazards require careful examination (see Chapter 2, Medical Tourism). Health care is quite variable in India and dependent on the location.

In general, travelers feel safe while in India. Peddlers and promoters are aggressive with tourists, however, and may require a firm "no." Travelers may want to avoid making eye contact with a peddler or his goods, or they may risk having someone follow them down the street trying to sell them something. The stress of negotiating one's way through India makes this destination a place where having a close traveling companion is important.

It is always wise to pay attention to Department of State advisories in case of issues that arise at some borders or occasional increases in religious tensions or terrorist activities.

BIBLIOGRAPHY

1. Bacaner N, Stauffer B, Boulware DR, Walker PF, Keystone JS. Travel medicine considerations for North American immigrants visiting friends and relatives. JAMA. 2004 Jun 16;291(23):2856–64.

2. Baggett HC, Graham S, Kozarsky PE, Gallagher N, Blumensaadt S, Bateman J, et al. Pretravel health preparation among US residents traveling to India to VFRs: importance of ethnicity in defining VFRs. J Travel Med. 2009 Mar–Apr;16(2):112–8.

3. Das K, Jain A, Gupta S, Kapoor S, Gupta RK, Chakravorty A, et al. The changing epidemiological pattern of hepatitis A in an urban population of India: emergence of a trend similar to the European countries. Eur J Epidemiol. 2000 Jun;16(6):507–10.

4. Kumarasamy KK, Toleman MA, Walsh TR, Bagaria J, Butt F, Balakrishnan R, et al. Emergence of a new antibiotic resistance mechanism in India, Pakistan, and the UK: a molecular, biological, and epidemiological study. Lancet Infect Dis. 2010 Sep;10(9):597–602.

5. Leder K, Tong S, Weld L, Kain KC, Wilder-Smith A, von Sonnenburg F, et al. Illness in travelers visiting friends and relatives: a review of the GeoSentinel Surveillance Network. Clin Infect Dis. 2006 Nov 1;43(9):1185–93.

6. Leder K, Torresi J, Brownstein JS, Wilson ME, Keystone JS, Barnett E, et al. Travel-associated illness trends and clusters, 2000–2010. Emerg Infect Dis. 2013 Jul;19(7):1049–73.

7. Shaw MT, Leggat PA, Chatterjee S. Travelling to India for the Delhi XIX Commonwealth Games 2010. Travel Med Infect Dis. 2010 May;8(3):129–38.

8. Steffen R, Tornieporth N, Clemens SA, Chatterjee S, Cavalcanti AM, Collard F, et al. Epidemiology of travelers' diarrhea: details of a global survey. J Travel Med. 2004 Jul–Aug;11(4):231–7.

9. Steinberg EB, Bishop R, Haber P, Dempsey AF, Hoekstra RM, Nelson JM, et al. Typhoid fever in travelers: who should be targeted for prevention? Clin Infect Dis. 2004 Jul 15;39(2):186–91.

NEPAL
David R. Shlim

DESTINATION OVERVIEW

Nepal is a country of >28 million people that stretches for 500 miles (805 km) along the Himalayan mountains that form the border of Nepal and Tibet. The topography rises from low plains with an altitude of 200 ft (70 m) to the highest point in the world at 29,029 ft (8,848 m), the summit of Mount Everest. Approximately 30% of tourists to Nepal come to trek into the mountains, while others come to experience the culture and stunning natural beauty. Kathmandu is the capital city, with a population of approximately 2.5 million people. It sits in a lush valley at 4,344 ft (1,324 m) in altitude. Nepal's latitude of 28° North (the same as Florida) means that the nonmountainous areas are temperate year round. Most of the annual rainfall comes during the monsoon season (June through September). The main tourist seasons are in the spring (March to May) and fall (October and November). The winter months, December through February, are pleasant in the lowlands but can be too cold to make trekking enjoyable in the high mountains.

There are 3 main trekking areas: the Mount Everest region east of Kathmandu, the Annapurna region to the west, and the Langtang region north of Kathmandu (see Map 4-12). Trekkers into the Mount Everest region routinely sleep at altitudes of 14,000–16,000 ft (4,267–4,876 m) and hike to altitudes >18,000 ft (5,486 m). This prolonged exposure to very high altitudes means that tourists must be knowledgeable about the risks of altitude illness and may need to carry specific medications to prevent and treat the problem (see Chapter 2, Altitude Illness). Most trekkers into the Mount Everest region arrive there by flying to a tiny airstrip at Lukla at 9,383 ft (2,860 m). The following day they reach Namche Bazaar at 11,290 ft (3,440 m). Acetazolamide prophylaxis can substantially decrease the chances of developing acute mountain sickness in Namche.

In the Annapurna region, short-term trekkers may choose to hike to viewpoints in the foothills without reaching any high altitudes. Others may undertake a longer trek around the Annapurna massif, going over a 17,769-ft (5,416-m) pass (the Thorung La). Roads have been constructed up the 2 major valleys of this trek, shortening the overall trekking distance and changing the nature of the experience (cars and motorcycles may be encountered along the trek). In response to this, new trails and teahouses are being constructed away from the roads

MAP 4-12. NEPAL DESTINATION MAP

in order to preserve the trekking experience. The total exposure to high altitude is less in this region than in the Everest region. Trekkers are also seeking out more remote treks, such as around Manaslu and the newly opened Tsum Valley.

In addition to trekking, Nepal has some of the best rafting and kayaking rivers in the world. Jungle lodges in Chitwan National Park allow tourists to view a wide range of wildlife, including tigers, rhinoceroses, bears, and crocodiles, and a huge variety of exotic birds. It is also possible to travel by road to comfortable lodges in the foothills that afford panoramic views of the Himalayas.

HEALTH ISSUES

Immunizations

Travelers to Nepal are at high risk for enterically transmitted diseases. Hepatitis A vaccine and typhoid vaccine are the 2 most important immunizations. The risk of typhoid fever and paratyphoid fever among travelers to Nepal is among the highest in the world, and the prevalence of fluoroquinolone resistance is high.

Japanese encephalitis (JE) is endemic in Nepal, with highest disease risk occurring in the Terai region during and immediately after the monsoon season (June through October). JE has been identified in local residents of the Kathmandu Valley, but no cases of JE acquired in Nepal have been reported in tourists or expatriates. JE vaccine is not routinely recommended for those trekking in higher altitude areas or spending short periods in Kathmandu or Pokhara on the way to such treks (see Chapter 3, Japanese Encephalitis).

Malaria

Malaria is not a risk for most travelers to Nepal. There is no transmission of malaria in Kathmandu or Pokhara, the 2 main cities in Nepal. All the main trekking routes in Nepal are free of malaria transmission. Chitwan National Park is a popular tourist destination for wildlife viewing in the Terai. Although the Nepalese Ministry of Health and other regional organizations regard the Terai to be a malaria transmission area, this author, in 30 years of treating travelers in Nepal, has not seen a single case of malaria in a traveler to Chitwan, including foreign workers living in the park.

Other Health and Safety Risks
Gastrointestinal Issues

Cyclospora cayetanensis is an intestinal protozoal pathogen that is highly endemic in Nepal. The risk for infection is distinctly seasonal: transmission occurs almost exclusively from May through October, with a peak in June and July. Because this is outside the main tourist seasons, the primary effect is on expatriates who stay through the monsoon. In addition to watery diarrhea, profound anorexia and fatigue are the hallmark symptoms of *Cyclospora* infection. The treatment of choice is trimethoprim-sulfamethoxazole; no highly effective alternatives have been identified.

Since many tourists are heading to remote areas that do not have medical care available, they should be provided with medications for self-treatment. Travelers' diarrhea is a risk, and the risk in the spring trekking season (March through May) is double that in the fall trekking season (October and November). *Campylobacter* is the main diarrheal pathogen seen in medical clinics in Kathmandu, and resistance to fluoroquinolones is >90%. Azithromycin may be a better choice than ciprofloxacin for empiric treatment of bacterial diarrhea.

Cholera epidemics occur in local people during the summer months, but no cases of severe cholera have ever been observed in expatriates or tourists.

Hepatitis E virus is endemic in Nepal, and several cases each year are diagnosed in tourists or expatriates. There is no vaccine commercially available against hepatitis E.

Respiratory Issues

The Kathmandu Valley often has air pollution. People with chronic respiratory diseases, such as asthma and chronic obstructive pulmonary disease, may suffer exacerbations in Kathmandu, particularly after a viral upper respiratory infection. Exacerbation of chronic respiratory disease has not been a problem for tourists outside Kathmandu.

Viral upper respiratory infections are extremely common, and the percentage of these that lead to bacterial sinusitis or bronchitis is high. Trekkers should consider carrying an antibiotic, such as azithromycin, to empirically treat a respiratory infection that lasts >7 days with no sign of improvement. More treks may have been ruined by prolonged respiratory infection than by gastrointestinal illness.

Rabies

Rabies is highly endemic among dogs in Nepal, but in recent years there are fewer stray dogs in Kathmandu. Half of all tourist exposures to a possibly rabid animal occur near Swayambunath, a beautiful hilltop shrine also known as the monkey temple. Tourists should be advised to be extra cautious with dogs and monkeys in this area. The monkeys can be aggressive if approached and can jump on a person's back if they smell food in a backpack. Clinics in Kathmandu that specialize in the care of foreigners almost always have complete postexposure rabies prophylaxis, including human rabies immune globulin. Trekkers who are bitten in the mountains should be able to return to Kathmandu within an average of 5 days.

Evacuation and Medical Care

Helicopter evacuation from most areas is readily available. Communication has improved from remote areas because of satellite and cellular telephones, and private helicopter companies accept credit cards and are eager to perform evacuations for profit. Evacuation can often take place on the same day as the request, if weather permits. Helicopter rescue is usually limited to morning hours because of afternoon winds in the mountains. Helicopter rescue is billed at $2,500 per hour, with an average total cost of $10,000.

Two main clinics in Kathmandu specialize in the care of foreigners in Nepal. Contact information is available on the International Society of Travel Medicine website (www.istm.org). Hospital facilities have improved steadily over the years, and general and orthopedic emergency surgery are reliable and available in Kathmandu. The closest evacuation point for definitive care is Bangkok.

Travelers should be made aware that many hospitals and clinics in Kathmandu pay a commission to tour guides who bring foreign patients to them; therefore, ill travelers may not be brought to the best institution for their care. Travel health professionals are advised to research the best clinics and hospitals in Nepal and make a recommendation to their patients before they travel to Nepal.

The Political Situation

The political situation in Nepal has been in transition since 1990, when a mainly peaceful democratic revolution led to a multiparty parliamentary system under a constitutional monarch. Frustration with the rate of progress in rural areas led to a Maoist insurrection and 10 years of low-grade but violent civil war. A peace agreement was reached and the monarchy abolished in 2008, but an effective government has yet to remain in place. The main effect on tourists can be disruptions to their schedule by demonstrations and strikes, but none of the political tension has been aimed at foreigners; Nepal remains a safe destination to visit. However, visitors should monitor the political situation while planning their journey.

BIBLIOGRAPHY

1. Cave W, Pandey P, Osrin D, Shlim DR. Chemoprophylaxis use and the risk of malaria in travelers to Nepal. J Travel Med. 2003 Mar–Apr;10(2):100–5.
2. Hoge CW, Shlim DR, Echeverria P, Rajah R, Herrmann JE, Cross JH. Epidemiology of diarrhea among expatriate residents living in a highly endemic environment. JAMA. 1996 Feb 21;275(7):533–8.
3. Schwartz E, Shlim DR, Eaton M, Jenks N, Houston R. The effect of oral and parenteral typhoid vaccination on the rate of infection with *Salmonella typhi* and *Salmonella paratyphi* A among foreigners in Nepal. Arch Intern Med. 1990 Feb;150(2):349–51.

THAILAND
Gabrielle A. Benenson, Michael W. Benenson

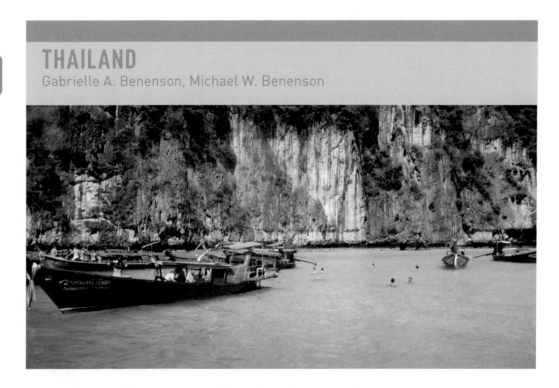

DESTINATION OVERVIEW

Thailand, known as "the Land of Smiles," is a popular travel destination because of its warm and welcoming reception of tourists and expatriates, beautiful beaches, delicious cuisine, excellent shopping, fabulous golf courses, exciting nightlife, and exotic adventure opportunities. Many travelers also visit Thailand for business, and the country is quickly becoming a regional business hub. In 2011, >19 million visitors spent more than 1 night in Thailand, and the number of visitors continues to grow. Thai is a melodic, tonal language that can be difficult to learn. Luckily, most popular destinations in Thailand feature Thai people who speak English and road signs, maps, and tourist guides that provide information in English and Thai.

With close to 67 million people, divided into 76 political provinces, Thailand is a geographically diverse country a little smaller than the state of Texas (Map 4-13). Thailand's geography includes the following:

> Sandy beaches and rocky shores along its 2,000-mile coastline and >1,400 islands
> Central plains made up of extensive rice fields along the Chao Phraya River

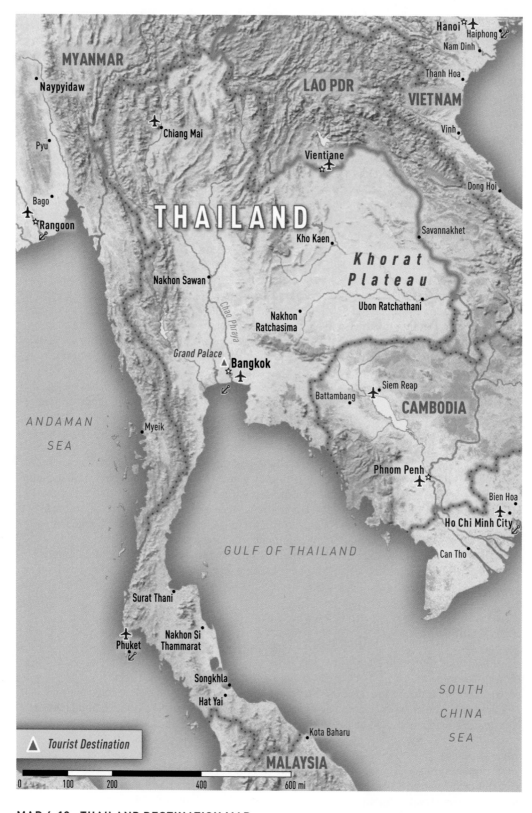

MAP 4-13. THAILAND DESTINATION MAP

> Mountainous areas in northern, western, and eastern Thailand
> The dry Khorat Plateau in northeastern Thailand.

Because Thailand is close to the equator, the climate is tropical and often hot and humid. Flooding is always a possibility in Thailand, and various regions are prone to flash floods. Monsoon rains fall from May through July and can last until cooler, drier weather comes in November, making November through February a popular time of year to visit Thailand. Thailand's central location and major international airport in Bangkok make it an easy access point for other destinations in Asia.

More than 9 million people live in the capital city of Bangkok, a major metropolis and center of commerce. Bangkok is a mix of old and new—skyscrapers and waterways, bustling city streets full of people, vendors, dogs, uneven sidewalks, and lots of traffic, in contrast to the fast, quiet, and cool modern monorail and subway systems. Tourists visit historic sites of glittering grandeur such as the Grand Palace to catch a glimpse of the Emerald Buddha or one of Bangkok's 400 Buddhist temples. The main artery of Bangkok is the Chao Phraya River and its canals, which provide access to tourist sites, boat tours, the floating market, and restaurants. Bangkok is a paradise of culinary delights, from local fare at a sidewalk noodle stand to a fancy 4-star meal in a restaurant. Rounding off a visit to Bangkok, many tourists will enjoy the pleasures of Thai nightlife, which includes a variety of bars and pubs, dance clubs, drag shows, and the famous red light districts of Soi Cowboy, Nana, and Patpong.

Visitors to Thailand will also likely visit Chiang Mai, in northern Thailand. The city, surrounded by a moat and defensive wall, has >300 temples, a popular night bazaar for great shopping, and easy access to the handicraft villages, elephant nature parks, and outdoor adventures that are popular in the region.

A popular reason to visit Thailand is for rest and relaxation on sandy beaches along the coast or on one of the many islands. Beach destinations include plenty of opportunities for snorkeling, scuba diving, windsurfing, sailing, swimming, and dining on fresh seafood. A growing number of tourists seek out such relaxation opportunities as part of their recovery from medical or dental procedures.

Over the years, medical tourism to Thailand has increased, as the costs for treatment are much lower and the quality of care is generally good. Thailand is frequently listed as one of the top medical tourist destinations worldwide; 27 Thai hospitals were accredited by the Joint Commission International in 2014. For example, Thailand's Bumrungrad Hospital has a special section of their website for medical tourists in addition to an office, with translators, to facilitate services for foreigners seeking treatment and care at their facility.

Thailand has a large expatriate community and has also become a popular destination for retirees from around the world. The warm climate and low cost of living make Thailand an attractive place to live.

HEALTH ISSUES

Immunizations
All travelers should be up-to-date on their routine vaccinations. In addition, travelers to Thailand should also be vaccinated against hepatitis A and hepatitis B. Typhoid and Japanese encephalitis vaccines should be considered based on potential risk.

Rabies vaccine
Government-sponsored mass vaccination campaigns for dogs and cats have reduced the prevalence of rabies in Thailand, but rabies is still a risk, particularly in Bangkok, where dogs roam the streets. Preexposure vaccination is only recommended for travelers who have an occupation that puts them at risk for exposure (such as veterinarians) or will be traveling for long periods of time. Hospitals and clinics in Bangkok cater to the expatriate

community and medical tourists, and rabies vaccine is readily available for preexposure and postexposure prophylaxis, although not all hospitals in Thailand carry human rabies immune globulin.

Japanese Encephalitis vaccine

Japanese encephalitis (JE) is endemic throughout Thailand (see Chapter 3, Japanese Encephalitis). Transmission occurs year-round, with seasonal epidemics from May through October in the northern provinces. JE vaccine is recommended for travelers who plan to visit Thailand for ≥1 month and should be considered for those visiting for a shorter period but who have an increased risk of JE virus exposure due to their itineraries or activities. The highest rates of human disease have been reported from the Chiang Mai Valley. Several cases have been reported among travelers who visited resort or coastal areas of southern Thailand.

Malaria

Malaria is endemic in specific areas of Thailand, particularly the rural, forested areas that border Burma (Myanmar), Cambodia, and Laos, as well as the rural, forested areas of Phang Nga and Phuket. Prophylaxis is recommended for travelers visiting any of these areas (see Chapter 3, Malaria). Transmission in Thailand occurs year-round, and most cases are due to *Plasmodium falciparum*, with the rest due to *P. vivax* or mixed infection. Atovaquone-proguanil or doxycycline are the recommended antimalarial drugs for travelers in Thailand.

Dengue

Dengue is endemic throughout Thailand (see Chapter 3, Dengue) with large epidemics that occur every several years. Peak transmission occurs during the rainy season, although cases occur year-round even in non-epidemic years. Travelers to Thailand should take measures to protect themselves from daytime mosquito bites to prevent dengue (see Chapter 2, Protection against Mosquitoes, Ticks, & Other Arthropods).

Travelers' Diarrhea

Although the Thai government and several nongovernmental organizations are leading projects to provide clean water across Thailand, and some hotels use their own filtration systems, water and food may still contain harmful bacteria and other contaminants. Travelers should practice food and water precautions and bring an antibiotic for self-treatment. Because fluoroquinolone resistance is widespread in Thailand and other areas of Southeast Asia, azithromycin may be preferred (see Chapter 2, Travelers' Diarrhea).

Water and Soil Diseases

Melioidosis is highly endemic in northeast Thailand, and the highest number of leptospirosis cases can be found in the southern and northeastern regions of the country. For both diseases, most cases occur during the rainy season. Travelers who visit endemic areas should avoid contact with soil and water that could be contaminated and ensure that any open wounds are covered to prevent exposure. When contact cannot be avoided, travelers should wear protective clothing and footwear to reduce the risk of exposure. Skin lacerations, abrasions, or burns that have been contaminated with soil or surface water should be immediately and thoroughly cleaned.

Other Health and Safety Risks

Medical Tourism

As one of the top destinations for medical travel, travelers who plan to seek medical care in Thailand should be advised to research facilities and develop a plan before departure, learn about health insurance coverage, and evaluate their health before making the trip (see Chapter 2, Medical Tourism).

Sexually Transmitted Diseases and HIV/AIDS

Thailand is a popular destination for sex tourism (see Chapter 3, *Perspectives*: Sex & Tourism), and although illegal, sex work is practiced openly across the country. A 100% condom program with sex workers helped slow the spread of HIV and other sexually transmitted diseases; however, approximately 450,000 people are living with HIV/AIDS in Thailand. Although the number of new HIV infections has been decreasing, HIV remains concentrated in key populations. Travelers should be aware of these risks and always use condoms during sex with partners whose HIV status is unknown.

Safety and Security

Approximately 13,000 people are killed on the roads in Thailand each year, and a substantial proportion (74% in 2010) are killed in motorcycle accidents. Motorcycles are a cheap, easy, and popular mode of transportation, but they are also the most vulnerable vehicles on the road. Travelers should avoid riding motorcycles. If they must ride, they should wear a helmet.

Since 2006, Thailand has experienced intermittent periods of political unrest. Travelers should be aware of the possibility of demonstrations, pay attention to the local news, and monitor the US embassy website (bangkok.usembassy.gov) and social media outlets to find out if and where protests and demonstrations may occur. Travelers should avoid these locations, since no one can predict whether protests will stay peaceful or turn violent.

BIBLIOGRAPHY

1. Bumrungrad International Hospital [Internet]. Plan your visit-overview. Bangkok, Thailand: Bumrungrad International Hospital; 2014 [cited 2014 Sep 18]. Available from: http://www.bumrungrad.com/en/plan-your-visit/overview.
2. Bureau of Epidemiology, Ministry of Public Health, Thailand. National disease surveillance (report 506): Leptospirosis. Bangkok: Ministry of Public Health Thailand; 2014 [cited 2014 Sep 22]. Available from: http://www.boe.moph.go.th/boedb/surdata/506wk/y57/en/d43_0957_en.pdf.
3. Chanlett-Avery E, Dolven B. Thailand: background and US relations. Washington, DC: Congressional Research Service; 2014 [cited 2014 Sep 22]. Available from: http://fas.org/sgp/crs/row/RL32593.pdf.
4. Gongal G, Wright AE. Human rabies in the WHO Southeast Asia Region: forward steps for elimination. Adv Prev Med. 2011;Article ID 383870:1–5.
5. Joint Commission International (JCI) [Internet]. JCI-accredited organizations. Oak Brook, IL: JCI; 2014 [cited 2014 Sep 18]. Available from: www.jointcommissioninternational.org/about-jci/jci-accredited-organizations/.
6. Joint United Nations Programme on HIV/AIDS (UNAIDS). HIV in Asia and the Pacific: UNAIDS report 2013. Geneva: UNAIDS; 2013 [cited 2014 Sep 22]. Available from: http://www.unaids.org/en/media/unaids/contentassets/documents/unaidspublication/2013/2013_HIV-Asia-Pacific_en.pdf.
7. Wiwanitkit V. Rate of malarial infection among foreigners in a tertiary hospital of Thailand: change of epidemiology and importance of travel medicine (1996–2005). J Vector Borne Dis. 2007 Sep;44(3):219–22.
8. World Bank [Internet]. International tourism, number of arrivals. Washington, DC: The World Bank Group; 2014 [cited 2014 Sep 22]. Available from: http://data.worldbank.org/data-catalog/world-development-indicators.
9. World Health Organization. WHO global status report on road safety 2013: supporting a decade of action Geneva: World Health Organization; 2013 [cited 2014 Sep 19]. Available from: http://www.who.int/violence_injury_prevention/road_safety_status/2013/en/.

VIETNAM

James C. Kile, Sheryl Lyss

DESTINATION OVERVIEW

Vietnam has a population of approximately 90 million people, making it the 13th most populous nation, of whom about 70% live in rural areas. The total size of Vietnam is 127,243 mi^2 (331,114 km^2), making it the 67th largest country in the world, comparable to Finland and Malaysia, or the combined size of Ohio, Kentucky, and Tennessee. It is located in Southeast Asia and borders China, Laos, and Cambodia. Vietnam is divided into 63 provinces. The terrain and climate vary, particularly between the north and the south and the mountainous and coastal areas.

Vietnam is an increasingly popular travel destination for business and tourism. Travelers often try to get a flavor for the entire country with a trip of at least 10 days or combine their Vietnam travels with other nearby Southeast Asia destinations such as Angkor Wat in Cambodia or Luang Prabang in Laos. There is no shortage of attractions in Vietnam, regardless of whether a traveler is interested in touring historical sites, shopping in ethnic markets or traditional trade villages, trekking or biking in hills or valleys, seeing native wildlife, cruising on the Mekong River, scuba diving in the sea, relaxing at a spa resort, visiting art galleries, or taking cooking lessons to understand the regional variations of Vietnam's cuisine.

A typical itinerary might start in the north and include visiting the capital, Hanoi; touring the UNESCO World Heritage site, Ha Long Bay, aboard a junk boat; and experiencing the rice fields and ethnic minorities in Sapa or Mai Chau. In the coastal region, travelers often go to Hue, Hoi An, Danang, Dalat, and Nha Trang, each with their own charms and unique personalities. In the south, travelers often choose to see Vietnam's largest, busiest, and most modern city, Ho Chi Minh City. From there, Phu Quoc Island, the Cu Chi tunnels, and floating markets of the Mekong Delta are easy trips (see Map 4-14).

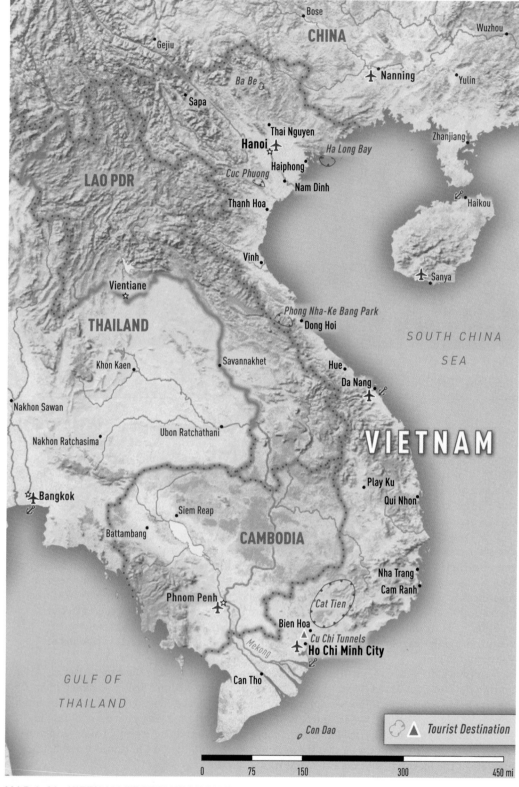

MAP 4-14. VIETNAM DESTINATION MAP

Immunizations

Travelers to Vietnam should be up-to-date on routine vaccines, such as measles-mumps-rubella, diphtheria-pertussis-tetanus, and seasonal influenza. Travelers should also protect themselves by getting vaccinated against typhoid and hepatitis A. Hepatitis B protection is advised, especially for long-term travelers and expatriates, given the high prevalence of chronic HBV infection in the population.

Japanese Encephalitis Vaccine

Because Japanese encephalitis (JE) is endemic throughout Vietnam, JE vaccination is recommended for all travelers who spend ≥1 month or more in the country and should be considered for short-term travelers who plan on spending time outside urban areas and may be involved in activities that expose them to the mosquitoes that transmit JE virus. Such activities may include camping, hiking, biking or other outdoor activities, or staying in accommodations without air conditioning, screens, or bed nets (see Chapter 3, Japanese Encephalitis). JE has seasonal peaks from May through October, and the highest rates of JE disease occur in the northern provinces around Hanoi and the northwestern and northeastern provinces bordering China. Personalized advice during a thorough pre-travel consultation is important.

Rabies Vaccine

Travelers should receive preexposure immunizations against rabies if they will be spending a lot of time outdoors, have direct contact with dogs and cats or with wildlife, or will be in Vietnam for a prolonged period of time. Dog rabies is a concern in Vietnam. Most dogs are not routinely vaccinated in Vietnam and are numerous even in urban areas where dogs are typically not leashed. Special consideration should be given to vaccinating children. Care should also be taken to avoid contact with nonhuman primates, as several tourist destinations (for example, islands in Ha Long Bay and off Nha Trang) have macaques that are not afraid of humans and may be infected with B virus as well as rabies. Human rabies immune globulin is usually available in larger cities, such as Hanoi and Ho Chi Minh City. Travelers should be encouraged to purchase travel health insurance that includes medical evacuation insurance in the event that postexposure prophylaxis is unavailable.

Malaria

Most tourist itineraries do not include malaria-endemic areas of Vietnam. Malaria is primarily a concern in rural areas and is mostly caused by *Plasmodium falciparum*. There are rare cases in the Mekong Delta and none in the Red River Delta, the coast north of Nha Trang, or in larger cities such as Da Nang, Haiphong, Hanoi, Ho Chi Minh City, Nha Tran, and Qui Nhon. Travelers to the Mekong Delta should take precautions to avoid mosquito bites, such as wearing loose-fitting clothing (long pants and long-sleeved shirts) and using insect repellent, but do not need to take antimalarial drugs. Travelers to other parts of Vietnam where malaria is known to be circulating should take chemoprophylaxis appropriate to the specific places they will be visiting. Mefloquine resistance has been reported in some areas, so travel health clinicians may feel more comfortable recommending atovaquone-proguanil or doxycycline to travelers (see Chapter 3, Malaria).

Dengue

Dengue is endemic in Vietnam and, although peak transmission occurs during the summer rainy season, dengue virus transmission occurs year-round. Travelers to Vietnam should take measures to protect themselves from daytime mosquito bites to prevent dengue (see Chapter 2, Protection against Mosquitoes, Ticks, & Other Arthropods).

Avian Influenza

Vietnam continues to report sporadic cases of human infection with avian influenza A (H5N1) virus or "bird flu," as it is commonly known. H5N1 is endemic in domestic poultry in Vietnam, with continued sporadic and geographically dispersed outbreaks. Most people who have become infected had direct contact or close exposure to sick or dead poultry by visiting live bird or poultry markets or preparing or eating uncooked or undercooked bird products (such as poultry meat, eggs, or blood). In extremely rare situations, a few people were infected as a result of close, prolonged contact with another person who was sick with avian influenza.

A novel avian influenza A (H7N9) virus was identified in China in 2013, including in a province bordering Vietnam. To date, no animals or humans have been identified in Vietnam with this strain of avian influenza virus.

To avoid infection with avian influenza viruses, travelers to an area affected by avian influenza should avoid direct contact with birds, including poultry (such as chickens and ducks) and wild birds; avoid touching surfaces that have bird droppings (feces) or other bird fluids on them; and avoid places where live birds are raised, kept, or sold, such as live bird markets.

Travelers should eat only bird meat or products that have been thoroughly cooked. Any dishes that contain uncooked (raw) or undercooked bird meat or products such as eggs and poultry blood should be avoided. For example, egg yolks should not be runny or liquid. Travelers should also practice healthy habits to help stop the spread of germs by washing hands often with soap and clean water or using an alcohol-based hand sanitizer (containing at least 60% alcohol) when soap and clean water are not available and hands are not visibly dirty.

Other Health and Safety Risks
Foodborne Illnesses

Drinking tap water should be avoided, as should beverages with ice. Travelers should avoid eating food or drinking beverages from street vendors and should avoid eating raw or undercooked meat or seafood, uncooked vegetables, and raw fruits that cannot be peeled by the traveler. Travelers with seafood allergies should be particularly cautious in Vietnam, given the common use of fish and other seafood sauces in many dishes.

Skin Diseases

Skin rashes may result from the combination of heat and humidity or fungal infections. Efforts should be made to keep clothes, shoes, and linens clean and dry and to minimize sun exposure by using sunscreen (SPF ≥15), clothing, hats, and umbrellas.

Noise and Air Pollution

Construction sounds and frequent honking of motorbike and car horns can be an annoyance. Travelers with allergies or asthma may find their conditions are exacerbated because of high levels of particulate matter and indoor air pollution, especially in Hanoi and Ho Chi Minh City.

Road Safety

To avoid motor vehicle–related injuries, travelers should fasten seat belts when riding in cars and wear a safety helmet when riding bicycles and motorbikes. Pedestrians may find road conditions in Vietnam to be challenging because of an apparent lack of rules and many vehicles and motorcycles sharing the road. Travelers are advised to walk facing traffic and, when crossing the street, to proceed at a consistent walking pace with no sudden movement changes, such as suddenly turning back. Pedestrians will observe that motorbikes and cars will go around them much like a school of fish will part when it encounters an object and then regroup. Note that motorbikes and sometimes cars will travel on the wrong sides of the street (against oncoming traffic) as well as on sidewalks, so travelers should be urged to always look in both directions.

Medical Care in Vietnam

Several private medical practices, clinics, and hospitals that serve foreigners are available in Hanoi and Ho Chi Minh City. However, blood transfusion services, inpatient care, and specialty services are generally not of high quality. Thus, travelers should ensure that they have adequate medical evacuation insurance in case they need to be evacuated to Singapore or Bangkok where high-quality specialty services are provided (see Chapter 2, Travel Insurance, Travel Health Insurance, & Medical Evacuation Insurance). To ensure the quality of any needed medications, travelers may want to consider purchasing them through an expatriate or international travel clinic, even if the price is higher. If a traveler is taking prescription medicine, he or she should bring enough medication for the entire trip, in the original bottle and with the prescription.

BIBLIOGRAPHY

1. Carrique-Mas JJ, Bryant JE. A review of foodborne bacterial and parasitic zoonoses in Vietnam. EcoHealth. 2013 Dec;10(4):465–89.

2. CDC. Japanese encephalitis among three US travelers returning from Asia, 2003–2008. MMWR Morb Mortal Wkly Rep. 2009 Jul 17;58(27):737–40.

3. Cuong HQ, Vu NT, Cazelles B, Boni MF, Thai KT, Rabaa MA, et al. Spatiotemporal dynamics of dengue epidemics, southern Vietnam. Emerg Infect Dis. 2013 Jun;19(6):945–53.

4. Hanoi International Women's Club. Hanoi Guide. Hanoi: Hanoi Publishing House; 2008.

5. Hsu A, Emerson J, Levy M, de Sherbinin A, Johnson L, Malik O, et al. The 2014 Environmental Performance Index: country profiles, Viet Nam. New Haven, CT: Yale Center for Environmental Law and Policy; 2014 [cited 2014 Sep 18]. Available from: http://epi.yale.edu/epi/country-profile/viet-nam.

6. Phan HYT, Yano T. Road traffic noise policy in Vietnam. J Temporal Des Arch Environ. 2009;9(1):150–3.

7. Sniadack DH, Mendoza-Aldana J, Huyen DT, Van TT, Cuong NV, Olive JM, et al. Epidemiology of a measles epidemic in Vietnam 2008–2010. J Infect Dis. 2011 Jul;204 Suppl 1:S476–82.

8. World Bank [Internet]. Vietnam overview. Washington, DC: The World Bank Group; 2014 [accessed 2014 Sep 22]. Available from: http://www.worldbank.org/en/country/vietnam/overview.

9. World Health Organization Western Pacific Region [Internet]. WHO representative office in Vietnam. Hanoi: World Health Organization; 2014 [cited 2014 Sep 18]. Available from: http://www.wpro.who.int/vietnam/en.

10. Yen NT, Duffy MR, Hong NM, Hien NT, Fischer M, Hills SL. Surveillance for Japanese encephalitis in Vietnam, 1998–2007. Am J Trop Med Hyg. 2010 Oct;83(4):816–9.

THE MIDDLE EAST & NORTH AFRICA

EGYPT & NILE RIVER CRUISES
Ann M. Buff

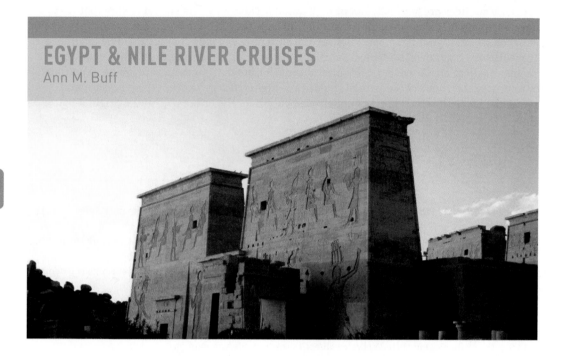

DESTINATION OVERVIEW

The Arab Republic of Egypt covers a land area >1,000,000 km², approximately the same size as Texas and New Mexico combined, and >95% of the country is desert. With an estimated 84 million people, Egypt accounts for one-fourth of the Arab world's population. Egypt has long been considered the cradle of civilization and may be the oldest tourist destination on earth. Throughout the world, Egypt is synonymous with the legends of the Pharaohs, the Great Pyramids, treasure-laden tombs, and hieroglyphs. Travelers visit Egypt to see the ancient monuments and timeless river vistas along the Nile Valley. However, since the 2011 Arab Spring revolution and ongoing civil unrest, tourism has declined sharply, and travel in certain parts of the country is officially prohibited for tourists due to safety concerns.

A typical visit to Egypt includes arrival in the capital city of Cairo, the largest city in Africa and the Middle East, with a population of over 17 million. Considered the "Mother of the World" by Arabs, Cairo today is a modern, cosmopolitan mix of Arab, African, and European influences. Travelers generally spend at least a few days in Cairo seeing the Egyptian Antiquities Museum, Pyramids at Giza, Citadel and Mosque of Al-Azhar, and Khan al-Khalili bazaar.

Most travelers include an Upper Nile River cruise as part of their itineraries. Nile River cruises are usually 3–7 days, with embarkation in either Luxor or Aswan. Even before 2011, riverboats did not sail through middle Egypt because of security concerns; therefore, most travelers take short domestic flights or trains from Cairo to Luxor or Aswan. Approximately 200 riverboats are based on the Nile, and the average boat accommodates 120 passengers. The largest boats accommodate upwards of 300 passengers; chartered yachts might have just a few cabins. Riverboats have a range of accommodations from basic to 5-star luxury, and nights aboard are generally spent cruising from one port to the next.

Virtually all Nile cruises sail between Luxor and Aswan. There are 3 usual Nile cruise durations and itineraries: a 3-night cruise from Aswan to Luxor (or the reverse), a 4-night cruise from Luxor to Aswan (or the reverse), and a 7-night cruise roundtrip from Luxor or Aswan (see Map 4-15). A standard itinerary is as follows:

> Day 1: Fly from Cairo to Aswan or Luxor. Stay in a hotel for the first night or board the boat directly and spend the afternoon and early the next morning visiting the sites (High Dam and Philae Temple in Aswan or Karnak Temple, Luxor Temple, Valley of the Kings, and Hapshepsut Temple in Luxor).
> Days 2–6: Visit temples of Edfu, Esna, and Kom Ombo and enjoy the passing riverside scenes of ancient villages, minarets, farmers in *galabiyas*, and traditional *feluccas*. Most travelers have an early breakfast aboard and then depart the boat for sightseeing early in the day to avoid the crowds and heat. Most travelers will be back aboard by mid- to late afternoon. Dinner and entertainment follow in the evening.
> Final day: Disembark and return to Cairo or travel to a Red Sea resort.

Egypt is also a beach destination, with thousands of miles of Mediterranean and Red Sea coastlines. Alexandria, Egypt's second largest city, with >5 million people, is located on the Mediterranean Sea and has a string of beaches and seafood restaurants. The World War II battlefield of El-Alamein lies along the Mediterranean coast, and divers will find an array of sunken cities and wartime wrecks to explore offshore. Egypt's Red Sea coast has reefs offshore, with diving and snorkeling traditionally centered in Hurghada.

Edged by coral reefs and teeming with tropical fish, the Sinai Peninsula has excellent diving, snorkeling, and beaches; Sharm el Sheikh is the most developed and visited area of the Sinai. Visits to Mount Sinai (7,497 ft [2,285 m] above sea level) and Saint Catherine's Monastery in the mountainous interior are popular destinations, especially with religious pilgrims.

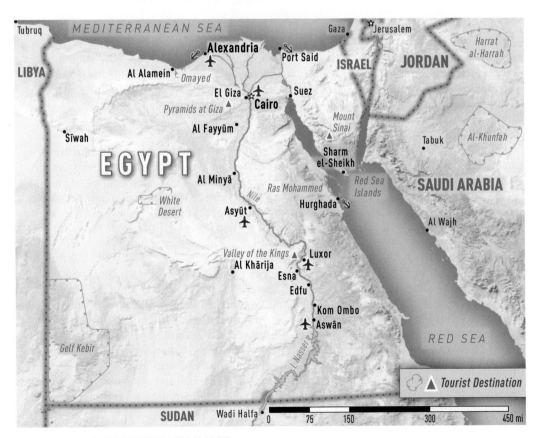

MAP 4-15. EGYPT DESTINATION MAP

Adventure travelers favor desert jeep safaris and camel treks to remote oases and spectacular *wadis*. Travelers start in Cairo or Assyut and follow the "Great Desert Circuit" through 4 oases and the White Desert. Tourists might be banned from travel to remote locations, including the interior of the Sinai Peninsula, for safety reasons. Military and police road checkpoints are common, and security services enforce official travel restrictions.

HEALTH ISSUES

In addition to being up-to-date on routine vaccines, hepatitis A and B and typhoid vaccines are recommended for travelers to Egypt. Egypt has the highest prevalence of hepatitis C virus infection (approximately 10%) in the world and a high estimated prevalence of hepatitis B virus infection (2%–7%). Travelers should be cautioned to protect themselves from all bloodborne pathogens by avoiding unprotected sex, invasive medical and dental procedures, injection drug use, and tattooing. Modern hospitals and clinics cater to the expatriate communities in Cairo and Alexandria and to tourists in the Red Sea resort areas.

Travelers' Diarrhea
In most large international tourist hotels, the tap water is adequately chlorinated, but bottled water is generally provided for drinking. Tap water is not safe to drink in other locations. Eating thoroughly cooked meat and vegetables in tourist hotels, on Nile River cruise ships, and in tourist restaurants is generally safe. Eating raw or undercooked ground meat or shellfish should be avoided. As in many developing countries, the safety of uncooked vegetables and salads is questionable. The risk of diarrhea in Egypt is high. Clinicians should consider prescribing an antibiotic for travelers to Egypt to empirically self-treat diarrhea.

Schistosomiasis
Schistosoma mansoni and *S. haematobium* are endemic in Egypt. Travelers to Egypt should avoid wading, swimming, or other contact with freshwater, including the Nile River and irrigation canals. Swimming in saline pools of desert oases, chlorinated swimming pools, the Mediterranean Sea, or Red Sea does not pose a risk for acquiring schistosomiasis.

Rabies
As in most other developing countries, rabies is endemic throughout Egypt. For most travelers on a package tour, the risk will be minimal. However, travelers should be aware that there are large numbers of stray dogs and cats in urban and tourist areas and should be advised to avoid contact with domestic or wild mammals. Rabies vaccine is available for preexposure and postexposure prophylaxis, and human rabies immune globulin (HRIG) is also available. Both rabies vaccine and HRIG are produced locally.

Environmental Concerns
Temperature and weather conditions vary widely in Egypt. The desert is extremely hot in summer (>100°F; >38°C) and can be cold in winter (<32°F; <0°C). Thirst is a late indicator of dehydration, and travelers should drink fluids regularly in the heat. Because sweat evaporates immediately, people can become dehydrated without realizing it. Travelers who are elderly or take diuretic, anticholinergic, or neuroleptic medications are at increased risk of heat-associated illnesses. To stay cool and protect themselves from sun exposure, travelers should wear a hat and lightweight, loose-fitting clothing and use sunscreen.

Sandstorms occur sporadically in the desert. Desert sand, dust, and smog can cause eye irritation and exacerbate asthma or other lung disorders. Travelers who wear contact lenses should ensure that they pack eyeglasses and contact lens care supplies.

Motion Sickness

Generally, the Nile is a slow, smooth river. However, the combination of diesel fuel, heat, and motion can cause distress for travelers. Most travelers do not consider the possibility of motion sickness on a river, so they are unprepared. Onboard medical services vary greatly. Travelers who know that they are sensitive to motion should carry anti–motion sickness medication.

Insects

Mosquitoes and other biting insects can be problematic for travelers. Avoiding insect bites will prevent local discomfort and irritation and reduce the risk of vectorborne diseases. Dengue has been reported rarely in travelers who visited Egypt. Although West Nile virus seroprevalance rates are high (24%) and transmission widely distributed, infections in returning travelers appear to be rare.

In 2014, local transmission of malaria was reported in a village in Aswan Governorate. These were the first cases of malaria seen in Egypt since 1998. Although malaria prophylaxis is not recommended, travelers should practice insect precautions (see Chapter 2, Protection against Mosquitoes, Ticks, & Other Arthropods). Vectorborne diseases should be considered in travelers with fever returning from Egypt.

BIBLIOGRAPHY

1. Burdino E, Milia MG, Sergi G, Gregori G, Allice T, Cazzato ML, et al. Diagnosis of dengue fever in North West Italy in travelers from endemic areas: a retrospective study. J Clin Virol. 2011 Aug;51(4):259–63.
2. El-Zanaty F, Way A. Egypt: demographic and health survey, 2008. Cairo: Ministry of Health, El-Zanaty and Associates, Macro International; 2009 [cited 2014 Sep 22]. Available from: http://www.measuredhs.com/pubs/pdf/FR220/FR220.pdf.
3. Gautret P, Schlagenhauf P, Gaudart J, Castelli F, Brouqui P, von Sonnenburg F, et al. Multicenter EuroTravNet/GeoSentinel study of travel-related infectious diseases in Europe. Emerg Infect Dis. 2009 Nov;15(11):1783–90.
4. Hatzakis A, Van Damme P, Alcorn K, Gore C, Benazzouz M, Berkane S, et al. The state of hepatitis B and C in the Mediterranean and Balkan countries: report from a summit conference. J Viral Hepat. 2013 Aug;20 Suppl 2:1–20.
5. Lehman EM, Wilson ML. Epidemiology of hepatitis viruses among hepatocellular carcinoma cases and healthy people in Egypt: a systematic review and meta-analysis. Int J Cancer. 2009 Feb 1;124(3):690–7.
6. Soliman A, Mohareb E, Salman D, Saad M, Salama S, Fayez C, et al. Studies on West Nile virus infection in Egypt. J Infect Public Health. 2010;3(2):54–9.

SAUDI ARABIA: HAJJ PILGRIMAGE

Christopher S. Bowron, Salahudin M. Maalim

DESTINATION OVERVIEW

They will come to thee on foot and (mounted) on every kind of camel, lean on account of journeys through deep and distant mountain highways...(Quran 22:27)

The Hajj is the annual pilgrimage to Mecca, Saudi Arabia, and the largest mass gathering in the world. Every able-bodied adult Muslim who can afford to do so is required to make Hajj at least once in his or her lifetime. Hajj takes place from the 8th through the 12th days of Dhu al-Hijja, the last month of the Islamic year. Because the Islamic calendar is lunar, the timing of Hajj varies with respect to the Gregorian calendar (for example, it was October 1–6 in 2014 and will be September 20–25 in 2015).

More than 2 million Muslims from >183 countries make Hajj each year (approximately 2.8 million in 2010), >11,000 of whom travel from the United States.

Most international pilgrims fly into Jeddah and take a bus to Mecca. By foot or by bus, the pilgrim then travels 8 km to the massive tent city of Mina, where most pilgrims are housed in air-conditioned tents.

At dawn on the 9th day of Dhu al-Hijja, pilgrims begin a 14.4-km walk to the plain of Arafat, passing Muzdalifah along the way (Map 4-16). The route is littered with cool mist sprinklers to counteract the oppressive daytime temperatures, but the risk of heat-related illnesses during this part of the journey is high. Hajj ambulances and medical stations along the route are available for medical assistance. Hajj culminates on the Plain of Arafat, a few miles east of Mecca, where the Prophet Muhammad delivered his final sermon. Pilgrims spend the day in supplication, praying and reading the Quran; it is the pinnacle of most pilgrims' spiritual lives. After sunset, pilgrims begin the 9-km walk back to Muzdalifah, where they sleep in the open air.

At sunrise on the 10th day of Dhu al-Hijja, pilgrims collect small pebbles at Muzdalifah and carry them to Mina. This day's ritual is called the Stoning of the Devil at Jamaraat. During this ritual, pilgrims throw 7 tiny pebbles (specifically, no larger than a chickpea) at each of

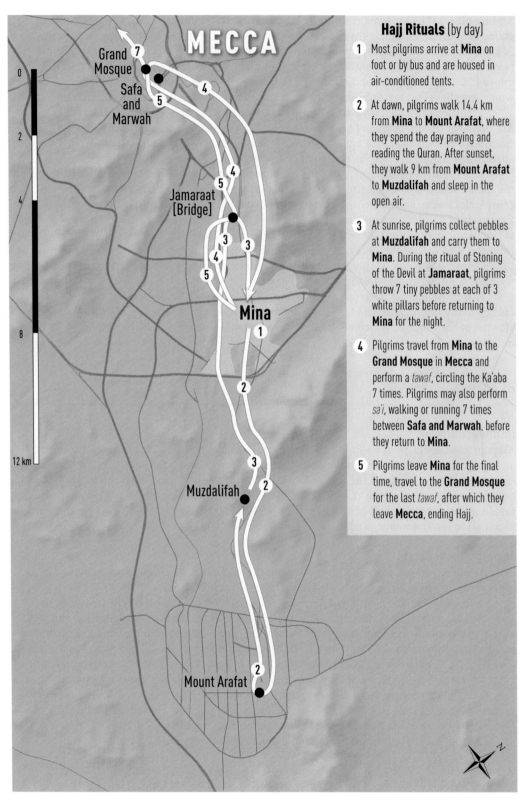

MECCA

Grand Mosque ⑦

Safa and Marwah ⑤

④

Jamaraat [Bridge] ④ ⑤

③ ③

④

⑤

Mina ①

②

③

②

Muzdalifah ②

Mount Arafat ②

0
2
4
8
12 km

Hajj Rituals (by day)

① Most pilgrims arrive at **Mina** on foot or by bus and are housed in air-conditioned tents.

② At dawn, pilgrims walk 14.4 km from **Mina** to **Mount Arafat**, where they spend the day praying and reading the Quran. After sunset, they walk 9 km from **Mount Arafat** to **Muzdalifah** and sleep in the open air.

③ At sunrise, pilgrims collect pebbles at **Muzdalifah** and carry them to **Mina**. During the ritual of Stoning of the Devil at **Jamaraat**, pilgrims throw 7 tiny pebbles at each of 3 white pillars before returning to **Mina** for the night.

④ Pilgrims travel from **Mina** to the **Grand Mosque** in **Mecca** and perform a *tawaf*, circling the Ka'aba 7 times. Pilgrims may also perform *sa'i*, walking or running 7 times between **Safa and Marwah**, before they return to **Mina**.

⑤ Pilgrims leave **Mina** for the final time, travel to the **Grand Mosque** for the last *tawaf*, after which they leave **Mecca**, ending Hajj.

4

MAP 4-16. HAJJ DESTINATION MAP

 SAUDI ARABIA: HAJJ PILGRIMAGE 491

3 white pillars. The crowded conditions at this site pose potential hazards; multiple deadly stampedes occurred from 1994 to 2004. In 2004, after 251 pilgrims were killed and another 244 injured, the Saudi government replaced the round pillars with wide, elliptical columns to reduce crowd densities. However, after another stampede in 2006 that killed 380 pilgrims and injured 289, the single-tiered Jamaraat pedestrian bridge was demolished and replaced with a wider, multilevel bridge. Subsequently, no further incidents have occurred at Jamaraat.

Traditionally after Jamaraat, pilgrims sacrifice an animal to symbolize the ram that Abraham sacrificed instead of his son. More recently, pilgrims are required to purchase a "sacrifice voucher" in Mecca and have this sacrifice performed by proxy. Centralized, licensed abattoirs perform the sacrifice on behalf of the pilgrim.

After returning to Mecca, pilgrims go immediately to the Grand Mosque, which contains the Ka'aba, the most sacred site in Islam, and perform a *tawaf*, circling the Ka'aba 7 times counterclockwise. Because of the vast number of people (each floor of the 3-level mosque has a capacity of 750,000), a single *tawaf* can take hours. In addition to *tawaf*, pilgrims may perform *sa'i*, walking or running 7 times between the hills of Safa and Marwah and then drinking water from the Well of Zamzam. Previously performed in open air, this route is now enclosed by the Grand Mosque and can be traversed via air-conditioned tunnels, with separate sections for walkers, runners, and disabled pilgrims.

After a final *tawaf*, pilgrims leave Mecca, ending Hajj. Although it is not required as part of Hajj, many pilgrims extend their trips to travel to Medina. In Medina, pilgrims visit the Mosque of the Prophet, which contains the tomb of Mohammed and is the second holiest site in Islam.

HEALTH ISSUES

Immunizations

All pilgrims should be up-to-date with routine immunizations. In addition, hepatitis A and B and typhoid vaccines are recommended. Although a requirement for polio vaccine does not include adult pilgrims from the United States, it is best to ensure full vaccination against polio before travel. Children up to 15 years of age must show proof of vaccination with quadrivalent meningococcal vaccine and polio vaccine. Children older than 15 years of age have the same vaccination requirements as adults.

Meningococcal Vaccine

Because of the intensely crowded conditions of the Hajj and high carrier rates of *Neisseria meningitidis* among pilgrims, outbreaks of meningococcal disease have historically been a problem during Hajj. In the aftermath of outbreaks in 2000 and 2001 that affected 1,300 and 1,109 people, respectively, the Saudi Ministry of Health began requiring all pilgrims and local at-risk populations to receive the meningococcal vaccine. Hajj visas cannot be issued without proof of meningococcal vaccination. All adults and children >2 years of age must have received a single dose of quadrivalent A/C/Y/W-135 vaccine and must show proof of vaccination on a valid International Certificate of Vaccination or Prophylaxis. Children between 3 months and 2 years of age must show proof of vaccination with 2 doses of meningococcal A monovalent vaccine with a 3-month interval between the doses. Hajj pilgrims must have had the meningococcal vaccine ≤3 years and ≥10 days before arriving in Saudi Arabia.

Current Hajj vaccination requirements are available from the following sources:

> Saudi Arabian Ministry of Hajj (www.haj.gov.sa/en-us/Pages/default.aspx)
> Saudi Arabian Ministry of Health (www.moh.gov.sa/en/Hajj/HealthGuidelines/Pages/BeforeHajj.aspx)
> Saudi Arabian Embassy (www.saudiembassy.net/services/hajj_requirements.aspx)

Respiratory Infections

Respiratory tract infections are common during Hajj; the most common cause of hospital admission is pneumonia. These risks underscore the need to follow the Advisory Committee on Immunization Practices' recommendations for pneumococcal polysaccharide vaccine for pilgrims aged ≥65 years and for younger pilgrims with comorbidities. Seasonal influenza vaccine, including H1N1, is strongly recommended for all pilgrims. Behavioral interventions such as hand hygiene, wearing a face mask, cough etiquette, social distancing, and contact avoidance can be effective at mitigating respiratory illness among Hajj pilgrims. Pre-Hajj travel advice about common respiratory conditions should include a general assessment for respiratory fitness, necessary vaccinations, and prescription of adequate supplies of portable respiratory medications (prefer inhalers over nebulizers).

The crowded conditions during Hajj increase the probability of tuberculosis transmission. Pilgrims are advised to see their doctors if they develop signs of active tuberculosis: cough with sputum and blood at times, chest pains, weakness, weight loss, fever, and night sweats.

Middle East respiratory syndrome (MERS) was first identified in Saudi Arabia in 2012. The illness is caused by a novel coronavirus that is similar to the virus responsible for the 2003 global outbreak of severe acute respiratory syndrome (SARS). Cases have been identified in and around the Arabian Peninsula, but cases have also been exported to other countries, including the United States. The most common symptoms include fever, cough, and shortness of breath. However, myalgias, diarrhea, vomiting, abdominal pain, thrombocytopenia, and leukopenia have also been reported. The severity of illness has ranged from mild to severe, and approximately 35% of reported cases have been fatal. The role of animal-to-human transmission is unclear, but the virus has been found in camels in this region. The diagnosis can be suspected on clinical grounds and confirmed by PCR testing. More information is available in Chapter 3, MERS.

Other Health and Safety Risks
Communicable Diseases

Diarrheal disease is common during Hajj, and travelers should be educated on usual prevention measures and self-treatment. A pre-travel visit should include discussions about prevention, oral rehydration strategies, antimotility agents, and emergency antibiotic use for treatment of traveler's diarrhea.

Chafing caused by long rituals of standing and walking in the heat can lead to fungal or bacterial skin infections. Clothing should be light, not restrictive, and changed often to maintain hygiene. Travelers should be advised to keep skin dry, use talcum powder, and be aware of any pain or soreness caused by garments. Any sores or blisters that develop should be disinfected and kept covered. Special attention should be paid to protect the feet, which are bare when inside the Grand Mosque.

Nasal ablution, called istinshaaq, is the practice of rinsing your nose with water before performing some rituals during the Hajj. Medical literature has identified rare cases of primary amebic meningoencephalitis (PAM) caused by Naegleria fowleri. Even though no cases of Hajj-related PAM have been reported, nasal ablution is common during Hajj, and pilgrims are advised to use safe water to protect themselves from this potential risk. When in doubt, they should use bottled water. Boiling or filtering the water are other ways to decrease the risk of PAM.

At the end of Hajj, Muslim men must shave their heads. The use of unclean blades can transmit bloodborne pathogens, such as hepatitis B, hepatitis C, and HIV. Licensed barbers are tested for these bloodborne pathogens and are required to use disposable, single-use blades. Unfortunately, unlicensed barbers continue to operate by the roadside, where they use nonsterile blades on multiple men. Male travelers should be advised to be shaved only at officially designated centers, which are clearly marked.

Noncommunicable Diseases and Other Hazards

Hajj is arduous even for young, healthy pilgrims, and many Muslims wait until they are older before making Hajj. Pilgrims who are caught up in the spiritual experience of Hajj may forget to take their usual medications. Travelers with chronic medical conditions should undergo a functional assessment before leaving for Hajj. The medical provider should identify each traveler's unique risks and tailor a plan on how to reduce them. The provider should make any adjustments to the usual medical regimen, ensure that the traveler has an adequate supply of medications, and educate the traveler about symptoms that should prompt urgent medical attention.

Heat exhaustion and heatstroke are leading causes of death, particularly when Hajj occurs during the summer months. Pilgrims should stay hydrated, wear sunscreen, and seek shade when possible. Umbrellas are frequently used to provide portable sun protection. Travelers should be counseled on minimizing the risk of heat-related injuries as well as sun avoidance. Some rituals may also be performed at night to avoid daytime heat. Pilgrims can be reassured that night rituals have been advocated as legitimate by religious clerics.

Fire is a potential risk at Hajj. In 1997, open stoves set tents on fire, and the resulting blaze killed 343 pilgrims and injured >1,500. As a result, makeshift tents were replaced with permanent fiberglass structures; no pilgrim is allowed to set up his own tent or prepare his own food. Cooking in the tents is also prohibited.

Trauma

Trauma is a major cause of injury and death during Hajj. Pilgrims may walk long distances through or near dense traffic, and motor vehicle accidents are inevitable. The most feared trauma hazard, however, is stampede. In such dense crowds, little can be done to avoid or escape a stampede once it has begun, but the physical environment of the Hajj has been engineered specifically to minimize this risk. Past stampedes have often begun as minor incidents; the 2006 Hajj stampede, for example, began when some pilgrims tripped over fallen luggage, but it resulted in hundreds of injuries and deaths. Death usually results from asphyxiation or head trauma, and providing prompt treatment is next to impossible in large crowds.

Special Health Considerations
Menstruation

Women are not permitted to perform *tawaf* around the Ka'aba stone if they are menstruating. The remainder of the rituals may be performed during menstruation if the *tawaf* was performed before the menstrual period began. Thus, a female Hajj pilgrim who suspects that she may be menstruating during the Hajj may request hormonal suppression of menstrual bleeding.

Diabetes Mellitus

Muslims with diabetes planning to make Hajj should make a pre-Hajj travel clinic visit with enough advanced notice to carefully construct a diabetes management plan tailored to the health challenges of the Hajj. Diabetic patients should ensure adequate prescriptions for all medications, including syringes and needles. A diabetes emergency kit should include easily accessible carbohydrate sources to counter hypoglycemia, glucometer and test strips, urine ketone sticks to evaluate for ketoacidosis, a list of medications and care plans, and glucagon as indicated. Lastly, durable and protective footwear are necessary to avoid minor foot trauma that can lead to infections.

Epilepsy

Before making Hajj, a pilgrim's seizure disorder must be controlled on stable doses of medications. Before departure, Hajj travelers should ensure they have adequate supplies of routine medications, as well as a buccal or rectal formulation of antiseizure medications.

The Saudi government has created a Ministry of Hajj that collaborates with the Ministry of Health to improve pilgrims' experience, including mitigating health risks during Hajj. The hospitals and health centers in and around the holy sites are adequately staffed and equipped for the large gathering. The medical facilities offer high quality of care, and services are offered free to Hajj pilgrims.

To ensure efficient transport through the King Abdulaziz International Airport in Jeddah, the Saudi government has built a modern airport terminal solely dedicated to Hajj pilgrims. Furthermore, modern modes of transportation (light rail, 15,000 Hajj dedicated buses, and even high-speed rail lines) have been developed to safely transport pilgrims to the city of Mecca and other holy sites.

To mitigate the risk of heat exposure during this journey, the government provides complimentary water distributed from refrigerated trucks, more air conditioned sites (tents at Mina), large sun-blocking canopies, and thousands of fine mist sprinklers. To further protect themselves, travelers are urged to avoid the most densely crowded areas during Hajj. When the option exists, performance of rituals at nonpeak hours is encouraged. For example, most pilgrims prefer to perform the Stoning of the Devil at midday, but Saudi authorities have decreed that it may be performed anytime between sunrise and sunset or even by proxy, if the pilgrim cannot access the Jamaraat bridge.

BIBLIOGRAPHY

1. Ahmed QA, Arabi YM, Memish ZA. Health risks at the Hajj. Lancet. 2006 Mar 25;367(9515):1008–15.
2. Alsafadi H, Goodwin W, Syed A. Diabetes care during Hajj. Clin Med. 2011 Jun;11(3):218–21.
3. Alzahrani AG, Choudhry AJ, Al Mazroa MA, Turkistani AH, Nouman GS, Memish ZA. Pattern of diseases among visitors to Mina health centers during the Hajj season, 1429 H (2008 G). J Infect Public Health. 2012 Mar;5(1):22–34.
4. Assiri A, Al-Tawfiq JA, Al-Rabeeah AA, Al-Rabiah FA, Al-Hajjar S, Al-Barrak A, et al. Epidemiological, demographic, and clinical characteristics of 47 cases of Middle East respiratory syndrome coronavirus disease from Saudi Arabia: a descriptive study. Lancet Infect Dis. 2013 Sep;13(9):752–61.
5. Balaban V, Stauffer WM, Hammad A, Afgarshe M, Abd-Alla M, Ahmed Q, et al. Protective practices and respiratory illness among US travelers to the 2009 Hajj. J Travel Med. 2012 May–Jun;19(3):163–8.
6. Khan NA, Ishag AM, Ahmad MS, El-Sayed FM, Bachal ZA, Abbas TG. Pattern of medical diseases and determinants of prognosis of hospitalization during 2005 Muslim pilgrimage Hajj in a tertiary care hospital. A prospective cohort study. Saudi Med J. 2006 Sep;27(9):1373–80.
7. Memish ZA. The Hajj: communicable and non-communicable health hazards and current guidance for pilgrims. Euro Surveill. 2010 Sep 30;15(39):19671.
8. Memish ZA. Saudi Arabia has several strategies to care for pilgrims on the Hajj. BMJ. 2011;343:d7731.
9. Memish ZA, Al-Rabeeah AA. Health conditions of travellers to Saudi Arabia for the pilgrimage to Mecca (Hajj and Umra) for 1434 (2013). J Epidemiol Glob Health. 2013 Jun;3(2):59–61.
10. World Health Organization. Health conditions for travellers to Saudi Arabia pilgrimage to Mecca (Hajj). Wkly Epidemiol Rec. 2005 Dec 9;80(49–50):431–2.

Post-Travel Evaluation

GENERAL APPROACH TO THE RETURNED TRAVELER

Jessica K. Fairley

THE POST-TRAVEL EVALUATION

Travel-related health problems have been reported in as many as 22%–64% of travelers to developing countries. Although most of these illnesses are mild, up to 8% of travelers are ill enough to seek care from a health care provider. Most post-travel infections become apparent soon after travel, but because incubation periods vary, some syndromes can present months to years after initial infection. When evaluating a patient with a probable travel-related illness, the clinician should consider the items summarized in Box 5-1.

The Severity of Illness

It is important to assess the severity of illness in order to triage the patient and to distinguish certain infections from each other. Is this a potentially life-threatening infection, such as malaria? Some conditions, such as a severe respiratory syndrome or signs of hemorrhagic fever, may also necessitate prompt involvement of public health authorities. See Management below for more details.

Travel Itinerary

The itinerary is crucial to formulating a differential diagnosis, because potential exposures differ depending on the region of travel.

A febrile illness with nonspecific symptoms could be malaria, dengue, typhoid fever, or rickettsial disease, among others. Being able to exclude certain infections will avoid unnecessary testing. A 2013 study from the GeoSentinel Surveillance Network found a distinct pattern of diagnoses depending on the region of the world visited. In travelers to sub-Saharan Africa presenting with fever, malaria was the most common specific diagnosis. On the other hand, febrile patients who traveled to Latin America or Southeast Asia were much more likely to have dengue. The duration of travel is also important, since the risk of a travel-related illness increases with the length of the trip. A travel or tropical medicine specialist can assist with the differential diagnosis and may be aware of outbreaks or the current prevalence of an infectious disease in a specific area.

Timing of Illness in Relation to Travel

Most ill travelers will seek medical attention within 1 month of return from their destination, because most common travel-related infections have short incubation periods. Occasionally, however, infections such as schistosomiasis, leishmaniasis, or tuberculosis can manifest months or even years later. Therefore, a detailed history that extends beyond a few months before presentation can be helpful. The most common travel-related infections with short incubation periods are listed in Table 5-1.

Underlying Medical Illness

Comorbidities can affect the susceptibility to infection, as well as the clinical manifestations and severity of illness. An increasing number of immunosuppressed people (due to organ transplants, immune-modulating medications, HIV infection, or other primary or acquired immunodeficiencies) are international travelers (see Chapter 8, Immunocompromised Travelers).

Vaccines Received and Prophylaxis Used

The history of vaccinations and malaria chemoprophylaxis should be reviewed when evaluating an ill returned traveler. Less than half of US travelers to developing countries seek pre-travel medical advice and may not have received vaccines or taken antimalarial drugs. Although adherence to malaria chemoprophylaxis does not rule out the possibility of malaria, it reduces the risk and increases the chance of an alternative diagnosis. Fever and a rash in a traveler without an up-to-date measles

vaccination would raise concern about measles. The most common vaccine-preventable diseases found in a large 2010 GeoSentinel study of returned travelers included enteric fever (typhoid and paratyphoid), viral hepatitis, and influenza. More than half of these patients with vaccine-preventable diseases were hospitalized.

Individual Exposure History

Knowledge of the patient's exposures during travel, including insect bites, contaminated food or water, or freshwater swimming, can also assist with the differential diagnosis. In addition to malarial parasites, mosquitoes can transmit viruses (such as dengue virus, yellow fever virus, and chikungunya virus) and filarial parasites (such as *Wuchereria bancrofti*). Depending on the clinical syndrome and location of exposure, a history of a tick bite could suggest a diagnosis of tickborne encephalitis, African tick-bite fever, or other rickettsial infections. Tsetse flies are large, and their bites are painful and often recalled by the patient. They can carry *Trypanosoma brucei*, the protozoan that causes African sleeping sickness. Freshwater swimming or other water contact can put the patient at risk for schistosomiasis, leptospirosis, and other diseases.

Table 5-1. Illnesses associated with fever presenting in the first 2 weeks after travel

SYNDROME	POSSIBLE CAUSE
Systemic febrile illness with initial nonspecific symptoms	Malaria Dengue Typhoid fever Rickettsial diseases (such as scrub typhus, relapsing fever) East African trypanosomiasis Acute HIV infection Leptospirosis
Fever with central nervous system involvement	Meningococcal meningitis Malaria Arboviral encephalitis (such as Japanese encephalitis virus, West Nile virus) East African trypanosomiasis Angiostrongyliasis Rabies
Fever with respiratory complaints	Influenza Bacterial pneumonia Acute histoplasmosis or coccidioidomycosis *Legionella* pneumonia Q fever Malaria Tularemia Pneumonic plague
Fever and skin rash	Dengue Measles Varicella Spotted-fever or typhus group rickettsiosis Typhoid fever Parvovirus B19 Mononucleosis Acute HIV infection

The purpose of the patient's trip and the type of accommodations can also influence the risk for acquiring certain diseases. Travelers who visit friends and relatives are at higher risk of malaria, typhoid fever, and certain other diseases because, compared with tourists, they stay longer, travel to more remote destinations, have more contact with local water sources, and are less likely to seek pre-travel advice (see Chapter 8, Immigrants Returning Home to Visit Friends & Relatives [VFRs]). Someone backpacking and camping in rural areas will also have a higher risk

of certain diseases than those staying in air-conditioned hotels.

COMMON SYNDROMES

The most common clinical presentations after travel to developing countries include systemic febrile illness, acute diarrhea, and dermatologic conditions. These are described in more detail in the following sections of this chapter (Fever in Returned Travelers, Persistent Travelers' Diarrhea, and Skin & Soft Tissue Infections in Returned Travelers). Respiratory complaints and eosinophilia are also conditions of importance in returning travelers. Fever in a traveler returning from a malaria-endemic country needs to be evaluated immediately.

Respiratory Complaints

Respiratory complaints are frequent among returned travelers and are typically associated with common respiratory viruses (see Chapter 2, Respiratory Infections). Influenza is among the most common vaccine-preventable diseases associated with international travel. Severe respiratory symptoms—especially associated with fever—in a returned traveler should alert the physician to common infectious diseases such as seasonal influenza, bacterial pneumonia, and malaria but could also suggest more unusual entities, such as Legionnaires' disease. Emerging respiratory infections such as Middle East respiratory syndrome (MERS) and H7N9 avian influenza should be in the differential if the travel history is appropriate and respiratory symptoms do not have a clear alternative diagnosis. In these suspected cases, local public health authorities and CDC should be alerted immediately. Refer to Chapter 2, Respiratory Infections for more details.

Delayed onset and chronic cough after travel could be tuberculosis, especially in a long-term traveler or health care worker. Other uncommon infections causing respiratory illness after travel to specific regions are histoplasmosis, coccidioidomycosis, Q fever, plague, tularemia, and melioidosis. Helminth infections that produce pulmonary disease include strongyloidiasis, paragonimiasis, and schistosomiasis.

Eosinophilia

Eosinophilia in a returning traveler suggests a possible helminth infection. Allergic diseases, hematologic disorders, and some viral, fungal, and protozoan infections can also cause eosinophilia. Fever and eosinophilia can be present during pulmonary migration of parasites, such as hookworm, *Ascaris*, and *Strongyloides*. Acute schistosomiasis, or Katayama syndrome, is also a cause of fever and eosinophilia and can be associated with pulmonary infiltrates. Other parasitic infections associated with eosinophilia include chronic strongyloidiasis, visceral larval migrans, lymphatic filariasis, and acute trichinellosis. Findings in a recent outbreak of sarcocystosis in travelers returning from Tioman Island, Malaysia, included myalgia and eosinophilia. The affected travelers had eosinophilic myositis on muscle biopsy.

MANAGEMENT

Most post-travel illnesses can be managed on an outpatient basis, but some patients, especially those with systemic febrile illnesses, may need to be hospitalized. In a 2007 analysis of GeoSentinel data, 46% of returned travelers with systemic febrile illness were hospitalized. Severe presentations, such as acute respiratory distress, mental status change, and hemodynamic instability, require inpatient care. Clinicians should have a low threshold for admitting febrile patients if malaria is suspected. Confirmation of diagnosis can be delayed, and complications can occur rapidly. Management in an inpatient setting is especially important if the patient may not reliably follow up or when no one is at home to assist if symptoms worsen quickly. Consultation with an infectious disease physician is recommended in severe travel-related infections, when management is complicated, or when the diagnosis remains unclear. A travel medicine or infectious disease specialist should be involved in cases that require specialized treatment, such as neurocysticercosis, severe malaria, and leishmaniasis, among others. CDC provides on-call assistance with the diagnosis and management of parasitic infections at 404-718-4745 for parasitic infections other than malaria or 770-488-7788 (toll-free at 855-856-4713) for malaria, during business hours. After business hours, call the CDC Emergency Operations Center at 770-488-7100.

BIBLIOGRAPHY

1. Boggild AK, Castelli F, Gautret P, Torresi J, von Sonnenburg F, Barnett ED, et al. Vaccine preventable diseases in returned international travelers: results from the GeoSentinel Surveillance Network. Vaccine. 2010 Oct 28;28(46):7389–95.
2. CDC. Notes from the field: acute muscular sarcocystosis among returning travelers—Tioman

Island, Malaysia, 2011. MMWR Morb Mortal Wkly Rep. 2012 Jan 20;61(2):37–8.

3. Chen LH, Wilson ME, Davis X, Loutan L, Schwartz E, Keystone J, et al. Illness in long-term travelers visiting GeoSentinel clinics. Emerg Infect Dis. 2009 Nov;15(11):1773–82.

4. Franco-Paredes C, Jacob JT, Hidron A, Rodriguez-Morales AJ, Kuhar D, Caliendo AM. Transplantation and tropical infectious diseases. Int J Infect Dis. 2010 Mar;14(3):e189–96.

5. Hamer DH, Connor BA. Travel health knowledge, attitudes and practices among United States travelers. J Travel Med. 2004 Jan–Feb;11(1):23–6.

6. Hendel-Paterson B, Swanson SJ. Pediatric travelers visiting friends and relatives (VFR) abroad: illnesses, barriers and pre-travel recommendations.

Travel Med Infect Dis. 2011 Jul;9(4): 192–203.

7. Leder K, Torresi J, Libman MD, Cramer JP, Castelli F, Schlagenhauf P et al. GeoSentinel surveillance of illness in returned travelers, 2007–2011. Ann Intern Med. 2013 Mar 19;158(6):456–68.

8. Ryan ET, Wilson ME, Kain KC. Illness after international travel. N Engl J Med. 2002 Aug 15;347(7):505–16.

9. Schulte C, Krebs B, Jelinek T, Nothdurft HD, von Sonnenburg F, Loscher T. Diagnostic significance of blood eosinophilia in returning travelers. Clin Infect Dis. 2002 Feb 1;34(3):407–11.

10. Wilson ME, Weld LH, Boggild A, Keystone JS, Kain KC, von Sonnenburg F, et al. Fever in returned travelers: results from the GeoSentinel Surveillance Network. Clin Infect Dis. 2007 Jun 15;44(12):1560–8.

FEVER IN RETURNED TRAVELERS

Mary Elizabeth Wilson

INITIAL FOCUS

Fever commonly accompanies serious illness in returned travelers. Because it can signal a rapidly progressive infection such as malaria, the clinician must initiate early evaluation, especially in people who have visited areas with malaria in recent months (see Chapter 3, Malaria). The initial focus in evaluating a febrile returned traveler should be on identifying infections that are rapidly progressive, treatable, or transmissible. In some instances, public health officials must be alerted if the traveler may have been contagious while traveling or infected with a pathogen of public health importance (such as yellow fever) at the origin or destination.

USE OF HISTORY, LOCATION OF EXPOSURE, AND INCUBATION TO LIMIT DIFFERENTIAL DIAGNOSIS

Often the list of potential diagnoses is long, but multiple recent studies help to identify more common diagnoses. A large proportion of illnesses in returned travelers is caused by common, cosmopolitan infections (such as bacterial pneumonia or pyelonephritis), so these must be considered along with unusual infections. Because the geographic area of travel determines the relative likelihood of major causes of fever, it is essential to identify where the febrile patient has traveled and lived (Table 5-2). Details about activities (such as freshwater exposure in schistosomiasis-endemic areas, animal bites, sexual activities, tattoos, or local medical care with injections) and accommodations in areas with malaria (bed nets, window screens, air conditioning) during travel may provide useful clues. Preparation before travel (such as hepatitis A vaccine or yellow fever vaccine) will markedly reduce the likelihood of some infections, so this is a relevant part of the history. A history of travel and residence should be an integral part of every medical history.

Because each infection has a characteristic incubation period (although the range is extremely wide with some infections), the time of exposures needs to be defined in different geographic areas (Table 5-3). This knowledge will allow the clinician to exclude some infections from the differential diagnosis. Most serious febrile infections manifest within the first month after return from tropical travel, yet infections related to travel exposures can occasionally occur months or even >1 year after return.

Table 5-2. Common causes of fever, by geographic area

GEOGRAPHIC AREA	COMMON TROPICAL DISEASE CAUSING FEVER	OTHER INFECTIONS CAUSING OUTBREAKS OR CLUSTERS IN TRAVELERS
Caribbean	Dengue, malaria (Haiti)	Acute histoplasmosis, leptospirosis, chikungunya
Central America	Dengue, malaria (primarily *Plasmodium vivax*)	Leptospirosis, histoplasmosis, coccidioidomycosis
South America	Dengue, malaria (primarily *P. vivax*)	Bartonellosis, leptospirosis, enteric fever, histoplasmosis
South-central Asia	Dengue, enteric fever, malaria (primarily non-falciparum)	Chikungunya
Southeast Asia	Dengue, malaria (primarily non-falciparum)	Chikungunya, leptospirosis
Sub-Saharan Africa	Malaria (primarily *P. falciparum*), tickborne rickettsiae (main cause of fever in southern Africa), acute schistosomiasis, dengue	African trypanosomiasis, chikungunya, enteric fever, filariasis

5

Table 5-3. Common infections, by incubation period

DISEASE	USUAL INCUBATION PERIOD (RANGE)	DISTRIBUTION
Incubation <14 Days		
Chikungunya	2–4 days (1–14 days)	Tropics, subtropics
Dengue	4–8 days (3–14 days)	Tropics, subtropics
Encephalitis, arboviral (Japanese encephalitis, tickborne encephalitis, West Nile virus, other)	3–14 days (1–20 days)	Specific agents vary by region
Enteric fever	7–18 days (3–60 days)	Especially in Indian subcontinent
Acute HIV	10–28 days (10 days to 6 weeks)	Worldwide

continued

 FEVER IN RETURNED TRAVELERS | 501

TABLE 5-3. COMMON INFECTIONS, BY INCUBATION PERIOD (continued)

DISEASE	USUAL INCUBATION PERIOD (RANGE)	DISTRIBUTION
Influenza	1–3 days	Worldwide, can also be acquired while traveling
Legionellosis	5–6 days (2–10 days)	Widespread
Leptospirosis	7–12 days (2–26 days)	Widespread, most common in tropical areas
Malaria, *Plasmodium falciparum*	6–30 days (98% onset within 3 months of travel)	Tropics, subtropics
Malaria, *P. vivax*	8 days to 12 months (almost half have onset >30 days after completion of travel)	Widespread in tropics and subtropics
Spotted-fever rickettsiae	Few days to 2–3 weeks	Causative species vary by region
Incubation 14 Days to 6 Weeks		
Encephalitis, arboviral; enteric fever; acute HIV; leptospirosis; malaria	See above incubation periods for relevant diseases	See above distribution for relevant diseases
Amebic liver abscess	Weeks to months	Most common in developing countries
Hepatitis A	28–30 days (15–50 days)	Most common in developing countries
Hepatitis E	26–42 days (2–9 weeks)	Widespread
Acute schistosomiasis (Katayama syndrome)	4–8 weeks	Most common in sub-Saharan Africa
Incubation >6 Weeks		
Amebic liver abscess, hepatitis E, malaria, acute schistosomiasis	See above incubation periods for relevant diseases	See above distribution for relevant diseases
Hepatitis B	90 days (60–150 days)	Widespread
Leishmaniasis, visceral	2–10 months (10 days to years)	Asia, Africa, Latin America, southern Europe, and the Middle East
Tuberculosis	Primary, weeks; reactivation, years	Global distribution, rates and levels of resistance vary widely

5

In the United States, >90% of reported cases of *Plasmodium falciparum* malaria manifest within 30 days of return, but almost half of cases of *P. vivax* malaria manifest >30 days after return.

FINDINGS REQUIRING URGENT ATTENTION

Presence of associated signs, symptoms, or laboratory findings can focus attention on specific infections (Table 5-4). Findings that should prompt urgent attention include hemorrhage, neurologic impairment, and acute respiratory distress. Even if an initial physical examination is unremarkable, it is worth repeating the examination, as new findings may appear that will help in the diagnostic process (such as skin lesions or tender liver). Although most febrile illnesses in returned travelers are related to infections, the clinician should bear in mind that other problems, including pulmonary emboli and drug hypersensitivity reactions, can be associated with fever.

Table 5-4. Common clinical findings and associated infections

COMMON CLINICAL FINDINGS	INFECTIONS TO CONSIDER AFTER TROPICAL TRAVEL
Fever and rash	Dengue, chikungunya, rickettsial infections, enteric fever (skin lesions may be sparse or absent), acute HIV infection, measles
Fever and abdominal pain	Enteric fever, amebic liver abscess
Undifferentiated fever and normal or low white blood cell count	Dengue, malaria, rickettsial infection, enteric fever, chikungunya
Fever and hemorrhage	Viral hemorrhagic fevers (dengue and others), meningococcemia, leptospirosis, rickettsial infections
Fever and eosinophilia	Acute schistosomiasis, drug hypersensitivity reaction, fascioliasis and other parasitic infections (rare)
Fever and pulmonary infiltrates	Common bacterial and viral pathogens, legionellosis, acute schistosomiasis, Q fever, leptospirosis
Fever and altered mental status	Cerebral malaria, viral or bacterial meningoencephalitis, African trypanosomiasis, scrub typhus
Mononucleosis syndrome	Epstein-Barr virus infection, cytomegalovirus infection, toxoplasmosis, acute HIV
Fever persisting >2 weeks	Malaria, enteric fever, Epstein-Barr virus infection, cytomegalovirus infection, toxoplasmosis, acute HIV, acute schistosomiasis, brucellosis, tuberculosis, Q fever, visceral leishmaniasis (rare)
Fever with onset >6 weeks after travel	*Plasmodium vivax* or *ovale* malaria, acute hepatitis (B, C, or E), tuberculosis, amebic liver abscess

FEVER IN RETURNED TRAVELERS   503

Fever accompanied by any of the following syndromes deserves further scrutiny, because it may indicate a disease of public health importance:

- Skin rash
- Difficulty breathing
- Shortness of breath
- Persistent cough
- Decreased consciousness
- Bruising or unusual bleeding (without previous injury)
- Persistent diarrhea
- Persistent vomiting (other than air or motion sickness)
- Jaundice
- Paralysis of recent onset

People who travel to visit friends and relatives (VFRs) often do not seek pre-travel medical advice and are at higher risk for some diseases than other travelers. A review of GeoSentinel Surveillance Network data showed that a larger proportion of immigrant VFRs than tourist travelers presented with serious (requiring hospitalization), potentially preventable travel-related illnesses.

CHANGE OVER TIME

Clinicians have access to resources on the Internet that provide information about geographic-specific risks, disease activity, and other useful information, such as drug-susceptibility patterns for pathogens. Infectious diseases are dynamic, as demonstrated by a review of adult returned travelers with fever and rash seen in 2006 and 2007 at a Paris hospital. The most common diagnosis was chikungunya, followed by dengue and African tick-bite fever. In contrast, because of the wide use of vaccine, hepatitis A infection is becoming less common in travelers.

Common infections in returned travelers may be seen at unexpected times of the year. Because influenza transmission can occur throughout the year in tropical areas, and the peak season in the Southern Hemisphere is May to August, clinicians in the Northern Hemisphere must be alert to the possibility of influenza outside the usual influenza season.

Travelers may acquire infections caused by common bacteria that are unusually resistant. Bacteria that produce the enzyme NDM-1, which confers resistance to virtually all available antibiotics, have been found in infections acquired during travel, most often related to medical care (both elective and emergency). These bacteria have been most commonly reported after exposures in the Indian subcontinent. Enteric fever, the term used to describe either typhoid or paratyphoid fever, has also become increasingly resistant to fluoroquinolones (see Chapter 3, Typhoid & Paratyphoid Fever).

The tables in this section identify some common infections by presenting findings or other characteristics, by area of travel and by incubation periods. These highlight only the most common infections. The listed references and websites should be consulted for more detailed information. In most studies, a specific cause for fever is not identified in about 25% of returned travelers.

KEEP IN MIND

- Initial symptoms of life-threatening and self-limited infections can be identical.
- Fever in returned travelers is often caused by common, cosmopolitan infections, such as pneumonia and pyelonephritis, which should not be overlooked in the search for more exotic diagnoses.
- Patients with malaria may be afebrile at the time of evaluation but typically give a history of fever or chills.
- Malaria is the most common cause of acute undifferentiated fever after travel to sub-Saharan Africa and to some other tropical areas.
- Malaria, especially P. falciparum, can progress rapidly. Diagnostic studies should be done promptly and treatment instituted immediately if malaria is diagnosed (see Chapter 3, Malaria).
- A history of taking malaria chemoprophylaxis does not exclude the possibility of malaria.
- Patients with malaria can have prominent respiratory (including acute respiratory distress syndrome), gastrointestinal, or central nervous system findings.
- Dengue is the most common cause of febrile illness among people who seek medical care after travel to Latin America or Asia.
- Viral hemorrhagic fevers are important to identify but are rare in travelers; bacterial

5

infections, such as leptospirosis, meningococcemia, and rickettsial infections, can also cause fever and hemorrhage and should be always be considered because of the need to institute prompt, specific treatment.

- Sexually transmitted diseases, including acute HIV, can cause acute febrile infections.
- Consider infection control, public health implications, and requirements for reportable diseases.

BIBLIOGRAPHY

1. Bottieau E, Clerinx J, Schrooten W, Van den Enden E, Wouters R, Van Esbroeck M, et al. Etiology and outcome of fever after a stay in the tropics. Arch Intern Med. 2006 Aug 14–28;166(15):1642–8.
2. Hochedez P, Canestri A, Guihot A, Brichler S, Bricaire F, Caumes E. Management of travelers with fever and exanthema, notably dengue and chikungunya infections. Am J Trop Med Hyg. 2008 May;78(5):710–3.
3. Jensenius M, Davis X, von Sonnenburg F, Schwartz E, Keystone JS, Leder K, et al. Multicenter GeoSentinel analysis of rickettsial diseases in international travelers, 1996–2008. Emerg Infect Dis. 2009 Nov;15(11):1791–8.
4. Kumarasamy KK, Toleman MA, Walsh TR, Bagaria J, Butt F, Balakrishnan R, et al. Emergence of a new antibiotic resistance mechanism in India, Pakistan, and the UK: a molecular, biological, and epidemiological study. Lancet Infect Dis. 2010 Sep;10(9):597–602.
5. Leder K, Torresi J, Libman MD, Cramer JP, Castelli F, Schlagenhauf P, et al. GeoSentinel surveillance of illness in returned travelers, 2007–2011. Ann Intern Med 2013 Mar 19;158(6):456–68.
6. Mendelson M, Han PV, Vincent P, von Sonnenburg F, Cramer JP, Loutan L, et al. Regional variation in travel-related illness acquired in Africa, March 1997–May 2011. Emerg Infect Dis. 2014 Apr;20(4):532–41.
7. Patel TA, Armstrong M, Morris-Jones SD, Wright SG, Doherty T. Imported enteric fever: case series from the Hospital for Tropical Diseases, London, United Kingdom. Am J Trop Med Hyg. 2010 Jun;82(6):1121–6.
8. Ryan ET, Wilson ME, Kain KC. Illness after international travel. N Engl J Med. 2002 Aug 15;347(7):505–16.
9. Wilson ME, Weld LH, Boggild A, Keystone JS, Kain KC, von Sonnenburg F, et al. Fever in returned travelers: results from the GeoSentinel Surveillance Network. Clin Infect Dis. 2007 Jun 15;44(12):1560–8.

PERSISTENT TRAVELERS' DIARRHEA

Bradley A. Connor

Although most cases of travelers' diarrhea are acute and self-limited, a certain percentage of travelers will develop persistent (>14 days) gastrointestinal symptoms (see Chapter 2, Travelers' Diarrhea). The pathogenesis of persistent travelers' diarrhea generally falls into one of the following broad categories: 1) persistent infection or coinfection with a second organism not targeted by initial therapy, 2) previously undiagnosed gastrointestinal disease unmasked by the enteric infection, or 3) a postinfectious phenomenon.

PERSISTENT INFECTION

Most cases of travelers' diarrhea are the result of bacterial infection and are short-lived and self-limited. Travelers may experience prolonged diarrheal symptoms if they are immunosuppressed, are infected sequentially with diarrheal pathogens, or are infected with protozoan parasites. Parasites as a group are the pathogens most likely to be isolated from patients with persistent diarrhea, and their probability relative to bacterial infections increases with increasing duration of symptoms. Parasites may also be the cause of persistent diarrhea in patients already treated for a bacterial pathogen.

Giardia is by far the most likely persistent pathogen to be encountered. Suspicion for giardiasis should be particularly high when upper gastrointestinal symptoms predominate. Untreated, symptoms may last for months, even in immunocompetent hosts.

The diagnosis can often be made through stool microscopy, antigen detection, or immunofluorescence. However, as *Giardia* infects the proximal small bowel, even multiple stool specimens may fail to detect it, and a duodenal aspirate may be necessary for definitive diagnosis. Given the high prevalence of *Giardia* in persistent travelers' diarrhea, empiric therapy is a reasonable option in the clinical setting after negative stool microscopy and in lieu of duodenal sampling. Other intestinal parasites that may cause persistent symptoms include *Cryptosporidium* species, *Entamoeba histolytica*, *Isospora belli*, *Microsporidia*, *Dientamoeba fragilis*, and *Cyclospora cayetanensis*.

Individual bacterial infections rarely cause persistence of symptoms, although persistent diarrhea has been reported in children infected with enteroaggregative or enteropathogenic *Escherichia coli* and among people with diarrhea due to *Clostridium difficile*. *C. difficile*–associated diarrhea may follow treatment of a bacterial pathogen with a fluoroquinolone or other antibiotic, or may even follow malaria chemoprophylaxis. This is especially important to consider in the patient with persistent travelers' diarrhea that seems refractory to multiple courses of empiric antibiotic therapy. The initial work-up of persistent travelers' diarrhea should always include a *C. difficile* stool toxin assay. Treatment of *C. difficile* infection is with metronidazole, oral vancomycin, or fidaxomicin, although increasing reports of resistance to the first 2 drugs have been noted.

Persistent travelers' diarrhea has also been associated with tropical sprue and Brainerd diarrhea. These syndromes are suspected to result from infectious diseases, but specific pathogens have not been identified. Tropical sprue is associated with deficiencies of vitamins absorbed in the proximal and distal small bowel and most commonly affects long-term travelers to tropical areas. Investigation of an outbreak of Brainerd diarrhea among passengers on a cruise ship to the Galápagos Islands of Ecuador revealed that diarrhea persisted from 7 to more than 42 months and did not respond to antimicrobial therapy.

UNDERLYING GASTROINTESTINAL DISEASE

In some cases, persistence of gastrointestinal symptoms relates to chronic underlying gastrointestinal disease or susceptibility unmasked by the enteric infection. Most prominent among these is celiac disease, a systemic disease manifesting primarily with small bowel changes. In genetically susceptible people, villous atrophy and crypt hyperplasia are seen in response to exposure to antigens found in wheat, leading to malabsorption. The diagnosis is made by obtaining serologic tests, including tissue transglutaminase antibodies. A biopsy of the small bowel showing villous atrophy confirms the diagnosis. Treatment is with a wheat (gluten)-free diet.

Idiopathic inflammatory bowel disease, both Crohn disease and ulcerative colitis, may be seen after acute bouts of travelers' diarrhea. One prevailing hypothesis is that an initiating endogenous pathogen triggers inflammatory bowel disease in genetically susceptible people.

Depending on the clinical setting and age group, it may be necessary to do a more comprehensive search for other underlying causes of chronic diarrhea. Colorectal cancer should be considered, particularly in patients passing occult or gross blood rectally or with the onset of a new iron-deficiency anemia.

POSTINFECTIOUS PHENOMENA

In a certain percentage of patients who present with persistent gastrointestinal symptoms, no specific source will be found. Patients may experience temporary enteropathy following an acute diarrheal infection, with villous atrophy, decreased absorptive surface area, and disaccharidase deficiencies. This can lead to osmotic diarrhea, particularly when large amounts of lactose, sucrose, sorbitol, or fructose are consumed. Use of antimicrobial medications during the initial days of diarrhea may also lead to alterations in intestinal flora and diarrhea symptoms.

Occasionally, the onset of symptoms of irritable bowel syndrome (IBS) can be traced to an acute bout of gastroenteritis. IBS that develops after acute enteritis has been termed postinfectious (PI)-IBS. To be labeled PI-IBS, symptoms should follow an episode of gastroenteritis or travelers' diarrhea if the work-up for microbial pathogens and underlying gastrointestinal disease is negative. The role of small intestinal bacterial overgrowth in the pathogenesis of PI-IBS, especially when gas and bloating predominate, is being investigated.

EVALUATION

Three or more stool examinations should be performed for ova and parasites, including acid-fast stains for *Cryptosporidium*, *Cyclospora*, and *Isospora*; *Giardia* antigen testing; *C. difficile* toxin assay; and a D-xylose absorption test to determine if nutrients are being properly absorbed. Patients may also be given empiric treatment for *Giardia* infection. If underlying gastrointestinal disease is suspected, an initial evaluation should include serologic tests for celiac and inflammatory bowel disease. Subsequently, other studies to visualize both the upper and lower gastrointestinal tracts, with biopsies, may be indicated.

MANAGEMENT

Dietary modifications may help those with malabsorption. If stools are bloody or when disease is caused by *C. difficile*, antidiarrheal medications such as loperamide or diphenoxylate should not be used in children and should be used cautiously, if at all, in adults. Probiotic medications have been shown to reduce the duration of persistent diarrhea among children in some settings. Antimicrobial medications may be useful in treating persistent diarrhea caused by parasites. Nonabsorbable antibiotics may help if small intestinal bacterial overgrowth accompanies the symptom complex.

BIBLIOGRAPHY

1. Connor BA. Chronic diarrhea in travelers. Curr Infect Dis Rep. 2013 Jun;15(3):203–10
2. Connor BA. Sequelae of traveler's diarrhea: focus on postinfectious irritable bowel syndrome. Clin Infect Dis. 2005 Dec 1;41 Suppl 8:S577–86.
3. Ford AC, Spiegel BM, Talley NJ, Moayyedi P. Small intestinal bacterial overgrowth in irritable bowel syndrome: systematic review and meta-analysis. Clin Gastroenterol Hepatol. 2009 Dec;7(12):1279–86.
4. Green PH, Jabri B. Coeliac disease. Lancet. 2003 Aug 2;362(9381):383–91.
5. Guerrant RL, Van Gilder T, Steiner TS, Thielman NM, Slutsker L, Tauxe RV, et al. Practice guidelines for the management of infectious diarrhea. Clin Infect Dis. 2001;32:331–50.
6. Mintz ED, Weber JT, Guris D, Puhr N, Wells JG, Yashuk JC, et al. An outbreak of Brainerd diarrhea among travelers to the Galapagos Islands. J Infect Dis. 1998 Apr;177(4):1041–5.
7. Norman FF, Perez-Molina J, Perez de Ayala A, Jimenez BC, Navarro M, Lopez-Velez R. *Clostridium difficile*-associated diarrhea after antibiotic treatment for traveler's diarrhea. Clin Infect Dis. 2008 Apr 1;46(7):1060–3.
8. Porter CK, Tribble DR, Aliaga PA, Halvorson HA, Riddle MS. Infectious gastroenteritis and risk of developing inflammatory bowel disease. Gastroenterology. 2008 Sep;135(3):781–6.
9. Spiller R, Garsed K. Postinfectious irritable bowel syndrome. Gastroenterology. 2009 May;136(6):1979–88.

SKIN & SOFT TISSUE INFECTIONS IN RETURNED TRAVELERS

Jay S. Keystone

Skin problems are among the most frequent medical problems in returned travelers. The largest case series of dermatologic problems in returned travelers from the GeoSentinel Surveillance Network showed that cutaneous larva migrans, insect bites, and bacterial infections were the most frequent skin problems in ill travelers who sought medical care, making up 30% of the 4,742 diagnoses (Table 5-5). In another review of 165 travelers who returned to France with skin problems, cellulitis, scabies, and pyoderma led the list

Table 5-5. Ten most common skin lesions in returned travelers, by cause[1]

SKIN LESION	PERCENTAGE OF ALL DERMATOLOGIC DIAGNOSES (N = 4,742)
Cutaneous larva migrans	9.8
Insect bite	8.2
Skin abscess	7.7
Superinfected insect bite	6.8
Allergic rash	5.5
Rash, unknown origin	5.5
Dog bite	4.3
Superficial fungal infection	4.0
Dengue	3.4
Leishmaniasis	3.3
Myiasis	2.7
Spotted-fever group rickettsiae	1.5
Scabies	1.5
Cellulitis	1.5

[1] Modified from Lederman ER, Weld LH, Elyazar IR, et al. Dermatologic conditions of the ill returned traveler: an analysis from the GeoSentinel Surveillance Network. Int J Infect Dis. 2008;12(6):593–602.

of skin conditions. These data are biased in that they do not include skin problems that were diagnosed and, in many cases, easily managed during travel or that were self-limited.

Skin problems generally fall into either of the following categories: 1) those associated with fever, usually a rash or secondary bacterial infection (cellulitis, lymphangitis, bacteremia, toxin-mediated) and 2) those not associated with fever. Most skin problems are minor and are not accompanied by fever. Diagnosis of skin problems in returned travelers is based on the following:

- Pattern recognition of the lesions: papular, macular, nodular, linear, or ulcerative
- Location of the lesions: exposed versus unexposed skin surfaces
- Exposure history: freshwater, ocean, insects, animals, or human contact
- Associated symptoms: fever, pain, pruritus

It is important to recognize that skin conditions in returned travelers may not have a travel-related cause.

PAPULAR LESIONS

Insect bites, the most common cause of papular lesions, may be associated with secondary infection or hypersensitivity reactions. Bed bug and flea bites may produce grouped papules (see Box 2-4 for more information about bed bugs). Flea bites tend to have hemorrhagic centers. Scabies infestation usually manifests as a generalized or regional pruritic, papular rash. Scabies burrows may present as papules or pustules in a short linear pattern on the skin.

Onchocerciasis may occur in long-stay travelers living in rural sub-Saharan Africa and, rarely, Latin America. It usually manifests as a generalized pruritic, papular dermatitis.

NODULAR OR SUBCUTANEOUS LESIONS, INCLUDING BACTERIAL SKIN INFECTIONS

Bacterial skin infections may occur more frequently after bites and other wounds in the tropics, particularly when good hygiene cannot be maintained. Organisms responsible are commonly *Staphylococcus aureus* or *Streptococcus pyogenes*. The presentations can include abscess formation, cellulitis, lymphangitis, or ulceration. Furunculosis, or recurrent pyoderma, may be the result of colonization of the skin and nasal mucosa with *S. aureus*. Boils may continue to occur weeks or months after a traveler returns and, if associated with *S. aureus*, definitive treatment usually involves decolonization with nasal mupirocin, a skin wash with an antimicrobial skin cleanser, and less often, an oral antibiotic combination including rifampin.

In addition to pyodermas, cellulitis or erysipelas may complicate excoriated insect bites or any trauma to the skin. Cellulitis and erysipelas manifest as areas of skin erythema, edema, and warmth in the absence of an underlying suppurative focus. Unlike cellulitis, erysipelas lesions are raised, there is a clear line of demarcation at the edge of the lesion, and the lesions are more likely to be associated with fever. Cellulitis, on the other hand, is more likely to be associated with lymphangitis. Cellulitis and erysipelas are usually caused by β-hemolytic streptococci; *S. aureus* (including methicillin-resistant strains) and gram-negative aerobic bacteria may also cause cellulitis. A recent study from France of 60 returned travelers with skin and soft tissue infections found 35% had impetigo and 23% had cutaneous abscesses. Methicillin-susceptible *S. aureus* was detected in 43%, group A *Streptococcus* in 34%, and both in 23%.

Another common bacterial skin infection, especially in children in the tropics, is impetigo, due to *S. aureus* or *S. pyogenes*. Impetigo is a highly contagious superficial skin infection that generally appears on the arms, legs, or face as "honey-colored" or golden crustings formed from dried serum. Local care and a topical antibiotic such as mupirocin may be used, although a systemic antibiotic may be required. Emerging antibiotic resistance among staphylococci and streptococci complicates antimicrobial options.

Myiasis presents as a painful lesion similar to a boil. It is caused by infestation with the larval stage of the African tumbu fly (*Cordylobia anthropophaga*) or the Latin American bot fly (*Dermatobia hominis*). At the center of the lesion is a small punctum that allows the larva to breathe. Extraction of the fly larva can be difficult, especially of the bot fly; extraction may be facilitated by first asphyxiating the larvae, usually with an occlusive dressing or covering (such as a bottle cap filled with petroleum jelly) for several hours and then squeezing the larva out.

Tungiasis is caused by a sand flea (*Tunga penetrans*). The female burrows into the skin, usually the foot, and produces a nodular, pale, subcutaneous lesion with a central dark spot. The painful or pruritic lesion expands as the female produces eggs in her uterus. Treatment involves extraction.

Loa loa filariasis occurs rarely in long-term travelers living in rural sub-Saharan Africa. The traveler may present with transient, migratory, subcutaneous, painful, or pruritic swellings produced by the adult nematode migration (Calabar swelling). Rarely, the worm can be visualized crossing the conjunctiva of the eye or eyelid. Eosinophilia is common. Loaiasis can be diagnosed by finding microfilariae in blood collected during daytime.

Gnathostomiasis is a nematode infection found primarily in Southeast Asia and less commonly in Africa and Latin America. Infection results from eating undercooked or raw freshwater fish. Infected travelers may experience transient, migratory, subcutaneous, pruritic, or painful swellings that may occur weeks or even years after exposure. The symptoms are due to migration of the worm through the body, and the central nervous system may be involved. Eosinophilia is common, and the diagnosis can be made by serology.

MACULAR LESIONS

Macular lesions are common and often nonspecific and may be due to drug reactions or viral exanthems. Superficial mycoses, such as tinea versicolor and tinea corporis, may also present as macular lesions.

Tinea versicolor, due to *Malassezia furfur* (previously *Pityrosporumovale*), is characterized by asymptomatic hypopigmented or hyperpigmented oval, slightly scaly patches measuring 1–3 cm that are found on the upper chest, neck, and back. Diagnosis may be made by examination with a Wood's lamp or by placing a drop of methylene blue on a slide onto which clear cellulose acetate tape is placed sticky side down, after it has been touched briefly to the skin lesions to pick up superficial scales. Detection of hyphae ("spaghetti") and spores ("meatballs") suggest the diagnosis. Treatment with topical or systemic azoles (ketoconazole, fluconazole), terbinafine, or selenium sulfide (present in some shampoos) is recommended.

Tinea corporis (ringworm) may be caused by a number of different superficial fungi. The lesion is often a single lesion with an expanding red, raised ring, with a central area of clearing in the middle. Treatment is usually several weeks' application of a topical antifungal agent.

Lyme disease, a tickborne infection with *Borrelia burgdorferi*, is common in North America, Europe, and Russia (see Chapter 3, Lyme Disease). An infected traveler may present with ≥1 large erythematous patches, with or without central clearing, often surrounding a prior tick bite. The patient may not have noticed the tick bite.

LINEAR LESIONS

Cutaneous larva migrans, a skin infection with the larval stage of dog or cat hookworm (*Ancylostoma braziliense*), manifests as an extremely pruritic, serpiginous, linear lesion that advances in the epidermis of the skin relatively slowly (see Chapter 3, Cutaneous Larva Migrans). A similar lesion that may be more urticarial and that rapidly progresses may be due to **larva currens** (running larva) due to cutaneous migration of filariform larvae of *Strongyloides stercoralis*.

Lymphocutaneous spread of infection occurs when organisms spread along superficial cutaneous lymphatics, producing raised, linear, cordlike lesions; nodules or ulcers may also be found. Examples include sporotrichosis, *Mycobacterium marinum* infection (associated with exposure to water), leishmaniasis, bartonellosis (cat-scratch disease), *Nocardia* infection, tularemia, melioidosis, and blastomycosis.

Phytophotodermatitis is a noninfectious condition that results from interaction of natural psoralens, most commonly from spilled lime juice, and ultraviolet radiation from the sun. The result is an exaggerated sunburn that gives rise to a linear, asymptomatic lesion that later develops hyperpigmentation. The hyperpigmentation may take weeks or months to resolve.

SKIN ULCERS

Ulcerated skin lesions may result from *Staphylococcus* infections or may be the direct result of an unseen spider bite. The necrotic ulcer of anthrax is often surrounded by edema and usually results from handling animal hides or products. Rarely, a painless destructive ulcer with undermining edges may result from infection with *Mycobacterium ulcerans* (Buruli ulcer). Of particular concern is the ulcer (or less commonly, nodule) caused by **cutaneous leishmaniasis**. The main areas of risk are Latin America, the Mediterranean, the Middle East, Asia, and parts of Africa. The lesion is a chronic, usually painless ulcer, unless superinfected, with heaped-up margins on exposed skin surfaces. Special diagnostic techniques are necessary to confirm the diagnosis. Both topical and systemic treatments may be effective; the species of the infection often determines the treatment modality. If cutaneous leishmaniasis

5

is suspected, clinicians can contact CDC for further advice about diagnosis and treatment at 404-718-4745 or parasites@cdc.gov (see Chapter 3, Leishmaniasis, Cutaneous).

MISCELLANEOUS SKIN INFECTIONS

Skin Infections Associated with Water

Soft tissue infections can occur after both freshwater and saltwater exposure, particularly if there is associated trauma. Puncture wounds due to fishhooks and fish spines, lacerations from inanimate objects during wading and swimming, and bites or stings from fish or other sea creatures may be the source of the trauma leading to waterborne infections. Soft tissue infections associated with exposure to water or water-related animals include *M. marinum, Aeromonas* spp., *Plesiomonas* spp., *Edwardsiella tarda, Erysipelothrix rhusiopathiae,* and *Vibrio vulnificus*. A variety of skin and soft tissue manifestations may occur in association with these infections, including cellulitis, abscess formation, ecthyma gangrenosum, and necrotizing fasciitis. *V. vulnificus* infection may be especially severe in those with underlying liver disease and may manifest as a dramatic cellulitis with hemorrhagic bullae and sepsis. In general, infections caused by these organisms may be more severe in those who are immunosuppressed. Acute infections related to aquatic injury should be treated with an antibiotic that provides both gram-positive and gram-negative coverage (such as a fluoroquinolone or third-generation cephalosporin) until a specific organism has been identified. *M. marinum* lesions are usually indolent and usually appear as solitary nodules or papules on an extremity, especially on the dorsum of feet and hands; subsequent progression to shallow ulceration and scar formation may occur. Occasionally, "sporotrichoid" spread may occur as the lesions spread proximally along superficial lymphatics.

"Hot tub folliculitis" due to *Pseudomonas aeruginosa* may result from the use of spa pools or whirlpools or exposure to inadequately chlorinated swimming pools and hot tubs. Folliculitis typically develops 8–48 hours after exposure in contaminated water and consists of tender, pruritic papules, papulopustules, or nodules. Most patients have malaise, and some have low-grade fever. The condition is self-limited in 2–12 days; typically no antibiotic therapy is required.

Skin Infections Associated with Bites

Wound infections after dog and cat bites are caused by a variety of microorganisms. *S. aureus*; α-, β-, and γ-hemolytic streptococci; several genera of gram-negative organisms; and a number of anaerobic microorganisms have been isolated. The prevalence of *Pasteurella multocida* isolates from dog bite wounds is 20%–50%; *P. multocida* is a major pathogen in cat bite infections. Splenectomized patients are at particular risk of severe cellulitis and sepsis due to *Capnocytophaga canimorsus* after a dog bite. Management of dog and cat bites includes consideration of rabies postexposure prophylaxis, tetanus immunization, and antibiotic prophylaxis. Primary closure of puncture wounds and dog bites to the hand should be avoided. Antibiotic prophylaxis for dog bites is controversial, although most experts would treat splenectomized patients with amoxicillin-clavulanate prophylactically. Since *P. multocida* is a common accompaniment of cat bites, prophylaxis with amoxicillin-clavulanate or a fluoroquinolone for 3–5 days should be considered. Management of monkey bites includes wound care, tetanus immunization, rabies postexposure prophylaxis, and consideration of antimicrobial prophylaxis. Bites and scratches from Old World macaque monkeys have also been associated with fatal encephalomyelitis due to B virus infection in humans (see Chapter 3, B virus). Valacyclovir postexposure prophylaxis is recommended after a high-risk macaque exposure.

FEVER AND RASH

Fever and rash in returned travelers are most often due to a viral infection.

Dengue is caused by 1 of 4 strains of dengue viruses (see Chapter 3, Dengue). The disease is transmitted by a primarily day-biting *Aedes* mosquito often found in urban areas, and its incidence continues to increase. The disease is characterized by the abrupt onset of high fever, frontal headache (often accompanied by retroorbital pain), myalgia, and a faint macular rash (containing islands of pallor) that becomes evident on the second to fourth day of illness. A petechial rash may be found in classical dengue, as well as severe dengue (such as dengue hemorrhagic fever). Antigen and antibody detection tests, as well as PCR assays are available to diagnose dengue; detecting IgM in the appropriate clinical scenario would support the diagnosis.

Chikungunya, a virus transmitted by a primarily day-biting *Aedes* mosquito, has recently caused major outbreaks of illness in southeast Africa, South Asia, the Americas, and the Caribbean (see Chapter 3, Chikungunya). Chikungunya fever is similar to dengue clinically, including the rash, although hemorrhage, shock, and death are not typical of chikungunya. A major distinguishing feature is that arthritis or arthralgia is common with chikungunya (and may persist for months), whereas in dengue, myalgia is the major clinical feature. Similar to dengue, serologic tests are available. Treatment of the arthritis is with nonsteroidal anti-inflammatory drugs.

South African tick typhus, or African tick-bite fever (*Rickettsia africae*), is the most frequent cause of fever and rash in southern Africa. Transmitted by ticks, the disease is characterized by fever and a papular or vesicular rash associated with localized lymphadenopathy and the presence of an eschar (a mildly painful 1- to 2-cm black necrotic lesion with an erythematous margin). Satellite lesions may be present. Diagnosis is usually through clinical recognition and is confirmed by serologic testing. Treatment is with doxycycline.

Rocky Mountain spotted fever (RMSF), although uncommon in travelers, is an important cause of fever and rash because of its potential severity and the need for early treatment. This tickborne infection is found in the United States, Mexico, and parts of Central and South America. Most patients with RMSF develop a rash between the third and fifth days of illness. The typical rash of RMSF begins on the ankles and wrists and spreads both centrally and to the palms and soles. The rash commonly begins as a maculopapular eruption and then becomes petechial, although in some patients it begins with petechiae. Doxycycline is the treatment of choice.

The category of fever with rash is large, and providers caring for ill travelers should also consider the following diagnoses: enteroviruses, such as echovirus and coxsackievirus; hepatitis B virus; measles; Epstein-Barr virus; cytomegalovirus; typhus; leptospirosis; syphilis; and HIV.

BIBLIOGRAPHY

1. Ansart S, Perez L, Jaureguiberry S, Danis M, Bricaire F, Caumes E. Spectrum of dermatoses in 165 travelers returning from the tropics with skin diseases. Am J Trop Med Hyg. 2007 Jan;76(1):184–6.

2. Bernard P. Management of common bacterial infections of the skin. CurrOpin Infect Dis. 2008 Apr;21(2):122–8.

3. Diaz JH. The epidemiology, diagnosis, management, and prevention of ectoparasitic diseases in travelers. J Travel Med. 2006 Mar–Apr;13(2):100–11.

4. Hochedez P, Canestri A, Lecso M, Valin N, Bricaire F, Caumes E. Skin and soft tissue infections in returning travelers. Am J Trop Med Hyg. 2009 Mar;80(3):431–4.

5. Jensenius M, Davis X, von Sonnenburg F, Schwartz E, Keystone JS, Leder K, et al. Multicenter GeoSentinel analysis of rickettsial diseases in international travelers, 1996–2008. Emerg Infect Dis. 2009 Nov;15(11):1791–8.

6. Klion AD. Filarial infections in travelers and immigrants. Curr Infect Dis Rep. 2008 Mar;10(1):50–7.

7. Lederman ER, Weld LH, Elyazar IR, von Sonnenburg F, Loutan L, Schwartz E, et al. Dermatologic conditions of the ill returned traveler: an analysis from the GeoSentinel Surveillance Network. Int J Infect Dis. 2008 Nov;12(6):593–602.

8. Nordlund JJ. Cutaneous ectoparasites. Dermatol Ther. 2009 Nov–Dec;22(6):503–17..

9. Solomon M, Benenson S, Baum S, Schwartz E. Tropical skin infections among Israeli travelers. Am J Trop Med Hyg. 2011 Nov;85(5):868–72.

10. Wilson ME, Chen LH. Dermatologic infectious diseases in international travelers. Curr Infect Dis Rep. 2004 Feb;6(1):54–62.

SCREENING ASYMPTOMATIC RETURNED TRAVELERS

Michael Libman

CDC has no official guidelines or recommendations for screening asymptomatic international travelers. (For recommendations regarding the screening of newly arrived immigrants and refugees, see Chapter 8, Newly Arrived Immigrants & Refugees.) Nevertheless, the screening of travelers returning from developing countries represents a substantial portion of the activity of many travel and tropical medicine clinics. The scientific literature on the cost-effectiveness of screening asymptomatic travelers is sparse. It is clear that asymptomatic travelers can harbor many infections acquired during travel, some of which have the potential to cause serious sequelae or have public health implications. In some cases, these will include pathogens rarely found in the traveler's country of origin. Local medical practitioners will have little familiarity with the associated diseases, and specific diagnostic tests may not be readily available or may have poorly defined operating characteristics. The decision to screen for particular pathogens will depend on the type of travel, itinerary, and exposure history. However, exposure history is often unreliable and poorly predictive of infection, the value of a detailed itinerary is limited by incomplete information on where pathogens are endemic, and the type of travel often does not provide a practical assessment of risk.

Screening traditionally has been viewed as a secondary prevention intervention, that is, an attempt to identify existing occult illnesses or health risks. The cost effectiveness of screening involves a consideration of the natural history of the problem, the predictive value of the test, the direct and indirect costs of the test, and the effectiveness of prevention or therapy. Because of convenience and the susceptibility to suggestion at the time of screening, the screening visit may also offer an opportunity to promote primary prevention by discussing behavioral or other risk factors predisposing to ill health. These may include, for example, counseling on sexual health or the avoidance of schistosomiasis or malaria.

PARASITIC INFECTION

Travelers and their sponsors are often most concerned with the possibility of occult parasitic infection. Unfortunately, when screening for parasitic disease, the literature shows that patient questionnaires and common laboratory testing have poor sensitivity and specificity. Studies have shown that even an exhaustive risk-factor history in asymptomatic patients is unable to reliably detect those who would or would not have evidence of parasitic infection. Physical examination is equally unrewarding.

Most commonly, a stool examination is performed, typically microscopy, although a variety of pathogen-specific antigenic and molecular tests are also in use or in development. Travelers are often concerned about "worms," by which they mean intestinal nematodes. However, probably because of hygiene and short duration of exposure, infections with large numbers of the common nematodes, such as *Ascaris*, *Trichuris*, or hookworm, are rare. Questioning returning expatriates infected with intestinal helminths has disclosed no attributable symptoms compared with uninfected controls, although there have been case reports of complications, such as migration of *Ascaris* into the biliary system. The life cycles of almost all helminths preclude any real risk of ongoing transmission from asymptomatic hosts in developed countries. Helminths generally have a natural lifespan of months to a few years, which ensures eventual spontaneous cure. The exception to this rule is *Strongyloides*. For this helminth, serious complications are well known, nonspecific symptoms may easily be overlooked, duration of carriage after infection is unlimited, and the original burden of infection is irrelevant. Unfortunately, diagnosis by stool examination is notoriously insensitive, and serologic methods are often required, as discussed below.

The finding of pathogenic protozoa in asymptomatic patients is of questionable significance (with the possible exception of *Entamoeba histolytica*, a rare finding in these travelers). History of exposure to contaminated food or water has poor predictive value. There is no evidence to suggest that these carriers are likely to develop symptoms at a later time, although minor, unreported symptoms could be alleviated. Certainly, the medications used to treat pathogens have their own adverse effects. In theory, these carriers pose a public health risk, although transmission by asymptomatic travelers appears to be rare. This is further complicated by the fact that stool microscopy for protozoa is expensive, not very sensitive, and not highly reproducible, and many laboratories have limited expertise. *Entamoeba histolytica* cannot be distinguished from *E. dispar* by microscopy, requiring further specimen collection and testing, and studies reveal that most travelers with *Entamoeba* on microscopy are carrying *E. dispar*. Antigen testing for *E. histolytica* and *Giardia* (among others) is fairly reliable but lacks the potential to screen for all intestinal parasites with a single test. Advances in molecular methods for screening stool specimens for multiple pathogens simultaneously will likely mitigate some of these problems, although costs will remain high. Discovery of questionably pathogenic organisms, such as *Blastocystis*, is common and may lead to patient anxiety and unnecessary treatment.

Among the extra-intestinal helminths theoretically capable of causing eventual illness in asymptomatic travelers, most emphasis has been given to *Strongyloides* and the parasites that cause schistosomiasis and filariasis. There is no evidence that the low-burden schistosomal infections typically found in travelers are likely to lead to the types of complications commonly found in endemic areas, such as liver fibrosis or malignancy. Nevertheless, this possibility cannot be entirely ruled out, particularly in those who may have more intense exposures. Even brief exposures to freshwater lakes and rivers in known endemic foci

in Africa are associated with substantial seroconversion rates. In addition, complications due to ectopic egg migration can occur in light infections and without warning. On the other hand, reports of travelers with late complications from asymptomatic filarial infections are virtually nonexistent. Traditional tests for the parasites that cause all 3 of these infections, including stool examination for *Strongyloides* and *Schistosoma* spp., urine for *S. haematobium*, and blood or skin snips for microfilaria, all lack sensitivity, particularly in low-burden infection. For this reason, serologic testing has been advocated as the best screening tool. The problems with serologic screening include expense, lack of easy availability, and lack of standardization. Serologic tests are often designed to maximize sensitivity, typically at the expense of specificity. Unfortunately, specificity is almost impossible to define. Seropositivity in the absence of direct pathogen detection is common, and its clinical significance can be difficult to determine. Fortunately, for strongyloidiasis and schistosomiasis, treatment is cheap, easy, and effective. While it is not clear who should be screened, it is logical to at least perform serologic tests on travelers with a high duration and risk of exposure and to treat all those found to be positive. Since asymptomatic filarial infections appear least likely to have sequelae, and treatment is often neither very effective nor easy, the threshold for filarial serology (or antigen testing in the case of *W. bancrofti*) should be higher. Serology usually only becomes positive after adult forms have matured, which means waiting for 3 months or so after exposure.

Screening for eosinophilia is another common test, since it is quick and universally available and theoretically of value in detecting invasive helminths, if not protozoa. However, multiple studies have shown eosinophilia to have poor sensitivity. Specificity can be high; however, the low prevalence of infection in asymptomatic travelers means positive predictive value is low. In addition, the finding of eosinophilia may lead to an extensive and often fruitless search for a cause, generating high costs. Many cases of eosinophilia resolve spontaneously, possibly because of infection with nonpathogenic organisms or a noninfectious cause, such as allergy or drug reaction. Eosinophil counts may be repeated after several weeks or months before embarking on an extensive investigation. Counts may be highly variable, even within single day, and are suppressed by endogenous or exogenous steroids. Evaluation of absolute counts, rather than by percentage of leukocytes, is more reproducible and predictive.

Immigrants with frequent and regular exposure to malaria may gradually develop partial immunity. This may result in low-level parasitemia with few or no symptoms. They may later recrudesce with more severe illness. This phenomenon is rare in other travelers. There is no justification for screening most asymptomatic travelers, whether by blood film, serologic tests, or molecular methods. No tests can detect latent infections with *Plasmodium vivax* or *P. ovale*. Travelers should be reminded to seek evaluation for unexplained fever and notify practitioners of any recent travel.

Recently, concern about occult trypanosomiasis has increased. Infection in asymptomatic travelers (as opposed to immigrants) appears to be extremely rare. Screening tests, such as serology and molecular diagnostics, are of unknown value. For travel to endemic areas of Latin America, testing might be considered in cases of prolonged residence in primitive housing, such as mud walls and thatched roofs, especially if the large reduviid bugs have been seen. East African trypanosomiasis has affected travelers but typically causes symptoms. West African disease is generally not reported in travelers.

NONPARASITIC ILLNESS

Sexual activity and travel seem to be linked. High rates of contact with new partners, including sex workers, have been documented in volunteers, expatriate workers, backpackers, and military personnel. Of concern are the low rates of reported condom use. Returning travelers with acute HIV or hepatitis B infection pose public health risks. Travelers may be hesitant to volunteer a relevant history. Screening for sexually transmitted infections should always be considered.

The incidence of tuberculosis related to travel is difficult to estimate. Estimates of exposure based on skin test (Mantoux) conversions suggest rates of exposure of the same general magnitude as the local population. Work in high-prevalence settings such as health care institutions or refugee camps merits screening. Traditionally, this has been done using pre- and post-travel skin tests. This is cumbersome, requiring as many as 4 pre-travel visits for a 2-step test and 2 visits after potential exposure. This number can be reduced by using the more expensive interferon-γ release assay (IGRA), which also is less subject to false-positive results related to BCG vaccination. Unfortunately, recent data suggest that IGRA results show inadequate reproducibility, leading to false "conversions" on follow-up testing. In most patients born and raised in low-prevalence countries, a case can be made for omitting the pre-travel test, because results are rarely positive.

For many long-term travelers, such as expatriate workers and some missionary and aid workers, the visits for asymptomatic screening may also be their only interludes from a continuing assignment abroad allowing for a general health evaluation. The usual recommendations for the periodic health exam, which may include screening for hypertension, diabetes, and malignancy, would apply.

SUMMARY

Recommendations for screening the asymptomatic traveler are necessarily based on opinion and common sense, rather than convincing evidence. The following may serve as a general guideline.

For the asymptomatic short stay (<3–6 months) traveler, the yield of screening is low and should be directed by specific risk factors revealed in the history. A history of prolonged (>2 weeks) digestive symptoms during travel can suggest protozoal infection. Exposure to fresh water in a region endemic for schistosomiasis, especially in Africa, merits serologic screening, with the addition of stool and urine examination in the case of high-intensity exposure. Serology for *Strongyloides* should be considered in those who have a high risk of skin exposure to soil likely to be contaminated with human feces, usually those with a history of frequently walking barefoot outdoors. A sexual history should be obtained. Work in a health care setting or other area at high risk for TB may merit screening.

For longer-stay travelers, as the overall yield of screening increases it becomes less useful to rely on history for selective testing. The emphasis should be on those with the longest stays and the most problematic sanitary conditions. In some cases, employers may require certain tests, partly for reasons of liability. Stool examinations are usually done, although they serve mostly to provide a psychological reassurance. Serologic testing for schistosomiasis and strongyloidiasis should be done in those reporting some level of risk. Eosinophil counts are usually done, although results should be interpreted cautiously. Screening for sexually transmitted infections should be offered to all except those with the most convincing absence of risk. Mantoux or IGRA tests should be limited to those who have worked in a health care or similar setting, or who have had intimate and prolonged contact with residents of an endemic area for ≥6 months. Possible exposure to bloodborne pathogens should be assessed. Any other screening should be guided by exceptional exposures or knowledge about local outbreaks.

BIBLIOGRAPHY

1. Baaten GG, Sonder GJ, van Gool T, Kint JA, van den Hoek A. Travel-related schistosomiasis, strongyloidiasis, filariasis, and toxocariasis: the risk of infection and the diagnostic relevance of blood eosinophilia. BMC Infect Dis. 2011 Apr 5;11:84.
2. MacLean JD, Libman M. Screening returning travelers. Infect Dis Clin North Am. 1998 Jun;12(2):431–43.
3. Soonawala D, van Lieshout L, den Boer MA, Claas EC, Verweij JJ, Godkewitsch A, et al. Post-travel screening of asymptomatic long-term travelers to the tropics for intestinal parasites using molecular diagnostics. Am J Trop Med Hyg. 2014 May;90(5):835–9.

5

Conveyance & Transportation Issues

AIR TRAVEL

Petra A. Illig, Karen J. Marienau, Phyllis E. Kozarsky

Worldwide, >1 billion people travel by commercial aircraft every year, and this number is expected to double in the next 20 years. Travelers often have concerns about the health risks of flying in airplanes. Those with underlying illness need to be aware that the entire point-to-point travel experience, including buses, trains, taxis, and public waiting areas, can pose challenges. While illness may occur as a direct result of air travel, it is uncommon; the main concerns are as follows:

- Exacerbations of chronic medical problems due to changes in air pressure and humidity
- Relative immobility during flights (risk of thromboembolic disease, see Chapter 2, Deep Vein Thrombosis & Pulmonary Embolism)
- Close proximity to other passengers with certain communicable diseases

CONTRAINDICATIONS TO FLIGHT

The Aerospace Medical Association publishes guidelines for preflight medical evaluation (www.asma.org). People with the following conditions are thought to be at higher risk for flight:

- Myocardial infarction (MI) within 2 weeks (or complicated MI within 6 weeks)
- Coronary artery bypass within 2 weeks

The following conditions may also pose a risk if uncontrolled:

- Congestive heart failure
- Seizures
- Hypertension
- Diabetes
- Mental illness
- Exacerbation of chronic disease

For information on contraindications and precautions related to pregnancy, see Chapter 8, Pregnant Travelers.

EXACERBATION OF CHRONIC DISEASE

During flight, the aircraft cabin pressure is usually maintained at the equivalent of 6,000–8,000 ft (1,829–2,438 m) above sea level. Most healthy travelers will not notice any effects. However, for travelers with cardiopulmonary diseases (especially those who normally require supplemental oxygen), cerebrovascular disease, anemia, or sickle cell disease, conditions in an aircraft can exacerbate underlying medical conditions. Aircraft cabin air is typically dry, usually 10%–20% humidity, which can cause dryness of the mucous membranes of the eyes and airways.

People with chronic illnesses, particularly those whose conditions may be unstable, should be evaluated by a health care provider to ensure they are fit for air travel. Certain surgeries or procedures may require delaying travel. For more information, see Chapter 8, Travelers with Chronic Illnesses.

Specific information for travelers with disabilities and medical conditions that may affect security screening can be found at www.tsa.gov/traveler-information/travelers-disabilities-and-medical-conditions.

For those who require supplemental in-flight oxygen, the following must be taken into consideration:

- Federal regulations prohibit airlines from allowing passengers to bring their own oxygen aboard; passengers requiring in-flight supplemental oxygen should notify the airline ≥72 hours before departure.
- Airlines might not offer in-flight supplemental oxygen on all aircraft or flights; some airlines permit only Federal Aviation Administration–approved portable oxygen concentrators (http://www.faa.gov/about/initiatives/cabin_safety/portable_oxygen/).
- Information regarding the screening of portable oxygen concentrators at airports in the United States can be found at http://www.tsa.gov/traveler-information/portable-oxygen.
- Travelers must arrange their own oxygen supplies while on the ground, at departure, during layovers, and on arrival. The National Home Oxygen Patients Association (www.homeoxygen.org/airline-travel-with-oxygen) and the Airline Oxygen Council of America (www.airlineoxygencouncil.org) provide information to assist people who require supplemental oxygen during travel.

BAROTRAUMA DURING FLIGHT

Barotrauma may occur when the pressure inside an air-filled, enclosed body space (such as the middle ear, sinuses, or abdomen) is not the same as air pressure inside the aircraft cabin. It most commonly occurs during rapid changes in environmental pressure, such as during ascent, when cabin pressure rapidly decreases, and during descent, when cabin pressure rapidly increases. Barotrauma most commonly affects the middle ear; it occurs when the eustachian tube is blocked and

thus unable to equalize the air pressure in the middle ear with the outside cabin pressure. Middle ear barotrauma is usually not severe or dangerous and can usually be prevented or self-treated. It may rarely cause complications such as a perforated tympanic membrane, dizziness, permanent tinnitus, or hearing loss. The following suggestions may help avoid potential barotrauma:

- People with ear, nose, and sinus infections or severe congestion may wish to temporarily avoid flying to prevent pain or injury.
- Oral pseudoephedrine 30 minutes before flight departure, or a decongestant nasal spray, may alleviate symptoms.
- Travelers with allergies should continue their regular allergy medication.
- Travelers should stay hydrated to help avoid irritation of nasal passages and pharynx and to promote better function of the eustachian tubes.
- Travelers sensitive to abdominal bloating should avoid carbonated beverages and foods that can increase gas production.
- People who have had recent surgery, particularly intra-abdominal, neurologic, intrapulmonary, or intraocular procedures, should consult with their physicians before flying.

VENTILATION AND AIR QUALITY

All commercial jet aircraft built after the late 1980s and a few modified older aircraft recirculate 10%–50% of the air in the cabin mixed with outside air. The recirculated air passes through a series of filters 20–30 times per hour. In most newer-model airplanes, the recycled air passes through high-efficiency particulate air (HEPA) filters, which capture 99.9% of particles (bacteria, fungi, and larger viruses or virus clumps) 0.1–0.3 μm in diameter. Air flow occurs transversely across the plane in limited bands, and air is not forced up and down the length of the plane. As a result, the air cabin environment is not conducive to the spread of most infectious diseases. However, some diseases may be spread by contact with infected secretions, such as when an ill person sneezes or coughs and the secretions land on someone's face (mouth, nose, eyes) or by touching a contaminated surface, then touching one's face with contaminated hands. Practicing good handwashing and respiratory hygiene (covering mouth when coughing or sneezing) decreases the risk of disease spread by direct or indirect contact.

IN-FLIGHT MEDICAL EMERGENCIES

Increasingly large aircraft, combined with an aging flying population, makes the incidence of onboard medical emergencies likely to increase. Approximately 1 in 10,000–40,000 passengers has a medical incident during air transport. Of these, approximately 1 in 150,000 requires use of in-flight medical equipment or drugs. The most commonly encountered in-flight medical events, in decreasing order of frequency, are the following:

- Vasovagal syncope
- Gastrointestinal events
- Respiratory events
- Cardiac events
- Neurologic events

Deaths aboard commercial aircraft have been estimated at 0.3 per 1 million passengers; approximately two-thirds of these are caused by cardiac problems. Air carriers in the United States that fly with a maximum payload capacity of >7,500 pounds and with ≥1 flight attendant (typically those aircraft with a capacity of ≥30 passengers) are now required to carry ≥1 approved automatic external defibrillator and an emergency medical kit. The kit is required to have the items specified by the Federal Aviation Administration (for contents, see www.faa. gov/regulations_policies/advisory_circulars/ index.cfm/go/document.information/ documentID/22516).

Although flight attendants receive training in basic first aid procedures, they are generally not certified in emergency medical response. Many airlines use ground-based medical consultants via radio or phone communication to assist volunteer passenger responders and flight attendants in managing medical cases.

The goal of managing in-flight medical emergencies is to stabilize the passenger until ground-based medical care can safely be reached; it should not be considered a

method of maintaining the original flight route in order to reach the scheduled destination. The captain must, therefore, weigh the needs of the ill passenger with other safety considerations such as weather, landing conditions, and terrain. Certain routes, such as transoceanic flights, may severely restrict diversion options, while others may present a number of safe landing choices. In the latter circumstance, consideration should be given to choosing an airport that has timely access to a medical facility.

IN-FLIGHT TRANSMISSION OF COMMUNICABLE DISEASES

Communicable diseases may be transmitted to other travelers during air travel; therefore, people who are acutely ill, or still within the infectious period for a specific disease, should delay their travel until they are no longer contagious. Travelers should be up-to-date on routine vaccinations and receive destination-specific vaccinations before travel. Travelers should be reminded to wash their hands frequently and thoroughly (or use an alcohol-based hand sanitizer containing ≥60% alcohol), especially after using the toilet and before preparing or eating food, and to cover their noses and mouths when coughing or sneezing.

If a passenger with a communicable disease is identified as having flown on a particular flight (or flights), passengers who may have been exposed may be contacted by public health authorities for possible screening or prophylaxis. When necessary, public health authorities will obtain contact information from the airline for potentially exposed travelers so they may be contacted and offered intervention. Notifying a passenger of potential exposure to a communicable disease during a flight is facilitated if he or she has provided the airline with accurate and up-to-date contact information.

CDC has the authority to restrict travel for people who are contagious with a communicable disease that poses a public health threat during travel if 1) they plan to travel by commercial air (domestically or internationally) or travel internationally by other means and 2) are not adhering to or are unaware of public health recommendations. For information regarding CDC's travel restrictions, see www. cdc.gov/quarantine/QuarantineIsolation.html.

To request a consultation, public health authorities may contact the CDC quarantine station of jurisdiction (see www.cdc.gov/quarantine/quarantinestations.html) or the CDC Emergency Operations Center by calling 770-488-7100.

Tuberculosis

Mycobacterium tuberculosis is transmitted from person to person via airborne respiratory droplet nuclei. Although the risk of transmission onboard aircraft is low, CDC recommends conducting passenger contact investigations for flights ≥8 hours if the person with tuberculosis (TB) is sputum smear positive for acid-fast bacilli and has cavitation on chest radiograph or has multidrug-resistant TB. People known to have active TB disease should not travel by commercial air (or any other commercial means) until they are determined to be noninfectious. State health department TB controllers are valuable resources for advice (www.tbcontrollers.org/community/statecityterritory).

Neisseria meningitidis

Meningococcal disease (caused by *Neisseria meningitidis*) is transmitted by direct contact with respiratory droplets and secretions and can be rapidly fatal. Therefore, close contacts need to be quickly identified and provided with prophylactic antimicrobial agents. Antimicrobial prophylaxis should be considered for any of the following:

- Household member traveling with the ill traveler
- Travel companion with very close contact
- Passenger seated directly next to the ill traveler on flights ≥8 hours

Measles

Measles (rubeola) is a viral illness transmitted by respiratory droplets or direct contact, but it can also be spread via airborne routes. Most measles cases diagnosed in the United States are imported from countries where measles is endemic. Travelers should ensure they are immune to measles before travel. Infants aged 6–11 months who will be traveling overseas should receive 1 dose of measles-mumps-rubella (MMR) vaccine before travel. However, this dose will not count as part of the recommended immunization schedule of 2 doses, which begins at age 12–15 months. An ill traveler is considered infectious during a flight of any duration if he or she traveled during the 4 days before rash onset through 4 days after rash onset. Flight-related contact investigations are initiated as quickly as possible so postexposure prophylaxis may be provided to susceptible travelers. MMR vaccine given within 72 hours of exposure or immune globulin given within 6 days of exposure may prevent measles or decrease its severity.

Influenza

Transmission of the influenza virus aboard aircraft has been documented, but data are limited. Transmission is thought to be primarily due to large droplets; therefore, passengers seated closest to the source patient are believed to be most at risk for exposure. Influenza vaccine is routinely recommended each year for all people aged ≥6 months who do not have contraindications.

DISINSECTION

To reduce the accidental spread of mosquitoes and other vectors via airline cabins and luggage compartments, a number of countries require disinsection of all inbound flights. The World Health Organization (WHO) and the International Civil Aviation Organization specify 2 approaches for aircraft disinsection:

- Spraying the aircraft cabin with an aerosolized insecticide (usually 2% phenothrin) while passengers are on board
- Treating the aircraft's interior surfaces with a residual insecticide while the aircraft is empty

Some countries use a third method, in which aircraft are sprayed with an aerosolized insecticide while passengers are not on board.

Disinsection is not routinely done on incoming flights to the United States. Although disinsection, when done appropriately, was declared safe by WHO in 1995, there is still much debate about the safety of the agents and methods used. Guidelines for disinsection have been updated for the revised International Health Regulations (www.who.int/ihr/en). Many countries, including the

 AIR TRAVEL

United States, reserve the right to increase the use of disinsection in case of increased threat of vector or disease spread. An updated list of countries that require disinsection and the types of methods used is available at the Department of Transportation website (http://www.dot.gov/office-policy/aviation-policy/aircraft-disinsection-requirements).

INFORMATION FOR AIR CREW

On occasion, flight crews may encounter passengers with potential infectious diseases. For additional information, see Chapter 8, Advice for Air Crews; the CDC Airline Guidance web page (www.cdc.gov/quarantine/air/index.html); and the CDC Travelers' Health website (www.cdc.gov/travel).

BIBLIOGRAPHY

1. Aerospace Medical Association Task Force. Medical guidelines for airline travel, 2nd ed. Aviat Space Environ Med. 2003 May;74(5 Suppl):A1–19.

2. Bagshaw M, Nicolls DN. The aircraft cabin environment. In: Keystone JS, Freedman DO, Kozarsky PE, Connor BA, Nothdurft HO, editors. Travel Medicine. 3rd ed. Philadelphia: Saunders Elsevier; 2013. p. 405–12.

3. CDC. Exposure to patients with meningococcal disease on aircrafts—United States, 1999–2001. MMWR Morb Mortal Wkly Rep. 2001 Jun 15;50(23):485–9.

4. CDC. Notes from the field: Multiple cases of measles after exposure during air travel—Australia and New Zealand, January 2011. MMWR Morb Mortal Wkly Rep. 2011 Jul 1;60(25):851.

5. CDC. Public health interventions involving travelers with tuberculosis—US ports of entry, 2007–2012. MMWR Morb Mortal Wkly Rep. 2012 Aug 3;61:570–3.

6. Delaune EF 3rd, Lucas RH, Illig P. In-flight medical events and aircraft diversions: one airline's experience. Aviat Space Environ Med. 2003 Jan;74(1):62–8.

7. Illig P. Passenger health. In: Curdt-Christiansen C, Draeger J, Kriebel J, Antunano M, editors. Principles and Practice of Aviation Medicine. Hackensack, NJ: World Scientific; 2009. p. 667–708.

8. Marienau KJ, Cramer EH, Coleman MS, Marano N, Cetron MS. Flight related tuberculosis contact investigations in the United States: comparative risk and economic analysis of alternate protocols. Travel Med Infect Dis. 2014 Jan–Feb;12(1):54–62.

9. Neatherlin J, Cramer EH, Dubray C, Marienau KJ, Russell M, Sun H, et al. Influenza A(H1N1)pdm09 during air travel. Travel Med Infect Dis. 2013 Mar–Apr;11(2):110–8.

10. Nelson K, Marienau K, Schembri C, Redd S. Measles transmission during air travel, United States, December 1, 2008–December 31, 2011. Travel Med Infect Dis. 2013 Mar–Apr;11(2):81–9.

11. World Health Organization. Tuberculosis and Air Travel: Guidelines for Prevention and Control. 3rd ed. Geneva: World Health Organization; 2008 [cited 2014 Jun 30]. Available from: http://whqlibdoc.who.int/publications/2008/9789241547505_eng.pdf?ua=1.

CRUISE SHIP TRAVEL

Krista Kornylo Duong, Kiren Mitruka, Susan A. Lippold

INTRODUCTION

Cruise ships bring together large numbers of people from a variety of communities and backgrounds. Communicable diseases can be introduced onboard by embarking passengers and crew members or acquired during visits to seaports. The crowded, semi-enclosed environment of the cruise ship can facilitate transmission of infectious diseases from person to person or from contaminated food, water, air, or environmental surfaces. Crew members who remain onboard during successive sailings can sustain transmission of communicable diseases. Certain groups, such as pregnant women, the elderly, and those who are immunocompromised, might be more seriously affected by infectious diseases. In addition, the stress of travel can worsen chronic conditions in any population.

CRUISE SHIP MEDICAL CAPABILITIES

Medical facilities on cruise ships can vary widely depending on ship size, itinerary, length of cruise, and passenger demographics. Generally, shipboard medical clinics can provide medical care comparable to that of ambulatory care centers. Although no official agency regulates medical practice aboard cruise ships, consensus-based guidelines for cruise ship medical facilities were published by the American College of Emergency Physicians (ACEP) in 1995, most recently updated in 2013. The ACEP guidelines (www.acep.org/content.aspx?id=29500), which are followed by most major cruise lines, state that the cruise ship medical facilities should maintain the following minimum capabilities:

- Provide emergency medical care for passengers and crew
- Stabilize patients and initiate reasonable diagnostic and therapeutic interventions
- Facilitate the evacuation of seriously ill or injured patients

ILLNESSES AND INJURY ABOARD CRUISE SHIPS

Cruise ship medical clinics deal with a wide variety of illnesses and injuries. Approximately 3%–11% of conditions reported to cruise ship infirmaries are urgent or an emergency. Approximately 95% of illnesses are treated or managed onboard, and 5% require evacuation and shoreside consultation for medical, surgical, and dental problems. Approximately half of passengers who seek medical care are older than 65 years. Most (69%–88%) passenger dispensary visits are due to medical conditions, of which respiratory (19%–29%) and gastrointestinal (GI) (9%–10%) illnesses are the most frequently reported diagnoses. Approximately 10%–25% of passengers report seasickness, and injuries (typically from slips, trips, or falls) account for 12%–18% of medical visits. Death rates for cruise ship passengers, most often from cardiovascular events, range from 0.6 to 9.8 deaths per million passenger-nights.

The most frequently documented cruise ship outbreaks involve respiratory infections (influenza and Legionnaires' disease), GI infections (norovirus), and vaccine-preventable diseases other than influenza, such as rubella and varicella (chickenpox). To reduce the risk of onboard introduction of communicable diseases by embarking passengers, ships may conduct preembarkation medical screening to identify ill passengers before boarding.

US federal quarantine regulations require ships destined for a US port to immediately report to CDC all shipboard deaths and certain illnesses. CDC guidance for management of common infectious diseases on ships (including varicella, influenzalike illness, and GI illness) and reporting to CDC is available at www.cdc.gov/quarantine/cruise/index.html and www.cdc.gov/nceh/vsp.

The following measures should be encouraged to limit the introduction and spread of communicable diseases on cruise ships:

- Passengers and their clinicians should consult CDC's Travelers' Health website (www.cdc.gov/travel) before travel for updates on outbreaks and travel health notices.
- Passengers ill with communicable diseases before a voyage should delay travel until they are no longer contagious.
- Passengers who become ill during the voyage should seek care in the ship's infirmary to receive clinical management, facilitate infection control measures, and maximize reporting of potential public health events.

SPECIFIC HEALTH RISKS
GI Illness

CDC's Vessel Sanitation Program (VSP) conducts twice-yearly, unannounced inspections of ships carrying ≥13 passengers with international itineraries that call on US seaports. In spite of good cruise ship environmental health standards and high VSP inspection scores, outbreaks of gastroenteritis on cruise ships continue to occur. Updates of outbreaks are posted on VSP's website at www.cdc.gov/nceh/vsp/surv/gilist.htm. More than 90% of GI outbreaks investigated by VSP with a confirmed cause are due to norovirus. Characteristics of norovirus that facilitate outbreaks are a low infective dose, easy person-to-person transmissibility, prolonged viral shedding, no long-term immunity, and the organism's ability to survive routine cleaning procedures. From 2005 through 2009, approximately 27 outbreaks of norovirus infections occurred on cruise ships each year. To reduce the spread of norovirus on cruise ships, passengers should be counseled on the following:

- Information on cruise ship norovirus outbreaks is available at www.cdc.gov/nceh/vsp.
- Passengers should wash their hands with soap and water often, especially before eating and after using the restroom.
- Passengers who develop a GI illness, even if symptoms are mild, should promptly call the ship's medical center and follow cruise ship guidance regarding isolation and other infection control measures (see Chapter 3, Norovirus). If no medical center exists, contact the ship's master to report GI illness

GI outbreaks on cruise ships from food and water sources have also been associated with *Salmonella* spp., enterotoxigenic *Escherichia coli*, *Shigella* spp., *Vibrio* spp., *Staphylococcus aureus*, *Clostridium perfringens*, *Cyclospora cayetanensis*, and hepatitis A and E viruses.

Respiratory Illness
Influenza

Influenza seasons in the Northern and Southern Hemispheres typically occur at opposite times of the year. Since passengers and crew originate from all regions of the world, shipboard outbreaks of influenza A and B can occur year-round, and travelers on cruise ships can be exposed to strains circulating in different parts of the world. Using 2008–2011 surveillance data, CDC found a mean rate of influenzalike illness (defined as temperature ≥100°F plus cough or sore throat) of 0.065 cases per 1,000 person-nights, without a detectable seasonal pattern.

During outbreaks, travelers can expect onboard control measures such as isolation of ill people, antiviral treatment of ill people, surveillance for new cases, and prophylaxis of contacts who are at high risk for complications. The following measures are recommended to reduce the spread of influenza aboard cruise ships:

- Clinicians should provide cruise travelers, particularly those at high risk for influenza complications, with the current seasonal influenza vaccine (if available) ≥2 weeks before travel.
- Passengers at high risk for influenza complications should discuss antiviral treatment and chemoprophylaxis with their health care provider before travel.
- Passengers should practice good respiratory hygiene and cough etiquette.
- Passengers should report their respiratory illness to the infirmary promptly and follow isolation recommendations, if indicated.

Additional guidance on the prevention and control of influenza on cruise ships is available at www.cdc.gov/quarantine/cruise/management/guidance-cruise-ships-influenza-updated.html. For more information, see Chapter 3, Influenza.

Legionnaires' Disease

Legionnaires' disease is a severe pneumonia caused by inhalation or possibly aspiration of warm, aerosolized water containing *Legionella* organisms. The organism is not transmitted from person to person. Contaminated ships' whirlpool spas and potable water supply systems are the most commonly implicated sources of shipboard *Legionella* outbreaks. Improvements in ship design and standardization of water disinfection have reduced the risk of *Legionella* growth and colonization.

Symptom onset is typically 2–10 days after exposure, and older travelers (≥65 years) and those with underlying medical conditions are at increased risk for infection. Most cruise ships can perform *Legionella* urine antigen testing. People with suspected Legionnaires' disease require prompt antibiotic treatment. See Chapter 3, Legionellosis (Legionnaires' Disease & Pontiac Fever) for more information.

More than 20%–25% of all Legionnaires' disease reported to CDC is travel-associated. Clusters of Legionnaires' disease associated with hotel or cruise ship travel are difficult to identify, because travelers often disperse from the source of infection before symptoms begin. In evaluating cruise travelers for Legionnaires' disease, clinicians should do the following:

- Obtain a thorough travel history of all destinations from 10 days before symptom onset (to assist in the identification of potential source of exposure)

- Collect urine for antigen testing
- Collect respiratory secretions for culture, which is essential for identifying the pathogen
- Inform CDC of any travel-associated Legionnaires' disease cases by sending an email to travellegionella@cdc.gov

Vaccine-Preventable Diseases (VPDs)

Although most cruise ship passengers are from countries with routine vaccination programs (such as the United States and Canada), many crew members originate from developing countries with low immunization rates. Outbreaks of measles, rubella, and, most commonly, varicella have been reported on cruise ships. Preventive measures to reduce the spread of VPDs aboard cruise ships should be followed:

- Crew members should have documented proof of immunity to VPDs.
- Passengers, especially older passengers (>65 years) and immunocompromised people, should be up-to-date with routine vaccinations before travel, as well as any required or recommended vaccinations specific for their destinations.
- Women of childbearing age should be immune to rubella before cruise ship travel.

Vectorborne Diseases

Cruise ship port visits may include countries where vectorborne diseases, such as malaria, dengue, yellow fever, and Japanese encephalitis are endemic. New diseases might surface in unexpected locations. For example, chikungunya was reported in late 2013 for the first time in the Caribbean (with subsequent spread throughout the Caribbean and in several North, Central, and South American countries), and outbreaks of Zika were reported in the Western Pacific in the first half of 2014. Yellow fever vaccination certificates may be required by some countries for entry.

Passengers should follow recommendations for avoiding mosquito bites and vectorborne infections:

- Use an effective insect repellent (see Chapter 2, Protection against Mosquitoes, Ticks, & Other Arthropods)
- While indoors, remain in well-screened or air-conditioned areas
- When outdoors, wear long-sleeved shirts, long pants, boots, and hats
- Take antimalarial chemoprophylaxis if needed (see Chapter 3, Yellow Fever & Malaria Information, by Country)

Other Health Concerns

Stresses of cruise ship travel include varying weather and environmental conditions, as well as unaccustomed changes in diet and physical activity. Foreign travel may increase the likelihood of risk-taking behaviors such as alcohol misuse, drug use, and unsafe sex. In spite of modern stabilizer systems, seasickness is a common complaint (affecting up to one-fourth of travelers) (see Chapter 2, Motion Sickness).

PREVENTIVE MEASURES FOR CRUISE SHIP TRAVELERS

Cruise ship travelers often have complex itineraries due to multiple, short port visits. Although most of these port visits do not include overnight stays off the cruise ship, many exotic trips have options for travelers to venture off the ship for ≥1 nights. Therefore, cruise ship travelers may be uncertain about potential exposures and which antimicrobial prophylaxis, immunizations, and preventive measures should be considered. Box 6-1 summarizes recommendations for cruise travelers and clinicians advising cruise travelers in pre-travel preparation and healthy behaviors during travel. Travelers with special medical needs, such as wheelchairs, oxygen tanks, or dialysis, should inform their cruise line before traveling. Travelers with health conditions should carry a written summary of essential health information (electrocardiogram, chest radiograph if abnormal, blood type, chronic conditions, allergies, and medication list) that would facilitate their care during a medical emergency. In addition, all prospective cruise travelers should verify coverage with their health insurance carriers and consider purchasing additional insurance to cover medical evacuation and health services in foreign countries (see Chapter 2, Travel Insurance, Travel Health Insurance, & Medical Evacuation Insurance).

BOX 6-1. CRUISE TRAVEL HEALTH PRECAUTIONS

Advice for Clinicians Giving Pre-Travel Cruise Consultations
Risk Assessment and Risk Communication
- Discuss itinerary, including season, duration of travel, and activities at port stops.
- Review the traveler's medical and immunization history, allergies, and special health needs.
- Discuss relevant travel-specific health hazards and risk reduction.
- Provide the traveler with documentation of his or her medical history, immunizations, and medications.

Immunization and Risk Management
- Provide immunizations that are routinely recommended (age-specific), required (yellow fever), and recommended based on risk.
- Discuss food and water precautions and insect bite prevention.
- Older travelers, especially those with a history of heart disease, should carry a baseline electrocardiogram to facilitate onboard or overseas medical care.

Medications Based on Risk and Need
- Consider malaria chemoprophylaxis if itinerary includes port stops in malaria-endemic areas.
- Consider motion sickness medications for self-treatment (see Chapter 2, Motion Sickness).

Precautions for Cruise Ship Travelers
Pre-Travel
- Evaluate the type and length of the planned cruise in the context of personal health requirements.
- Consult medical and dental care providers before cruise travel.
- Notify cruise line of special needs (such as wheelchair access, dialysis, oxygen tank).
- Consider additional insurance for overseas health care and medical evacuation.
- Carry prescription medications in their original containers, with a copy of the prescription and accompanying physician's letter.
- Bring insect repellent and sunscreen.
- Defer travel while acutely ill.
- Consult www.cdc.gov/travel for travel health notices.
- Check www.cdc.gov/nceh/vsp/surv/gilist.htm for gastrointestinal outbreaks.

During Travel
- Wash hands frequently with soap and water. If soap and water are not available, use an alcohol-based sanitizer that contains ≥60% alcohol.
- Follow safe food and water precautions when eating off the ship at ports of call.
- Use measures to prevent insect bites during port visits, especially in malaria- or dengue-endemic areas or in areas where outbreaks of vectorborne diseases, such as chikungunya and Zika, are occurring.
- Use sun protection.
- Maintain good fluid intake, but avoid excessive alcohol consumption.
- Avoid contact with ill people.
- If sexually active, practice safe sex.
- Report illness to ship's infirmary and follow medical recommendations.

REPORTING ILLNESS AFTER TRAVEL

Travelers who become ill after returning home should inform their health care providers of where they have traveled. Clinicians should report suspected communicable diseases in recently returned cruise ship travelers to public health authorities:

- Report GI illnesses related to cruise ship travel to the CDC VSP by calling 800-CDC-INFO (800-232-4636) or by visiting www.cdc.gov and clicking on "Contact CDC-INFO")
- Inform CDC of any travel-associated Legionnaires' disease cases by sending an e-mail to travellegionella@cdc.gov.
- Report communicable diseases to the public health authority of jurisdiction. Health departments should notify the CDC quarantine station of jurisdiction (www.cdc.gov/quarantine/quarantinestations.html) for communicable diseases of public health concern during travel.

BIBLIOGRAPHY

1. Bell TR, Kornylo Duong K, Finelli L, Slaten DD. Influenza surveillance on cruise ships. Am J Prev Med. 2014 Mar;46(3):327–9.
2. Cramer EH, Slaten DD, Guerreiro A, Robbins D, Ganzon A. Management and control of varicella on cruise ships: a collaborative approach to promoting public health. J Travel Med. 2012 Jul;19(4):226–32.
3. Guyard C, Low DE. Legionella infections and travel associated legionellosis. Travel Med Infect Dis. 2011 Jul;9(4):176–86.
4. Hill CD. Cruise ship travel. In: Keystone JS, Freedman DO, Kozarsky PE, Connor BA, Nothdurft HD, editors. Travel Medicine. 3rd ed. Philadelphia: Saunders Elsevier; 2013. p. 349–55.
5. Kornylo K, Henry R, Slaten D. Respiratory disease on cruise ships. Clin Infect Dis. 2012 Mar 1;54(5):v–vi.
6. Lanini S, Capobianchi MR, Puro V, Filia A, Del Manso M, Karki T, et al. Measles outbreak on a cruise ship in the western Mediterranean, February 2014, preliminary report. Euro Surveill. 2014;19(10):2–6.
7. Lawson CJ, Dykewicz CA, Molinari NA, Lipman H, Alvarado-Ramy F. Deaths in international travelers arriving in the United States, July 1, 2005 to June 30, 2008. J Travel Med. 2012 Mar–Apr;19(2):96–103.
8. Mitruka K, Felsen CB, Tomianovic D, Inman B, Street K, Yambor P, et al. Measles, rubella, and varicella among the crew of a cruise ship sailing from Florida, United States, 2006. J Travel Med. 2012 Jul;19(4):233–7.
9. Peake DE, Gray CL, Ludwig MR, Hill CD. Descriptive epidemiology of injury and illness among cruise ship passengers. Ann Emerg Med. 1999 Jan;33(1):67–72.
10. Tomaszewski R, Nahorski WL. Interpopulation study of medical attendance aboard a cruise ship. Int Marit Health. 2008;59(1–4):61–8.
11. Uyeki TM, Zane SB, Bodnar UR, Fielding KL, Buxton JA, Miller JM, et al. Large summertime influenza A outbreak among tourists in Alaska and the Yukon Territory. Clin Infect Dis. 2003 May 1;36(9):1095–102.
12. Wikswo ME, Cortes J, Hall AJ, Vaughan G, Howard C, Gregoricus N, et al. Disease transmission and passenger behaviors during a high morbidity norovirus outbreak on a cruise ship, January 2009. Clin Infect Dis. 2011 May;52(9):1116–22.
13. World Health Organization. Sanitation on ships: compendium of outbreaks of foodborne and waterborne disease and Legionnaires' diseases associated with ships, 1997–2001. Geneva: World Health Organization; 2001 [cited 2014 Sep 18]. Available from: http://www.who.int/water_sanitation_health/hygiene/ships/en/shipsancomp.pdf?ua=1.

Perspectives

WHAT TO EXPECT WHEN TRAVELING DURING AN INTERNATIONAL OUTBREAK

Todd W. Wilson, Nicole J. Cohen

OVERVIEW

Outbreaks of communicable diseases have occurred throughout history, dramatically shaping the human experience. One of the most recognizable examples of an outbreak with terrible consequences for both human health and culture was the 14th-century plague epidemic, or "Black Death," thought to have been caused by *Yersinia pestis*, which killed up to 60% of Europe's population and also spread to Asia and Africa, possibly reducing the global population by 17%.

In recent times, diseases such as Middle East respiratory syndrome (MERS), Ebola virus disease, and severe acute respiratory syndrome (SARS) have appeared, seemingly from nowhere, and resulted in high numbers of deaths and illness among those infected. And throughout history new strains of influenza have emerged, circled the globe, and caused social disruption and economic upheaval. These diseases and others like them, which emerge, spread rapidly via travel across international borders, and have serious or initially unknown health effects, have led countries to take public health measures at borders that affect travelers.

TRAVELER HEALTH SCREENING IS ALWAYS IN PLACE

When disease threats emerge, countries may take border measures that range from minimal to invasive, regardless of available evidence of the efficacy of those measures. These interventions vary between and within countries and can change rapidly without official notification to the public.

To understand what to expect during an emergency, it is important to know that health screening of travelers is always in place at international ports of entry into most countries. Usually, the form of screening is minimal and routine, since the risk for major health threats is low most of the time. Emergence of a contagious disease with the potential for spread through travel may lead to enhanced screening and the implementation of control measures when potentially infected travelers are identified. Below is a list of public health measures, ranked in order from the least to the most invasive, that may be used internationally to detect or control infection in travelers, depending on the situation:

- Visual screening—observation of travelers for signs of illness, typically without direct interaction with travelers, usually in place at all times

---

Perspectives sections are written as editorial discussions aiming to add depth and clinical perspective to the official recommendations contained in the book. The views and opinions expressed in this section are those of the authors and do not necessarily represent the official position of CDC.

- Health education for travelers—health communications (such as printed material handed to travelers, announcements or posted messages in transit areas, or use of social media or websites) intended to educate international travelers about a particular disease, recommended actions, and border screening measures in place
- Travel warning—a notice published by government health authorities advising people to avoid nonessential travel to an area where a disease outbreak has been identified
- Passenger locator form—a form used by health officials to gather contact information for potentially exposed travelers, for the purpose of locating the travelers for evaluation or to provide information
- Traveler's health declaration form—a form used by customs or health officials at ports of entry to gather information related to a traveler's health, prior itinerary, and exposure to infection
- Direct questioning—interview of travelers by customs or health officials to assess the risk of disease exposure or infection
- Fever screening—measurement of travelers' temperatures, either remotely by using thermal imaging cameras or through use of thermometers
- Detention—holding in custody a traveler suspected of being infected with a communicable disease of concern, to allow further medical evaluation
- Isolation—separating and restricting the movement of an ill person who has a communicable disease of concern from those who are healthy, to minimize disease spread by preventing further transmission
- Quarantine—separating and restricting the movement of people who are well but may have been exposed to a communicable disease, to monitor their health and prevent possible transmission to others, until it is determined that they are not infected

Ultimately, for a given outbreak, the decision on which health measures to use, and how extensively each measure is implemented, will depend on a number of factors, including the transmissibility and severity of the disease in question, local customs, and governmental public health regulations and policies.

WHAT TO EXPECT DURING AN INTERNATIONAL DISEASE OUTBREAK

Whether a person is a first-time or seasoned international traveler, chances are he or she has planned the itinerary carefully to make the trip an enjoyable travel experience. Factoring in some amount of risk and being aware of as many chance variables as possible can help mitigate some of the negative repercussions, should an outbreak of illness occur that impacts travel. The following situations have been observed in nearly all international outbreaks of disease during the modern travel era since the 1960s:

- Travel delays—Travel into, out of, or within certain regions may be affected by border health measures or behavior of travelers.
- Inconsistent information—Early in an outbreak, information may change rapidly, be conflicting, or later be determined to be incorrect, while governments, health officials, and the travel industry work to define the situation and provide reliable information.

- Canceled flights, ship voyages, trains, buses, or routes—Travel cancellations can occur suddenly, especially for air travel, which can be particularly sensitive to shifts in passenger demand and is often unpredictable during outbreaks.
- Voluntary cessation of travel—Travelers may choose to postpone their travel because of official travel warnings, travel advisories, or concerns about their health, border measures, or the possibility of being stranded in a foreign country. Large decreases in travel volume can decrease travel options and disrupt travel schedules, especially to and from the countries most affected by the outbreak.
- Increase in travel—People traveling in affected countries in the early stages of an emerging outbreak may seek unplanned return journeys, as people try to avoid infection or seek health care in their home countries.
- Grounding of flights—In extreme circumstances, flights may be unavailable in a region for a period of time.
- Entry or exit screening—The set of border health measures described earlier in this section may be applied, in whole or in part, at international borders, either to prevent the introduction of infection into the country (entry screening) or to prevent infected people from leaving and spreading infection to other countries (exit screening).

Guidelines and practices for what governments ask of travelers on arrival or exit may differ markedly from country to country. Some countries maintain national control over all ports of entry and exit, while in other countries such control is delegated to state, provincial, or local authorities. In either case, requirements and procedures may differ widely and change over time. Flexibility, honesty, and compliance are essential to a successful interaction with public health and other government officials during international travel.

Below is a list of actions travelers might experience upon arrival in or exit from a country during a communicable disease outbreak. This list is not comprehensive or exhaustive. Travelers may be asked or forced to comply with ≥1 of the following:

- Have their temperatures taken either by thermal imaging camera or thermometer
- Provide personal contact information and details about their travel itineraries
- Respond to questions regarding symptoms of illness or exposure to ill people
- Undergo a medical evaluation for infection, including diagnostic testing
- Be isolated from other people until they are determined to be noncontagious
- Be hospitalized and given medical treatment if they test positive for or are otherwise diagnosed with a communicable disease of public health concern
- Be quarantined for a specified period of time if they were exposed to someone who is suspected or confirmed to be infected
- Monitor their health during and after travel and report any symptoms they develop to health officials
- Forego communications with family, friends, or traveling companions for a certain period
- Be denied boarding on an airplane, ship, bus, or train, if it is determined they are contagious or may have been exposed to a communicable disease of public health concern

RECOMMENDATIONS AND RESOURCES

In the event of an outbreak or epidemic, any country has the right to enact measures to protect its citizens from ill travelers entering its borders or to protect global health from ill travelers exiting the country. These border measures may infringe on the individual rights of travelers. The ability of the US Department of State to intervene in such situations is limited.

Travelers can consult the embassies of the countries in their travel itineraries for information about health interventions and procedures that may affect their travel and for instructions on how to deal with being questioned by host country government officials regarding health or other issues. The Department of State website may be helpful (http://travel.state.gov). Up-to-date information regarding infectious disease risks related to travel may be found at the CDC website (www.cdc.gov/travel). Finally, because of the potential for delays and unexpected costs arising from an outbreak of communicable disease, CDC strongly recommends that travelers consider purchasing travel insurance to cover possible trip cancellations, requirements for health care abroad, or possible emergency medical evacuations (see Chapter 2, Travel Insurance, Travel Health Insurance, & Medical Evacuation Insurance).

BIBLIOGRAPHY

1. Barry JM. Observations on past influenza pandemics. Disaster Med Public Health Prep. 2009 Dec;3 Suppl 2:S95–9.

2. Berro A, Gallagher N, Yanni E, Lipman H, Whatley A, Bossak B. World Health Organization (WHO) travel recommendations during the 2003 SARS outbreak: lessons learned for mitigating influenza pandemic and globally emerging infectious diseases. Board 109. International Conference on Emerging Infectious Diseases; 2009 Mar 16–19; Atlanta, Georgia.

3. CDC. Update: outbreak of severe acute respiratory syndrome—worldwide, 2003. MMWR Morb Mortal Wkly Rep. 2003 Mar 28;52(12):241–6, 248.

4. Chan M. World now at the start of 2009 influenza pandemic. Geneva: World Health Organization; 2009 [cited 2014 Sep 23]. Available from: http://www.who.int/mediacentre/news/statements/2009/h1n1_pandemic_phase6_20090611/en/index.html.

5. Christian MD, Poutanen SM, Loutfy MR, Muller MP, Low DE. Severe acute respiratory syndrome. Clin Infect Dis. 2004 May 15;38(10):1420–7.

6. Hays JN. Epidemics and Pandemics: Their Impacts on Human History. Santa Barbara, CA: ABC-CLIO; 2005.

7. Snowden FM. Emerging and reemerging diseases: a historical perspective. Immunol Rev. 2008 Oct;225:9–26.

8. World Health Organization. International Health Regulations (2005). Geneva: World Health Organization; 2005 [cited 2014 Sep 23]. Available from: http://www.who.int/ihr/publications/9789241596664/en/.

9. World Health Organization. Public health measures taken at international borders during early stages of pandemic influenza A (H1N1) 2009: preliminary results. Wkly Epidemiol Rec. 2010 May 21;85(21):186–95.

DEATH DURING TRAVEL

Clare A. Dykewicz, Nicole J. Cohen

OBTAINING US DEPARTMENT OF STATE ASSISTANCE

When a US citizen dies outside the United States, the deceased person's family members, domestic partner, or legal representative should notify US consular officials at the Department of State. Consular personnel are available 24 hours a day, 7 days a week, to provide assistance to US citizens for overseas emergencies.

- If a family member, domestic partner, or legal representative is in the foreign country with the deceased US citizen, he or she should contact the nearest US embassy or consulate for assistance. Contact information for US embassies, consulates, and consular agencies overseas may be found at the Department of State website (www.usembassy.gov).
- If a family member, domestic partner, or legal representative is located in the United States or Canada, he or she should call the Department of State's Office of Overseas Citizens Services in Washington, DC, from 8 AM to 8 PM Eastern Time, Monday through Friday, at 888-407-4747 (toll-free) or 202-501-4444. For emergency assistance after working hours or on weekends and holidays, call the Department of State switchboard at 202-647-4000 and ask to speak with the Overseas Citizens Services duty officer. In addition, the US embassy closest to or in the country where the US citizen died can provide assistance (www.usembassy.gov).

Emergency services provided by US consular officials can include advising the family, domestic partner, or legal representative about disposing of the remains and personal effects of the deceased. Preparing and returning human remains to the United States can be an expensive and lengthy process. The Department of State does not pay for these expenses; they are the responsibility of the deceased person's family, domestic partner, or legal representative. Consular officials may also serve as provisional conservators of the deceased person's estate, if no other legal representative is present in the foreign country where the death occurred.

IMPORTATION OF HUMAN REMAINS FOR INTERMENT OR CREMATION

General Guidance

Except for cremated remains, human remains intended for interment (placement in a grave or tomb) or cremation after entry into the United States must be accompanied by a death certificate stating the cause of death. A death certificate is an official document signed by a coroner, health care provider, or other official authorized to make a declaration of cause of death. Death certificates written in a language other than English must be accompanied by an English translation.

Remains of a Person Known or Suspected to Have Died from a Quarantinable Communicable Disease

Federal quarantine regulations (42 CFR Part 71.55) state that the remains of a person who is known or suspected to have died from a quarantinable communicable disease may not be brought into the United States unless the remains are cremated, properly embalmed and placed in a hermetically sealed casket, or accompanied by a CDC permit to allow importation of human remains, issued by the CDC director.

Quarantinable communicable diseases include cholera, diphtheria, infectious tuberculosis, plague, smallpox, yellow fever, viral hemorrhagic fevers (Lassa, Marburg, Ebola, Crimean-Congo, or others not yet isolated or named), severe acute respiratory syndrome (SARS), and influenza caused by novel or re-emergent influenza viruses that are causing or have the potential to cause a pandemic. A hermetically sealed casket is one that is airtight and secured against the escape of microorganisms. It should be accompanied by valid documentation certifying that it is hermetically sealed.

If a CDC permit is obtained to allow importation of human remains, CDC may impose additional conditions for importation. Permits for the importation of human remains of a person known or suspected to have died from a quarantinable communicable disease may be obtained from CDC's Division of Global Migration and Quarantine by calling the CDC Emergency Operations Center at 770-488-7100. A copy of the CDC permit must accompany the human remains at all times during shipment.

Remains of a Person Who Died of Any Cause Other than a Quarantinable Communicable Disease

When the cause of death is anything other than a quarantinable communicable disease, the remains may be cleared, released, and authorized for entry into the United States if one of the following conditions is met:

1. The remains meet the standards for importation found in 42 CFR 71.55: the remains are cremated or properly embalmed and placed in a hermetically sealed casket or are accompanied by a permit issued by the CDC director.

2. The remains are shipped in a leakproof container. A leakproof container is one that is puncture resistant and sealed so that there is no leakage of fluids outside the container during handling, storage, transport, or shipping.

CDC may also require additional measures, including detention, disinfection, disinfestation, fumigation, or other related measures, if there is evidence that the human remains are or may be infected or contaminated with a communicable disease and that such measures are necessary to prevent the introduction, transmission, or spread of communicable diseases into the United States.

EXPORTATION OF HUMAN REMAINS

CDC places no restrictions on the exportation of human remains outside the United States, although other state and local regulations may apply. Exporters of human remains and travelers taking human remains out of the United States should be aware that the importation requirements of the destination country and the air carrier must be met. Information regarding these requirements may be obtained from the appropriate foreign embassy or consulate (www.state/gov/s/cpr/rls/fco/index.htm) and the air carrier.

BIBLIOGRAPHY

1. CDC. Guidance for importation of human remains into the United States for interment or subsequent cremation. Atlanta: CDC; 2014 [cited 2014 Sep 23]. Available from: http://www.cdc.gov/quarantine/human-remains.html.

2. CDC. Quarantine station contact list, map, and fact sheets. Atlanta: CDC; 2013 [cited 2014 Sep 23]. Available from: http://www.cdc.gov/quarantine/quarantinestationcontactlistfull.html.

3. CDC. Specific laws and regulations governing the control of communicable diseases. Atlanta: CDC; 2014 [cited 2014 Sep 23]. Available from: http://www.cdc.gov/quarantine/SpecificLawsRegulations.html.

4. National Funeral Directors Association. Shipping remains from the United States to a foreign country. Brookfield, WI: National Funeral Directors Association; c2014 [cited 2014 Sep 23]. Available from: http://nfda.org/additional-tools-shipping/2257-shipping-remains-from-the%20united-states%20to%20a%20foreign-country.html.

5. US Customs and Border Protection. Requirements for importing bodies in coffins/ashes in urns. Washington, DC: US Department of Homeland Security; 2013 [cited 2014 Sep 23]. Available from: https://help.cbp.gov/app/answers/detail/a_id/237/kw/importation%20of%20human%20remains.

6. US Department of State. Death abroad. Washington, DC: US Department of State; 2014 [cited 2014 Sep 23]. Available from: http://travel.state.gov/content/passports/english/abroad/events-and-records/death.html.

7. US Department of State. Return of remains of deceased US citizens. Washington, DC: US Department of State; 2014 [cited 2014 Sep 23]. Available from: http://travel.state.gov/content/passports/english/abroad/events-and-records/death/return-remains.html.

TAKING ANIMALS & ANIMAL PRODUCTS ACROSS INTERNATIONAL BORDERS

G. Gale Galland, Robert J. Mullan, Heather Bair-Brake

CDC restricts the importation of animals and animal products that might pose an infectious disease threat to humans. Any animal or animal product can be restricted from entry if there is reasonable knowledge or suspicion that it poses a human health risk. However, CDC has explicit restrictions for specific animals such as dogs, cats, turtles, nonhuman primates, African rodents, civets, and bats, as well as products made from them. Importers must meet stringent requirements in order to import these animals and items into the United States. Many of these animals are also regulated by other federal agencies or by individual state governments. Travelers should check with the US Department of Agriculture (USDA), the US Fish and Wildlife Service (FWS), and their destination state for specific rules about importation. Importers should research applicable requirements as soon as they know they will be importing an animal or animal product into the United States. Veterinary exams or certifications, vaccinations, or permits may be needed.

It is important to know that animals taken out of the United States are subject, upon their return, to the same regulations as those entering for the first time.

ANIMAL HEALTH CERTIFICATES

CDC regulations do not require general health certificates for animals entering the United States. However, some states may require health certificates for entry, and some airlines may require these certificates for transport. Before departure, travelers should check with the departments of health and of agriculture in their destination states and with the airline for any certificate requirements. The department of environmental protection or department of natural resources of some states

and local governments may have additional requirements.

INTERNATIONAL PET RESCUE AND ADOPTION

Although done with the best of intentions, rescuing and importing stray animals from foreign countries can create human health risks. Travelers are at an increased risk for possible bites and scratches among fearful and stressed animals, which may result in injury or exposure to infectious disease. Animals that are infected with zoonotic diseases might not show any outward signs of being ill. Therefore, all rescued animals should be examined by a licensed veterinarian both before departure and after arrival in the United States. If the intent of travel is to rescue animals, participants should discuss rabies preexposure prophylaxis with their health care providers.

IMPORTATION OF LIVE ANIMALS
Dogs

Dogs are subject to inspection upon entry into the United States if they have evidence of being infected with a communicable disease or if they have not been vaccinated against rabies. If a dog appears to be ill, further examination by a licensed veterinarian may be required before entry is permitted. If necessary, this examination will be at the owner's expense.

Rabies vaccination is required for all dogs entering the United States from a country where rabies is present. Dogs must be accompanied by a current, valid rabies vaccination certificate that includes the following information:

- Name and address of owner
- Breed, sex, age, color, markings, and other identifying information for the dog
- Date of rabies vaccination and vaccine product information

- Date of expiration of vaccination
- Name, license number, address, and signature of veterinarian
- Rabies certificates have expiration dates that range from 1 to 3 years from the date of vaccination, depending on the type of vaccine given. All dogs must be >3 months of age before receiving their first rabies vaccination. Rabies vaccinations must occur at least 30 days before the date of arrival, as it takes 30 days for these vaccines to be fully effective.
- Routine rabies vaccination of dogs is recommended in the United States and required by most state and local health authorities in the United States. Check with state authorities at the final destination to determine any state requirements for rabies vaccination. State-specific information is found at http://www.aphis.usda.gov/wps/portal/aphis/ourfocus/animalhealth/sa_import_into_us/sa_entry_requirements/ct_us%20state_and_territory_animal_import_regulations/.
- Under certain limited circumstances, CDC may allow exceptions to the standard importation requirements as outlined. For further information, see www.cdc.gov/animalimportation/dogs.html. People seeking to import dogs that do not meet CDC's requirements should contact CDC in advance at CDCAnimalImports@cdc.gov to discuss their particular situation.

Cats

Cats are subject to inspection at US ports of entry and may be denied entry into the United States if they have evidence of being infected with a communicable disease. If a cat appears to be ill, further examination by a licensed veterinarian may be required before entry is permitted. This examination, if necessary, is conducted at the owner's expense. CDC does not require cats to have proof of rabies vaccination for importation into the United States. However, many states have rabies vaccination requirements for cats. Check with state and local health authorities at the final destination to determine any state requirements for rabies vaccination of cats. For more information about importing cats, see www.cdc.gov/animalimportation/cats.html.

All dogs and cats arriving in the state of Hawaii and the territory of Guam, even from the US mainland, are subject to locally imposed quarantine requirements. This requirement also applies to dogs and cats from the US mainland. For more information about animal importation in Hawaii, consult http://hdoa.hawaii.gov/ or call 808-483-7151. For more information about animal importation in Guam, see www.guamcourts.org/CompilerofLaws/GAR/09GAR/09GAR001-1.pdf.

Nonhuman Primates

Nonhuman primates can transmit a variety of serious diseases to humans, including Ebola virus disease and tuberculosis. Nonhuman primates may only be imported into the United States by a CDC-registered importer and only for scientific, educational, or exhibition purposes. All nonhuman primates are considered endangered or threatened and require additional FWS permits for importation. Nonhuman primates that leave the United States may only return through a registered importer and only for the purpose of science, education, or exhibition. Nonhuman primates may not be imported as pets. Nonhuman primates that are kept as pets in the United States and travel outside of the United States will not be allowed to reenter the United States as pets. For more information on CDC's importation requirements, see www.cdc.gov/animalimportation/monkeys.html.

Turtles

Although often kept as pets, turtles can transmit *Salmonella* to humans. For this reason, CDC restricts the importation of some turtles. A person may import up to 6 viable turtle eggs or live turtles with a shell length of <4 in (10 cm) for noncommercial purposes. More live turtles or viable turtle eggs may be imported with CDC permission but only for science, education, or exhibition. CDC does not restrict the importation of live turtles with a shell length >4 inches. Check with USDA or FWS regarding additional requirements to import turtles. More information is available at www.cdc.gov/animalimportation/turtles.html.

African Rodents

African rodents are a known source of communicable diseases, such as monkeypox. Thus, CDC does not allow the importation of these animals. Exceptions may be made for animals imported for science, education, or exhibition purposes, with permission from CDC. Check with USDA or FWS regarding additional requirements to import African rodents. For additional information, see www.cdc.gov/animalimportation/africanrodents.html.

Civets and Related Animals

To reduce the risk of introducing the severe acute respiratory syndrome (SARS) coronavirus, civets and related animals (family Viverridae) may not be imported into the United States. Exceptions may be made for animals imported for science, education, or exhibition purposes, with permission from CDC. Check with USDA or FWS regarding additional requirements to import civets and related animals. For more information, see www.cdc.gov/animalimportation/civets.html.

Bats and Other Vectors

Bats are reservoirs of many viruses that can infect humans, including rabies virus, Nipah virus, and SARS coronavirus. To reduce the risk of introducing these viruses, the importation of all live bats requires a CDC permit. Many bats require additional permits issued by FWS. The application for a CDC import permit for bats can be found at www.cdc.gov/animalimportation/bats.html.

In some circumstances, known vectors of human disease such as ticks or mosquitoes may be imported into the United States with a permit from CDC for science, education, or exhibition. For additional information, see www.cdc.gov/od/eaipp.

Other Animals

Travelers planning to import horses, ruminants, swine, poultry or other birds, or dogs used for handling livestock should contact National Import Export Services, a part of USDA's Animal Plant Health Inspection Service, at 301-851-3300 or visit www.aphis.usda.gov to learn about additional requirements.

Travelers planning to import fish, reptiles, spiders, wild birds, rabbits, bears, wild members of the cat family, or other wild or endangered animals should contact FWS at 800-344-9453 (toll-free general number), 703-358-1949 (FWS Office of Law Enforcement), or visit www.fws.gov/le/travelers.html.

IMPORTATION OF ANIMAL PRODUCTS

Trophies and Animal Products

Travelers often want to import animal skins, hunting trophies, or other items made from animals when returning from a trip. Many of these items must either be rendered noninfectious (see www.cdc.gov/animalimportation/animalproducts.html) or be accompanied by an import permit. CDC restricts products made from nonhuman primates, African rodents, civets, and bats. These products may also be regulated by other US federal agencies. CDC has the right to restrict other items known to carry infectious diseases. For example, CDC restricts goatskin souvenirs, such as goatskin drums, from entry into the United States because they have been associated with cases of anthrax in humans. Travelers who want to import hunting trophies or other products made from animals should check with CDC, USDA, and FWS to make sure they are complying with federal regulations.

Bushmeat

Animal products may also include items intended for human consumption. Bushmeat, for example, is an animal product that is an important aspect of West and Central African culture. This product, generally raw, smoked, or partially processed meat from wild animals, might harbor infectious and zoonotic agents that can cause human and animal disease. Bushmeat has been linked to deadly diseases like HIV/AIDS and Ebola. Recent studies have found evidence of simian foamy viruses, which are known to cause infections in humans but have not been associated with human disease. As people migrate around the world, bushmeat has become a growing commodity in the global wildlife trade. CDC prohibits the importation of bushmeat into the United States from CDC-restricted species. Bushmeat importation may also be restricted under USDA or FWS regulations. In addition to the human and animal health risks, many of the wild animals commonly hunted for bushmeat are threatened or endangered species protected

6

by international wildlife laws and treaties such as the Convention on International Trade of Endangered Species (CITES).

TRAVELING ABROAD WITH A PET

Travelers planning to take a companion animal to a foreign country should be advised to meet the entry requirements of the destination country and transportation guidelines of the airline. To obtain this information, travelers should contact the country's embassy in Washington, DC or the nearest consulate (see www.state.gov/s/cpr/rls/fco). Travelers should be aware that long flights can be hard on pets, particularly older animals with chronic health conditions. Additionally, upon reentering the United States, US pets that traveled abroad are subject to the same import requirements as animals that have never lived in the United States.

For additional information about importing animals and animal products into the United States and for permit applications, travelers should visit www.cdc.gov/animalimportation/index.html or contact 1-800-CDC INFO (1-800-232-4636). To request CDC permission to import a CDC-regulated animal or product, send a message to CDCAnimalImports@cdc.gov.

BIBLIOGRAPHY

1. Bair-Brake H, Bell T, Higgins A, Bailey N, Duda M, Shapiro S, et al. Is that a rodent in your luggage? A mixed method approach to describe bushmeat importation into the United States. Zoonoses Public Health. 2014 Mar;61(2):97–104.
2. CDC. Multistate outbreak of monkeypox—Illinois, Indiana, and Wisconsin, 2003. MMWR Morb Mortal Wkly Rep. 2003 Jun 13;52(23):537–40.
3. CDC. Rabies in a dog imported from Iraq—New Jersey, June 2008. MMWR Morb Mortal Wkly Rep. 2008 Oct 3;57(39):1076–8.
4. DeMarcus TA, Tipple MA, Ostrowski SR. US policy for disease control among imported nonhuman primates. J Infect Dis. 1999 Feb;179 Suppl 1:S281–2.
5. Dobson AP. What links bats to emerging infectious diseases? Science. 2005 Oct 28;310(5748):628–9.
6. Editorial: bongo-drum disease. Lancet. 1974 Jun 8;1(7867):1152.
7. McQuiston JH, Wilson T, Harris S, Bacon RM, Shapiro S, Trevino I, et al. Importation of dogs into the United States: risks from rabies and other zoonotic diseases. Zoonoses Public Health. 2008 Oct;55(8–10):421–6.
8. National Association of State Public Health Veterinarians, Inc. Compendium of animal rabies prevention and control, 2009. MMWR Recomm Rep. 2009;58(RR-1):1–15.
9. Stam F, Romkens TE, Hekker TA, Smulders YM. Turtle-associated human salmonellosis. Clin Infect Dis. 2003 Dec 1;37(11):e167–9.
10. Wu D, Tu C, Xin C, Xuan H, Meng Q, Liu Y, et al. Civets are equally susceptible to experimental infection by two different severe acute respiratory syndrome coronavirus isolates. J Virol. 2005 Feb;79(4):2620–5.

International Travel with Infants & Children

TRAVELING SAFELY WITH INFANTS & CHILDREN

Nicholas Weinberg, Michelle S. Weinberg, Susan A. Maloney

OVERVIEW

The number of children who travel or live outside their home countries has increased dramatically. In 2010, an estimated 2.2 million US resident children aged ≤18 years traveled internationally. Although data about the incidence of pediatric illnesses associated with international travel are limited, the risks that children face while traveling are likely similar to those their parents face. However, children are less likely to receive pre-travel advice. In a review of children with post-travel illnesses seen at clinics in the GeoSentinel Surveillance Network, only 51% of all children and 32% of the children visiting friends and relatives (VFRs) had received pre-travel medical advice, compared with 59% of adults. The most commonly reported health problems among child travelers are as follows:

- Diarrheal illnesses
- Dermatologic conditions, including animal and arthropod bites, cutaneous larva migrans, and sunburn
- Systemic febrile illnesses, especially malaria
- Respiratory disorders

Motor vehicle and water-related injuries are also major health problems for child travelers. In assessing a child who is planning international travel, clinicians should

- Review routine childhood and travel-related vaccinations. The pre-travel visit is an opportunity to ensure that children are up-to-date on routine vaccinations.
- Assess all anticipated travel-related activities.
- Provide preventive counseling and interventions tailored to specific risks, including special travel preparations and treatment that may be required for infants and children with underlying conditions, chronic diseases, or immunocompromising conditions. Older adolescents traveling in a student group or program may require counseling about disease prevention and the risks of sexually transmitted infections, empiric treatment and management of common travel-related illnesses, sexual assault, and drug and alcohol use during international travel (see Chapter 8, Study Abroad & Other International Student Travel).

- Give special consideration to the risks of children who are VFR travelers in developing countries. Conditions may include increased risk of malaria, intestinal parasites, and tuberculosis.
- Consider counseling adults and older children to take a course in basic first aid before travel.

DIARRHEA

Diarrhea and associated gastrointestinal illness are among the most common travel-related problems affecting children. Infants and children with diarrhea can become dehydrated more quickly than adults. The etiology of travelers' diarrhea (TD) in children is similar to that in adults (see Chapter 2, Travelers' Diarrhea).

Prevention

For infants, breastfeeding is the best way to reduce the risk of foodborne and waterborne illness. Infant formulas available abroad may not be the same as in the United States; parents feeding their child formula should consider whether they need to bring formula from home.

Water served to young children, including water used to prepare infant formula, should be disinfected (see Chapter 2, Water Disinfection for Travelers). In some parts of the world, bottled water may also be contaminated and should be disinfected before consumption.

Similarly, food precautions should be followed diligently. Foods served to children should be thoroughly cooked and eaten while still hot; fruits eaten raw should be peeled by the caregiver immediately before consumption. Additionally, caution should be used with fresh dairy products, which may not be pasteurized and may be diluted with untreated water. For short trips, parents may want to bring a supply of safe snacks from home for times when the children are hungry and the available food may not be appealing or safe. See Chapter 2, Food & Water Precautions for more information.

Scrupulous attention should be paid to handwashing and cleaning bottles, pacifiers, teething rings, and toys that fall to the floor or are handled by others; water used to clean these items should be potable. Parents should be particularly careful to wash hands well after diaper changes, especially for infants with diarrhea, to avoid spreading infection to themselves and other family members. When proper handwashing facilities are not available, an alcohol-based hand sanitizer (containing ≥60% alcohol) can be used as a disinfecting agent. However, because alcohol-based hand sanitizers are not effective against certain pathogens, hands should be washed with soap and water as soon as possible. Additionally, alcohol does not remove organic material; visibly soiled hands should be washed with soap and water.

Chemoprophylaxis with antibiotics is not generally used in children.

Treatment
Antiemetics and Antimotility Drugs

Because of potential side effects, antiemetics are generally not recommended for self- or family-administered treatment of children with vomiting and TD. Because of the association between salicylates and Reye syndrome, bismuth subsalicylate (BSS), the active ingredient in both Pepto-Bismol and Kaopectate, is not generally recommended to treat diarrhea in children aged <12 years. However, some clinicians use it off-label with caution in certain circumstances. Caution should be taken in administering BSS to children with viral infections, such as varicella or influenza, because of the risk for Reye syndrome. BSS is not recommended for children aged <3 years. A recent Cochrane Collaboration Review of the use of antiemetics for reducing vomiting related to acute gastroenteritis in children and adolescents showed some benefits with ondansetron, metoclopramide, or dimenhydrinate. However, the routine use of these medications for emesis associated with TD has not yet been determined and is not generally recommended.

Antimotility drugs, such as loperamide and diphenoxylate, are rarely given to small children. Loperamide is not recommended for children aged <6 years. Diphenoxylate and atropine combination tablets are not recommended for children aged <2 years. These drugs should be used with caution in children because of potential side effects (See Chapter 2, Travelers' Diarrhea).

Antibiotics

Few data are available regarding empiric treatment of TD in children. The antimicrobial options for empiric treatment of TD in children are limited. In practice, when an antibiotic is indicated for moderate to severe diarrhea, some clinicians prescribe azithromycin as a single daily dose (10 mg/kg) for 3 days. Clinicians can prescribe unreconstituted azithromycin powder before travel, with instructions from the pharmacist for mixing it into an oral suspension if it becomes necessary to use it. Although resistance breakpoints have not yet been determined, elevated minimum inhibitory concentrations for azithromycin have been reported for some gastrointestinal pathogens. Therefore, parents should be counseled to seek medical attention for their children if they do not improve after empiric treatment. Clinicians should review possible contraindications, such as QT prolongation and cardiac arrhythmias with azithromycin, before prescribing medications for empiric treatment of TD.

Although fluoroquinolones are frequently used for the empiric treatment of TD in adults, they are not approved by the Food and Drug Administration for this purpose among children aged <18 years because of cartilage damage seen in animal studies. The American Academy of Pediatrics suggests that fluoroquinolones be considered for the treatment of children with severe infections caused by multidrug-resistant strains of *Shigella* species, *Salmonella* species, *Vibrio cholerae*, or *Campylobacter jejuni*. Clinicians should be aware that fluoroquinolone resistance in gastrointestinal organisms has been reported from some countries, particularly in Southeast Asia. Routine use of fluoroquinolones for chemoprophylaxis or empiric treatment for TD among children is not recommended.

Management

The biggest threat to the infant with diarrhea and vomiting is dehydration. Fever or increased ambient temperature increases fluid loss and speeds dehydration. Adults traveling with children should be counseled about the signs and symptoms of dehydration and the proper use of oral rehydration salts (ORS). Medical attention may be required for an infant or young child with diarrhea who has

- Signs of moderate to severe dehydration
- Bloody diarrhea
- Temperature >101.5°F (38.6°C)
- Persistent vomiting (unable to maintain oral hydration)

The mainstay of management of TD is adequate hydration.

ORS Use and Availability

Parents should be advised that dehydration is best prevented and treated by use of ORS, in addition to the infant's usual food. ORS should be provided to the infant by bottle, cup, oral syringe (often available in pharmacies), or spoon while medical attention is obtained. Low-osmolarity ORS is the most effective in preventing dehydration, although other formulations are available and may be used if they are more acceptable to young children. Homemade sugar-salt solutions are not recommended. Adults traveling with children should be counseled that sports drinks, which are designed to replace water and electrolytes lost through sweat, do not contain the same proportions of electrolytes as the solution recommended by the World Health Organization for rehydration during diarrheal illness. However, if ORS is not readily available, children should be offered whatever safe, palatable liquid they will take until ORS is obtained.

ORS packets are available at stores or pharmacies in almost all developing countries. ORS is prepared by adding 1 packet to boiled or treated water (see Chapter 2, Water Disinfection for Travelers). Travelers should be advised to check packet instructions carefully to ensure that the salts are added to the correct volume of water. ORS solution should be consumed or discarded within 12 hours if held at room temperature or 24 hours if kept refrigerated.

A dehydrated child will usually drink ORS avidly; travelers should be advised to give it to the child as long as the dehydration persists. As dehydration lessens, the child may refuse the salty-tasting ORS solution, and another safe liquid can be offered. An infant or child who has been vomiting will usually keep ORS down if it is offered by spoon or oral syringe in small sips; these

7

small amounts must be offered frequently, however, so the child can receive an adequate volume of ORS. Older children will often drink well by sipping through a straw. Severely dehydrated children, however, often will be unable to drink adequately. Severe dehydration is a medical emergency that usually requires administration of fluids by intravenous or intraosseous routes.

In general, children weighing <22 lb (10 kg) who have mild to moderate dehydration should be administered 2–4 oz (60–120 mL) ORS for each diarrheal stool or vomiting episode. Children who weigh ≥22 lb (10 kg) should receive 4–8 oz (120–240 mL) of ORS for each diarrheal stool or vomiting episode. The American Academy of Pediatrics provides detailed guidance on rehydration for vomiting and diarrhea; see "Care Advice" at www.healthychildren.org/English/tips-tools/Symptom-Checker/Pages/Vomiting-With-Diarrhea.aspx.

ORS packets are available in the United States from Jianas Brothers Packaging Company (816-421-2880; http://rehydrate.org/resources/jianas.htm). ORS packets may also be available at stores that sell outdoor recreation and camping supplies. In addition, Cera Products (843-842-2600 or 888-237-2598; www.ceraproductsinc.com) markets a rice-based, rather than glucose-based, product.

Dietary Modification

Breastfed infants should continue nursing on demand. Formula-fed infants should continue their usual formula during rehydration. They should receive a volume that is sufficient to satisfy energy and nutrient requirements. Lactose-free or lactose-reduced formulas are usually unnecessary. Diluting formula may slow resolution of diarrhea and is not recommended. Older infants and children receiving semisolid or solid foods should continue to receive their usual diet during the illness. Recommended foods include starches, cereals, pasteurized yogurt, fruits, and vegetables, following safe food selection guidelines. Foods that are high in simple sugars, such as soft drinks, undiluted apple juice, gelatins, and presweetened cereals, can exacerbate diarrhea by osmotic effects and should be avoided. In addition, foods high in fat may not be tolerated because of their tendency to delay gastric emptying.

The practice of withholding food for ≥24 hours is not recommended. Early feeding can decrease changes in intestinal permeability caused by infection, reduce illness duration, and improve nutritional outcome. Highly specific diets (such as the BRAT [bananas, rice, applesauce, and toast] diet) have been commonly recommended; however, similar to juice-based and clear fluid diets, such severely restrictive diets have no scientific basis and should be avoided.

MALARIA

Malaria is among the most serious and life-threatening diseases that can be acquired by pediatric international travelers. Pediatric VFR travelers are at particularly high risk for acquiring malaria if they do not receive chemoprophylaxis.

Children with malaria can rapidly develop high levels of parasitemia. They are at increased risk for severe complications of malaria, including shock, seizures, coma, and death. Initial symptoms of malaria in children may mimic many other common causes of pediatric febrile illness and therefore may result in delayed diagnosis and treatment. Clinicians should counsel adults traveling with children in malaria-endemic areas to use preventive measures, be aware of the signs and symptoms of malaria, and seek prompt medical attention if they develop.

Antimalarial Drugs

Pediatric doses for malaria chemoprophylaxis are provided in Table 3-10. All dosing should be calculated on the basis of body weight. Medications used for infants and young children are the same as those recommended for adults, except under the following circumstances:

- Doxycycline should not be given to children aged <8 years because of the risk of teeth staining.
- Atovaquone-proguanil should not be used for prophylaxis in children weighing <11 lb (<5 kg) because of lack of data on safety and efficacy.

Chloroquine, mefloquine, and atovaquone-proguanil have a bitter taste. Before departure, pharmacists can be asked to pulverize tablets and prepare gelatin capsules with calculated pediatric doses. Mixing the powder in a small amount of food or drink can facilitate the administration of antimalarial drugs to infants and children. Additionally, any compounding pharmacy can alter the flavoring of malaria medication tablets so that children are more willing to take them. Assistance with finding a compounding pharmacy is available on the International Academy of Compounding Pharmacists' website (www.iacprx.org). Because overdose of antimalarial drugs, particularly chloroquine, can be fatal, medication should be stored in childproof containers and kept out of the reach of infants and children.

Personal Protection Measures

Children should sleep in rooms with air conditioning or screened windows or sleep under bed nets, when available. Mosquito netting should be used over infant carriers. Children can reduce skin exposed to mosquitoes by wearing long pants and long sleeves while outdoors in areas where malaria is transmitted. Clothing and mosquito nets can be treated with insect repellents such as permethrin, a repellent and insecticide that repels and kills ticks, mosquitoes, and other arthropods. Permethrin remains effective through multiple washings. Clothing and bed nets should be retreated according to the product label. Permethrin should not be applied to the skin. Although permethrin provides longer duration protection, recommended repellents that can be applied to skin (DEET [N,N-diethyl-m-toluamide], picaridin, oil of lemon eucalyptus [OLE] or PMD [para-menthane-3,8-diol], and IR3535) can also be used on clothing and mosquito nets. See Chapter 2, Protection against Mosquitoes, Ticks, & Other Arthropods for more details about these protective measures.

Repellent Use

CDC recommends the use of repellents containing one of the following active ingredients, which are registered with the US Environmental Protection Agency, according to the product labels: DEET, picaridin, OLE or PMD, and IR3535 (http://cfpub.epa.gov/oppref/insect/). Most repellents can be used on children aged >2 months, with the following considerations:

- Products containing OLE specify that they should not be used on children aged <3 years.
- Repellent products must state any age restriction. If none is stated, the Environmental Protection Agency has not required a restriction on the use of the product.
- Many repellents contain DEET as the active ingredient. The concentration of DEET varies considerably among products. The duration of protection varies with the DEET concentration: higher concentrations protect longer. Products with DEET concentration above 50% do not offer a marked increase in protection time. The American Academy of Pediatrics recommends that
  > ≤30% DEET should be used on children aged >2 months.
  > Repellents with DEET should not be used on infants aged <2 months.

Repellents can be applied to exposed skin and clothing; however, they should not be applied under clothing. Repellents should never be used over cuts, wounds, or irritated skin. Young children should not be allowed to handle the product. When using repellent on a child, an adult should apply it to his or her own hands and then rub them on the child, with the following considerations:

- Avoid the child's eyes and mouth, and apply sparingly around the ears.
- Do not apply repellent to children's hands, since children tend to put their hands in their mouths.
- Heavy application and saturation are generally unnecessary for effectiveness. If biting insects do not respond to a thin film of repellent, then apply a bit more.
- After returning indoors, wash treated skin with soap and water or bathe. This is particularly important when repellents are used repeatedly in a day or on consecutive days.

Products that contain both repellents and sunscreen are generally not recommended, because instructions for use are different and the need to reapply sunscreen is usually more frequent than with repellent alone. In general, apply sunscreen first, and then apply repellent.

Mosquito coils should be used with caution in the presence of children to avoid burns and inadvertent ingestion. For more information about repellent use and other protective measures, see Chapter 2, Protection against Mosquitoes, Ticks, & Other Arthropods.

DENGUE AND OTHER ARBOVIRUSES

Pediatric VFR travelers who may have frequent and prolonged travel may have risk similar to children living in areas where dengue or other arboviruses (such as chikungunya, Japanese encephalitis, yellow fever, or Zika viruses) are endemic. Among 8 children who were diagnosed with acute dengue infection after visiting friends and relatives in the Caribbean, 3 developed either dengue hemorrhagic fever or dengue shock syndrome. Children traveling to areas with dengue or other arboviruses should use the same mosquito protection measures described for malaria. However, families should be counseled that, unlike the mosquitoes that transmit malaria, the *Aedes* mosquitoes that transmit dengue, chikungunya, yellow fever, and Zika bite during the daytime. Clinicians should consider dengue or other arboviral infections in children with fever if they have recently been in an endemic area. For more information about these diseases, see their respective sections in Chapter 3.

INFECTION AND INFESTATION FROM SOIL CONTACT

Children are more likely than adults to have contact with soil or sand, and, therefore, they may be exposed to diseases caused by infectious stages of parasites present in soil, including ascariasis, hookworm infestation, cutaneous or visceral larva migrans, trichuriasis, and strongyloidiasis. Children and infants should wear protective footwear and play on a sheet or towel rather than directly on the ground. Clothing should not be dried on the ground. In countries with a tropical climate, clothing or diapers dried in the open air should be ironed before use to prevent infestation with fly larvae.

ANIMAL BITES AND RABIES

Worldwide, rabies is more common in children than adults. In addition to the potential for increased contact with animals, children are also more likely to be bitten on the head or neck, leading to more severe injuries. Children and their families should be counseled to avoid all stray or unfamiliar animals and to inform adults of any contact or bites. Bats throughout the world are considered to have the potential to transmit rabies virus. Mammal-associated injuries should be washed thoroughly with water and soap (and povidone iodine if available), and the child should be evaluated promptly to assess the need for rabies postexposure prophylaxis. Because rabies vaccine and rabies immune globulin may not be available in certain destinations, families should seriously consider purchasing medical evacuation insurance.

AIR TRAVEL

Although air travel is safe for healthy newborns, infants, and children, a few issues should be considered in preparation for travel. Children with chronic heart or lung problems may be at risk for hypoxia during flight, and a clinician should be consulted before travel. Making sure that children can be safely restrained during a flight is a safety consideration. Severe turbulence or crash can create enough momentum that a parent cannot hold onto a child:

- Children should be placed in a rear-facing Federal Aviation Authority–approved child-safety seat until they are aged ≥1 year and weigh ≥20 lb.
- Children aged ≥1 year and 20–40 lb should use a forward-facing Federal Aviation Authority–approved child-safety seat.
- Children who weigh >40 lb can be secured in the aircraft seat belt.

Ear pain can be troublesome for infants and children during descent. Pressure in the middle ear can be equalized by swallowing or chewing:

- Infants should nurse or suck on a bottle.
- Older children can try chewing gum.
- Antihistamines and decongestants have not been shown to be of benefit.

There is no evidence that air travel exacerbates the symptoms or complications associated with otitis media. Travel to different time zones, jet lag, and schedule disruptions can disturb sleep patterns in infants and children, as well as adults (Chapter 2, Jet Lag).

INJURIES
Vehicle-Related
Vehicle-related injuries are the leading cause of death in children who travel. While traveling in automobiles and other vehicles, children weighing ≤40 lb should be restrained in age-appropriate car seats or booster seats, as described above. These seats often must be carried from home, since availability of well-maintained and approved seats may be limited abroad. In general, children are safest traveling in the rear seat; no one should ever travel in the bed of a pickup truck. Families should be counseled that in many developing countries, cars may lack front or rear seatbelts. They should attempt to arrange transportation in vehicles or rent vehicles with seatbelts and other safety features.

Drowning and Water-Related Illness and Injuries
Drowning is the second leading cause of death in young travelers. Children may not be familiar with hazards in the ocean or in rivers. Swimming pools may not have protective fencing to keep toddlers from falling into the pool. Close supervision of children around water is essential. Water safety devices such as life vests may not be available abroad, and families should consider bringing these from home. Protective footwear is important to avoid injury in many marine environments. Schistosomiasis is a risk to children and adults in endemic areas. While in schistosomiasis-endemic areas (Map 3-12), children should not swim in fresh, unchlorinated water such as lakes or ponds.

Accommodations
Conditions at hotels and other lodging may not be as safe as those in the United States, and accommodations should be carefully inspected for exposed wiring, pest poisons, paint chips, or inadequate stairway or balcony railings.

ALTITUDE
Children are as susceptible to altitude illness as adults. Young children who cannot talk can show nonspecific symptoms, such as loss of appetite and irritability. They may have unexplained fussiness and change in sleep and activity patterns. Older children may complain of headache or shortness of breath. If children demonstrate unexplained symptoms after an ascent, it may be necessary to descend to see if they improve. Acetazolamide is not approved for pediatric use for altitude illness, but it is generally safe in children when used for other indications.

SUN EXPOSURE
Sun exposure, and particularly sunburn before age 15 years, is strongly associated with melanoma and other forms of skin cancer (see Chapter 2, Sun Exposure). Exposure to UV light is highest near the equator, at high altitudes, during midday (10 AM–4 PM), and where light is reflected off water or snow. Sunscreens are generally recommended for use in children aged >6 months. Sunscreens (or sun blocks), either physical (such as titanium or zinc oxides) or chemical (sun protection factor [SPF] ≥15 and providing protection from both UVA and UVB), should be applied as directed and reapplied, as needed, after sweating and water exposure. Babies aged <6 months require extra protection from the sun because of their thinner and more sensitive skin; severe sunburn for this age group is considered a medical emergency. Babies should be kept in the shade and wear clothing that covers the entire body. A minimal amount of sunscreen can be applied to small exposed areas, including the infant's face and hands.

Sun-blocking shirts are available that are made for swimming and preclude having to rub sunscreen over the entire trunk. Hats and sunglasses also reduce sun injury to skin and eyes. If both sunscreen and a DEET-containing insect repellent are applied, the SPF of the sunscreen may be diminished by one-third, and covering clothing should be worn or time in the sun decreased accordingly.

OTHER GENERAL CONSIDERATIONS
Travel Stress
Changes in schedule, activities, and environment can be stressful for children. Including children in planning for the trip and

7

bringing along familiar toys or other objects can decrease these stresses. For children with chronic illnesses, decisions regarding timing and itinerary should be made in consultation with the child's health care providers.

Insurance

As for any traveler, insurance coverage for illnesses and injuries while abroad should be verified before departure. Consideration should be given to purchasing special medical evacuation insurance for airlifting or air ambulance to an area with adequate medical care (see Chapter 2, Travel Insurance, Travel Health Insurance, & Medical Evacuation Insurance).

Identification

In case family members become separated, each infant or child should carry identifying information and contact numbers in his or her own clothing or pockets. Because of concerns about illegal transport of children across international borders, if only 1 parent is traveling with the child, he or she may need to carry relevant custody papers or a notarized permission letter from the other parent.

BIBLIOGRAPHY

1. Bradley JS, Jackson MA, Committee on Infectious Diseases. The use of systemic and topical fluoroquinolones. Pediatrics. 2011 Oct;128(4):e1034–45.
2. DuPont HL, Ericsson CD, Farthing MJ, Gorbach S, Pickering LK, Rombo L, et al. Expert review of the evidence base for prevention of travelers' diarrhea. J Travel Med. 2009 May–Jun;16(3):149–60.
3. Fedorowicz Z, Jagannath VA, Carter B. Antiemetics for reducing vomiting related to acute gastroenteritis in children and adolescents. Cochrane Database Syst Rev. 2011(9):1–71.
4. Hagmann S, Neugebauer R, Schwartz E, Perret C, Castelli F, Barnett ED, et al. Illness in children after international travel: analysis from the GeoSentinel Surveillance Network. Pediatrics. 2010 May;125(5):e1072–80.
5. Han P, Balaban V, Marano C. Travel characteristics and risk-taking attitudes in youths traveling to nonindustrialized countries. J Travel Med. 2010 Sep–Oct;17(5):316–21.
6. Herbinger KH, Drerup L, Alberer M, Nothdurft HD, Sonnenburg F, Loscher T. Spectrum of imported infectious diseases among children and adolescents returning from the tropics and subtropics. J Travel Med. 2012 May–Jun;19(3):150–7.
7. Hunziker T, Berger C, Staubli G, Tschopp A, Weber R, Nadal D, et al. Profile of travel-associated illness in children, Zurich, Switzerland. J Travel Med. 2012 May–Jun;19(3):158–62.
8. Kamimura-Nishimura K, Rudikoff D, Purswani M, Hagmann S. Dermatological conditions in international pediatric travelers: epidemiology, prevention and management. Travel Med Infect Dis. 2013 Nov–Dec;11(6):350–6.
9. Krishnan N, Purswani M, Hagmann S. Severe dengue virus infection in pediatric travelers visiting friends and relatives after travel to the Caribbean. Am J Trop Med Hyg. 2012 Mar;86(3):474–6.
10. van Rijn SF, Driessen G, Overbosch D, van Genderen PJ. Travel-related morbidity in children: a prospective observational study. J Travel Med. 2012 May–Jun;19(3):144–9.

VACCINE RECOMMENDATIONS FOR INFANTS & CHILDREN

Michelle S. Weinberg

Vaccinating children for travel requires careful evaluation. Whenever possible, children should complete the routine immunizations of childhood on a normal schedule. However, travel at an earlier age may require accelerated schedules. **Not all travel-related vaccines are effective in infants, and some are specifically contraindicated.**

The recommended childhood and adolescent immunization schedule is available at www.cdc.gov/vaccines/schedules/downloads/child/0-18yrs-schedule.pdf. The catch-up schedule for children and adolescents who start their vaccination schedule late or who are >1 month behind can also be accessed at www.cdc.gov/vaccines/schedules/downloads/child/catchup-schedule-pr.pdf. This table also describes the recommended minimum intervals between doses for children who need to be vaccinated on an accelerated schedule, which may be necessary before international travel.

Country-specific vaccination recommendations and requirements for departure and entry vary over time. For example, at the time of this publication, proof of yellow fever vaccination is required for entry into certain countries. Meningococcal vaccination is required for travelers entering Saudi Arabia for the annual Hajj. The World Health Organization issued temporary vaccination requirements for residents of and long-term visitors to countries with active wild poliovirus transmission. Clinicians should check the CDC website for up-to-date requirements and recommendations (www.cdc.gov/travel).

Additional information about diseases and routine vaccination is available in the disease-specific sections in Chapter 3. Interactive tools for determining routine and catch-up childhood vaccination are available at www.cdc.gov/vaccines/schedules/hcp/child-adolescent.html.

MODIFYING THE IMMUNIZATION SCHEDULE FOR INADEQUATELY IMMUNIZED INFANTS AND YOUNGER CHILDREN BEFORE INTERNATIONAL TRAVEL

Several factors influence recommendations for the age at which a vaccine is administered, including age-specific risks of the disease and its complications, the ability of people of a given age to develop an adequate immune response to the vaccine, and potential interference with the immune response by passively transferred maternal antibodies.

The routine immunization schedules for infants and children in the United States do not provide specific guidelines for those traveling internationally before the age when specific vaccines and toxoids are routinely recommended. Recommended age limitations are based on potential adverse events (yellow fever vaccine), lack of efficacy

data or inadequate immune response (polysaccharide vaccines and influenza vaccine), maternal antibody interference (measles-mumps-rubella [MMR] vaccine), or lack of safety data. In deciding when to travel with a young infant or child, parents should be advised that the earliest opportunity to receive routinely recommended immunizations in the United States (except for the dose of hepatitis B vaccine at birth) is at age 6 weeks.

Routine Infant and Childhood Vaccinations

Children should receive routine vaccination for hepatitis A virus; hepatitis B virus; diphtheria, tetanus, pertussis; *Haemophilus influenzae* type b (Hib); human papillomavirus; influenza; MMR; *Neisseria meningitidis*; polio; rotavirus; *Streptococcus pneumoniae*; and varicella. In order to complete vaccine series before travel, vaccine doses can be administered at the minimum intervals. Parents should be informed that infants and children who have not received all recommended doses might not be fully protected. Rotavirus vaccine is unique among the routine vaccines given to US infants because it has maximum ages for the first and last doses; specific consideration should be given to the timing of an infant's travel so that the infant will still be able to receive the vaccine series, if at all possible.

Travel-specific vaccine considerations include the following:

- **Hepatitis A vaccine:** Although hepatitis A is often not severe in infants and children aged <5 years, infected children may transmit the infection to older children and adults, who are at risk for severe disease. Vaccination should be ensured for all children traveling to areas where there is an intermediate or high risk of hepatitis A. Because of the potential interference by maternal antibodies, the hepatitis A vaccine is not approved for children aged <1 year. The vaccine series consists of 2 doses ≥6 months apart. One dose of monovalent hepatitis A vaccine administered at any time before departure can provide adequate protection for most healthy children. The second dose is necessary for long-term protection.

7

- **Immune globulin (IG) for hepatitis A protection:** Children aged <1 year or who are allergic to a vaccine component and who are traveling to high-risk areas can receive IG. One dose of 0.02 mL/kg intramuscularly provides protection for up to 3 months, and 1 dose of 0.06 mL/kg IM provides protection for 3–5 months. Children should receive a second dose after 5 months if travel continues. For optimal protection, children aged ≥1 year who are immunocompromised or have chronic medical conditions and who are planning to depart to a high-risk area in <2 weeks should receive the initial dose of vaccine along with IG at a separate anatomic injection site. IG does not interfere with the response to yellow fever vaccine but can interfere with the response to other live injected vaccines (such as MMR and varicella vaccines). Administration of MMR and varicella vaccines should be delayed for >3 months after administration of IG for hepatitis A prophylaxis. IG should not be administered <2 weeks after MMR or varicella vaccines unless the benefits exceed those of vaccination. If IG is given during this time, the child should be revaccinated with the live MMR or varicella vaccines but not sooner than 3 months after IG administration. When travel plans do not allow adequate time to administer live vaccines and IG before travel, the severity of the diseases and their epidemiology at the destination will help determine the course of preparation.
- **Hepatitis B vaccine:** Vaccine can be administered with an accelerated schedule of 4 doses of vaccine given at 0, 1, 2, and 12 months; the last dose may be given on return from travel.
- **Influenza vaccine:** Influenza viruses circulate predominantly in the winter months in temperate regions (typically November–April in the Northern Hemisphere and April–September in the Southern Hemisphere) but can occur year-round in tropical climates. Since influenza viruses may be circulating at any time of the year, travelers aged ≥6 months who were not vaccinated during the influenza season of their country of residence should be vaccinated ≥2 weeks before departure if vaccine is available. Children aged 6 months through 8 years who are receiving influenza vaccine for the first time require 2 doses administered ≥4 weeks apart. For 2014–2015, Advisory Committee on Immunization Practices (ACIP) has recommended that live, attenuated influenza vaccine is preferred for healthy children 2–8 years if it is readily available. Check the CDC website annually for updated recommendations about seasonal influenza vaccination.
- **MMR or MMRV vaccine:** Children traveling abroad may need to be vaccinated at an earlier age than is routinely recommended. Infants aged 6–11 months should receive 1 dose of MMR vaccine before departure, then be vaccinated with MMR or MMRV (measles-mumps-rubella-varicella) vaccine at 12–15 months (≥28 days after the initial dose) and again at 4–6 years, according to the routinely recommended schedule. Children aged ≥12 months need 2 doses of MMR vaccine before traveling overseas. Children who have received 1 dose should receive their second dose before departure, provided the 2 doses are separated by ≥28 days.
- **Meningococcal vaccine:** Epidemics of meningococcal disease, caused by the bacterium *Neisseria meningitidis*, occur in sub-Saharan Africa during the dry season, December through June (see Map 3-11). CDC recommends that travelers be vaccinated before traveling to this region. Meningococcal vaccination is a requirement to enter Saudi Arabia when traveling to Mecca during the annual Hajj. Health requirements and recommendations for US travelers to the Hajj are available each year on the CDC Travelers' Health website (www.cdc.gov/travel). Meningococcal vaccine is also recommended for children aged 2 months through 18 years who travel to or reside in areas where *N. meningitidis* is hyperendemic or epidemic; for these children, providers should take care to use a meningococcal vaccine that is licensed for the child's age group and contains all 4 serotypes (A, C, Y, W-135). The schedule for the primary series and booster doses varies depending on which meningococcal vaccine is administered (see CDC's Immunization Schedules webpage at www.cdc.gov/vaccines/schedules for additional information).

- **Polio vaccine:** Polio vaccine is recommended for travelers to countries with evidence of wild poliovirus (WPV) circulation (during the last 12 months) and for travelers with a high risk of exposure to someone with imported WPV infection when traveling to some countries that border areas with WPV circulation. Refer to the CDC Travelers' Health website destination pages for the most up-to-date polio vaccine recommendations (wwwnc.cdc.gov/travel/destinations/list). Clinicians should ensure that travelers have completed the recommended age-appropriate polio vaccine series and have received a single lifetime booster dose, if necessary. See Chapter 3, Poliomyelitis and CDC's Immunization Schedules webpage (www.cdc.gov/vaccines/schedules) for information about accelerated schedules for completing the routine series. Young adults (≥18 years of age) who are traveling to areas where polio vaccine is recommended and who have received a routine series with either inactivated polio vaccine (IPV) or live oral polio vaccine in childhood should receive a single lifetime booster dose of IPV before departure. Available data do not indicate the need for more than a single lifetime booster dose with IPV. However, requirements for long-term travelers may apply when departing certain countries.
- In May 2014, the World Health Organization (WHO) declared the international spread of polio to be a Public Health Emergency of International Concern (PHEIC) under the authority of the International Health Regulations (2005). To prevent further spread of disease, WHO issued temporary polio vaccine recommendations for long-term travelers (staying >4 weeks) and residents departing from countries with WPV transmission ("exporting WPV" or "infected with WPV"). Clinicians should be aware that long-term travelers and residents may be required to show proof of polio vaccination when departing from these countries. All polio vaccination administration should be documented on an International Certificate of Vaccination or Prophylaxis (ICVP). The polio vaccine must be received between 4 weeks and 12 months before the date of departure from the polio-infected country. Country requirements may change, so clinicians should check for updates on the CDC Travelers' Health website. Refer to the Clinical Update: Interim CDC Guidance for Travel to and from Countries Affected by the New Polio Vaccine Requirements (wwwnc.cdc.gov/travel/news-announcements/polio-guidance-new-requirements) for a list of affected countries, guidance on meeting the vaccination requirements, and instructions on how to order and fill out the ICVP.

Other Vaccines

Japanese Encephalitis Vaccine

Japanese encephalitis (JE) virus is transmitted by mosquitoes and is endemic throughout Asia. The risk can be seasonal in temperate climates and year-round in more tropical climates. The risk to short-term travelers and those who confine their travel to urban centers is low. JE vaccine is recommended for travelers who plan to spend a month or longer in endemic areas during the JE virus transmission season. JE vaccine should be considered for short-term (<1 month) travelers whose itinerary or activities might increase their risk for exposure to JE virus. The decision to vaccinate a child should follow the more detailed recommendations in Chapter 3, Japanese Encephalitis.

An inactivated Vero cell culture–derived JE vaccine (Ixiaro [Valneva]) was licensed by the Food and Drug Administration in 2009 for use in the United States for travelers aged ≥17 years. In 2013, the recommendations were expanded and the vaccine was licensed for use in children starting at age 2 months.

The primary series is 2 intramuscular doses administered 28 days apart. Information on age-appropriate dosing is available at www.cdc.gov/japaneseencephalitis/vaccine/vaccineChildren.html. For people aged ≥17 years, ACIP recommends that if the primary series was administered >1 year previously, a booster dose may be given before potential JE virus exposures. Although studies are being conducted on the need for a booster dose following a primary series of Ixiaro in children, data are not yet available.

7

Rabies Vaccine

Rabies virus causes an acute viral encephalitis that is virtually 100% fatal. Traveling children may be at increased risk of rabies exposure, mainly from dogs who roam the streets in developing countries. Bat bites carry a potential risk of rabies throughout the world. There are 2 strategies to prevent rabies in humans:

- Avoiding animal bites or scratches.
- A 3-shot preexposure immunization series on days 0, 7, and 21 or 28. In the event of a subsequent possible rabies virus exposure, the child will require 2 more doses of rabies vaccine on days 0 and 3. The decision whether to obtain preexposure immunization for children should follow the recommendations in Chapter 3, Rabies.

For children who have not received preexposure immunization and may have been exposed to rabies, a weight-based dose of human rabies immune globulin and a series of 4 rabies vaccine injections are required on days 0, 3, 7, and 14.

Typhoid Vaccine

Typhoid fever is caused by the bacterium *Salmonella enterica* serotype Typhi. Vaccination is recommended for travelers to areas where there is a recognized risk of exposure to *Salmonella* Typhi.

Two typhoid vaccines are available: Vi capsular polysaccharide vaccine (ViCPS) administered intramuscularly and oral live attenuated vaccine (Ty21a). Both vaccines induce a protective response in 50%–80% of recipients. The ViCPS vaccine can be administered to children who are aged ≥2 years, with a booster dose 2 years later if continued protection is needed. The Ty21a vaccine, which consists of a series of 4 capsules (1 taken every other day) can be administered to children aged ≥6 years. A booster series for Ty21a should be taken every 5 years, if indicated. The capsule cannot be opened for administration but must be swallowed whole. All 4 doses should be taken ≥1 week before potential exposure.

Yellow Fever Vaccine

Yellow fever, a disease transmitted by mosquitoes, is endemic in certain areas of Africa and South America (see Maps 3-15 and 3-16). Proof of yellow fever vaccination is required for entry into some countries (see Chapter 3, Yellow Fever & Malaria Information, by Country). Infants and children aged ≥9 months can be vaccinated if they travel to countries within the yellow fever–endemic zone. More information, including how to access yellow fever vaccine in the United States, is available in Chapter 3, Yellow Fever.

Infants aged <9 months are at higher risk for developing encephalitis from yellow fever vaccine, which is a live virus vaccine. Studies conducted during the early 1950s identified 4 cases of encephalitis out of 1,000 children aged <6 months vaccinated with yellow fever vaccine. An additional 10 cases of encephalitis associated with yellow fever vaccine administered to infants aged <4 months were reported worldwide during the 1950s.

Travelers with infants aged <9 months should be advised against traveling to areas within the yellow fever–endemic zone. ACIP recommends that yellow fever vaccine *never* be given to infants aged <6 months. Infants aged 6–8 months should be vaccinated only if they must travel to areas of ongoing epidemic yellow fever and if a high level of protection against mosquito bites is not possible. Clinicians considering vaccinating infants aged 6–8 months may contact their respective state health departments or CDC toll-free at 800-CDC-INFO (800-232-4636) or www.cdc.gov/cdc-info/requestform.html.

BIBLIOGRAPHY

1. CDC. General recommendations on immunization—recommendations of the Advisory Committee on Immunization Practices (ACIP). MMWR Recomm Rep. 2011 Jan 28;60(2):1–64.

2. CDC. Interim CDC guidance for polio vaccination for travel to and from countries affected by wild poliovirus. MMWR Morb Mortal Wkly Rep. 2014 Jul 11;63(27):591–4.

3. CDC. Prevention and control of meningococcal disease: recommendations of the Advisory Committee on Immunization Practices (ACIP). MMWR Recomm Rep. 2013 Mar 22;62(RR-2):1–28.

4. CDC. Prevention of hepatitis A through active or passive immunization: recommendations of the Advisory Committee on Immunization Practices (ACIP). MMWR Recomm Rep. 2006 May 19;55(RR-7):1–23.

5. CDC. Prevention of varicella: recommendations of the Advisory Committee on Immunization Practices (ACIP). MMWR Recomm Rep. 2007 Jun 22;56(RR-4):1–40.

6. CDC. Use of a reduced (4-dose) vaccine schedule for postexposure prophylaxis to prevent human rabies: recommendations of the advisory committee on immunization practices. MMWR Recomm Rep. 2010 Mar 19;59(RR-2):1–9.

7. CDC. Use of Japanese encephalitis vaccine in children: recommendations of the Advisory Committee on Immunization Practices, 2013.

MMWR Morb Mortal Wkly Rep. 2013 Nov 15;62(45):898–900.

8. CDC. Yellow fever vaccine: recommendations of the Advisory Committee on Immunization Practices (ACIP). MMWR Recomm Rep. 2010 Jul 30;59(RR-7):1–27.

9. Global Polio Eradication Initiative. Polio public health emergency: temporary recommendations to reduce international spread of poliovirus. Geneva: Global Polio Eradication Initiative; 2014 [cited 2014 Sep 22]. Available from: http://www.polioeradication.org/infectedcountries/polioemergency.aspx.

10. Pickering LK, editor. Red Book: 2012 Report of the Committee on Infectious Diseases. 29th ed. Elk Grove Village, IL: American Academy of Pediatrics; 2012.

TRAVEL & BREASTFEEDING

Katherine R. Shealy

The medical preparation of a traveler who is breastfeeding differs only slightly from that of other travelers and depends in part on whether the mother and child will be separated or together during travel. Most mothers should be advised to continue breastfeeding their infants throughout travel. Before departure, mothers may wish to carry with them a list of local breastfeeding resources at their destination. Clinicians may be able to help breastfeeding mothers find out about available breastfeeding support experts at their destination through sources that include the following:

- International board-certified lactation consultants (IBCLCs)—health professionals in approximately 96 countries who specialize in the clinical management of breastfeeding (http://iblce.org). The Find a Lactation Consultant (FALC) tool can help clinicians and mothers identify in advance local IBCLCs worldwide (www.ilca.org/i4a/pages/index.cfm?pageid=3432).
- La Leche League leaders—accredited volunteer mothers in approximately 65 countries who provide mother-to-mother breastfeeding support and help (www.llli.org). La Leche League's interactive map lists location and contact information for La Leche League leaders and groups worldwide (www.llli.org/search/groups).

Mothers who plan to use a breast pump while traveling may need an electrical current adapter and converter and should have a back-up option available, including written instructions for hand expression (for more detailed instructions about hand expression, see www.workandpump.com/handexpression.htm).

TRAVELING WITH A BREASTFEEDING CHILD

Breastfeeding provides unique benefits to mothers and children traveling together. Health care providers should explain clearly to breastfeeding mothers the value of continuing breastfeeding during travel. For the first 6 months of life, exclusive breastfeeding is recommended. This is especially important during travel because exclusive breastfeeding means feeding only breast milk, no other foods or drinks, which protects infants from exposure to contamination and pathogens via foods or liquids. Additionally, feeding only at the breast protects infants from exposure to contamination from containers (bottles, cups, utensils).

Breastfeeding infants require no water supplementation, even in extreme heat environments. Breastfeeding protects children from eustachian tube pain and collapse during air travel, especially during ascent and descent, by allowing them to stabilize and gradually equalize internal and external air pressure, which cannot be replicated by sucking on a bottle or pacifier.

Clinicians should offer information to breastfeeding mothers so that they are better able to continue breastfeeding during travel. Frequent, unrestricted breastfeeding opportunities ensure the mother's milk supply remains ample and the child's nutrition and hydration are ideal. Safe use of a fabric infant carrier helps maintain breastfeeding by increasing breastfeeding opportunities and skin-to-skin contact with the child, while also protecting the child from environmental hazards and easing the burden of carrying a heavy child. Mothers who are concerned about breastfeeding away from home may feel more comfortable breastfeeding the child in a fabric carrier. In many countries around the world, breastfeeding in public places is more widely practiced than in the United States. US federal legislation protects mothers' and children's right to breastfeed anywhere they are otherwise authorized to be while on federal property, which includes US Customs areas, embassies, and consulates overseas.

AIR TRAVEL

X-rays used in airport screenings have no effect on breastfeeding, breast milk, or the process of lactation. Airlines typically consider breast pumps as personal items to be carried onboard, similar to laptop computers, handbags, and diaper bags.

Before departure, mothers who will be traveling by air and expect to have expressed milk with them during travel need to carefully plan how they will transport their milk. Airport security regulations for passengers carrying expressed milk vary internationally and are subject to change. In the United States, the Transportation Security Administration (TSA) recognizes expressed milk in the category of liquid medications that may be carried on, regardless of whether the breastfeeding child is also traveling, as long as it is declared before screening. TSA recommends that travelers carrying expressed milk have with them a printed copy of the TSA website page (www.tsa.gov/traveling-formula-breast-milk-and-juice) to help prevent problems at security checkpoints.

Travelers carrying expressed milk in checked luggage should refer to cooler pack storage guidelines in "Proper Handling and Storage of Human Milk" on CDC's website (www.cdc.gov/breastfeeding/recommendations/handling_breastmilk.htm) to protect milk during travel. Expressed milk is not considered a biohazard. International Air Transport Authority regulations for shipping category B biological substances (UN 3373) do not apply to expressed milk; it is considered a food for individual use. Travelers shipping frozen milk should follow guidelines for shipping other frozen foods and liquids. Expressed milk does not need to be declared at US Customs upon return to the United States.

IMMUNIZATIONS AND MEDICATIONS

In almost all situations, clinicians can and should select immunizations and medications for the nursing mother that are compatible with breastfeeding. In most circumstances, it is inappropriate to counsel mothers to wean in order to be vaccinated or to withhold vaccination due to breastfeeding status.

Breastfeeding and lactation do not affect maternal or infant dosage guidelines for any immunization or medication; children always require their own immunization or medication, regardless of maternal dose. In the absence of documented risk to the breastfeeding child of a particular maternal medication, the known risks of stopping breastfeeding generally outweigh a theoretical risk of exposure via breastfeeding.

Immunizations

Breastfeeding mothers and children should be vaccinated according to routine, recommended schedules. Administration of most live and inactivated vaccines does not affect breastfeeding, breast milk, or the process of

TRAVEL & BREASTFEEDING | 551

lactation. Only 2 vaccines, vaccinia (smallpox) and yellow fever, require special consideration. Preventive vaccinia (smallpox) vaccine is contraindicated for use in breastfeeding mothers.

Special Consideration: Yellow Fever Vaccination

Breastfeeding is a precaution for yellow fever vaccine administration. Three cases of yellow fever vaccine–associated neurologic disease (YEL-AND) have been reported in exclusively breastfed infants whose mothers were vaccinated with yellow fever vaccine. All 3 infants were diagnosed with encephalitis and aged <1 month at the time of exposure. Further research is needed to document the risk of potential vaccine exposure through breastfeeding. Data about possible excretion of vaccine virus and duration of excretion in breast milk are insufficient to make a recommendation about temporary suspension of breastfeeding, pumping, and discarding pumped milk. Until more information is available, yellow fever vaccine should be avoided in breastfeeding women. However, when nursing mothers must travel to a yellow fever–endemic area, these women should be vaccinated.

Medications

According to the American Academy of Pediatrics (AAP) 2013 Clinical Report: The Transfer of Drugs and Therapeutics into Human Breast Milk, many mothers are inappropriately advised to discontinue breastfeeding or avoid taking essential medications because of fears of adverse effects on their infants. The AAP advises that this cautious approach may be unnecessary in many cases because only a small proportion of medications are contraindicated in breastfeeding mothers or associated with adverse effects on their infants. The National Institutes for Health's database of information on drugs and lactation (LactMed) is an online database of clinical information about drugs and breastfeeding (http://toxnet.nlm.nih.gov/cgi-bin/sis/htmlgen?LACT). It provides information about maternal levels of drugs in breast milk, infant levels in blood, potential effects in breastfeeding infants and on lactation itself, the AAP category indicating the level of compatibility of the drug with

breastfeeding, and alternate drugs to consider. The pharmaceutical reference guide, Medications and Mothers' Milk, is updated every 2 years and provides a comprehensive review of the compatibility or effects on breastfeeding of approximately 1,000 drugs, including concerns such as risk categories, pharmacologic properties, interactions with other drugs, and suitable alternatives.

Special Consideration: Antimalarial Medications

Since chloroquine and mefloquine may be safely prescribed to infants, both are considered safe to prescribe to mothers who are breastfeeding. Most experts consider short-term use of doxycycline compatible with breastfeeding. Primaquine may be used for breastfeeding mothers and children with normal glucose-6-phosphate dehydrogenase (G6PD) levels. The mother and infant should be tested for G6PD deficiency before primaquine is given to the breastfeeding mother. Because data are not yet available on the safety of atovaquone-proguanil prophylaxis in infants weighing <11 lb (5 kg), CDC does not recommend it to prevent malaria in women breastfeeding infants who weigh <5 kg.

Special Consideration: Travelers' Diarrhea

Exclusive breastfeeding protects infants against travelers' diarrhea. Breastfeeding is ideal rehydration therapy. Children who are suspected of having travelers' diarrhea should breastfeed more frequently. Children in this situation should not be offered other fluids or foods that replace breastfeeding. Breastfeeding mothers with travelers' diarrhea should continue breastfeeding and increase their own fluid intake. The organisms that cause travelers' diarrhea do not pass through breast milk. Breastfeeding mothers should carefully check the labels of over-the-counter antidiarrheal medications to avoid using bismuth subsalicylate compounds, which can lead to the transfer of salicylate to the child via breast milk. Fluoroquinolones and macrolides, which are commonly used to treat travelers' diarrhea, are excreted in breast milk. The decision about the use of antibiotics such as fluoroquinolones and macrolides in nursing mothers should be made in consultation with the child's primary health care provider. Most experts consider the use of short-term azithromycin compatible with breastfeeding. Use of oral rehydration salts by breastfeeding mothers and their children is fully compatible with breastfeeding.

TRAVELING WITHOUT A BREASTFEEDING CHILD

A breastfeeding mother traveling without her breastfeeding infant or child may wish to express and store a supply of milk to be fed to the infant or child during her absence. Building a supply to be fed in her absence takes time and patience and is most successful when begun gradually, many weeks in advance of the mother's departure.

A mother's milk supply can diminish if she does not express milk while away from her nursing child, but this does not need to be a reason to stop breastfeeding. Clinicians should help mothers determine the best course for breastfeeding based on a variety of factors, including the amount of time she has to prepare for her trip, her flexibility of time while traveling, her options for expressing and storing milk while traveling, the duration of her travel, and her destination. A mother who returns to her nursing infant or child can continue breastfeeding and, if necessary, supplement as needed until her milk supply returns to its prior level. Often, after a mother returns from travel, her nursing infant or child will help bring her milk supply to its prior level. However, nursing infants or children who are separated from their mother for an extended time may have difficulty transitioning back to breastfeeding.

BIBLIOGRAPHY

1. Academy of Breastfeeding Medicine (ABM) Protocol Committee. ABM clinical protocol #8: human milk storage information for home use for full-term infants. Breastfeed Med. 2010 Jun;5(3):127–30.
2. CDC. Transmission of yellow fever vaccine virus through breast-feeding—Brazil, 2009. MMWR Morb Mortal Wkly Rep. 2010 Feb 12;59(5):130–2.
3. CDC. Perspectives in disease prevention and health promotion update: universal precautions for prevention of transmission of human immuno-deficiency virus, hepatitis B virus, and other blood-borne pathogens in health-care settings. MMWR Morb Mortal Wkly Rep. 1988 Jun 24;37(24):377–82, 387–88.
4. Hale TW, Rowe HE. Medications and Mothers' Milk 2014: A Manual of Lactational Pharmacology. 16th ed. Plane, TX: Hale Pub; 2014.
5. Kuhn S, Twele-Montecinos L, MacDonald J, Webster P, Law B. Case report: probable transmission of vaccine strain of yellow fever virus to an infant via breast milk. CMAJ. 2011 Mar 8;183(4):e243–5.
6. Sachdev HP, Krishna J, Puri RK, Satyanarayana L, Kumar S. Water supplementation in exclusively breastfed infants during summer in the tropics. Lancet. 1991 Apr 20;337(8747):929–33.
7. Section on Breastfeeding. Breastfeeding and the use of human milk. Pediatrics. 2012 Mar;129(3):e827–41.
8. Staples JE, Gershman M, Fischer M. Yellow fever vaccine: recommendations of the Advisory Committee on Immunization Practices (ACIP). MMWR Recomm Rep. 2010 Jul 30;59(RR-7):1–27.

INTERNATIONAL ADOPTION
Mary Allen Staat, Heather Burke

OVERVIEW

In the past 15 years, >250,000 children have come to the United States to join their families through international adoption. Families traveling to unite with their adopted child, siblings who wait at home for the child's arrival, extended family members, and childcare providers are all at risk for acquiring infectious diseases secondary to travel or resulting from contact with the newly arrived child. International adoptees may be under-immunized and are at increased risk for infections such as measles, hepatitis A, and hepatitis B because of crowded living conditions, malnutrition, lack of clean water, lack of immunizations, and exposure to endemic diseases that are not commonly seen in the United States. Challenges in providing care to internationally adopted children include the absence of a complete medical history, lack of availability of biological family history, questionable reliability of immunization records, variation in preadoption living standards, varying disease epidemiology in the countries of origin, the presence of previously unidentified medical problems, and the increased risk for developmental delays and psychological issues in these children.

TRAVEL PREPARATION FOR ADOPTIVE PARENTS AND THEIR FAMILIES

A pre-travel visit is strongly recommended for prospective adoptive parents. In preparation, the travel health provider must know the disease risks in the adopted child's country of origin and the medical and social histories of the adoptee (if available), as well as which family members will be traveling, their immunization and medical histories, the season of travel, the length of stay in the country, and the itinerary while in country.

Family members who remain at home, including extended family, should be current on their routine immunizations. Protection against measles, varicella, tetanus, diphtheria, pertussis, hepatitis A, hepatitis B, and polio must be ensured for everyone who will be in the household or in close contact by providing care for the adopted child. Measles immunity or 2 doses of measles-mumps-rubella (MMR) vaccine separated by ≥28 days should be documented for all people born in or after 1957. Varicella vaccine should be given to those without a history of varicella disease or documentation of 2 doses of varicella vaccine ≥3 months apart. Adults who have not received the tetanus-diphtheria-acellular pertussis (Tdap) vaccine, including adults >65 years old, should receive a single dose of Tdap to protect against *Bordetella pertussis* in addition to tetanus and diphtheria. Unprotected family members and close contacts of the adopted child should be immunized against hepatitis A virus (HAV) before the child's arrival.

Most adult family members and caretakers will need to be immunized with hepatitis B vaccine, since it has only been routinely given since 1990. If the adopted child is from a polio-endemic area, family members and caretakers should ensure they have completed the recommended age-appropriate polio vaccine series. A one-time inactivated polio booster for adults who have completed the primary series in the past is recommended if they are traveling to these areas and can be considered for adults who remain at home but who will be in close contact caring for the child.

Prospective adoptive parents and any children traveling with them should receive advice on travel safety, food safety, immunization, malaria chemoprophylaxis, diarrhea prevention and treatment, and other travel-related health issues, as outlined elsewhere in this book. Instructions on car seats, injury prevention, food safety, and air travel apply equally to the adoptive child, so the travel health provider should also be familiar with and provide information on these child-specific issues.

OVERSEAS MEDICAL EXAMINATION OF THE ADOPTED CHILD

All immigrants, including children adopted internationally by US citizens, must undergo a medical examination in their country of origin, performed by a physician designated by the Department of State. The medical examination is used primarily to detect diseases or risk behaviors that may make the immigrant ineligible for a visa. Prospective adoptive parents should not rely on this medical examination to detect all possible disabilities and illnesses. Laboratory results from the country of origin may be unreliable. This examination should not replace the evaluation that is recommended once the child comes to the United States.

Additional information about the medical examination and the vaccination exemption form for internationally adopted children are available on the Department of State website at http://travel.state.gov/content/adoptionsabroad/en/us-visa-for-your-child/medical-examination.html and www.state.gov/documents/organization/80002.pdf, respectively.

FOLLOW-UP MEDICAL EXAMINATION AFTER ARRIVAL IN THE UNITED STATES

The adopted child should have a medical examination within 2 weeks of arrival in the United States or earlier if the child has fever, anorexia, diarrhea, vomiting, or other medical concerns. Items to consider during medical examination of an adopted child include the following:

- Temperature (fever requires further investigation)
- General appearance: alert, interactive
- Anthropometric measurements: weight/age, height/age, weight/height, head circumference/age, body mass index
- Facial features: length of palpebral fissures, philtrum, upper lip (fetal alcohol syndrome: short palpebral fissures, thin upper lip, indistinct philtrum)
- Hair: texture, color
- Eyes: jaundice, pallor, strabismus, visual acuity screen
- Ears: hearing screen, otitis media
- Mouth: palate, teeth
- Neck: thyroid (enlargement secondary to hypothyroidism, iodine deficiency)
- Heart: murmurs
- Chest: symmetry, Tanner stage breasts
- Abdomen: liver or spleen enlargement
- Skin: Mongolian spots, scars, bacillus Calmette-Guérin (BCG) scar, birth marks, molluscum contagiosum, tinea capitis, tinea corporis
- Lymph nodes: enlargement suggestive of TB or other infections
- Back: scoliosis
- Genitalia: Tanner stage, presence of both testicles, findings of sexual abuse

In addition, all children should receive a developmental screening by a clinician with experience in child development to determine if immediate referrals should be made for a more detailed neurodevelopmental examination and therapies. Further evaluation will depend on the country of origin, the age of the child, previous living conditions, nutritional status, developmental status, and the adoptive family's specific questions. Concerns raised during the preadoption medical review may dictate further investigation.

SCREENING FOR INFECTIOUS DISEASES

The current panel of tests for infectious diseases recommended by the American Academy of Pediatrics (AAP) for screening internationally adopted children is as follows:

- HAV serologic testing (IgG and IgM)
- Hepatitis B virus (HBV) serologic testing (repeat at 6 months if negative)
- Hepatitis C antibody
- Syphilis serologic testing (treponemal and nontreponemal testing)
- HIV 1 and 2 serologic testing
- Complete blood cell count with differential and red blood cell indices
- Stool examination for ova and parasites (3 specimens)
- Stool examination for *Giardia intestinalis* and *Cryptosporidium* antigen (1 specimen)
- Tuberculin skin test (TST) (all ages) or interferon-γ release assay (IGRA) (for children >5 years of age) (repeat at 6 months if negative)

Additional screening tests may be useful, depending on the child's country of origin or specific risk factors. These screens may include Chagas disease serologic tests, malaria smears, or serologic testing for schistosomiasis, strongyloidiasis, and filariasis.

Gastrointestinal Parasites

Gastrointestinal parasites are commonly seen in international adoptees, but the prevalence varies by birth country and age. The highest rates of infection have been reported from Ukraine and Ethiopia and increase with older age. *G. intestinalis* is the most common parasite identified. Three stool samples collected in the early morning, 2–3 days apart and placed in a container with preservative are recommended for ova and parasite analysis. Only one of these samples needs to be analyzed for *Giardia* antigen and *Cryptosporidium* antigen. Although theoretically possible, transmission of intestinal parasites from internationally adopted children to family and school contacts has not been reported; however, good hand hygiene is recommended to prevent infection. Stool samples should be cultured for enteric bacterial pathogens for any child with fever and bloody diarrhea. Unlike refugees, internationally adopted children are not treated for parasites before departure.

Hepatitis A

HAV serology (IgG and IgM) should be considered for all internationally adopted children to identify children who may be acutely infected and shedding virus and to make decisions regarding HAV immunization. In 2007 and early 2008, multiple cases of hepatitis A secondary to exposure to newly arrived internationally adopted children were reported in the United States. Some of these cases involved extended family members who were not living in the household. Identification of acutely infected toddlers new to the United States is necessary to prevent further transmission. If a child is found to have acute infection, HAV vaccine or immunoglobulin can be given to close contacts to prevent infection. In addition, it is cost effective to identify children with past infection with serologic testing since they would not need to receive the HAV vaccine.

Hepatitis B

All internationally adopted children should be screened for HBV infection with serology for hepatitis B surface antigen (HBsAg) and hepatitis B surface antibody to determine past or current infection and protection from vaccination. HBV infection has been reported in 1%–5% of newly arrived adoptees. Because of widespread use of the HBV vaccine, the prevalence of HBV infection has decreased over the years. Children found to be positive for HBsAg should be retested 6 months later to determine if the child has a chronic infection. Results of a positive HBsAg test should be reported to the state health department. HBV is highly transmissible within the household. All members of households adopting children with chronic HBV infection must be immunized and should have follow-up antibody titers to determine whether levels consistent with immunity have been achieved. Children with chronic HBV infection should receive additional tests for HBV e antigen, HBV e antibody, hepatitis D virus antibody, viral load, and liver function. They should be vaccinated for hepatitis A if they are not immune. They should also

have a consultation with a pediatric gastroenterologist. Repeat screening at 6 months after arrival should be done on all children who initially test negative for HBV surface antibody.

Hepatitis C

Routine screening for hepatitis C virus (HCV) should be considered, since most children with HCV infection are asymptomatic, screening for risk factors is not possible, effective treatments are available, and close follow-up of infected patients is needed to identify long-term complications. Antibody testing with an EIA should be done for screening. Since maternal antibody may be present in children <18 months of age, PCR testing should be done if the EIA is positive. Children with HCV infection should be referred to a gastroenterologist for further evaluation, management, and treatment.

Syphilis

Screening for *Treponema pallidum* is recommended for all internationally adopted children. Initial screening is done with both nontreponemal and treponemal tests. Treponemal tests remain positive for life in most cases even after successful treatment and are specific for treponemal diseases, which include syphilis and other diseases (such as yaws, pinta, and bejel) that can be seen in some countries. In children with a history of syphilis, the child's initial evaluation, treatment (antibiotic type and treatment duration), and follow-up testing are rarely available; therefore, a full evaluation for disease must be undertaken and antitreponemal treatment given dependent upon the results.

HIV

HIV screening is recommended for all internationally adopted children. Positive HIV antibodies in children aged <18 months may reflect maternal antibody and not infection. Assaying for HIV DNA with PCR will confirm the diagnosis of HIV in the infant or child. Standard screening for HIV is with ELISA antibody testing, but some experts recommend PCR for any infant aged <6 months on arrival. If PCR testing is done, 2 negative results from assays administered 1 month apart, at least one of which is done after the age of 4 months, are necessary to exclude infection. Children with HIV infection should be referred to a specialist. Some experts recommend repeating the screen for HIV antibodies 6 months after arrival.

Chagas Disease

Screening for Chagas disease should be considered for children arriving from a country endemic for Chagas disease. Chagas disease is endemic throughout much of Mexico, Central America, and South America (Chapter 3, Trypanosomiasis, American [Chagas Disease]). The risk of Chagas disease varies by region within endemic countries. Although the risk of Chagas disease is likely low in adopted children from endemic countries, treatment of infected children is effective. Serologic testing when the child is aged 9–12 months will avoid possible false-positive results from maternal antibody. Testing by PCR can be done in children <9 months of age. If a child tests positive for Chagas disease, the child should be referred to a specialist for further evaluation and management.

Malaria

Routine screening for malaria is not recommended for internationally adopted children. However, thick and thin malaria smears should be obtained immediately for any febrile child newly arrived from a malaria-endemic area (See Chapter 3, Malaria).

Tuberculosis

All internationally adopted children should be screened for tuberculosis (TB) after arriving in the United States. Internationally adopted children are at 4–6 times the risk for TB than their US-born peers. The TST is indicated for all children, regardless of their BCG status. TST results must be interpreted carefully for internationally adopted children; guidelines may be found in the bibliography. For children aged ≥5 years, IGRA (such as QuantiFERON-TB Gold) is an acceptable screening alternative to the TST. IGRA has the advantage of not requiring a follow-up visit for testing or requiring individual interpretation of results (although results may be termed "indeterminate" by the laboratory). In addition, they appear to be more specific than the TST for *Mycobacterium tuberculosis* infection in children who have had BCG vaccination. The TST remains the most widely used screening test for TB in children. A chest radiograph and complete physical examination to assess for pulmonary and extrapulmonary TB are indicated for all children with positive TB screening results. Hilar lymphadenopathy is a more sensitive finding for TB in young children than are pulmonary infiltrates or cavitation. A repeat TST 3–6 months after arrival is recommended for children who initially test negative. Children who have a positive TST or IGRA result but have no evidence of active disease have latent tuberculosis infection (LTBI) and should generally be treated with isoniazid for 9 months. In consultation with TB experts, a shorter-course LTBI treatment regimen may be considered. Additional information is available at www.cdc.gov/tb/topic/treatment/ltbi.htm.

If active disease is found, every effort should be made to isolate the organism and determine sensitivities, particularly if the child is from a region of the world with a high rate of multidrug-resistant TB (see Chapter 3, Tuberculosis).

Eosinophilia

A complete blood count with a differential should be done on all internationally adopted children. An eosinophil count >450 cells/mm^3 in an internationally adopted child may warrant further evaluation. Intestinal parasite screening will identify some helminths that may cause eosinophilia. Further investigation of the eosinophilia might include serologic evaluation for *Strongyloides stercoralis, Toxocara canis, Ancylostoma* spp., and *Trichinella spiralis*. For children arriving from countries endemic for *Schistosoma* spp. and filariasis, serologic testing should be done for these diseases as well.

SCREENING FOR NONINFECTIOUS DISEASES

Several screening tests for noninfectious diseases should be performed in all or in select internationally adopted children. All children should have a complete blood count with a differential, hemoglobin electrophoresis, and G6PD deficiency screening. Serum levels of thyroid-stimulating hormone and lead should be measured in all internationally adopted children. Testing for serum levels of iron, iron-binding capacity, transferrin, ferritin, and total vitamin D 25 hydroxy should be considered. In certain circumstances, neurologic and psychological testing may also be considered.

IMMUNIZATIONS

The US Immigration and Nationality Act requires that any person seeking an immigrant visa for permanent residency must show proof of having received the Advisory Committee on Immunization Practices (ACIP)-recommended vaccines before immigration (www.cdc.gov/vaccines/schedules/downloads/child/0-18yrs-schedule.pdf). This requirement applies to all immigrant infants and children entering the United States, but internationally adopted children aged <10 years are exempt from the overseas immunization requirements. Adoptive parents are required to sign a waiver indicating their intention to comply with the immunization requirements within 30 days of the child's arrival in the United States.

Most children throughout the developing world receive BCG, oral polio, measles, diphtheria, tetanus, and pertussis vaccines per the original immunization schedule of the United Nations Expanded Programme of Immunizations (begun in 1974). In many developing countries, HBV, *Haemophilus influenzae* type b (Hib), and rotavirus vaccines have become more widely available. Upon arrival in the United States, >90% of newly arrived internationally adopted children need catch-up immunizations to meet ACIP guidelines. Hib, hepatitis A, mumps, pneumococcal conjugate, rotavirus, rubella, human papillomavirus, and varicella vaccines are often not available in developing countries. Reliability of vaccine records appears to differ by, and even within, country of origin. Some children may have an immunization record with documentation of the vaccines and dates they were given, and others may have incomplete documentation or no record at all. In addition, some children may be immune to vaccine-preventable diseases such as hepatitis A, measles, mumps, rubella, or varicella. A clinical diagnosis of any of these diseases should not be accepted as evidence of immunity.

Providers can choose 1 of 2 approaches for vaccination of internationally adopted children. The first is to reimmunize regardless of immunization record. The second, applicable to children aged ≥6 months, is to test antibody titers to the vaccines reportedly administered and reimmunize only for those diseases to which the child has no protective titers. Immunity to *B. pertussis* is an exception; antibody titers do not correlate with immune status to *B. pertussis*. However, protective antibody levels to diphtheria and tetanus imply protective antibody levels to *B. pertussis*. For children ≥6 months of age, testing can be done for diphtheria (IgG), tetanus (IgG), polio (neutralizing antibody to each serotype), hepatitis B (surface antibody), and Hib. Reimmunization for pneumococcus is recommended given that there are 13 serotypes in the vaccine. Most experts recommend serologic testing for infants and children aged ≥6 months. For children ≥12 months of age, testing can be done for measles, mumps, rubella, hepatitis A, and varicella. MMR is not given in most countries of origin; measles vaccine is administered as a single antigen.

Immunizations should be given according to the current ACIP schedule for catch-up vaccination. If the infant is <6 months old and there is uncertainty regarding immunization status or validity of the immunization record, the child should be reimmunized according to the ACIP schedule.

BIBLIOGRAPHY

1. American Academy of Pediatrics. Medical evaluation of internationally adopted children for infectious diseases. In: Pickering LK, editor. Red Book: 2012 Report of the Committee on Infectious Diseases. 29th ed. Elk Grove Village, IL: American Academy of Pediatrics; 2012. p. 191–3.

2. American Academy of Pediatrics Committee on Infectious Diseases. Recommendations for administering hepatitis A vaccine to contacts of international adoptees. Pediatrics. 2011 Oct;128(4):803–4.

3. CDC. CDC immigration requirements: technical instructions for tuberculosis screening and treatment: using cultures and directly observed therapy. 2009 [cited 2014 Jun 20]. Available from: http://www.cdc.gov/

7

immigrantrefugeehealth/pdf/tuberculosis-ti-2009. pdf.

4. CDC. Measles among adults associated with adoption of children in China—California, Missouri, and Washington, July–August 2006. MMWR Morb Mortal Wkly Rep. 2007 Feb 23;56(7):144–6.

5. CDC. Recommended immunization schedules for persons aged 0 through 18 years—United States, 2014. MMWR Morb Mortal Wkly Rep. 2014 Feb 7;63(5):108–9.

6. CDC, ACIP. Updated recommendations from the Advisory Committee on Immunization Practices (ACIP) for use of hepatitis A vaccine in close contacts of newly arriving international adoption. MMWR Morb Mortal Wkly Rep. 2009;58(36):1006–7.

7. Immigrant visas issued to orphans coming into the US [database on the Internet]. US Department of State. 1999– [cited 2014 Jun 20]. Available from: http://adoption.state.gov/about_us/statistics.php.

8. Mandalakas AM, Kirchner HL, Iverson S, Chesney M, Spencer MJ, Sidler A, et al. Predictors of *Mycobacterium tuberculosis* infection in international adoptees. Pediatrics. 2007 Sep;120(3):e610–6.

9. Staat MA, Rice M, Donauer S, Mukkada S, Holloway M, Cassedy A, et al. Intestinal parasite screening in internationally adopted children: importance of multiple stool specimens. Pediatrics. 2011 Sep;128(3):e613–22.

10. Staat MA, Stadler LP, Donauer S, Trehan I, Rice M, Salisbury S. Serologic testing to verify the immune status of internationally adopted children against vaccine preventable diseases. Vaccine. 2010 Nov 23;28(50):7947–55.

11. Stadler LP, Donauer S, Rice M, Trehan I, Salisbury S, Staat MA. Factors associated with protective antibody levels to vaccine preventable diseases in internationally adopted children. Vaccine. 2010 Dec 10;29(1):95–103.

Advising Travelers with Specific Needs

TRAVELERS WITH CHRONIC ILLNESSES
Deborah Nicolls Barbeau

GENERAL TRAVEL PREPARATION: PRACTICAL CONSIDERATIONS

Although traveling abroad can be relaxing and rewarding, the physical demands of travel can be stressful, particularly for travelers with underlying chronic illnesses. With adequate preparation, however, those with chronic illnesses can have safe and enjoyable trips. The following is a list of general recommendations for advising patients with chronic illnesses:

- Ensure that any chronic illnesses are well controlled. Patients with an underlying illness should see their health care providers to ensure that the management of their illness is optimized.
- Encourage patients to seek pre-travel consultation early, ≥4–6 weeks before departure, to ensure adequate time to respond to immunizations and, in some circumstances, to try medications before travel (see the Immunocompromised Travelers section later in this chapter).
- Advise patients to consider a destination that is not too remote.
- Ask about previous health-related issues encountered during travel, such as complications during air travel.

- Provide a clinician's letter. The letter should be on office letterhead stationery, outlining existing medical conditions, medications prescribed (including generic names), and any equipment required to manage the condition.
- Encourage travelers with underlying medical conditions to consider choosing a medical assistance company that allows them to store their medical history pre-departure so it can be accessed worldwide if needed (see Chapter 2, Obtaining Health Care Abroad for the Ill Traveler).
- Advise travelers to pack medications and medical supplies (such as pouching for ostomies) in their original containers in carry-on luggage and to carry a copy of their prescriptions. Ensure the traveler has sufficient quantities of medications for the entire trip, plus extra in case of unexpected delays. Since medications should be taken based on elapsed time and not time of day, travelers may need guidance on scheduling when to take medications during and after crossing time zones.
- Advise travelers to check with the American embassy or consulate to clarify medication restrictions in the destination

country. Some countries do not allow visitors to bring certain medications into the country.

- Educate travelers regarding drug interactions (see Chapter 2, Interactions among Travel Vaccines & Drugs). Medications (such as warfarin) used to treat chronic medical illnesses may interact with medications prescribed for self-treatment of travelers' diarrhea or malaria chemoprophylaxis. Discuss all medications used, either daily or on an as-needed basis.
- Suggest supplemental insurance. Three types of insurance policies can be considered: 1) trip cancellation in the event of illness; 2) supplemental insurance so that money paid for health care abroad may be reimbursed, since most medical insurance policies do not cover health care in other countries; and 3) medical evacuation insurance (see Chapter 2, Travel Insurance, Travel Health Insurance, & Medical Evacuation Insurance). Travelers may need extra help in finding supplemental insurance, as some plans will not cover costs for preexisting conditions.
- Help travelers devise a health plan. This plan should give instructions for managing minor problems or exacerbations of underlying illnesses and should include information about medical facilities available in the destination country (see Chapter 2, Obtaining Health Care Abroad for the Ill Traveler).
- Advise travelers to wear a medical alert bracelet or carry medical information on his or her person (various brands of jewelry or tags, even electronic, are available).
- Advise travelers to keep well-hydrated, wear loose-fitting clothing, and walk and stretch at regular intervals during long-distance travel (see Chapter 2, Deep Vein Thrombosis & Pulmonary Embolism).
- Always advise the traveler about packing a health kit (see Chapter 2, Travel Health Kits).

SPECIFIC CHRONIC ILLNESSES

Issues related to specific chronic medical illnesses are addressed in Table 8-1. These recommendations should be used in conjunction with the other recommendations given throughout this book. Below is a non-inclusive list of additional resources for information:

- American Association of Kidney Patients (www.aakp.org)
- American Diabetes Association (www.diabetes.org)
- American Heart Association (www.heart.org)
- American Lung Association (www.lungusa.org)
- American Society of Clinical Oncology, Cancer.Net (www.cancer.net)
- American Thoracic Society (www.thoracic.org)
- Anticoagulation Forum (www.acforum.org)
- British Thoracic Society (www.brit-thoracic.org.uk)
- Crohn's and Colitis Foundation of America (www.ccfa.org)
- Global Dialysis (www.globaldialysis.com)
- International Self-Monitoring Association of Oral Anticoagulated Patients (www.ismaap.org)
- National Multiple Sclerosis Society (www.nationalmssociety.org)
- Transportation Security Administration (www.tsa.gov)
- Department of State (www.state.gov)

Also, many health care facilities outside the United States are accredited by the Joint Commission International, an affiliate of the Joint Commission, which is the largest accreditor of US-based health care organizations. A list of accredited international facilities is available at their website (www.jointcommissioninternational.org).

If travelers or their health care providers have concerns about fitness for air travel or the need to obtain a medical certificate before travel, the medical unit affiliated with the specific airline is a valuable source for information. Remember to notify the airline in advance if oxygen or other equipment is needed on the plane. The TSA Cares Help Line (toll-free at 855-787-2227) can also provide information on how to prepare for the airport security screening process with respect to a particular disability or medical condition.

Table 8-1. Special considerations for travelers with chronic medical illnesses

CONDITION	ABSOLUTE AND RELATIVE CONTRAINDICATIONS TO AIRLINE TRAVEL	PRE-TRAVEL CONSIDERATIONS	IMMUNIZATION CONSIDERATIONS	MISCELLANEOUS
Cancer	Severe anemia Cerebral edema due to intracranial tumor ≤6 weeks since cranial surgery Cardiovascular, pulmonary, or gastrointestinal complications referred to below	Emphasize food and water precautions Plan for self-management of dehydration DVT precautions Supplemental oxygen Wear loose-fitting clothing to prevent worsening of lymphedema	Immunosuppressive medications may alter response to immunizations Live attenuated vaccines may be contraindicated Revaccination may be necessary following cancer treatment	Check for medication restrictions in the destination country, especially if controlled medications are required for pain management See the Immunocompromised Travelers section later in this chapter
Cardiovascular diseases	Following acute coronary syndrome: • those at very low risk—within 3 days after event • medium risk—within 10 days • high risk or awaiting further intervention or treatment—defer air travel until disease is stable Unstable angina CHF, severe, decompensated Uncontrolled hypertension CABG within 14 days CVA within 2 weeks Elective percutaneous coronary intervention within 2 days Uncontrolled arrhythmia Eisenmenger syndrome Severe symptomatic valvular heart disease	Supplemental oxygen Plan for self-management of dehydration and volume overload; may include adjusting medications Bring copy of recent EKG Bring pacemaker or AICD card DVT precautions	Influenza Pneumococcal Hepatitis B	Have sublingual nitroglycerine available in carry-on bag Mefloquine not recommended for people with cardiac conduction abnormalities, particularly for those with ventricular arrhythmias Self-monitoring and management of INR should be tailored to the individual patient by the anticoagulant primary provider

Condition			Vaccines	
Pulmonary diseases	Severe, labile asthma Recent hospitalization for acute respiratory illness Bullous lung disease Active lower respiratory infection Pneumothorax within 2–3 weeks Pleural effusion within 14 days High supplemental oxygen requirements at baseline Major chest surgery within 10–14 days	Supplemental oxygen Discuss with airline need for other equipment on plane (such as nebulizer) Plan for self-management of exacerbations (including COPD, asthma) DVT precautions	Influenza Pneumococcal Hepatitis B	Consider carrying a short course of antibiotics and steroids, as appropriate, for exacerbations Consider advising an inhaler be available in carry-on bag, even if not routinely used
Gastrointestinal diseases	Surgery, including laparoscopic, within 10–14 days Gastrointestinal bleed within 24 hours Colonoscopy within 24 hours Partial bowel obstruction Liver failure (especially cirrhosis or heavy alcohol use)	Emphasize food and water precautions Consider prescribing prophylactic antibiotic for TD Recommend avoiding undercooked seafood, if cirrhosis or heavy alcohol use (Vibrio vulnificus)	Influenza Pneumococcal Hepatitis A Hepatitis B	May experience increased colostomy output during air travel H₂ blockers and PPIs increase susceptibility to TD Use mefloquine with caution in any chronic liver disease For YF vaccine, see the Immunocompromised Travelers section later in this chapter
Renal failure and chronic renal insufficiency	None	Emphasize food and water precautions Plan for self-management of dehydration, which can worsen renal function Arrange dialysis abroad, if needed Adjust medications for CrCl	Influenza Pneumococcal Hepatitis B	Know HIV, hepatitis C, and hepatitis B status Atovaquone-proguanil contraindicated when CrCl <30 mL/min AAKP and Global Dialysis websites can help with finding dialysis centers; check for accreditation For YF vaccine, see the Immunocompromised Travelers section later in this chapter

continued

TRAVELERS WITH CHRONIC ILLNESSES

TABLE 8-1. SPECIAL CONSIDERATIONS FOR TRAVELERS WITH CHRONIC MEDICAL ILLNESSES (continued)

CONDITION	ABSOLUTE AND RELATIVE CONTRAINDICATIONS TO AIRLINE TRAVEL	PRE-TRAVEL CONSIDERATIONS	IMMUNIZATION CONSIDERATIONS	MISCELLANEOUS
Diabetes mellitus	None	Plan for self-management of dehydration, diabetic foot, and pressure sores Insulin adjustments Should check FSBG at 4- to 6-hour intervals during air travel Discuss changes in insulin regimen or oral agent with diabetes specialist Provide physician's letter stating need for all equipment, including syringes, glucose meter, and supplies	Influenza Pneumococcal Hepatitis B	Keep insulin and all glucose meter supplies in carry-on bag Bring food and supplies needed to manage hypoglycemia during travel Check feet daily for pressure sores For YF vaccine, see the Immunocompromised Travelers section later in this chapter
Severe allergic reactions	None	Plan for managing allergic reactions while traveling and consider bringing a short course of steroids for possible allergic reactions Should carry injectable epinephrine and antihistamines (H_1 and H_2 blockers)—always have on person		Many airlines already have policies in place for dealing with peanut allergies Make sure to carry injectable epinephrine in case of a severe reaction while in flight
Autoimmune and rheumatologic diseases	None	Should have a baseline TST or IGRA before starting TNF blockers.	Immunosuppressive medications and TNF blockers may alter response to immunizations Live attenuated vaccines may be contraindicated	Particular emphasis should be placed on food and water precautions and hand hygiene

Abbreviations: DVT, deep vein thrombosis; CHF, congestive heart failure; CABG, coronary artery bypass graft; CVA, cerebrovascular accident; EKG, electrocardiogram; AICD, automatic implantable cardioverter defibrillators; INR, international normalized ratio; COPD, chronic obstructive pulmonary disease; TD, travelers' diarrhea; PPIs, proton-pump inhibitors; YF, yellow fever; CrCl, creatinine clearance; AAKP, American Association of Kidney Patients; FSBG, fingerstick blood glucose; TST, tuberculin skin test; IGRA, interferon-γ release assay; TNF, tumor necrosis factor.

BIBLIOGRAPHY

1. Aerospace Medical Association. Medical Guidelines for Airline Travel. 2nd ed. Alexandria, VA: Aerospace Medical Association; 2003 [cited 2014 Apr 23]. Available from: http://www.asma.org/asma/media/asma/Travel-Publications/medguid.pdf.

2. Chandran M, Edelman SV. Have insulin, will fly: diabetes management during air travel and time zone adjustment strategies. Clin Diabetes. 2003;21(2):82–5.

3. Exemption from import/export requirements for personal medical use, 21 CFR Part 1301 (2004) [cited 2014 Sep 23]. Available from: http://www.deadiversion.usdoj.gov/fed_regs/rules/2004/fr0914.htm.

4. Josephs LK, Coker RK, Thomas M, British Thoracic Society Air Travel Working Group. Managing patients with stable respiratory disease planning air travel: a primary care summary of the British Thoracic Society recommendations. Prim Care Respir J. 2013 Jun;22(2):234–8.

5. McCarthy AE, Burchard GD. The travelers with pre-existing disease. In: Keystone JS, Freedman DO, Kozarsky PE, Connor BA, Nothdurft HD, editors. Travel Medicine. 3rd ed. Philadelphia: Saunders Elsevier; 2013. p. 258–63.

6. Perdue C, Noble S. Foreign travel for advanced cancer patients: a guide for healthcare professionals. Postgrad Med J. 2007 Jul;83(981):437–44.

7. Ringwald J, Strobel J, Eckstein R. Travel and oral anticoagulation. J Travel Med. 2009 Jul–Aug;16(4):276–83.

8. Simons FE. Anaphylaxis. J Allergy Clin Immunol. 2008 Feb;121(2 Suppl):S402–7.

9. Smith D, Toff W, Joy M, Dowdall N, Johnston R, Clark L, et al. Fitness to fly for passengers with cardiovascular disease. Heart. 2010 Aug;96 Suppl 2:ii1–16.

PREGNANT TRAVELERS
Diane F. Morof, I. Dale Carroll

INTRODUCTION

Pregnancy is an altered state of health that requires special considerations. With careful preparation, however, most pregnant women are able to travel safely.

PRE-TRAVEL EVALUATION

The pre-travel evaluation of a pregnant traveler (Box 8-1) should begin with a careful medical and obstetric history, with particular attention to gestational age and evaluation for high-risk conditions. A visit with an obstetrician should be a part of the pre-travel assessment, which should include an ultrasound—to establish the gestational age of the pregnancy and identify any potential problems—and evaluation of the mother's blood type and Rh status. The traveler should be provided with a copy of her prenatal records and physician's contact information. Checking for immunity to various infectious diseases may obviate the need for some vaccines.

A review of the pregnant woman's travel itinerary, including destinations, types of accommodation, and planned activities, should guide pre-travel health advice. Preparation includes educating the pregnant woman regarding avoidance of travel-associated risks, the management of minor pregnancy discomforts, and recognition of more serious complications. Bleeding, severe pelvic or abdominal pain, contractions or premature labor, premature rupture of the membranes, symptoms of preeclampsia (unusual swelling, severe headaches, nausea and vomiting, vision changes), severe vomiting, diarrhea, dehydration, and symptoms of potential deep vein thrombosis (unusual swelling of leg with pain in calf or thigh) or pulmonary embolism (unusual shortness of breath) are conditions that require urgent medical attention.

Pregnant travelers should pack a travel health kit that includes all prescription medications, hemorrhoid cream, antiemetic drugs, antacids, prenatal vitamins, medication for vaginitis or yeast infection, and support hose, in addition to the items recommended for all travelers (see Chapter 2, Travel Health Kits). Pregnant travelers should consider packing a blood pressure monitor if travel may limit access to a health center with blood pressure monitoring available.

 PREGNANT TRAVELERS | 565

BOX 8-1. PRE-TRAVEL CONSULTATION CHECKLIST FOR PREGNANT TRAVELERS

- Ultrasound to establish a reliable due date and to confirm normal pregnancy
- Check for immunity to infectious diseases, for example, hepatitis A and B, rubella, varicella, measles, pertussis
- Update routine immunizations: tetanus-diphtheria-pertussis, influenza (inactivated), and hepatitis A and B
- Destination risk considerations
  - > Infectious disease
    - > Malaria
    - > Outbreak of disease requiring a live virus vaccine
    - > Outbreak of a disease for which no vaccine is available but which has a high risk of maternal or fetal illness or death
    - > Sexually transmitted diseases
    - > Food and water precautions
    - > Insect exposure
  - > Environmental: altitude, heat, humidity, pollution
  - > Medical services available during transit and at destination
- Travel risk assessment
  - > Mode of travel, destination, length of travel, and style
  - > Planned activities such as climbing, water sports, snorkeling
- Supplemental travel insurance, travel health insurance, and medical evacuation insurance (research-specific coverage information and limitations for pregnancy-related health issues)
- Signs and symptoms for which care should be sought immediately
  - > Pelvic or abdominal pain
  - > Bleeding
  - > Rupture of membranes
  - > Contractions or preterm labor
  - > Symptoms of preeclampsia (unusual swelling, severe headaches, nausea and vomiting, vision changes)
  - > Vomiting, diarrhea, dehydration
  - > Symptoms of potential deep vein thrombosis or pulmonary embolism (unusual swelling of leg with pain in calf or thigh, unusual shortness of breath)
- Recommendations
  - > Immunizations that reflect actual risk of disease and probable benefit
  - > Prescription medications maintained in carry-on luggage
  - > Malaria chemoprophylaxis, if indicated
  - > Preventive measures to decrease the above potential risks
- Paperwork
  - > Check airline and cruise line policies
  - > Letter confirming due date and fitness to travel
  - > Copy of medical records
  - > Letter for customs regarding medications
  - > Exemption letter or waiver for required vaccines, if applicable
- Preparing for obstetric care
  - > Check coverage by medical insurance
  - > Arrange for obstetric care at destination, as needed
  - > Check availability of emergency medical assistance
- Comfort arrangements
  - > Loose clothing and comfortable shoes
  - > Pillows, support hose
  - > Bottled water
  - > Upgrade flight seating if possible
  - > Lighten itinerary if not accustomed to planned activities
- Postpone travel if risks outweigh benefits

CONTRAINDICATIONS FOR TRAVEL DURING PREGNANCY

Although travel is rarely contraindicated during a normal pregnancy, complicated pregnancies require extra consideration and may warrant a recommendation that travel be delayed (Box 8-2). Pregnant travelers should be advised that the risk of obstetric complications is highest in the first and third trimesters.

PLANNING FOR EMERGENCY CARE

Obstetric emergencies are often sudden and life-threatening. Travel to remote locations or areas in some developing countries where obstetric care may be less than the standard at home is inadvisable. For a woman in the third trimester of pregnancy, it is advisable to identify a medical facility in her destination that could manage complications of pregnancy, her delivery, a caesarean section, and neonatal problems. Some complications may be managed so that the mother could travel to a facility where she could receive advanced obstetric care, but some conditions are contraindications for any travel (Box 8-2). In such cases, it may be preferable to transport help to the patient rather than transport the patient.

Many general health insurance policies do not cover complications of pregnancy overseas. Supplemental travel health insurance should be strongly considered to cover both pregnancy-related problems and care of the neonate, as needed. Evacuation insurance with a policy that includes coverage of pregnancy-related complications is highly encouraged as well.

TRANSPORTATION CONSIDERATIONS

Pregnant women should be advised to wear seatbelts, when available, on all forms of transport, including airplanes, cars, and buses. A diagonal shoulder strap with a lap belt provides the best protection. The shoulder belt should be worn between the breasts with the lap belt low across the upper thighs. When only a lap belt is available, it should be worn low, between the abdomen and the pelvis.

Air Travel

Most commercial airlines allow pregnant travelers to fly until 36 weeks' gestation. Some limit international travel earlier in pregnancy, and some require documentation of gestational age. Travelers should check with the airline to find out their specific requirements or guidance for pregnant women. Air cabins of most commercial jetliners are pressurized to 6,000–8,000 ft (1, 829–2,438 m) above sea level; the lower oxygen tension should not cause fetal problems in a normal pregnancy, but women with preexisting cardiovascular problems, sickle cell disease, or severe anemia (hemoglobin <8.0 g/dL) may experience the effects of low arterial oxygen saturation. Risks of air travel include potential exposure to communicable diseases, immobility, and the common discomforts of flying. Abdominal distention and pedal edema frequently occur. The pregnant traveler may benefit from an upgrade in airline seating and should seek convenient and practical accommodations (such as close proximity to the toilet) and aisle seating so she can move about frequently. Loose clothing and comfortable shoes should be recommended.

PREGNANT TRAVELERS | 567

Some experts report that the risk of deep vein thrombosis in pregnancy is 5–10 times higher than for nonpregnant women. Preventive measures include frequent stretching, walking and isometric leg exercises, and wearing graduated compression stockings.

Cosmic radiation during air travel poses little threat, but may be a consideration for pregnant travelers who are frequent fliers (such as air crew). Older airport security machines are magnetometers and are not harmful to the fetus. Newer security machines use backscatter x-ray scanners, which emit low levels of radiation; most experts agree that the risk of radiation exposure from these scanners is extremely low.

Cruise Ship Travel

Most cruise lines restrict travel beyond 28 weeks of pregnancy, and some as early as 24 weeks. Pregnant travelers may be required to carry a physician's note stating that they are fit to travel and including the estimated date of delivery. Pregnant women should check with the cruise line to find out their specific requirements or guidance. The pregnant traveler planning a cruise should be advised regarding motion sickness, gastrointestinal and respiratory infections, and the risk of falls on a moving vessel.

ENVIRONMENTAL CONSIDERATIONS

Air pollution may cause more health problems during pregnancy, as ciliary clearance of the bronchial tree is slowed and mucus more abundant. Body temperature regulation is not as efficient during pregnancy, and temperature extremes can cause more stress on the gravid woman. In addition, an increase in core temperature, such as with heat prostration or heat stroke, may harm the fetus. The vasodilatory effect of a hot environment might also cause fainting. For these reasons, accommodation should be sought in air-conditioned quarters and activities restricted in hot environments.

Pregnant women should avoid activities at high altitude unless trained for and accustomed to such activities. Women unaccustomed to high altitudes may experience exaggerated breathlessness and palpitations. The common symptoms of acute mountain sickness (insomnia, headache,

and nausea) are frequently also associated with pregnancy, and it may be difficult to distinguish the cause of the symptoms. Most experts recommend a slower ascent with adequate time for acclimatization. No studies or case reports show harm to a fetus if the mother travels briefly to high altitudes during pregnancy. However, it may be prudent to recommend that pregnant women not stay at sleeping altitudes >12,000 ft (3,658 m), if possible. Probably the largest concern regarding high-altitude travel in pregnancy is that many high-altitude destinations are inaccessible and far from medical care (see Chapter 2, Altitude Illness).

ACTIVITIES

Pregnant travelers should be discouraged from undertaking unaccustomed vigorous physical activity. Swimming and snorkeling during pregnancy are generally safe, but waterskiing has resulted in falls that inject water into the birth canal. Most experts advise against scuba diving for pregnant women because of the risk of fetal gas embolism during decompression. Riding bicycles, motorcycles, or animals presents risk of trauma to the abdomen.

INFECTIOUS DISEASES

Pregnant women who develop travelers' diarrhea or other gastrointestinal infection may be more vulnerable to dehydration than are nonpregnant travelers. Strict hand hygiene and food and water precautions should be stressed (see Chapter 2, Food & Water Precautions). Bottled or boiled water is preferable to chemically treated or filtered water. Iodine-containing compounds should not be used to purify water for pregnant women because of potential effects on the fetal thyroid (see Chapter 2, Water Disinfection for Travelers). The treatment of choice for travelers' diarrhea is prompt and vigorous oral hydration; however, azithromycin may be given to pregnant women if clinically indicated. Use of bismuth subsalicylate is contraindicated.

Hepatitis A and E are both spread by the fecal-oral route. Hepatitis A has been reported to increase the risk of placental abruption and premature delivery. Hepatitis E is more likely to cause severe disease during pregnancy and may result in a case-fatality ratio of 15%–30%; when acquired during the third trimester, it is also associated with fetal complications and fetal death. Some foodborne illnesses of particular concern during pregnancy include toxoplasmosis and listeriosis. The risk during pregnancy is that the infection will cross the placenta and cause spontaneous abortion, stillbirth, or congenital or neonatal infection. Risk of fetal infection increases with the length of gestation, but severity of infection is decreased. The pregnant traveler should be warned, therefore, to avoid unpasteurized cheeses and undercooked meat products. Parasitic diseases are less common but may cause concern, particularly in women who are visiting friends and relatives in developing areas. In general, intestinal helminths rarely cause enough illness to warrant treatment during pregnancy. Most intestinal helminths, in fact, can safely be addressed with symptomatic treatment until the pregnancy is over. On the other hand, protozoan intestinal infections, such as *Giardia*, *Entamoeba histolytica*, and *Cryptosporidium*, often do require treatment. These parasites may cause acute gastroenteritis, severe dehydration, chronic malabsorption resulting in fetal growth restriction, and in the case of *E. histolytica*, invasive disease, including amebic liver abscess and colitis. Pregnant women are advised to avoid swimming or wading in freshwater lakes, streams, and rivers that may harbor schistosomes.

Pregnant women should avoid mosquito bites when traveling in areas endemic for arboviruses or malaria. Preventive measures include the use of bed nets and insect repellents and wearing protective clothing (see Chapter 2, Protection against Mosquitoes, Ticks, & Other Arthropods).

Respiratory and urinary infections and vaginitis are also more likely to occur and to be more severe in pregnancy.

MEDICATIONS

Various systems are used to classify drugs in regard to their safety in pregnancy. In most cases, it is preferable to refer to specific data regarding the effects of a given drug during pregnancy rather than simply to depend on a classification.

Analgesics that can be used during pregnancy include acetaminophen and some narcotics. Aspirin may increase the incidence of abruption, and other anti-inflammatory agents could cause premature closure of the ductus arteriosus. Constipation may require a mild bulk laxative. Several simple remedies are often effective in relieving the symptoms of morning sickness, and these may prevent motion sickness. Nonprescription remedies include ginger, which as a powder can be mixed with food or drinks such as tea. It is also available in candy, such as lollipops. Similarly, pyridoxine (vitamin B6) is effective in reducing symptoms of morning sickness and is available in tablet form, as well as lozenges and lollipops. Antihistamines, such as meclizine and dimenhydrinate, are often used in pregnancy for morning sickness and motion sickness and appear to have a good safety record.

VACCINES

In the best possible scenario, a woman should be up-to-date on routine vaccinations before she becomes pregnant. The most effective way of protecting the infant against many diseases is to immunize the mother. Tetanus, diphtheria, and pertussis (Tdap) vaccine should be given **during each pregnancy** irrespective of the woman's history of receiving Tdap. To maximize the maternal antibody response and passive antibody transfer to the infant, **optimal timing for Tdap administration is between 27 and 36 weeks of gestation,** although it may be given at any time during pregnancy. Annual influenza vaccine (inactivated) is recommended during any trimester for all women who are or will be pregnant (in any trimester) during influenza season; for travelers, vaccination is recommended ≥2 weeks before departure if vaccine is available. Certain vaccines, including meningococcal polysaccharide (MPSV4), and hepatitis A and B vaccines that are considered safe during pregnancy, may be indicated based on risk. No adverse effects of inactivated polio vaccine (IPV) have been documented among pregnant women or their fetuses; however, vaccination of pregnant women should be avoided because of theoretical concerns. IPV can be administered in accordance with the recommended schedules for adults if a pregnant woman is at increased risk for infection and requires immediate protection against polio. Rabies postexposure prophylaxis with rabies immune globulin and vaccine should be administered after any moderate- or high-risk exposure to rabies; preexposure vaccine may be considered for travelers when the risk of exposure is substantial.

Most live-virus vaccines, including measles-mumps-rubella vaccine, varicella vaccine, and live attenuated influenza vaccine, are contraindicated during pregnancy; the exception is yellow fever vaccine, for which pregnancy is considered a precaution by Advisory Committee on Immunization Practices (ACIP). If travel is unavoidable, and the risks for yellow fever virus exposure are felt to outweigh the risks of vaccination, a pregnant woman should be vaccinated. If the risks for vaccination are felt to outweigh the risks for yellow fever virus exposure, pregnant women should be issued a medical waiver to fulfill health regulations. Because pregnancy might affect immunologic function, serologic testing to document an immune response to yellow fever vaccine should be considered. Postexposure prophylaxis of a nonimmune pregnant woman exposed to measles or varicella may be provided by administering immune globulin (IG) within 6 days for measles or varicella-zoster IG within 10 days for varicella. Women planning to become pregnant should be advised to wait 4 weeks after receipt of a live-virus vaccine before conceiving. For certain travel-related vaccines, including Japanese encephalitis vaccine and typhoid vaccine, data are insufficient for a specific recommendation for use in pregnant women. A summary of current ACIP guidelines for vaccinating pregnant women is available at www.cdc.gov/vaccines/pubs/preg-guide.htm.

MALARIA CHEMOPROPHYLAXIS

Malaria may be much more serious in pregnant than in nonpregnant women and is associated with high risks of illness and death for both mother and child. Malaria in pregnancy may be characterized by heavy parasitemia, severe anemia, and sometimes profound hypoglycemia, and may be complicated by cerebral malaria and acute respiratory distress syndrome. Placental sequestration of parasites may result in fetal loss due to abruption, premature labor, or miscarriage. An infant born to an infected mother is apt to be of low birth weight, and, although rare, congenital malaria is a concern.

Because no prophylactic regimen provides complete protection, pregnant women should avoid or delay travel to malaria-endemic areas. However, if travel is unavoidable, pregnant women should take precautions to avoid mosquito bites, and use of an effective prophylactic regimen is essential.

Chloroquine and mefloquine are the drugs of choice for pregnant women for destinations with chloroquine-sensitive and chloroquine-resistant malaria, respectively. Doxycycline is contraindicated because of teratogenic effects on the fetus after the fourth month of pregnancy. Primaquine is contraindicated in pregnancy because the infant cannot be tested for glucose-6-phosphate dehydrogenase deficiency, putting the infant at risk for hemolytic anemia. Atovaquone-proguanil is not recommended because of lack of available safety data. A list of the available antimalarial drugs and their uses and contraindications during pregnancy can be found in Table 3-10 and in Chapter 3, Malaria.

BIBLIOGRAPHY

1. ACOG Committee on Obstetric Practice. ACOG Committee Opinion No. 443: Air travel during pregnancy. Obstet Gynecol. 2009 Oct;114(4):954–5.
2. Carroll ID, Williams DC. Pre-travel vaccination and medical prophylaxis in the pregnant traveler. Travel Med Infect Dis. 2008 Sep;6(5):259–75.
3. CDC. Guidelines for vaccinating pregnant women. Atlanta: CDC; 2014 [cited 2014 Sep 23]. Available from: http://www.cdc.gov/vaccines/pubs/preg-guide.htm.
4. Dotters-Katz S, Kuller J, Heine RP. Parasitic infections in pregnancy. Obstet Gynecol Surv. 2011 Aug;66(8):515–25.
5. Hezelgrave NL, Whitty CJ, Shennan AH, Chappell LC. Advising on travel during pregnancy. BMJ. 2011;342:d2506.
6. Irvine MH, Einarson A, Bozzo P. Prophylactic use of antimalarials during pregnancy. Can Fam Physician. 2011 Nov;57(11):1279–81.
7. Magann EF, Chauhan SP, Dahlke JD, McKelvey SS, Watson EM, Morrison JC. Air travel and pregnancy outcomes: a review of pregnancy regulations and outcomes for passengers, flight attendants, and aviators. Obstet Gynecol Surv. 2010 Jun;65(6):396–402.

8. Mehta P, Smith-Bindman R. Airport full-body screening: what is the risk? Arch Intern Med. 2011 Jun 27;171(12):1112–5.
9. Rasmussen SA, Watson AK, Kennedy ED, Broder KR, Jamieson DJ. Vaccines and pregnancy: past, present, and future. Semin Fetal Neonatal Med. 2014 Jun;19(3):161–9.
10. Roggelin L, Cramer JP. Malaria prevention in the pregnant traveller: a review. Travel Med Infect Dis. 2014 May–Jun;12(3):229–36.

TRAVELERS WITH DISABILITIES

Kira A. Barbre

OVERVIEW

According to the Americans with Disabilities Act, a person has a disability if he or she has a physical or mental impairment that substantially limits at least 1 major life activity. Some travelers with disabilities, including those experiencing reduced mobility, may require special attention and adaptation of transportation services. With proper preparation, many travelers with disabilities can travel internationally. The following recommendations may assist in ensuring safe, accessible travel:

- Assess each international itinerary on an individual basis, in consultation with specialized travel agencies or tour operators
- Consult travel health providers for additional recommendations
- Plan ahead to ensure that necessary accommodations are available throughout the entire trip

AIR TRAVEL
Regulations and Codes

In 1986, Congress passed the Air Carrier Access Act (ACAA) to ensure that people with disabilities are treated without discrimination in a way consistent with the safe carriage of all passengers. The regulations established by the Department of Transportation (DOT) apply to all flights of US airlines as well as flights to or from the United States by foreign carriers.

Because of the act, carriers may not refuse transportation on the basis of a disability. However, there are a few exceptions; for example, the carrier may refuse transportation if the person with a disability would endanger the health or safety of other passengers or if transporting the person would be a violation of Federal Aviation Administration safety rules. (Travelers and their clinicians can learn more about these exceptions and other aspects of the act at http://airconsumer.ost.dot.gov/publications/horizons.htm.) Air carriers are also obliged to accept a declaration by a passenger that he or she is self-reliant. A medical certificate, which is a written statement from the passenger's health care provider saying that the passenger is capable of completing the flight safely without requiring extraordinary medical care or endangering other passengers, can be required only in specific situations (for example, if a person intends to travel with a possible communicable disease, will require a stretcher or oxygen, or if the person's medical condition can be reasonably expected to affect the operation of the flight).

Many airlines voluntarily adhere to codes of practice that are similar to US legislation based on guidelines from the International Civil Aviation Organization. However, these guidelines are not identical to those outlined in US legislation, and the degree of implementation may vary by airline and location. If a traveler's plans include flying between foreign countries while abroad, one must check with the overseas airlines to ensure that the carriers adhere to accessibility standards that are adequate for that traveler's needs.

The Transportation Security Administration (TSA) has established a program for screening travelers with disabilities and their equipment, mobility aids, and devices. TSA permits prescriptions, liquid medications, and other liquids needed by people with disabilities and medical conditions. Travelers who have disabilities or medical conditions that may affect TSA screening may use notification cards to discreetly communicate with the officer. Notification cards are available at www.tsa.gov/traveler-information/notification-card. Travelers can learn more about the TSA guidelines for travelers with disabilities at www.tsa.gov/traveler-information/travelers-disabilities-and-medical-conditions.

Assistance and Accommodations

Under the guidelines of the ACAA, when a traveler with disability requests assistance, the airline is obliged to meet certain accessibility requirements. For example, carriers must provide access to the aircraft door (preferably by a level entry bridge), an aisle seat, and a seat with removable armrests. However, aircraft with <30 seats are generally exempt from these requirements. Any aircraft with >60 seats must have an onboard wheelchair, and personnel must help move the wheelchair from a seat to the lavatory area. However, airline personnel are not required to transfer passengers from wheelchair to wheelchair, wheelchair to aircraft seat, or wheelchair to lavatory seat. In addition, airline personnel are not obliged to assist with feeding, visiting the lavatory, or dispensing medication to travelers. Only wide-body aircraft with ≥2 aisles are required to have fully accessible lavatories. Travelers with disabilities who require assistance should travel with a companion or attendant. However, carriers may not, without reason, require a person with a disability to travel with an attendant.

Airlines may not require advance notice of a passenger with a disability; however, they may require up to 48 hours' advance notice and 1-hour advance check-in for certain accommodations that require preparation time, such as the following services (if they are available on the flight):

- Medical oxygen for use on board the aircraft
- Carriage of an incubator
- Hook-up for a respirator to the aircraft electrical power supply
- Accommodation for a passenger who must travel in a stretcher

- Transportation of an electric wheelchair on a flight scheduled on an aircraft with <60 seats
- Provision by the airline of hazardous material packaging for a battery used in a wheelchair or other assistive devices
- Accommodation for a group of ≥10 people with disabilities who travel as a group
- Provision of an onboard wheelchair to be used on an aircraft that does not have an accessible lavatory

DOT maintains a toll-free hotline (800-778-4838, available 9 AM to 5 PM Eastern Time, Monday through Friday, except federal holidays) to provide general information to consumers about the rights of air travelers with disabilities and to assist air travelers with time-sensitive disability-related issues.

Patients with Respiratory Conditions

Travelers with certain respiratory conditions that cause low blood oxygen levels may need supplemental oxygen to make up for the reduced air pressure in the cabin during flight. More information about air travel for people who may need supplemental oxygen is available at www.uptodate.com/contents/supplemental-oxygen-on-commercial-airlines-beyond-the-basics.

Service Animals

Under the ACAA, carriers must permit guide dogs or other service animals with identification to accompany a person with a disability on a flight. Carriers must permit a service animal to accompany a traveler with a disability to any assigned seat, unless the animal obstructs an aisle or other area that must remain clear to facilitate an emergency evacuation, in which case the passenger will be assigned another seat. However, service animals are not exempt from compliance with quarantine regulations and may not be allowed to travel to all international destinations. They are also subject to US animal import regulations on return (see Chapter 6, Taking Animals & Animal Products across International Borders).

CRUISE SHIPS

US companies or entities conducting programs or tours on cruise ships have obligations regarding access for travelers with disabilities, even if the ship itself is of foreign registry. However, all travelers with disabilities should check with individual cruise lines regarding availability of requested or needed items before booking. Cruise operators and travel agents that cater to travelers with special needs also exist, and a list of some of these can be found at www.disabledtravelers.com/accessible_cruises.htm.

USEFUL LINKS

- Department of Transportation, Aviation Consumer Protection Division
  > New Horizons Information for the Air Traveler with a Disability (http://airconsumer.ost.dot.gov/publications/horizons.htm)
  > Aviation Consumer Protection and Enforcement Rules (see links under Part 382, Passengers with Disabilities) (http://airconsumer.ost.dot.gov/rules/rules.htm)
  > Passengers with Disabilities (site provides a summary of the main points of the DOT rule, Title 14 CFR Part 382) (http://airconsumer.ost.dot.gov/publications/disabled.htm)
- Transportation Security Administration—travelers with disabilities and medical conditions (www.tsa.gov/traveler-information/travelers-disabilities-and-medical-conditions)
- MossRehab ResourceNet (www.mossrehab.com/Accessible-Travel/travel-resources.html)
- American Council of the Blind—lists cruises, books, useful telephone numbers, and links to products for purchase (www.acb.org)
- Society for Accessible Travel and Hospitality (www.sath.org)
- Aerospace Medical Association—medical publications for airline travel (www.asma.org/publications/medical-publications-for-airline-travel)
- Mobility International USA (www.miusa.org)
  > Collection of tipsheets for US travelers going abroad (www.miusa.org/resources?f[0]=field_resource_type%3A60&f[1]=field_resource_audience%3A9)

BIBLIOGRAPHY

1. Nondiscrimination on the basis of disability in air travel, 14 CFR Part 382 (2003) [cited 2014 Sep 23]. Available from: http://airconsumer.dot.gov/rules/382short.pdf.
2. International Civil Aviation Organization. Manual on access to air transport by persons with disabilities. Montréal: International Civil Aviation Organization; 2013 [cited 2014 Sep 23]. Available from: http://www.passepartouttraining. com/uploads/2013/03/ICAO-Manual-Doc-9 984-1st-Edition-alltext-en_published_March-2013.pdf.
3. Josephs LK, Coker RK, Thomas M, British Thoracic Society Air Travel Working Group. Managing patients with stable respiratory disease planning air travel: a primary care summary of the British Thoracic Society recommendations. Prim Care Respir J. 2013 Jun;22(2):234–8.

IMMIGRANTS RETURNING HOME TO VISIT FRIENDS & RELATIVES (VFRs)

Jay S. Keystone

DEFINITION OF VFR

A traveler categorized as a VFR is an immigrant, ethnically and racially distinct from the majority population of the country of residence (a higher-income country), who returns to his or her home country (lower-income country) to visit friends or relatives. Included in the VFR category are family members, such as the spouse or children, who were born in the country of residence.

Some experts have recommended that the term VFR refer to all those visiting friends and relatives regardless of the traveler's country of origin; however, this proposed definition may be too broad and not take into consideration cultural, economic, and attitudinal issues. Thus in this review, the more classic definition is used.

DISPROPORTIONATE INFECTIOUS DISEASE RISKS IN VFRs

Altered migration patterns to North America in the past 30 years have resulted in many immigrants originating from Asia, Southeast Asia, and Latin America instead of Europe. Although 13% of the US population is foreign born, in 2012, up to 40% of certain groups of international travelers from the United States (such as travelers to Asia) listed VFR as a reason for travel. VFRs experience a higher incidence of travel-related infectious diseases, such as malaria, typhoid fever, tuberculosis, hepatitis A, and sexually transmitted diseases, than do other groups of international travelers, for a number of reasons:

- Lack of awareness of risk
- ≤30% have a pre-travel health care encounter
- Financial barriers to pre-travel health care
- Clinics are not geographically convenient
- Cultural and language barriers with health care providers
- Lack of trust in the medical system
- Last-minute travel plans and longer trips
- Travel to higher-risk destinations, such as staying in homes and living the local lifestyle that often includes lack of safe food and water and bed net use
- Divergent health beliefs

Malaria

In 2011, 55% of imported malaria cases in US civilians occurred among VFRs. Data from GeoSentinel Surveillance Network show that among ill travelers who present for medical care, VFRs are 8 times more likely to be diagnosed with malaria than are tourist travelers. Reports from the United Kingdom show similar results for VFR versus tourist travelers to West Africa. Many VFRs assume they are immune; however, in most VFRs,

especially those who left their countries of origin years previously, immunity has waned and is no longer protective. In recent years, a number of VFRs have died of malaria on their return to North America; in 2011, 59% of those with severe malaria for whom the purpose of travel was known were VFRs, mostly returned from West Africa.

Other Infections

In the United States, 66% of typhoid cases occur in VFRs, mostly from South Asia and Latin America; 90% of paratyphoid A cases are imported from South Asia as well. A recent Canadian study showed that 94% of typhoid cases in Quebec were in VFRs, mostly from the Indian subcontinent.

VFR children aged <15 years are at highest risk for hepatitis A, and many are asymptomatic. The Quebec study cited above showed that 65% of hepatitis A cases were in VFRs aged <20 years, and in a Swedish study of 636 cases of imported infection, 52% were in VFRs, of whom 90% were <14 years old. Other diseases, such as tuberculosis, hepatitis B, cholera, and measles, occur more commonly in VFRs after travel.

PRE-TRAVEL HEALTH COUNSELING FOR VFRs

Table 8-2 summarizes VFR health risks and prevention recommendations. It is important to increase awareness among travelers regarding their unique risks for travel-related infections and the barriers to travel health services. If possible, clinics should incorporate culturally sensitive educational materials, provide language translators, and provide handouts in multiple languages.

Vaccinations

Travel immunization recommendations and requirements for VFRs are the same as those for US-born travelers. It is crucial, however, to first try to establish whether the immigrant traveler has had routine immunizations (such as measles and tetanus) or has a history of the diseases. Adult travelers, in the absence of documentation of immunizations, may be considered to be susceptible, and age-appropriate vaccinations (or serologic studies to check for antibody status) should be provided, with 2 caveats:

Table 8-2. Diseases for which VFR travelers are at increased risk, proposed reasons for risk variance, and recommendations to reduce risks specific to travelers visiting friends and relatives[1]

SPECIFIC DISEASES	REASON FOR RISK VARIANCE[2]	RECOMMENDATIONS TO STRESS WITH VFR TRAVELERS
Foodborne and waterborne illness	Social and cultural pressure (eat the meal served by hosts)	Frequent handwashing Avoid high-risk foods (dairy products, undercooked foods) Simplify treatment regimens (single dose, such as azithromycin, 1,000 mg, or ciprofloxacin, 500 mg) Discuss food preparation
Fish-related toxins and infections	Eating high-risk foods Less pre-travel advice	Avoidance counseling about specific foods (such as raw freshwater fish)
Malaria	Longer stays Higher-risk destinations Less pre-travel advice leading to less use of chemoprophylaxis and fewer personal protection measures Belief that one is already immune	Education on malaria, mosquito avoidance, and the need for chemoprophylaxis Consider cost of chemoprophylaxis Use of insecticide-treated bed nets
Tuberculosis (particularly multidrug-resistant)	Increased close contact with local population Increased contact with HIV-co-infected people	Check PPD 2–3 months after return if history of negative tuberculin skin test and long stay (>3 months) Educate about tuberculosis signs, symptoms, and avoidance
Blood borne and sexually transmitted diseases	More likely to seek substandard local care Cultural practices (tattoos, female genital mutilation) Longer stays and increased chance of blood transfusion Higher likelihood of sexual encounters with local population	Discuss high-risk behaviors, including tattoos, piercings, dental work, sexual encounters Encourage purchase of condoms before travel Consider providing syringes, needles, and intravenous catheters for long-term travel
Schistosomiasis and soil-transmitted helminths	Limited access to piped-in water in rural areas for bathing and washing clothes	Avoid freshwater exposure Use liposomal DEET preparation with freshwater exposures[3] Discourage children from playing in dirt Use ground cover Use protective footwear

continued

TABLE 8-2. DISEASES FOR WHICH VFR TRAVELERS ARE AT INCREASED RISK, PROPOSED REASONS FOR RISK VARIANCE, AND RECOMMENDATIONS TO REDUCE RISKS SPECIFIC TO TRAVELERS VISITING FRIENDS AND RELATIVES[1] (continued)

SPECIFIC DISEASES	REASON FOR RISK VARIANCE[2]	RECOMMENDATIONS TO STRESS WITH VFR TRAVELERS
Respiratory problems	Increased close exposure to fires, smoking, or pollution	Prepare for asthma exacerbations by considering stand-by bronchodilators and steroids
Zoonotic diseases (such as rickettsial infections, leptospirosis, viral fevers, leishmaniasis, anthrax, Chagas disease)	Rural destinations Staying with family where animals are kept Increased exposure to insects Increased exposure to mice and rats Sleeping on floors	Avoid animal contact Wash hands Wear protective clothing and use insect repellent Check for ticks daily Avoid thatched roofs and mud walled accommodation and fresh sugar cane juice in Latin America Avoid sleeping at floor level
Envenomations (snakes, spiders, scorpions)	Sleeping on floors	Avoid sleeping at floor level Wear shoes outdoors at night
Toxin ingestion (medication adverse events, heavy metal ingestion)	Purchase of local medications Use of traditional therapies Use of contaminated products (such as pottery with lead glaze) Eating contaminated freshwater fish	Anticipate need and purchase medications before travel Counsel avoidance of known traditional medications (such as Hmong bark tea with aspirin) and high-risk items (such as large reef fish)
Yellow fever and Japanese encephalitis (risk is decreased in adults)	Unclear, partial immunity from previous exposure or vaccination	Avoid mosquitoes by taking protective measures and receiving vaccination when appropriate
Dengue (especially risk of severe dengue)	Severe dengue occurs on repeat exposure to a different serotype of dengue; VFRs more likely to have had previous exposure	Avoid mosquitoes by taking protective measures

Abbreviations: VFR, visiting friends and relatives; PPD, tuberculin purified protein derivative; DEET, N,N-diethyl-m-toluamide.
[1] Adapted from: Bacaner N, Stauffer W, Boulware DR, Walker PF, Keystone JS. Travel medicine considerations for North American immigrants visiting friends and relatives. JAMA. 2004;291(23):2856–64.
[2] Hypothesis unless referenced to support assertions.
[3] In animal models, DEET (liposomal preparations) prevents *Schistosoma* cercariae from penetrating the skin.

- Immunity to hepatitis A should not be assumed; many young adults and adolescents from developing countries are still susceptible. Pre-travel serologic testing for both hepatitis A and B may be worthwhile.

- Consider varicella immunization for immigrants from South and Southeast Asia and Latin America. These travelers may be more susceptible, because infection occurs at an older age in tropical than in temperate regions. Also, rates of death and complications from varicella disease are higher in adults than in children.

Malaria Prevention

VFR travelers to endemic areas should not only be encouraged to take prophylactic medications, but also be reminded of the benefits of barrier methods of prevention, such as bed nets and insect repellents, particularly for children (see Chapter 2, Protection against Mosquitoes, Ticks, & Other Arthropods). VFRs should be advised that drugs such as chloroquine and pyrimethamine, as well as proguanil monotherapy, are no longer effective in most areas, especially in sub-Saharan Africa. These medications are often readily available and

inexpensive in their home countries but are not efficacious.

VFRs should also be encouraged to purchase their medications before traveling to ensure good drug quality. Studies in Africa and Southeast Asia show that one-third to half of antimalarial drugs purchased locally were counterfeit or substandard; a recently published study from Laos showed that 88% of oral artesunate sold in pharmacies was of poor quality.

How to reach VFRs to educate them about the need for travel advice is a perennial problem. Recently, in Australia, an approach to reach VFRs by using community-based initiatives included travel health messages through media, print, and community festivals.

BIBLIOGRAPHY

1. Angell SY, Cetron MS. Health disparities among travelers visiting friends and relatives abroad. Ann Intern Med. 2005 Jan 4;142(1):67–72.
2. Bacaner N, Stauffer B, Boulware DR, Walker PF, Keystone JS. Travel medicine considerations for North American immigrants visiting friends and relatives. JAMA. 2004 Jun 16;291(23):2856–64.
3. Barnett ED, Christiansen D, Figueira M. Seroprevalence of measles, rubella, and varicella in refugees. Clin Infect Dis. 2002 Aug 15;35(4):403–8.
4. Bate R, Coticelli P, Tren R, Attaran A. Antimalarial drug quality in the most severely malarious parts of Africa—a six country study. PLoS One. 2008;3(5):e2132.
5. Greenaway C, Dongier P, Boivin JF, Tapiero B, Miller M, Schwartzman K. Susceptibility to measles, mumps, and rubella in newly arrived adult immigrants and refugees. Ann Intern Med. 2007 Jan 2;146(1):20–4.
6. Hendel-Paterson B, Swanson SJ. Pediatric travelers visiting friends and relatives (VFR) abroad: illnesses, barriers and pre-travel recommendations. Travel Med Infect Dis. 2011 Jul;9(4):192–203.
7. Leder K, Lau S, Leggat P. Innovative community-based initiatives to engage VFR travelers. Travel Med Infect Dis. 2011 Sep;9(5):258–61.
8. Leder K, Tong S, Weld L, Kain KC, Wilder-Smith A, von Sonnenburg F, et al. Illness in travelers visiting friends and relatives: a review of the GeoSentinel Surveillance Network. Clin Infect Dis. 2006 Nov 1;43(9):1185–93.
9. Lynch MF, Blanton EM, Bulens S, Polyak C, Vojdani J, Stevenson J, et al. Typhoid fever in the United States, 1999–2006. JAMA. 2009 Aug 26;302(8):859–65.
10. Pavli A, Maltezou HC. Malaria and travellers visiting friends and relatives. Travel Med Infect Dis. 2010 May;8(3):161–8

HEALTH CARE WORKERS

Henry M. Wu, V. Ramana Dhara, Alan G. Czarkowski, Eric J. Nilles

RISKS FOR HEALTH CARE WORKERS TRAVELING OUTSIDE THE UNITED STATES

Health care workers practicing outside the United States may face unique health hazards. Numerous infectious risks are associated with patient contact or handling clinical

specimens. Various types of health care workers may be at risk:

- Physicians, nurses, and other ancillary clinical staff providing care in international settings, including, clinics, hospitals, and field locations

- Medical students and other health trainees participating in clinical rotations overseas
- Others working in clinics, hospitals, or laboratories, including researchers, laboratory technicians, ancillary staff, and public health workers

Health care workers in all settings are at risk for exposure to numerous infectious diseases, including infections spread through blood and bodily fluids (such as HIV or hepatitis B) or through airborne or respiratory droplet routes (such as tuberculosis [TB] or influenza). Risks vary depending on the duties of the worker, the geographic location, and the practice setting. Increased risks are due to multiple factors including the following:

- Less stringent safety regulations or infection control standards
- Limited availability of personal protective equipment (PPE) or safety-engineered devices
- Unfamiliar practice conditions or equipment
- Challenging practice conditions that can prevent providers from adhering to standard precautions (such as extremely resource-limited settings, natural disasters, or conflict zones) (see Box 8-3, Health care workers in extreme circumstances)
- Unfamiliar medical procedures
- High prevalence of transmissible infections (such as HIV, hepatitis B, hepatitis C, or TB)
- Potentially high infectious burden and increased transmission risk from source patients (such as high HIV viral loads in untreated patients)
- Limited resources for evaluation and treatment after exposure to bloodborne pathogens
- Potential for outbreaks of uncommon infectious diseases that are transmissible in health care settings (such as Middle East respiratory syndrome [MERS] or viral hemorrhagic fevers)
- Increased psychological stress resulting from practicing in resource-limited settings, isolated areas, and long-term assignments

PRE-TRAVEL VACCINATION AND SCREENING

In addition to vaccinations specifically indicated for the country visited, all health care workers should be up-to-date on all routine and recommended vaccinations (or have documented immunity). These include the following:

- Measles, mumps, and rubella
- Influenza
- Varicella
- Tetanus, diphtheria, and pertussis
- Hepatitis B
- Other age-appropriate vaccines or those appropriate for travelers with certain underlying medical conditions (such as pneumococcal vaccine)

For hepatitis B, postvaccination serologic testing is recommended for health care workers; of people who do not respond to a primary vaccine series, 25%–50% respond to an additional vaccine dose, and 44%–100% respond to a 3-dose revaccination series. Inactivated polio vaccine (given as an adult booster dose) or meningococcal vaccine may be indicated for specific locations experiencing high incidence or outbreaks of these infections. Providers should consult country-specific recommendations and travel alerts on the CDC Travelers' Health website (www.cdc.gov/travel) for updated vaccination recommendations.

Regular screening for latent TB infection with tuberculin skin test or interferon-γ release assay is recommended for health care workers, and pre- and post-travel testing is particularly important when the provider is working in a country with a high prevalence of TB infection or in a setting of high TB exposure, such as in prisons (see Chapter 3, Tuberculosis). Routine vaccination of health care workers with bacillus Calmette-Guérin (BCG) is not recommended in the United States; however, BCG vaccination may be considered for some health care workers who will work in settings with high TB transmission risk and a high prevalence of strains resistant to isoniazid and rifampin. Baseline testing for HIV and hepatitis C before travel is not routinely recommended, although it should be considered if risk of exposure will be high and reliable testing will not be available at the destination in the event of an exposure.

PPE AND INFECTION CONTROL

Health care workers should consistently follow standard precautions whenever possible. These include the use of PPE such as gloves, gowns, aprons, surgical masks, and protective eyewear. Workers untrained in standard precautions should not participate in clinical activities, handle clinical specimens, or handle contaminated medical equipment. Needlestick injuries are a common mode

HEALTH CARE WORKERS

of percutaneous exposure to bloodborne pathogens, and practices known to increase risk of needlestick injuries, such as recapping syringes or using needles to transfer a bodily fluid between containers, should be avoided. For further details, guidelines, and training materials on standard precautions and PPE, see www.cdc.gov/HAI/prevent/ppe.html and www.cdc.gov/hicpac/2007IP/2007isolationPrecautions.html.

In preparation, traveling health care workers should

- Ensure they are properly trained for all anticipated procedures, considering the locally available equipment
- Maintain strict safety standards, even if local standards are less stringent
- Bring their own supply of PPE or safety-engineered medical devices if they are unsure of local availability
- Assess the local availability of reliable postexposure prophylaxis (PEP) for HIV, and consider bringing a supply for personal use if unavailable (see HIV PEP, below).

The traveling health care worker should consider the local practice environment, as limited use of PPE or even reuse of equipment that would not be acceptable in the United States is common. Although HIV antiretroviral medications are now available in much of the developing world, traveling health care workers should confirm availability of HIV PEP with their sponsoring institutions in advance of travel, or bring their own supply.

INFECTIONS TRANSMITTED BY AIRBORNE OR DROPLET ROUTES
Health care workers are at risk of acquiring numerous airborne and droplet-transmitted infections from patients. Although some of these pathogens are vaccine preventable (such as measles, influenza, and varicella), airborne or droplet isolation precautions for patients suspected of having some respiratory infections are a mainstay of infection control in the United States. These precautions include PPE such as fit-tested N95 respirator masks and negative-pressure isolation rooms for airborne precautions and surgical masks for droplet precautions. Health care

workers should inquire about the availability of PPE and isolation facilities when working internationally. Bringing a personal supply of PPE for use during travel might be prudent (see above, PPE and Infection Control).

TB is a particular concern for health care workers working overseas in high-incidence areas; however, routine use of N95 respirators in settings with limited diagnostic capabilities and suboptimal isolation facilities can be difficult. Pre- and post-travel screening for latent TB is recommended for workers traveling to highly endemic countries (see above, Pre-Travel Vaccination and Screening).

Traveling health care workers should be aware that they may encounter patients with unusual or novel pathogens, particularly when working in areas where epidemics have occurred (such as MERS in the Arabian Peninsula or avian influenza in Asia), and they should consult the disease-specific CDC websites at www.cdc.gov and the CDC Traveler's Health website (www.cdc.gov/travel) for updates and infection control recommendations.

INFECTIONS TRANSMITTED THROUGH BLOOD OR BODILY FLUIDS
Health care workers are at risk for numerous infections transmitted through exposure to blood or bodily fluids via percutaneous, mucous membrane, or nonintact skin exposures. The prevalence of HIV, hepatitis B (HBV), and hepatitis C virus (HCV) infections high in many countries. The global number of HIV infections among health care workers attributable to sharps injuries has been estimated to be 1,000 cases per year. The risk of HIV transmission is approximately 0.3% after a percutaneous exposure to HIV-infected blood and approximately 0.09% after a mucous membrane exposure. Other bodily fluids that may transmit HIV include cerebrospinal fluid, synovial fluid, pericardial fluid, pleural fluid, peritoneal fluid, amniotic fluid, semen, and vaginal secretions. Saliva, urine, sputum, nasal secretions, tears, feces, vomitus, and sweat are not considered infectious for HIV unless they are visibly bloody. Typically, exposures occur as a result of percutaneous exposure to contaminated sharps, including needles, lancets, scalpels, and broken glass (from capillary or test

tubes). The risk of infection after percutaneous exposures is considered increased with exposure to larger blood volumes (visible blood on the injuring device, hollow-bore needles, deeper injuries, or procedures that involved direct cannulation of an artery or vein). Skin exposures to potentially infectious bodily fluids are only considered to be at risk for HIV infection if there is evidence of compromised skin integrity (for example, dermatitis, abrasion, or open wound). Higher circulating viral load in the source patient is also thought to increase the risk of transmission, and this can be of particular concern in resource-poor settings where treatment for HIV and viral hepatitis is limited.

Hepatitis B vaccination, standard precautions, PPE, and safety-engineered devices are important preventative measures (see above sections, Pre-Travel Vaccination and Screening and PPE and Infection Control). Numerous other infections have also been transmitted to health care workers via blood or bodily fluids, including many that are uncommon or not endemic in the United States, such as viral hemorrhagic fevers, parasitic infections, and brucellosis.

Health care workers who may have been occupationally exposed to blood or bodily fluids should immediately perform the following steps:

- Wash the exposed area with soap and water thoroughly. If mucous membrane exposure has occurred, flush the area with copious amounts of water or saline.
- If possible, assess the HIV and HCV status of the source patient. HBV testing of the source patient may be indicated if the health care worker is not a documented responder to hepatitis B vaccination.
- Rapid HIV testing of the source patient is preferred. Exposures originating from source patients who test HIV negative are considered not to have HIV transmission risk, unless they have clinical evidence of primary HIV infection or HIV-related disease.
- Baseline HIV (and potentially HCV and HBV) testing of the exposed health care worker should be performed at the time of the exposure. Seek qualified medical evaluation as soon as possible to guide decisions on HIV PEP (see below).

Postexposure Prophylaxis (PEP)

A number of medication combinations are available for PEP (see the Updated US Public Health Service Guidelines for the Management of Occupational Exposures to HIV and Recommendations for Postexposure Prophylaxis at http://aidsinfo.nih. gov/guidelines). Expert consultation is important when considering PEP, since regimen choice should be made with consideration of exposed person's medical history, potential drug interactions, and the possibility of exposure to a drug-resistant strain. When expert advice is not immediately available, the National Clinicians' Postexposure Prophylaxis Hotline (PEPline) can be reached toll-free at 888-448-4911 (9 AM to 2 AM Eastern Time daily) for assistance in managing occupational exposures to HIV and hepatitis B and C (http://nccc.ucsf. edu/clinician-consultation/post-exposure-prophylaxis-pep/). When initiating HIV PEP, it must be started as soon as possible. PEP can be stopped if new information changes the assessment; however, waiting to start PEP until all information is gathered can decrease its efficacy.

Other potentially infectious exposures in the source material should be considered and managed as appropriate. If the health care worker is not a documented serologic responder to hepatitis B vaccination or is incompletely vaccinated, postexposure testing of the source patient and health care worker may be indicated, as well as PEP with hepatitis B immune globulin and vaccination. For further details, see www.cdc.gov/mmwr/preview/mmwrhtml/rr6210a1.htm.

Postexposure Testing and Counseling

Health care workers with occupational exposure to HIV should receive standard HIV testing as soon as possible after exposure as a baseline, with follow-up testing at 6 weeks, 3 months, and 6 months (follow-up to 4 months is acceptable if a fourth-generation combination HIV p24 antigen-HIV antibody test is used). Health care workers with known or potential exposure to HCV should also have baseline and follow-up testing for HCV. Extended HIV follow-up testing for up to 12 months is recommended for those who become infected with HCV after exposure to a source coinfected with HIV and HCV.

Postexposure counseling and medical evaluation should be provided, whether or not the exposed person receives PEP. During the first 12 weeks after exposure, health care workers should take precautions to avoid secondary transmission (such as abstaining from sexual contact, using barrier contraception, avoiding blood or tissue donations, and breastfeeding, if possible). When PEP is initiated, exposed health care workers should be counseled regarding drug toxicities, drug interactions, and the importance of adherence. Drug side effects are a common reason for PEP discontinuation, although newer regimens have improved tolerability. The emotional consequences of occupational exposures can be substantial and might be further exacerbated by stressors already present in the work environment. Psychological counseling should be considered an essential part of the management of exposures.

BIBLIOGRAPHY

1. CDC. Healthcare Infection Control Practices Advisory Committee (HICPAC). Atlanta: CDC; 2010 [cited 2014 Jul 31]. Available from: http://www.cdc.gov/hicpac/2007IP/2007isolationPrecautions.html.
2. CDC. Healthcare-associated infections (HAIs). Atlanta: CDC; 2014 [cited 2014 Jul 31]. Available from: http://www.cdc.gov/HAI/prevent/ppe.html.
3. CDC. Tuberculosis (TB). Atlanta: CDC; 2014 [cited 2014 Jul 31]. Available from: http://www.cdc.gov/tb/default.htm.
4. Clinicians Consultation Center. Post-exposure prophylaxis (PEP): timely answers for urgent exposure management. San Francisco: UCSF; 2014 [cited 2014 Sep 24]. Available from: http://nccc.ucsf.edu/clinician-consultation/post-exposure-prophylaxis-pep/.
5. Kuhar DT, Henderson DK, Struble KA, Heneine W, Thomas V, Cheever LW, et al. Updated US Public Health Service guidelines for the management of occupational exposures to human immunodeficiency virus and recommendations for postexposure prophylaxis. Infect Control Hosp Epidemiol. 2013 Sep;34(9):875–92.
6. Lee R. Occupational transmission of bloodborne diseases to healthcare workers in developing countries: meeting the challenges. J Hosp Infect. 2009 Aug;72(4):285–91.
7. Mohan S, Sarfaty S, Hamer DH. Human immunodeficiency virus postexposure prophylaxis for medical trainees on international rotations. J Travel Med. 2010 Jul–Aug;17(4):264–8.
8. Schillie S, Murphy TV, Sawyer M, Ly K, Hughes E, Jiles R, et al. CDC guidance for evaluating health-care personnel for hepatitis B virus protection and for administering postexposure management. MMWR Recomm Rep. 2013 Dec 20;62(RR-10):1–19.
9. Uslan DZ, Virk A. Postexposure chemoprophylaxis for occupational exposure to human immunodeficiency virus in traveling health care workers. J Travel Med. 2005 Jan–Feb;12(1):14–8.
10. Vaid N, Langan KM, Maude RJ. Post-exposure prophylaxis in resource-poor settings: review and recommendations for pre-departure risk assessment and planning for expatriate healthcare workers. Trop Med Int Health. 2013 May;18(5):588–95.

ADVICE FOR AIR CREWS

Phyllis E. Kozarsky

OVERVIEW

As airlines expand their reach and air crews are asked to travel to more exotic destinations, these travelers need to prepare ahead of time for the exposures they may encounter. To some degree, air crews are similar to all travelers to such destinations, but the differences require some modifications of travel health guidance for several reasons:

- Layovers are short, often 24–48 hours.
- Travel is frequent.
- Travel to new destinations may be on short notice.
- Despite short travel times, air crews may be more adventuresome and thus have more risk than typical tourists.
- Air crews interact with each other frequently, and misinformation spreads quickly.

- Air crews may perceive themselves to be low risk because of their generally healthy status and because their exposure time in-country is short.

Given these factors, it is worth noting some guidelines for this special group. In general, air carriers traveling to destinations in the developing world try to inform their crews about health issues they may face. However, airlines do not necessarily have available on their staff occupational health or other providers who are experts in travel medicine, and the airlines may not be aware of special risks at their destinations. Air crews and clinicians seeing such travelers should, therefore, encourage airlines to avail themselves of professionals who are knowledgeable in the field and who can help determine recommendations for the various destinations served.

Pilots often know some of the medications and classes of medications that are not permitted while flying, so clinicians should always discuss medication options. Medications with central nervous system adverse events should not be prescribed, and pilots should take a trial between trips of any new medications or those that could have side effects that may interfere with flying. Pilots and flight attendants should also be aware that certain foods and beverages contain trace amounts of products that could cause a drug screen to turn positive. If questions arise, an aeromedical examiner should be consulted (www.faa.gov/pilots/amelocator/) who will know the Federal Aviation Administration rules for what medications can and cannot be taken by pilots. These physicians are responsible for certifying that pilots are fit to fly, and they examine pilots regularly.

Although any travel health provider can see and advise flight crews, it is important to ask the crew member what the airline may require, in addition to what is required or recommended to maintain the person's health while traveling. If in doubt, the travel health provider should contact the airline medical director or occupational health department for guidance. For example, some air crews primarily fly domestic routes or routes to Western Europe or Japan, so would not fly to a region of yellow fever risk in their normal daily work. However, an airline may require that crew members without contraindications be vaccinated against yellow fever, so that the airline has flexibility to shift crews and be able to address any urgent need.

GENERAL HEALTH MEASURES

Although pilots are required to have periodic provider visits to ensure they are fit to fly, these may not address some issues that may affect them when they travel internationally, particularly to destinations in the developing world. Flight attendants and others should also consider asking their health care providers about these recommendations:

- Administering a periodic tuberculin skin test, if traveling frequently to destinations where the prevalence of tuberculosis is much higher than in the United States, where the incidence of antimicrobial resistance is higher, and where the crew member will be in close contact with crowds (www.who.int/tb/challenges/mdr/en)
- Checking at each visit to make sure that routine immunizations are up-to-date (see below)
- Immunizing against seasonal influenza every year when the vaccine becomes available

In addition, all medications for chronic conditions should be carried in extra quantities, as they may not be available at some locations, and even if available and less costly, may be counterfeit or be of poor quality (see Chapter 2, *Perspectives:* Pharmaceutical Quality & Counterfeit Drugs). The business of manufacturing counterfeit medications in developing countries is huge and growing; it is impossible to tell from the packaging or pills if they are counterfeit. Some counterfeit drugs contain little or no active ingredient, and others contain toxic contaminants.

Vaccinations

Because of the frequency of travel to international destinations, air crews may be exposed to various diseases that are not common in the United States. For example, measles can be a life-threatening illness for adults; it is more common in most of the world, including Europe, because of lack of mandatory childhood immunization against the disease in many countries. In addition, flight crews may not have had chickenpox as children and may not have been immunized. This illness often occurs at a later age in the tropics; thus, if there is interaction with local populations in these destinations, risk for infection will be higher. International flight crews should consider a travel health visit to ensure as complete protection as possible. Some may have short notice before traveling to new destinations; thus, air crew members should be asked about this possibility during their visit, so that vaccinations for an upcoming trip—that may not be imminent—may be given, or a series may be started early. Providers should educate travelers about health risks in the various destinations; whether certain vaccinations are administered will depend on the traveler's tolerance for risk.

Routine Vaccinations

All travelers should make sure they are up-to-date with routine vaccinations (see the separate sections on these diseases in Chapter 3):

- **Measles**—A person born in the United States before 1957 is assumed to be immune to measles. People born after 1957 should have documentation of having had the disease or having had 2 vaccine doses against measles. Measles vaccine is typically given as MMR (measles-mumps-rubella).
- **Varicella**—Strongly recommended for travelers with no history of chickenpox.
- **Polio**—A single booster is recommended as an adult. Although transmission of the polio virus is not a problem in the Western Hemisphere, it remains a risk in some countries in sub-Saharan Africa and in Asia.
- **Diphtheria-tetanus-pertussis**—Administered at 10-year intervals (a single booster of the triple combination, and thereafter Td) for complete protection.
- **Hepatitis B**—Administered to all children and adolescents in the United States, it is advisable for frequent travelers because of the unpredictability of exposure.

- **Hepatitis A**—Administered to all children in the United States, it is advisable for all travelers and may be stressed for air crews, since limited data suggest they have low rates of protection.
- **Influenza**—Recommended annually for all people who do not have a contraindication; should also be stressed for air crews.
- **Others**—Any age-related (such as varicella-herpes zoster) or health maintenance-related (such as pneumococcal) vaccinations should be considered.

Special Vaccinations for Travel

Although there are no established guidelines or recommendations for the use of travel vaccinations in pilots and other air crew members, for some it may be reasonable to offer meningococcal, Japanese encephalitis, yellow fever, and typhoid vaccines because of their frequent, short-stay, and at times unpredictable travel and destinations. As well, they are generally a group who travel frequently beyond work, so they should always be asked during a consultation whether they plan other travel itineraries that can be addressed at the same time.

Malaria Chemoprophylaxis

Crew members are typically informed by their airline as to which destinations harbor malaria. Some European and Asian air carriers have longer experience flying to destinations where malaria is endemic, and these airlines have various policies with respect to its prevention. Although there may be malaria transmission in some areas of destination countries, sometimes there is none in the capitals or the larger urban areas to which the major American carriers fly (such as in China or the Philippines). This is generally not the case in sub-Saharan Africa, where there can be substantial exposure during a short 24-hour layover (however, in Kenya, there is no malaria risk in Nairobi). Although there may be little risk at the hotels in the destination, risk may be increased at the international airports, during unpredictable delays in transit, and during outings on layovers. Even during short single stops (for example, in West Africa on the way to South Africa), there is some risk when the aircraft doors are open. Little published data are available on the risk of malaria for flight crews with short layovers, but some information suggests that it is less than that for tourists.

Unfortunately, experience in American and European air crews to malaria-endemic destinations has shown that air crews continue to acquire malaria, as well as develop severe and complicated disease. Some illness may result from lack of awareness of airline recommendations, failure to take precautions against mosquito bites, lack of compliance with antimalarial prophylaxis, and inaccurate information regarding toxicity of medication. Transmission can be focal and intermittent, so chemoprophylaxis for every trip to a highly endemic region should be stressed.

Flight crew members should have easy access to educational materials and chemoprophylaxis and, if desired, should be able to have an individual risk assessment for preventive measures. For destinations where the prevalence of malaria is high (countries in West Africa, for example), crew members should take prophylaxis for layovers. For other destinations where crews are thought to be at low risk based on local intensity of transmission, accommodations, and personal behaviors, they may be advised to use insect repellents and take no chemoprophylaxis. Flight crews should always

- Educate themselves as much as possible about malaria
- Understand the importance of personal protective measures such as repellents, and use them properly
- Take chemoprophylaxis if recommended.
- Know that if fever or chills occur after exposure, it is a medical emergency
- Know how they can get medical assistance at their destinations or at home in the event of symptoms or signs of malaria

There are several options for malaria chemoprophylaxis, depending on the destination city, although needed duration of prophylaxis and adverse effects profiles of some of the drugs make them less than desirable for air crews. Country-specific recommendations can be accessed either in this text (see Chapter 3, Yellow Fever & Malaria Information, by Country) or on the CDC Travelers' Health website (www.cdc.gov/travel). International airlines generally prefer the combination drug atovaquone-proguanil; its adverse effect profile and its dosing make it the most suitable.

Additional information on malaria prevention may be found in Chapter 3, Malaria.

Food and Water Precautions and Travelers' Diarrhea

Pilots and air crew members should follow the same safe food and water precautions and prevention and management of travelers' diarrhea as other travelers (see Chapter 2, Travelers' Diarrhea). They should also be well versed in the recognition and self-treatment of travelers' diarrhea to shorten the duration of illness that could affect their job performance.

Bloodborne and Sexually Transmitted Infections

Although these risks and preventions are addressed in more detail in other sections, it is worth reiterating that frequent travelers have an increased likelihood of engaging in casual and unprotected sex. It is common to think that people from Western countries would have the same risk of HIV and other sexually transmitted infections; however, travelers have far higher rates of such infections. The risk of acquisition may be higher not only for diseases such as gonorrhea and chlamydia, but also for chronic illnesses such as hepatitis B and C. Dental procedures and activities such as acupuncture, tattooing, and piercing also are ill-advised during travel to developing countries.

BIBLIOGRAPHY

1. Bagshaw M, Barbeau DN. The aircraft cabin environment. In: Keystone JS, Freedman DO, Kozarsky PE, Connor BA, Nothdurft HD, editors. Travel Medicine. 3rd ed. Philadelphia: Saunders Elsevier; 2013. p. 405–12.
2. Byrne N. Urban malaria risk in sub-Saharan Africa: where is the evidence? Travel Med Infect Dis. 2007 Mar;5(2):135–7.
3. Byrne NJ, Behrens RH. Airline crews' risk for malaria on layovers in urban sub-Saharan Africa: risk assessment and appropriate prevention policy. J Travel Med. 2004 Nov–Dec;11(6): 359–63.
4. CDC. Notes from the field: malaria imported from West Africa by flight crews—Florida and

ADVICE FOR AIR CREWS | 585

Pennsylvania, 2010. MMWR Morb Mortal Wkly Rep. 2010 Nov 5;59(43):1412.

5. Schwartz MD, Macias-Moriarity LZ, Schelling J. Professional aircrews' attitudes toward infectious diseases and aviation medical issues. Aviat Space Environ Med. 2012 Dec;83(12):1167–70.

6. Selent M, de Rochars VMB, Stanek D, Bensyl D, Martin B, Cohen NJ, et al. Malaria prevention knowledge, attitudes, and practices (KAP) among international flying pilots and flight attendants of a US commercial airline. J Travel Med. 2012 Dec;19(6):366–72.

HUMANITARIAN AID WORKERS

Brian D. Gushulak

OVERVIEW

Through organizations and agencies or individual activities, many thousands of people are involved in the delivery of humanitarian and disaster relief aid in diverse locations every year. After large-scale events such as earthquakes or tsunamis, the number of those traveling to provide humanitarian aid and assistance can increase. Additionally, many others already engaged in international missionary or faith-based activities often become involved in humanitarian and disaster relief efforts. Maintaining the health of humanitarian aid workers is important to ensure that they are able to deliver care to those in need and avoid additional strain on local health services.

In common with other travelers, people who travel to provide humanitarian aid or disaster relief must first address their personal health and welfare before, during, and after travel. This includes knowledge of and preparation for all the usual elements associated with travel to the area. In addition, aid workers can experience specific risks and situations related to the provision of humanitarian care, such as

- Exposure to the environment that precipitated or sustains a crisis or event, such as a natural disaster or conflict
- Working long hours under adverse or extreme conditions, often in close contact with the affected population
- Damaged or absent infrastructure, including limits in the availability of food, water, lodging, transportation, and health services

- Reduced levels of security and protection
- Stress, ethical, and moral challenges related to the event and the resource capacities of the situation

Humanitarian service can damage personal health. Studies involving long-term humanitarian workers have noted that >35% report that their personal health status deteriorated during the mission. Accidents and violence are documented risks for humanitarian aid workers and cause more deaths than disease and natural causes. Recent estimates place the risk of violence-related deaths, medical evacuations, and hospitalizations at approximately 6 per 10,000 person-years among aid workers. Conditions and outcomes vary by location, nature of the humanitarian event, and time spent in the field.

A study of American Red Cross workers noted a 10% ratio of injury or accident and an exposure to violence of 16%. The same study also showed that >40% found the experience more stressful than expected. An earlier study of deaths among Peace Corps volunteers noted that unintentional injuries were the cause of nearly 70% of deaths, followed by homicide at 17%. Illness was responsible for 14% of the Peace Corps fatalities.

However, risks to humanitarian aid workers are not uniformly distributed across the spectrum of humanitarian aid. Ongoing surveillance of violence directed against humanitarian and disaster relief aid workers continues to demonstrate that a small number of insecure locations (Afghanistan, Pakistan, Sudan, and Somalia) account for most of these events.

PRE-TRAVEL CONSIDERATIONS
Evaluation and Pre-Travel Medical Care

Giving careful attention to pre-travel evaluation, both medical and psychological, in addition to educating travelers, can reduce the likelihood of illness and the need for repatriation. Comprehensive medical examinations can prepare travelers by helping identify previously unrecognized disease and allowing for treatment before travel. Careful evaluation of risk factors (family history, history of alcohol or substance abuse, sexually transmitted diseases, and psychiatric illness) may direct additional evaluation and identify previously unrecognized psychological problems or chronic conditions. Identifying alcohol or substance dependence, depression, or other psychiatric illness is important, as these conditions may be exacerbated by the stress of the mission and are often the reason for emergency repatriation. People planning long-term assignments should have their dental condition assessed and any problems dealt with before departure.

Missionaries and faith-based workers may have additional issues that need to be considered by health care providers. Their service may involve extended periods of time abroad, possibly their entire professional lives, so the provider must consider the implications of long-term residence in areas of health risk. Additionally, they may be accompanied by family members, including young children. Both of these factors engender additional travel health considerations that may be different than those encountered by short-term humanitarian and disaster relief workers. For more information, see the next section in this chapter, Long-Term Travelers & Expatriates.

Those who will be providing medical care or participating in clinical research as part of their humanitarian activities should be evaluated in terms of occupational risk and the need for preventive preexposure or postexposure interventions. Disaster relief and humanitarian aid workers destined for areas of active conflict or limited police presence may benefit from specialized security briefings, either provided by the employing agency or private sources. Medical facilities may be compromised by the disaster or overwhelmed in responding to it. Therefore,

volunteers with underlying conditions or pregnant women should be counseled against travel and encouraged to support the response in other ways. Travelers planning to participate in animal rescue should review information available in Chapter 6, Taking Animals and Animal Products across International Borders, and discuss rabies preexposure prophylaxis with a health care provider.

Travelers who will be caring for people sick with Ebola or other diseases spread by contact with blood or other body fluids should ensure that their organization provides personal protective equipment (PPE), such as masks, gloves, gowns, and eye protection. If the organization does not provide it, travelers must pack PPE and bring it with them, since these items may not be available at the destination.

Regardless of the area of the world in which the aid worker will be deployed, certain basics should be addressed in the pre-travel encounter, including routine vaccinations, malaria chemoprophylaxis (if appropriate), food and water precautions, self-treatment for travelers' diarrhea, risks from insect bites, and injury prevention.

Counseling and Advice

Predeployment education and training are essential, as personal illness or injury burdens the community the worker has come to support. Injuries and motor vehicle accidents are common risks for travelers anywhere in the world; thus, travelers should be sensitive to their surroundings and carefully select the type of transportation and hour of travel, if possible. In disaster and emergency situations, the traveler should also be aware of physical hazards such as debris, unstable structures, downed power lines, environmental hazards, and extremes of temperature. Although rare, emergency situations in developed nations may involve unusual exposures, such as radiation exposures observed after damage to nuclear facilities in Japan in 2011.

Travelers to conflict areas should be aware of landmines and other potential hazards associated with unexploded ordnance. In situations associated with damage or destruction to local services and facilities, humanitarian aid workers should

 HUMANITARIAN AID WORKERS

expect, anticipate, and plan for limited accommodations, logistics, and personal support. Disaster relief and humanitarian aid workers destined for low-resource areas or situations may benefit from pre-travel training and counseling regarding the moral complexities of providing service in these environments.

Preparation
Health Items
The traveler should be advised to prepare a travel health kit that is more extensive than the typical kit and should also be familiar with basic first aid to self-treat any injury until medical attention can be obtained. Aid workers may need to disinfect their own water and may want to carry high-energy, nonperishable food items for emergency use. Humanitarian and disaster relief workers should research the available resources in the destination to tailor how extensive their packed supplies should be.

Those with underlying medical conditions requiring treatment should ensure that, if possible, they travel with prescriptions and medications sufficient for the duration of their service. It is a good practice to separate and store medications in 2 separate allotments in case of loss or theft. People with dental crowns or bridgework may wish to carry temporary dental adhesive for short-term management of a dislodged dental appliance. In addition to a basic travel health kit (see Chapter 2, Travel Health Kits), humanitarian aid workers should consider bringing the following items:

Toiletries
- Toothbrush and toothpaste
- Skin moisturizer
- Soap, shampoo
- Lip balm
- If corrective lenses are used:
  > Extra pair of prescription glasses in a protective case and a copy of the prescription
  > Eyeglasses cleaning supplies and repair kit
  > Extra contact lenses and lens cleaner
- Disposable razor, extra cartridges

- Nail clippers
- Toilet paper
- Menstrual supplies

Protective clothing
- Comfortable, lightweight clothing
- Long pants
- Long-sleeved shirts
- Hat
- Boots
- Shower shoes
- Rain gear
- Bandana or handkerchief
- Towel (highly absorbent travel towel if possible)
- Gloves (leather gloves if physical labor will be performed; rubber gloves if handling blood or body fluids)
- Safety goggles

Items for daily living
- Sunglasses
- Sunscreen
- Insect repellent
- Waterproof watch
- Flashlight
- Spare batteries
- Sewing kit
- Laundry detergent
- Small clothesline and clothespins
- Travel plug or voltage adapters for electronics
- Knife, such as a Swiss Army knife or Leatherman[1]
- If traveling to an area where food and water may be contaminated:
  > Bottled water or water filters/ purification system/water purification tablets
  > Nonperishable food items
- If traveling to malaria-endemic areas:
  > Personal bed net (insecticide-impregnated)

Safety and security
- Money belt
- Cash
- Cellular telephone, equipped to work internationally, or satellite telephone (with charger)

[1] Pack these items in checked baggage, since they are considered sharp objects and will be confiscated by airport or airline security if packed in carry-on bags.

- Candles, matches, and lighter in a zip-top bag[2]
- Extra zip-top bags

Personal Items

Because of the loss of life, serious injuries, missing and separated families, and destruction often associated with disasters, humanitarian aid workers should recognize that situations they encounter may be extremely stressful. Keeping a personal item nearby, such as a family photo, favorite music, or religious material, can offer comfort in such situations. Checking in with family members and close friends from time to time is another means of support. Satellite telephones are small, can work almost anywhere in the world, and can be rented for <$10 per day.

Important Documents

In uncertain circumstances, extra passport-style photos may be required for certain types of visas or for additional work permits. Travelers should bring photocopies of important documents, such as passports and credit cards, as well as copies of their medical, nursing, or other professional license, if applicable. Medical information, such as immunization records and blood type, is also helpful to have. The traveler should carry these copies and also leave copies with someone back home. In addition, they should carry contact information for the person who should be notified in an emergency.

Registration with Embassies

Travelers should enroll in the Department of State's Smart Traveler Enrollment Program (STEP, https://step.state.gov/step/) to register with the US embassy in the destination country before departure. This will ensure that the local consulate is aware of their presence, they can receive notifications, and they may be accounted for and included in evacuation plans. They should also consider supplemental travel, travel health, and medical evacuation insurance to cover medical care and evacuation should they become ill or injured.

POST-TRAVEL CONSIDERATIONS

Returning disaster relief and humanitarian aid workers should be advised to seek medical care if they sustained injuries during their travel or become ill after returning. To ensure proper evaluation, they should advise their providers of the nature of their recent travel.

Depending upon the length of time away or their activities (such as working in health care), returning aid workers may benefit from a complete medical review. Homecoming has also been identified as a risk period for difficulties in psychological adjustment, and treatment or counseling should be sought. Workers who witnessed or were involved in situations of mass casualties, deaths, or serious injuries or who have been victims of violence (assault, kidnapping, or serious road traffic crash) should be considered for referral for critical incident counseling.

Studies have indicated that >30% of aid workers report depression shortly after returning home. The adjustment process can be assisted by a skilled debriefing. Generally, humanitarian aid and disaster relief workers are able to adapt to the acute and chronic stressors of their work and demonstrate considerable resilience, but they will also benefit from proper rest and support to help them fully adjust back into the home environment.

BIBLIOGRAPHY

1. Aid Worker Security Database (AWSD) [database on the Internet]. London: Humanitarian Outcomes. 1997–present. Total incidents by country; [cited 2014 Sep 24]. Available from: https://aidworkersecurity. org/incidents/report/country.
2. Callahan MV, Hamer DH. On the medical edge: preparation of expatriates, refugee and disaster relief workers, and Peace Corps volunteers. Infect Dis Clin North Am. 2005 Mar;19(1):85–101.
3. CDC. Coping with a traumatic event: information for the public. Atlanta: CDC; 2009 [cited 2012 Sep 23]. Available from: http://www.bt.cdc.gov/masscasualties/copingpub.asp.

[2] See www.tsa.gov for restrictions on traveling with lighters and matches.

 HUMANITARIAN AID WORKERS

4. Connorton E, Perry MJ, Hemenway D, Miller M. Humanitarian relief workers and trauma-related mental illness. Epidemiol Rev. 2012 Jan;34(1):145–55.

5. Gamble K, Lovell D, Lankester T, Keystone JS. Aid workers, expatriates and travel. In: Zuckerman J, editor. Principles and Practice of Travel Medicine. Hoboken, NJ: Wiley; 2001. p. 448–66.

6. Kortepeter MG, Seaworth BJ, Tasker SA, Burgess TH, Coldren RL, Aronson NE. Health care workers and researchers traveling to developing-world clinical settings: disease transmission risk and mitigation. Clin Infect Dis. 2010 Dec 1;51(11):1298–305.

7. McFarlane CA. Risk associated with the psychological adjustment of humanitarian aid workers. The Australas J Disaster Trauma Stud [serial on the Internet]. 2004 [cited 2012 Sep 23]. Available from: http://www.massey.ac.nz/~trauma/issues/2004-1/mcfarlane.htm.

8. Mitchell AM, Sakraida TJ, Kameg K. Critical incident stress debriefing: implications for best practice. Disaster Manag Response. 2003 Apr–Jun;1(2):46–51.

9. Nurthen NM, Jung P. Fatalities in the Peace Corps: a retrospective study, 1984 to 2003. J Travel Med. 2008 Mar–Apr;15(2):95–101.

10. Peytremann I, Baduraux M, O'Donovan S, Loutan L. Medical evacuations and fatalities of United Nations High Commissioner for Refugees field employees. J Travel Med. 2001 May–Jun;8(3):117–21.

LONG-TERM TRAVELERS & EXPATRIATES

Lin H. Chen, Davidson H. Hamer

The risk of illness or injury increases with duration of travel, so special consideration should be given to travelers who are planning long-term visits (≥6 months is a common definition) to low- or middle-income countries, whether they are expatriates with definite plans or are adventurers with open itineraries. Points to discuss in the pre-travel consultation include accessing care at the destination, vaccines, infectious diseases not prevented by vaccines, injury, and psychological and cultural issues that long-term travelers may encounter.

ACCESSING CARE ABROAD

Before departure, all long-term travelers should undergo complete medical and dental examinations. Travelers should anticipate that they will need care at some point during their stay, and they should plan where they will get it and how they will pay for it. Those traveling for work or with an organization (such as a university or the Peace Corps) may have a predetermined source of care; other travelers should identify a source in advance (see Chapter 2, Obtaining Health Care Abroad for the Ill Traveler). Long-term travelers should also determine if they will need supplemental travel health insurance and evacuation insurance (see Chapter 2, Travel Insurance, Travel Health Insurance, & Medical Evacuation Insurance), since health insurance can be a challenge to procure locally.

In some countries, travelers are likely to encounter counterfeit or low-quality medications. Because the pills and packaging may be nearly indistinguishable from their legitimate counterparts, travelers should bring a sufficient supply of their routine medications (antihypertensive or antihyperlipidemic drugs, for example) from the United States (see Chapter 2, *Perspectives: Pharmaceutical Quality & Counterfeit Drugs*).

VACCINES

Routine vaccines, including influenza vaccine, should be updated. In addition, long-term travelers should be aware of any vaccine requirements at their destination, either for employment, schooling, or entry. A number of travel-related vaccines warrant consideration:

- Hepatitis A and typhoid vaccines are appropriate given the cumulative risk, although the traveler should be aware that the latter does not provide full protection.
- Travel-associated hepatitis B infections are rare, but the risk for travelers may

be higher than for nontravelers, and the vaccine should be considered for all long-term travelers and expatriates.

- Meningococcal disease is more likely in travelers with prolonged exposure to local populations in endemic or epidemic areas; quadrivalent vaccine should be considered for those at risk.
- According to the Advisory Committee on Immunization Practices recommendations, Japanese encephalitis vaccine is recommended for travelers who plan to reside in endemic areas or who plan to visit ≥1 month during the virus transmission season (see Chapter 3, Japanese Encephalitis).
- Rabies preexposure immunoprophylaxis is an important consideration for people spending a prolonged time in endemic countries, especially in areas where rabies immune globulin is not available (which is true of many resource-limited countries). Vaccinating children who will be living in high-risk areas is a priority.
- Yellow fever vaccine should be considered for travelers who will be staying in an endemic area or a country with a vaccine requirement, or who may be traveling to one.

In addition to the intended destination, consider disease risk in surrounding areas, since long-term travelers may be likely to travel locally. For example, a short-term traveler to Seoul would not be considered at risk for Japanese encephalitis, but an expatriate living in Seoul may have opportunities to visit the Korean countryside or other areas in Asia where he or she could be exposed.

INFECTIOUS DISEASES NOT PREVENTED BY VACCINES
Malaria

Data suggest that the incidence of malaria increases and the use of preventive measures decreases with increasing length of stay. For instance, malaria incidence in British travelers returning from West Africa after a stay of 6–12 months was 80 times that of the incidence in travelers who had stayed only 1 week. Among expatriate corporate employees in Ghana, adherence to malaria chemoprophylaxis deteriorated with increasing duration of stay, and all

those who had been on the site for >1 year had abandoned chemoprophylaxis. About half of the cohort used insect repellent only intermittently, and more than one-third never used repellent. Even though most British expatriates from the UK Foreign and Commonwealth Office had good knowledge about malaria and its prevention strategies, they adhered to malaria chemoprophylaxis <25% of the time; only 25% reported rigorous compliance, and 13% reported having contracted malaria. Given the high relative risk of malaria for travelers in Africa, these data on long-term travelers and expatriates highlight worrisome risks and practices.

A traveler who will be residing in an area of continuous malaria transmission should continue to use malaria chemoprophylaxis for his or her entire stay. It is important to reassure the traveler that the drugs are safe and effective. Doxycycline has been well-tolerated for long-term malaria chemoprophylaxis in the military, and CDC has no recommended limits on its duration of use for malaria chemoprophylaxis. Mefloquine has been well-tolerated during prolonged stays by Peace Corps volunteers, with a discontinuation rate of 0.9%, and showed no evidence of accumulation after long-term use. Mefloquine may be appropriate for long-term chemoprophylaxis for chloroquine-resistant areas because of its convenient weekly dosing, but concern has increased regarding its neuropsychiatric side-effect profile. The new Food and Drug Administration label indicating that neurologic side effects may persist might limit drug acceptability among travelers. Atovaquone-proguanil has shown good long-term tolerability in postmarketing surveillance, with a discontinuation rate of only 1% because of diarrhea. Long-term use of chloroquine raises concern for retinal toxicity when a cumulative dose of 100 g is reached, which may occur after 5–6 years of weekly dosing. A baseline ophthalmic examination is recommended, with follow-up every 6–12 months after 5 years of use. Except for ophthalmologic evaluation when taking chloroquine long-term, no specific testing is recommended for the long-term use of other antimalarial drugs.

The possibility of pregnancy requires careful consideration for long-term female travelers to malarious areas (see the

Pregnant Travelers section earlier in this chapter). Malaria infection during pregnancy can result in severe complications to both mother and fetus. When pregnancy is anticipated, chemoprophylaxis options may need to be adjusted. Ideally, this possibility should be explored before travel with all female long-term travelers of childbearing age. For women who are pregnant or plan to become pregnant during long-term travel, mefloquine is considered safe in all trimesters. Data from published studies in pregnant women have shown no increase in the risk of teratogenic effects or adverse pregnancy outcomes after mefloquine prophylaxis during pregnancy. Chloroquine has also been used long-term without ill effect on pregnancy. If a woman traveling long-term is taking atovaquone-proguanil, doxycycline, or primaquine, she should discontinue her medication and begin weekly mefloquine (or chloroquine in those areas where it remains efficacious) and wait at least 3–4 weeks to conceive so that a therapeutic blood level of mefloquine can build up.

Women who become pregnant while taking antimalarial drugs do not need a therapeutic abortion but should be advised during the pre-travel consultation of potential risks. The effect of atovaquone-proguanil on the fetus is unknown, but doxycycline is associated with fetal toxicity in animals and is contraindicated in pregnant women. Primaquine may harm a glucose-6-phosphate dehydrogenase–deficient fetus, so it should not be used in pregnancy.

For long-term travelers, the need for adjuncts to chemoprophylaxis should also be stressed, such as personal protection measures to avoid mosquito bites (sleeping under a bed net, using screens, and applying repellents). Travelers should bring a sufficient supply of antimalarial drugs from the United States, since drugs purchased at the destination may be of poor quality or counterfeit. Even with urging to adhere to personal protective measures and reassurance that long-term chemoprophylaxis is safe and effective, adherence is likely to decline over time. Consequently, the pre-travel consultation for a long-term traveler to a malarious area should stress the severity of malaria, its signs and symptoms, and the need to seek care immediately if they develop. Travelers could consider bringing a reliable supply of drugs to treat malaria if they are diagnosed with malaria. For additional discussion, see the next section in this chapter, *Perspectives:* Malaria in Long-Term Travelers & Expatriates.

Other Diseases

Because diarrhea and gastrointestinal diseases are common in long-term travelers, they should be educated about the management of acute diarrhea, including rehydration, the use of antimotility agents, empiric antimicrobial therapy, and when to seek care.

Tuberculosis risk may rise to the level of the local population if the traveler or expatriate has a longer stay and intimate contact with the local population. A baseline tuberculin test or interferon-γ release assay, followed by the same test after travel, should be considered, especially for health care workers or those who may be working in hospitals, refugee camps, or in prisons.

Likewise, dengue seroconversion occurred at a rate of 3.4/1,000 people per month of stay in endemic areas among development aid workers. Other mosquitoborne viral illnesses are also a risk, so long-term travelers and expatriates should be advised to protect themselves from the mosquito vectors.

Risk for HIV and sexually transmitted infections are increased in travelers and expatriates, and the consistent use of condoms in expatriates is low (approximately 20%). Long-term travelers should be educated about the risk of HIV and sexually transmitted diseases in their destination, as well as preventive measures. The potential for occupational exposure to HIV is important to consider in health care workers; postexposure prophylaxis with highly active antiretroviral therapy and risk avoidance should be included in the pre-travel consultation (see the Health Care Worker section earlier in this chapter).

Transfusion is a potential source of hepatitis C infection in expatriates. The risk of hepatitis E, spread by the fecal-oral route, is highest in Asia, although it has been transmitted in many different tropical locations. Pregnant women are at highest risk of fulminant disease.

ADVISING TRAVELERS WITH SPECIFIC NEEDS

Other infections vary with location and include giardiasis, amebiasis, strongyloidiasis, schistosomiasis, cutaneous leishmaniasis, and filariasis. *Strongyloides stercoralis* infections can be prevented by not walking barefoot through soil, and schistosomiasis may be prevented by not swimming or wading in fresh water. This latter risk is difficult to communicate to long-term travelers who, for example, may be living in sub-Saharan Africa and who look forward to river rafting or vacationing at a lake. The risks of strongyloidiasis and schistosomiasis increase with long-term travel, so screening on return should also be discussed. Cutaneous leishmaniasis and filariasis should be reviewed if a traveler has the potential geographic exposure risk. Compared with short-term travelers, long-term travelers also experience more chronic diarrhea and postinfectious irritable bowel syndrome (possibly because of complacency), and should be advised to continue food and water precautions in order to reduce the risk for these conditions.

INJURY

Injuries are the leading cause of preventable death in travelers, so long-term travelers should be educated about safety. Road and vehicle safety should be stressed, and travelers should choose the safest vehicle options available. Roads are often poorly constructed and maintained, traffic laws may not be enforced, vehicles may not have seatbelts or be properly maintained, and drivers may be reckless and poorly trained. See Chapter 2, Injury Prevention for strategies to reduce the risk of traffic and other injuries.

PSYCHOLOGICAL ISSUES

The stress of long-term travel can trigger or exacerbate psychiatric reactions. A long-term traveler should be assessed for preexisting psychiatric diagnosis, depressed mood, recent major life stressors, and use of medications that may have psychiatric effects. These conditions may suggest a need for further screening. All long-term travelers should be urged to take care of their physical and mental health by exercising regularly and eating healthfully. They should be able to recognize signs of anxiety and depression and have a plan for coping with them. Having photographs or other mementoes of friends and family at hand and staying in close contact with loved ones at home can alleviate the stress of long-term travel. For more information, see Chapter 2, Mental Health.

LONG-TERM TRAVELERS WITH OPEN ITINERARIES

Offering pre-travel care to travelers with no itinerary (or those who present with only vague travel plans) presents unique challenges. These travelers benefit from broad immunization coverage for all potential exposures to vaccine-preventable diseases, although some prioritization may be necessary. Because their plans are unclear, these travelers must understand that they may need to diagnose and treat themselves for common ailments, including travelers' diarrhea, upper respiratory tract infections, urinary tract infections, vaginitis, skin disorders, and musculoskeletal problems (see Chapter 2 for details on a variety of self-treatable conditions). In addition to strategies to prevent health problems and injuries during their long sojourns, traveler education is imperative regarding health resources, signs and symptoms that require urgent medical evaluation, and medical evacuation.

SCREENING LONG-TERM TRAVELERS AND EXPATRIATES AFTER RETURN

Long-term travelers, whether they are expatriate workers, Peace Corps volunteers, or highly adventurous travelers, need a thorough medical interview to assess potential infectious exposures after return to their country of origin. A careful itinerary-specific history with detailed questioning about potential high-risk exposures, including food, water, animal, and human contact, is the foundation of the post-travel evaluation. A physical examination focused on specific signs and symptoms and a selected array of laboratory tests, including a complete blood count with differential, hepatic transaminases, and serologic markers depending on types of exposure, are helpful to detect subclinical infections and determine whether seroconversion to common pathogens has occurred (see Chapter 5, Screening Asymptomatic Returned Travelers). A benefit of the post-travel evaluation is preventive counseling for potential future travel.

BIBLIOGRAPHY

1. Chen LH, Wilson ME, Davis X, Loutan L, Schwartz E, Keystone J, et al. Illness in long-term travelers visiting GeoSentinel clinics. Emerg Infect Dis. 2009 Nov;15(11):1773–82.

2. Chen LH, Wilson ME, Schlagenhauf P. Prevention of malaria in long-term travelers. JAMA. 2006 Nov 8;296(18): 2234–44.

3. Clerinx J HD, von Gompel A. Post-travel screening. In: Keystone J, Kozarsky P, Freedman DO, Nothdurft HD, Connor BA, editors. Travel Medicine. 3rd ed. Philadelphia: Saunders Elsevier; 2013. p. 467–74.

4. Cockburn R, Newton PN, Agyarko EK, Akunyili D, White NJ. The global threat of counterfeit drugs: why industry and governments must communicate the dangers. PLoS Med. 2005 Apr;2(4):e100.

5. Cunningham J, Horsley J, Patel D, Tunbridge A, Lalloo DG. Compliance with long-term malaria prophylaxis in British expatriates. Travel Med Infect Dis. 2014 Jul–Aug;12(4):341–8.

6. Hamer DH, Ruffing R, Callahan MV, Lyons SH, Abdullah AS. Knowledge and use of measures to reduce health risks by corporate expatriate employees in western Ghana. J Travel Med. 2008 Jul–Aug;15(4):237–42.

7. Lim PL, Han P, Chen LH, MacDonald S, Pandey P, Hale D, et al. Expatriates ill after travel: results from the Geosentinel Surveillance Network. BMC Infect Dis. 2012;12:386.

8. Pierre CM, Lim PL, Hamer DH. Expatriates: special considerations in pretravel preparation. Curr Infect Dis Rep. 2013 Aug;15(4):299–306.

9. Toovey S, Moerman F, van Gompel A. Special infectious disease risks of expatriates and long-term travelers in tropical countries. Part II: infections other than malaria. J Travel Med. 2007 Jan–Feb;14(1):50–60.

10. Visser JT, Edwards CA. Dengue fever, tuberculosis, human immunodeficiency virus, and hepatitis C virus conversion in a group of long-term development aid workers. J Travel Med. 2013 Nov–Dec;20(6): 361–7.

Perspectives

MALARIA IN LONG-TERM TRAVELERS & EXPATRIATES

Lin H. Chen

Long-term travelers and expatriates in malarious areas are at risk for severe malaria throughout their stay, but sometimes they do not recognize the continued need for reducing risk through chemoprophylaxis and personal protective measures. Even those with knowledge of the need for preventive practices may be unable to adhere to them or may opt to discontinue them. Guidelines for malaria prevention might be interpreted as focusing on preventing *Plasmodium falciparum* malaria in short-term travelers. Optimal malaria prevention in long-term travelers poses dilemmas because of diverse traveler

Perspectives sections are written as editorial discussions aiming to add depth and clinical perspective to the official recommendations contained in the book. The views and opinions expressed in this section are those of the author and do not necessarily represent the official position of CDC.

characteristics and itineraries (including traveling in and out of malarious areas), the heterogeneous quality of and access to medical care, and the limited reports on long-term safety and efficacy of antimalarial drugs. Moreover, parasite resistance, seasonality, and the intensity of transmission evolve with environmental and population alterations.

For this discussion, long-term travelers are defined as nonimmune travelers staying in malaria-endemic countries for ≥6 months. A recent review summarized published data on the risk of malaria in long-term travelers, evidence for personal protective measures, and safety and tolerability of malaria chemoprophylaxis during long-term use (Box 8-4).

INDIVIDUALIZED RISK CONSIDERATIONS

Some travelers have preconceived notions about malaria prevention for their long-term journey or stay in an endemic region that may shape their acceptance of standard recommendations. Even when educational efforts appear successful in convincing such travelers to take chemoprophylaxis, they often meet other travelers or locals who convince them that the medication is either not necessary or is in some way detrimental to their health. Nonetheless, taking a detailed assessment of the traveler's risk and attitude may help the clinician determine the traveler's likelihood of adherence to preventive actions during long-term travel. Consider asking about the following:

- Traveler's beliefs regarding personal protective measures
- Traveler's knowledge and preferences toward continuous chemoprophylaxis

BOX 8-4. KEY FINDINGS FROM A REVIEW OF STUDIES RELEVANT TO LONG-TERM TRAVELERS AND EXPATRIATES[1]

- Long-term travelers are at higher risk for malaria than short-term travelers.
- Long-term travelers underuse personal protective measures and often abandon continuous chemoprophylaxis.
- Travelers use a variety of unproven strategies during long stays: discontinuing chemoprophylaxis after the initial period of stay, using different medications for chemoprophylaxis in succession, relying on standby emergency self-treatment, or taking chemoprophylaxis intermittently during high-transmission periods or locations.
- All the chemoprophylaxis strategies have advantages and disadvantages, but chemoprophylaxis is recommended for at least high-transmission destinations and seasons. People who elect to take chemoprophylaxis only for high-transmission destinations and seasons should ensure they have access to a reliable supply of a full course of an approved malaria treatment regimen (Box 3-3 and Table 3-8).
- Counterfeit drugs (including antimalarial drugs) threaten the health of long-term travelers who obtain their medications in developing countries.
- Primaquine (in people with adequate levels of glucose-6-phosphate dehydrogenase) can be used as presumptive antirelapse therapy after long exposures in areas with high *Plasmodium vivax* prevalence.

[1] Adapted from: Chen LH, Wilson ME, Schlagenhauf P. Prevention of malaria in long-term travelers. JAMA. 2006;296(18):2234–44.

- Travel characteristics, including the quality of accommodations, activities, and social support and network
- Economic considerations
- Destination-specific infrastructure, including medical service, access to high-quality care, medication supply, and availability of repellents, insecticides, and nets

PRACTICAL RECOMMENDATIONS
Personal Protective Measures
Preventing malaria in all travelers is a complex issue and particularly so for long-term travelers and expatriates, who require personalized expert advice. For long-term travelers and expatriates, malaria prevention must stress the role of personal protective measures as an adjunct to chemoprophylaxis, including adapting behaviors to minimize mosquito exposure, staying in housing with screened windows and doors, using air conditioning, sleeping under an insecticide-treated bed net, applying insecticide sprays in the residence, managing the environment to reduce vector breeding, using effective repellent, and wearing long sleeves and pants when practical (Box 8-5).

Malaria Chemoprophylaxis
Chemoprophylaxis decreases the risk of illness, hospitalization, and death. However, some travelers may disregard chemoprophylaxis recommendations. Working with the traveler to overcome his or her concerns, providing insight into the severity of malaria, and deriving a feasible and sensible chemoprophylaxis plan are recommended (Box 8-6). For example, a long-term traveler or expatriate based in a malaria-endemic country with highly seasonal or geographically focal malaria transmission may rely primarily on personal protective measures at some times and target periods of chemoprophylaxis during the transmission season or when venturing into endemic areas. However, a traveler who will be staying in an area of high continuous malaria transmission should continue to use malaria chemoprophylaxis for the entire stay.

Another scenario that may arise and merits discussion with long-term travelers is whether they should continue malaria chemoprophylaxis if they develop fever during travel. Rapid diagnostic tests are unreliable for

BOX 8-5. PRACTICAL ADVICE ON PERSONAL PROTECTIVE MEASURES FOR CLINICIANS COUNSELING LONG-TERM TRAVELERS AND EXPATRIATES

- Instruct on treating clothing and bed nets with a pyrethroid insecticide
- Discuss the effectiveness of applying repellent
- Review experience regarding efficacy and safety of repellents: in >60 years since DEET came into wide use, no adverse effects attributed to long-term use have been published
- Discuss mosquito-proofing methods for use in accommodations, including maintenance of drains, elimination of mosquito breeding sites, installation of screens, and applying insecticide indoors
- Advise on the biting habits of the local *Anopheles* mosquito populations

self-diagnosis in travelers because most travelers are not able to use and read the test correctly. (In the United States, rapid diagnostic tests are only approved for laboratory use.) Because fever has numerous possible causes besides malaria, travelers should continue their recommended chemoprophylaxis provided that they are tolerating it well. In addition, they should be tested for malaria, even if taking prophylaxis. Obviously, the possibility of other treatable causes of fever should be explored. Travelers who will be >24 hours from adequate medical care should consider carrying a full course of malaria medication for emergency self-treatment when malaria is suspected, regardless of whether they take continuous chemoprophylaxis. Travelers who might self-administer treatment should be told that they still require follow-up care as soon as they are able to access it.

Unfortunately, in many countries, malaria is a frequent diagnosis in people who do not have malaria. In addition to receiving unnecessary treatment, long-term travelers and expatriates who are misdiagnosed with malaria may stop taking their chemoprophylaxis because they erroneously believe that it did not work. It is difficult to relay such a concept during the pre-travel consult, but the attempt should be made.

SUMMARY

Recommendations for malaria prevention in all travelers must be personalized. Tailoring advice by assessing the traveler's preferences and determining the traveler's possible adherence, along with education regarding malaria, will likely result in better adherence than simply prescribing a course of chemoprophylaxis. The following messages should be conveyed to the long-term traveler regarding malaria prevention:

- Adherence to chemoprophylaxis is essential.
- Use of personal protective measures, such as bed nets and screens, is critical (as many will not use repellents long term).
- Reliable medical facilities at the destination should be located as soon as feasible.
- Data support the safety of long-term use of chemoprophylaxis.
- Supplies of antimalarial drugs should be brought from home, because counterfeit and poor-quality drugs are prevalent in malaria-endemic countries.
- Fever is a worrisome sign, and malaria must be considered and ruled out (see Chapter 5, Fever in Returned Travelers).
- A medical evacuation insurance policy should be purchased if the traveler will be in an area with inadequate medical facilities.
- Although individual use of rapid diagnostic tests is not advised, carrying standby treatment with follow-up medical care may be appropriate for some.
- Presumptive antirelapse therapy may be appropriate for exposure in areas with intense *P. vivax* transmission (after a normal level of glucose-6-phosphate dehydrogenase is documented).
- Misconceptions regarding malaria are pervasive in malaria-endemic countries among expatriates and local residents, and long-term travelers should trust health advice only from reputable and respected sources.

BIBLIOGRAPHY

1. Berg J, Visser LG. Expatriate chemoprophylaxis use and compliance: past, present and future from an occupational health perspective. J Travel Med. 2007 Sep–Oct;14(5):357–8.
2. Chen LH, Wilson ME, Davis X, Loutan L, Schwartz E, Keystone J, et al. Illness in long-term travelers visiting GeoSentinel clinics. Emerg Infect Dis. 2009 Nov;15(11):1773–82.
3. Chen LH, Wilson ME, Schlagenhauf P. Controversies and misconceptions in malaria chemoprophylaxis for travelers. JAMA. 2007 May 23;297(20):2251–63.
4. Chen LH, Wilson ME, Schlagenhauf P. Prevention of malaria in long-term travelers. JAMA. 2006 Nov 8;296(18):2234–44.
5. Cunningham J, Horsley J, Patel D, Tunbridge A, Lalloo DG. Compliance with long-term malaria prophylaxis in British expatriates. Travel Med Infect Dis. 2014 Jul–Aug;12(4):341–8.
6. Keiser J, Singer BH, Utzinger J. Reducing the burden of malaria in different eco-epidemiological settings with environmental management: a systematic review. Lancet Infect Dis. 2005 Nov;5(11):695–708.
7. Lengeler C. Insecticide-treated bed nets and curtains for preventing malaria. Cochrane Database Syst Rev. 2004(2):CD000363.
8. Newton PN, Green MD, Fernandez FM, Day NP, White NJ. Counterfeit anti-infective drugs. Lancet Infect Dis. 2006 Sep;6(9):602–13.
9. Pluess B, Tanser FC, Lengeler C, Sharp BL. Indoor residual spraying for preventing malaria. Cochrane Database Syst Rev. 2010(4):CD006657.
10. Toovey S, Moerman F, van Gompel A. Special infectious disease risks of expatriates and long-term travelers in tropical countries. Part I: malaria. J Travel Med. 2007 Jan–Feb;14(1):42–9.

LAST-MINUTE TRAVELERS

Gail A. Rosselot

Ideally, travelers should seek medical advice at least 4–6 weeks before departure, but clinicians are frequently asked to provide pre-travel care to travelers leaving on short notice, sometimes within days or even hours. "Last-minute travelers" can refer to people who are leaving on short notice (such as some business travelers or immigrants returning to their home country for a family emergency), or it may refer to people who have planned a trip for some time but delayed seeking pre-travel care. Regardless of the reason, clinicians can offer travelers support for their upcoming trip even on short notice. This support could include vaccination with standard or accelerated immunization schedules, health counseling, prescriptions, and referrals to services at the destination.

VACCINATIONS

Consider the traveler's itinerary and activities at the destination when assessing which vaccines might be indicated. Note that immunity generally takes approximately 2 weeks to develop after vaccination (although this duration is shorter after booster vaccinations), so travelers might not be adequately protected if they are vaccinated immediately before travel. Counsel travelers to adhere to preventive behaviors regarding food, water, and insects (see the Food & Water Precautions and Protection against Mosquitoes, Ticks, & Other Arthropods sections in Chapter 2) in case they are incompletely protected, as well as to prevent diseases for which no vaccine is available.

Routine Vaccinations

Most travelers who attended school in the United States have received standard routine vaccinations. If the traveler is not completely up-to-date on age-appropriate routine vaccines, administer first or additional doses of these. Depending on the age and medical conditions of the traveler, pneumococcal, meningococcal, and Haemophilus influenzae

type b vaccines may also be indicated. Note that if the traveler needs >1 live-virus vaccine (yellow fever, measles-mumps-rubella, varicella, intranasal influenza), they must be given on the same day or separated by ≥28 days.

Recommended Vaccinations: Single-Dose Protection

Even when a traveler has limited time before departure, research supports the use of certain single-dose vaccines, if indicated, to initiate protection. These include hepatitis A (monovalent), typhoid (injectable), polio (inactivated), and meningococcal meningitis vaccines. The second dose in the hepatitis A vaccine series should be completed ≥6 months after the first dose is administered.

Recommended Vaccinations: Multiple Doses Needed

Last-minute travelers often cannot complete the full course of vaccines that require multiple doses to induce full protection. If a traveler needs protection against hepatitis B, Japanese encephalitis, or rabies, the clinician can consider alternative approaches.

Hepatitis B

As time allows, complete the accelerated monovalent hepatitis B (Engerix-B) schedule (0, 1, and 2 months, plus a 12-month booster) or the super-accelerated combination hepatitis A/B (Twinrix) schedule (0, 7, 21–30 days, plus a 12-month booster). If an accelerated schedule cannot be completed before travel, start the vaccination series and schedule a follow-up visit to complete it, or, for extended-stay travelers or expatriates, help them identify resources at the destination to complete the series.

Japanese Encephalitis

At present, no accelerated schedule is available for Japanese encephalitis vaccine (Ixiaro). In one study, 22 of 23 people who received 2 doses of Ixiaro on days 0 and 14 had protective antibody titers at day 28, which suggests that a shorter dosing interval may provide reasonable short-term protection, but more studies are needed. People who receive only 1 dose may have a suboptimal response and may not be protected. Travelers who cannot complete the primary vaccine series ≥1 week before travel should be counseled to adhere rigidly to mosquito precautions if they will be at risk for Japanese encephalitis. Alternatively, the clinician can help them identify resources for vaccination at their destination.

Rabies

Because of the multiple immunizations required to complete a primary rabies vaccine series (0, 7, and 21 or 28 days), it may be difficult for last-minute travelers to complete the series before departure. A person who starts but does not complete a primary series and is potentially exposed should receive the same postexposure prophylaxis as a completely unimmunized person. Counsel travelers about the importance of avoiding animals, washing any bite thoroughly with soap and water, and seeking immediate medical care. Travelers to developing or remote destinations should consider medical evacuation insurance in case evacuation is needed to receive postexposure prophylaxis.

Required Vaccinations

Documentation of a yellow fever vaccine becomes valid 10 days after administration. If a yellow fever vaccine is required by a country in the traveler's itinerary and the traveler lacks sufficient time, it may be necessary to rearrange the order of travel or reschedule the trip. Otherwise, the traveler risks entry problems at the country's border or risks yellow fever vaccination at the border. Additionally, the traveler who receives the yellow fever vaccine <10 days before entering a yellow fever risk area risks yellow fever infection. Travelers for whom the yellow fever vaccination is contraindicated can be issued a medical waiver letter.

Meningococcal vaccine is required of all adults and children aged >2 years traveling to Saudi Arabia for religious pilgrimage, including Hajj. Hajj visas cannot be issued without proof that applicants received meningococcal vaccine ≥10 days and ≤3 years before arriving in Saudi Arabia.

The World Health Organization has asked certain countries to require travelers leaving those countries to show proof of polio vaccination before they leave, if they have been in the country >4 weeks. The proof of vaccination should be documented on an International Certificate of Vaccination or Prophylaxis and is valid from 4 weeks to 1 year after the vaccine is administered. This requirement should not present a problem to travelers receiving the vaccine at the last minute, since if they stay for >4 weeks, the vaccination will be valid, even if administered on the day of travel. However, if travelers stay in the country for >1 year, they should be advised to get revaccinated >4 weeks before they plan to leave. For more information, see Chapter 3, Poliomyelitis.

MALARIA

Effective malaria chemoprophylaxis is possible for the last-minute traveler. The choice of antimalarial agent depends on a number of factors, including itinerary, drug resistance at the destination, medication contraindications and precautions, cost, and patient preference. Chloroquine and mefloquine should be initiated 1–2 weeks before departure, so most clinicians recommend doxycycline or atovaquone-proguanil for travelers who are departing in <1–2 weeks. Both doxycycline and atovaquone-proguanil can be started 1–2 days before arriving in an endemic area. Instruct the traveler to purchase malaria medication before departure, and reinforce the importance of minimizing insect bites and of seeking medical care if illness occurs.

HEALTH COUNSELING

Pre-travel counseling is critical for last-minute travelers. Determine prior knowledge and experience with travel health risks, and direct your advice accordingly. Focus on major risks of the trip, and deliver simple, customized messages about prevention and self-care. Provide travelers with education and prescriptions for travelers' diarrhea, such as a fluoroquinolone or macrolide, as well as education and prescriptions for altitude illness, if indicated. Last-minute travelers may be tempted to buy medications at their destination. Encourage them to purchase all medications in the United States before departure to avoid buying medications that may be counterfeit.

Counsel the traveler on these topics (see related in-depth discussions on the following topics in Chapters 2 and 3):

- Unintentional injuries, including motor vehicle accidents (the leading cause of preventable death in healthy travelers), and personal safety
- Accessing health care abroad and the need to consider travel health and evacuation insurance
- Packing a travel health kit that includes an extra supply of usual prescriptions and over-the-counter medications
- Insect precautions
- Rabies avoidance and what to do in the event of an animal bite
- Food and water safety
- Sexually transmitted diseases
- Issues related to long flights, including venous thromboembolism (for at-risk travelers) and jet lag
- Consider enrolling in the State Department's Smart Traveler Enrollment Program (STEP), registering their trip to receive alerts and notifications (https://step.state.gov/step/)
- Pertinent literature and Internet resources for further travel health information, including the CDC travel health program (www.cdc.gov/travel)

Clinicians should also encourage last-minute travelers to schedule an appointment after the trip to complete any needed vaccinations and to initiate preparation for the next potential "spur of the moment" trip. For travelers likely to have future last-minute trips, preemptive vaccinations or "pre-loading" for certain itineraries might also be considered.

SPECIAL CHALLENGES AND ADDITIONAL CONSIDERATIONS

The Traveler Leaving in a Few Hours: If time does not permit an appointment, the clinician can still provide general prevention messages by telephone or e-mail. Refer the traveler to useful websites such as CDC (www.cdc.gov/travel), the Department of State (www.travel.state.gov), and the International Society of Travel Medicine clinic directory (www.istm.org). Recommend travel health kit items that can be bought at the airport, if necessary. Some international airports now have travel health or vaccination clinics; suggest the traveler try to visit one before departure.

The Traveler with Preexisting Medical Conditions: These patients may be at increased risk for travel-related illness if they have inadequate time for preparation. They should consider purchasing travel health insurance, and possibly medical evacuation insurance, and should carry a sufficient supply of all medications and a portable medical record. Emphasize the importance of a pre-travel appointment or conversation with their treating clinician. Some conditions, such as pregnancy and immunosuppression, often require additional discussion and advance planning and may warrant delaying departure.

The Last-Minute, Extended-Stay Traveler: Advise these travelers to arrange an early visit with a qualified clinician at their destination for additional evaluation and education. A last-minute consultation does not provide an expatriate with adequate time for a full medical and psychological evaluation.

Requests for Off-Label Vaccine Dosing: Because of time constraints, some travelers may ask for a vaccine to be administered off-label (different schedule, double dosing, partial series). Using a vaccine in a nonstandard manner can have consequences that include medical-legal issues and inducing a false sense of protection in the traveler.

Recurring Last-Minute Travelers: Any clinic that frequently sees last-minute travelers may want to address this as a management issue. One option is to build some flexibility into the appointment schedule. Another option, which may be particularly relevant for clinics that are part of a corporation or university, is to attempt early identification of people who are likely to travel internationally and to intervene proactively.

BIBLIOGRAPHY

1. CDC. Epidemiology and Prevention of Vaccine-Preventable Diseases. 12th ed. Washington, DC: Public Health Foundation; 2012 [cited 2014 Sep 24]. Available from: http://www.cdc.gov/vaccines/pubs/pinkbook/index.html.

2. CDC. General recommendations on immunization—recommendations of the Advisory Committee on Immunization Practices (ACIP). MMWR Recomm Rep. 2011 Jan 28;60(2):1–64.

3. Chen LH, Leder K, Wilson ME. Business travelers: vaccination considerations for this population. Expert Rev Vaccines. 2013 Apr;12(4):453–66.

4. Chiodini J. The challenging traveler. Practice Nurse. 2008 Apr 11;35(7):41–8.

5. Connor BA. Hepatitis A vaccine in the last-minute traveler. Am J Med. 2005 Oct;118 Suppl 10A:58S–62S.

6. Erra EO, Askling HH, Yoksan S, Rombo L, Riutta J, Vene S, et al. Cross-protective capacity of Japanese encephalitis (JE) vaccines against circulating heterologous JE virus genotypes. Clin Infect Dis. 2013 Jan;56(2):267–70.

7. Grieve S. Duty of care, part 1: the pre-travel consultation. Practice Nursing. 2011;22(6):298–303.

8. Lankester T. Health care of the long-term traveller. Travel Med Infect Dis. 2005 Aug;3(3):143–55.

9. Ross MH, Kielkowski D, de Frey A, Brink G. Travelling for work: seeking advice in South Africa. Travel Med Infect Dis. 2008 Jul;6(4):187–9.

10. Zuckerman JN, Van Damme P, Van Herck K, Loscher T. Vaccination options for last-minute travellers in need of travel-related prophylaxis against hepatitis A and B and typhoid fever: a practical guide. Travel Med Infect Dis. 2003 Nov;1(4):219–26.

SPECIAL CONSIDERATIONS FOR US MILITARY DEPLOYMENTS

Alan J. Magill

The US military, as a matter of policy, follows most of the recommendations in the CDC Yellow Book. However, certain situations apply only to the US military, and some policies or recommendations differ from what is recommended in the Yellow Book for civilian travel. Active-duty military physicians generally manage pre-deployment medicine, but civilian physicians may interact with people who are on reserve status, home on leave, recently discharged from active duty, or veterans. Predeployment and postdeployment information, policies, and guidelines for clinicians, service members and their families, and veterans can be found on the Deployment Health Clinical Center website (www.pdhealth.mil). The purpose of this section is to inform US military medical corps officers, who routinely consult the Yellow Book, about these differences and also make civilian clinicians, who frequently see military personnel, aware of them.

In many countries, one of the largest traveling populations is their military personnel. The military should be considered a special population with demographics, destinations, and needs that may differ from those of civilian travelers. This section focuses on the unique aspects of using pre-travel vaccines and malaria chemoprophylaxis in the military population. The specific examples will be from the US military, but the concepts may be applicable to other militaries. In 2014, approximately 1.2 million US military members were on active duty, and approximately 1.0 million were in the reserve forces.

Several characteristics of the military force differ from those of the civilian population (Table 8-3). In general, the active duty military population is younger and in better health than the population at large, and is predominately male.

FORCE HEALTH PROTECTION

Force Health Protection (FHP) is an important concept in military medicine. FHP is defined as all measures taken by commanders,

Table 8-3. Differences between military populations and civilian traveling populations

CHARACTERISTIC	TRAVEL MEDICINE	MILITARY MEDICINE
Primary focus	Individual	Unit
Goal	Optimizing advice and interventions for individual travelers	Ensuring mission success; optimizing advice and interventions for each person is difficult
Adherence	Strongly encouraged but travelers are free to choose	Required; vaccines and malaria chemoprophylaxis are part of Force Health Protection (FHP)
Education	One-on-one encounters	Unit education
Population	Not prescreened; travel health providers see all ages and people with preexisting medical conditions	Prescreened; people with serious medical problems are not allowed to join the military or be deployed
Special populations	Infants, children, pregnant women, elderly people, people with renal or hepatic impairment and often taking other medications	Less frequent in military population or deployments
Disease comorbidity	Similar to civilian population	Limited, generally healthy
Sex	50% male, 50% female	85% male
Unusual activities	Adventure activities, such as trekking, climbing, scuba diving, spelunking	Housed in barracks or other group settings, aviators, Special Forces, operating complex weapons systems, hostile and extreme environments, stress of combat operations, night operations, and use of night-vision goggles
Duration of malaria chemoprophylaxis use	Mostly short term, 2–3 weeks	The US military often uses chemoprophylaxis for longer periods of time than do short-term travelers. Many deployments are for 1 year or longer.

supervisors, individual service members, and the military health system to promote, protect, improve, conserve, and restore the mental and physical well-being of service members across the range of military activities and operations. Delivery of vaccines and the use of malaria chemoprophylaxis agents are 2 aspects of FHP.

Medical interventions for FHP are the responsibility of the unit commander, with advice from the unit medical officer. When pre-deployment vaccines or malaria chemoprophylaxis are indicated, the commander includes such requirements in the mission plan. Service members are then required to receive these interventions under proper medical supervision. If a particular vaccine or drug is medically contraindicated, alternative agents may be employed if they are available. The unit medical officer documents which military personnel have not received standard preventive measures, so these people may receive additional monitoring or treatment if they become ill.

FHP policy positions in the Department of Defense (DoD) are issued as directives and instructions. All directives and instructions can be found online at www.dtic.mil/whs/directives. The Policy and Program for Immunizations to Protect the Health of Service Members and Military Beneficiaries is found in directive 6205.O2E (September 19, 2006) at www.dtic.mil/whs/directives/corres/pdf/620502p.pdf. Although policy may be made at higher levels in Washington, DC, the final decision to use vaccines or malaria chemoprophylaxis under FHP is made by commanders in the field, guided by their medical staff. In certain circumstances, individual service members may be exempt from vaccination. There are 2 types of exemptions from immunization: medical and administrative. Granting medical exemptions is a medical function that can only be validated by a health care professional. Granting administrative exemptions is a nonmedical function, usually controlled by the person's unit commander. Further information on exemption from vaccination may be found at www.vaccines.mil/VHC/ExemptionGuidance.aspx.

ROUTINE AND TRAVEL-RELATED IMMUNIZATION

DoD policy states that the recommendations for immunization from CDC and the Advisory Committee for Immunization Practices shall generally be followed, consistent with requirements and guidance of the Food and Drug Administration (FDA) and with consideration for the unique needs of military settings and exposure risks. The Military Vaccine Agency (MILVAX) supports all 5 branches of the US Armed Services to enhance military medical readiness by coordinating DoD immunization (vaccination) programs worldwide. A valuable source of service-specific information on immunizations for all branches of the US military is found at the MILVAX website (www.vaccines.mil).

In particular, the quick reference tab of the MILVAX website (www.vaccines.mil/QuickReference) provides an easily accessible and complete source of information with product specifics and policy documents that both military and civilian providers will find useful. DoD and service-specific policies for vaccines and geographic-specific vaccine recommendations can also be downloaded from this site.

GEOGRAPHIC AREAS OF RESPONSIBILITY

The US military issues FHP recommendations based on geographic areas of responsibility (AOR) (www.vaccines.mil/QuickReference). Command and control over US military personnel in each AOR are under a unified combatant command, which is a joint (all branches of the US military) command that provides recommendations for all service members being deployed to that AOR. For example, Afghanistan is in the Central Command (CENTCOM) AOR. All personnel on orders to deploy or travel to Afghanistan should receive the vaccines listed in the "Vaccine Recommendations" tab of the above quick reference web page unless there is a medical contraindication.

MALARIA CHEMOPROPHYLAXIS

Preventing malaria in military units deployed to endemic areas is an essential objective of FHP. Malaria can be prevented through 1) education and training; 2) use of personal protection measures, which include individual bed nets, permethrin-impregnated uniforms, and insect repellents; and 3) use of chemoprophylaxis where indicated. The joint instruction on immunization and chemoprophylaxis stipulates that medical commanders designate trained staff to provide comprehensive malaria prevention counseling to military and civilian personnel considered to be at risk of contracting malaria and that such counseling "include instruction on how to take prescribed antimalarial medications, the importance of compliance with the prescribed medication schedule, information about potential adverse effects, and the need to seek medical care if these adverse effects occur" (www.vaccines.mil/documents/1682_Joint_Instruction_Immunization_2013.pdf).

Malaria cases seen in returning US military personnel reflect the current deployments around the world. In 2013, the number of malaria cases had declined with the drawdown of deployed personnel to Afghanistan. The risk of *Plasmodium falciparum* malaria is substantial for people with frequent training and development missions to sub-Saharan Africa.

Several features of malaria chemoprophylaxis under FHP that are unique to the US military are derived from the activities and stressors of military deployments. When antimalarial drugs are used for chemoprophylaxis as part of FHP, the military can only use FDA-approved chemoprophylaxis agents in accordance with the specific FDA-approved indications. Off-label use of drugs is not allowed when given under FHP. If off-label use is felt to be in the best interest of the person or unit, trained and knowledgeable clinicians must provide one-on-one medical evaluations, document in the medical record the rationale for such use, and provide a by-name prescription for the drug or vaccine to each person.

In September 2011, United States Africa Command (AFRICOM) issued a policy change recommending atovaquone-proguanil (Malarone) as the recommended malaria chemoprophylaxis option for all personnel for both short- and long-term deployments in high-transmission areas of Africa. High-transmission areas for the purpose of this policy are defined by the National Center for Medical Intelligence. For practical purposes, this includes most of sub-Saharan Africa. For people who are unable to receive atovaquone-proguanil because of intolerance or contraindication, doxycycline is the preferred second-line therapy. Use of mefloquine as prophylaxis is a third-line recommendation for those unable to receive either atovaquone-proguanil or doxycycline. Before prescribing mefloquine for prophylaxis, absolute and relative contraindications as described in the approved product label must be considered.

In April 2013, the Assistant Secretary of Defense (Health Affairs) issued new guidance on medications to prevent malaria. Atovaquone-proguanil and doxycycline are both first-line choices in areas other than sub-Saharan Africa. Mefloquine should be reserved for people with intolerance or contraindications to both first-line medications. Before using mefloquine for prophylaxis, care should be taken to identify any contraindications on an individual basis and ensure required FDA mefloquine medication guide (www.accessdata.fda.gov/drugsatfda_docs/label/2013/076523s007lbl.pdf) is given to people prescribed mefloquine.

As a matter of policy, the US military routinely uses primaquine for presumptive antirelapse treatment (PART) in returning military populations to prevent the late relapse of *P. vivax* malaria or *P. ovale* malaria. PART is also referred to as "terminal prophylaxis." In PART, primaquine is given to otherwise healthy people on their departure from an endemic area. Primaquine is used for this indication much more frequently in the military than in most civilian travelers.

The FDA-approved regimen for PART is 15 mg (base) given daily for 14 days. This regimen was approved in 1952 and has not been revisited since. In the intervening decades, an overwhelming amount of data has accumulated to show that the total dose of primaquine to eliminate the dormant hypnozoite stages responsible for late relapses is dependent on the infecting *P. vivax* strain and the weight of the patient; therefore, the optimal human dose should be based on weight and adjusted for the infecting *P. vivax* strain.

In 2003, CDC recommended 30 mg (base) of primaquine daily for 14 days for PART based on available evidence, but the FDA-approved regimen remains the lower dose. Adherence to the daily 14-day regimen is poor unless primaquine is given under directly observed therapy, which is rarely done. As a result of noncompliance and subtherapeutic dosing with the 15 mg (base) for 14 days regimen, periodic outbreaks of relapsed *P. vivax* malaria continue to occur in returning military personnel. Use of the higher-dose primaquine regimen for PART is now recommended for military personnel. This recommendation is consistent with the spirit of DoD issuance 6200.02 (February 17, 2008), in that the higher-dose recommendation for primaquine when used as PART is "standard medical practice in the United States."

Although primaquine is included as an acceptable alternative by CDC for primary prophylaxis in some countries where the risk of malaria is exclusively or mostly *P. vivax* malaria, primaquine is not FDA-approved for primary prophylaxis. Because use of primaquine for primary prophylaxis constitutes off-label use, it cannot be prescribed for a deploying group under FHP, but it can be prescribed by a licensed medical provider on an individual basis as part of medical practice.

The most important risk of using primaquine is hemolytic anemia in those who are deficient in glucose-6-phosphate dehydrogenase (G6PD). Current policy is for all US military personnel to be screened for G6PD deficiency on entry into military service. However, some people, such as reservists, may have deployed without testing, or clinicians may not be able to confirm results for all people in a unit requiring PART. Clinicians should be aware that hemolytic reactions to primaquine may occur in those with unrecognized G6PD deficiency.

A recurrent issue for military medicine is the correct timing of primaquine when given as PART in conjunction with the standard chemoprophylaxis drug being taken. Primaquine can be given at any time after personnel leave an endemic area. For convenience and for enhancing adherence to the 14-day regimen of primaquine, it is often best for military units to prescribe primaquine in the immediate 2 weeks after deployment. During this time, the units are often still at their home base completing their in-processing before block leave. Once personnel depart on leave, adherence and monitoring for side effects are more difficult.

Under FHP, military personnel are required to take their chemoprophylaxis agents as prescribed to maintain mission readiness. Individual soldiers do not have the right to refuse an order given under FHP. There is great variability in practice as to how seriously individual commanders enforce these policies, however, and continued outbreaks of malaria occur in military populations because of poor compliance.

Differences between civilian and US military use of chemoprophylaxis drugs are summarized in Table 8-4.

Table 8-4. Differences between CDC recommendations and US military's use of malaria chemoprophylaxis

	CDC RECOMMENDATION	US MILITARY POLICY
Choice of malaria chemoprophylaxis agent	Chemoprophylaxis guidelines do not recommend one drug versus another, but rather emphasize the goal of tailoring the recommendation for the individual traveler on the basis of past experience, itinerary, possible drug interaction, potential side effects, costs, and medical contraindications such as drug allergies.	Individualizing advice and recommendations for large military deployments is rarely logistically possible or feasible. Recognizing this reality, in April 2013, the US military adopted a new policy on the use of malaria chemoprophylaxis in the US military. Atovaquone-proguanil and doxycycline are now the first-line drugs of choice to prevent malaria in deployed US military forces in all areas other than sub-Saharan Africa. Atovaquone-proguanil is the drug of choice for short-term travel (up to 2 or 3 weeks) and for people who travel frequently, to minimize long postexposure prophylaxis treatment courses. In September 2011, AFRICOM policy changed to recommending atovaquone-proguanil for most destinations in sub-Saharan Africa.

continued

ADVISING TRAVELERS WITH SPECIFIC NEEDS

TABLE 8-4. DIFFERENCES BETWEEN CDC RECOMMENDATIONS AND US MILITARY'S USE OF MALARIA CHEMOPROPHYLAXIS (continued)

	CDC RECOMMENDATION	US MILITARY POLICY
Doxycycline	An option for chemoprophylaxis in all areas.	Recommended first-line chemoprophylaxis choice in all areas other than sub-Saharan Africa.
Mefloquine	An option for chemoprophylaxis in all areas except Southeast Asia.	Mefloquine is not recommended as a primary option. It should be reserved for people with intolerance or contraindications to atovaquone-proguanil and doxycycline. Before using mefloquine for prophylaxis, care should be taken to identify any contraindications on an individual basis and ensure the required FDA mefloquine medication guide (www.accessdata.fda.gov/drugsatfda_docs/label/2013/076523s007lbl.pdf) is given to people prescribed mefloquine.
Atovaquone-proguanil	An option for chemoprophylaxis in all areas.	Atovaquone-proguanil is the drug of choice for sub-Saharan Africa and a first-line option in all other areas.
Primaquine chemoprophylaxis	CDC recommends the use of primaquine as primary chemoprophylaxis in geographic areas with mainly *Plasmodium vivax* malaria.	There is no FDA-approved indication for the use of primaquine to prevent malaria. Therefore, the US military cannot use primaquine as a chemoprophylaxis agent under current FHP guidelines.
PART	Primaquine at 30 mg (base) for 14 days.	There is no FDA-approved indication for the use of primaquine at the higher dose of 30 mg (base) for 14 days. However, primaquine is an FDA-approved drug with an indication for PART. The CDC-recommended (higher) dose is recommended, as it is the standard of medical practice in the United States.

Abbreviations: AFRICOM, African Command; FDA, Food and Drug Administration; FHP, Force Health Protection; PART, presumptive antirelapse treatment.

UNIQUE NEEDS FOR THE MILITARY

US military personnel may encounter threats, such as biological warfare agents, that are not usually considered for civilian travelers. Vaccines, immunoglobulins, drug prophylaxis, and drug treatment regimens can be given under FHP, but only in accordance with FDA-licensed products and regimens and for FDA-approved indications.

Products not approved by the FDA are given to soldiers only with voluntary informed consent under an institutional review board-approved protocol and in accordance with a current and FDA-approved investigational new drug application.

Only under exceptional circumstances would products not approved by the FDA be given to soldiers without informed consent. This circumstance is governed by emergency use authorization procedures. Section 564 of the Federal Food, Drug, and Cosmetic Act (21 USC 360bbb-3), as amended by the Project

BioShield Act of 2004 (Public Law 108–276), permits the FDA commissioner to authorize the use of an unapproved medical product or an unapproved use of an approved medical product during a declared emergency involving a heightened risk of attack on the public or US military forces, or when there is a potential to affect national security.

BIBLIOGRAPHY

1. Armed Forces Health Surveillance Center. Update; malaria, US Armed Forces, 2013. MSMR. 2014 Jan;21(1):4–7.
2. Brisson M, Brisson P. Compliance with antimalaria chemoprophylaxis in a combat zone. Am J Trop Med Hyg. 2012 Apr;86(4):587–90.
3. Carr ME Jr, Fandre MN, Oduwa FO. Glucose-6-phosphate dehydrogenase deficiency in 2 returning Operation Iraqi Freedom soldiers who developed hemolytic anemia while receiving primaquine prophylaxis for malaria. Mil Med. 2005 Apr;170(4):273–6.
4. Food and Drug Administration. Emergency use authorization of medical products. Rockville, MD: Food and Drug Administration; 2007 [cited 2014 Sep 13]. Available from: http://www.fda.gov/RegulatoryInformation/Guidances/ucm125127.htm.
5. Office of the Assistant Secretary of Defense (Health Affairs). HA-Policy 13-002. Guidance on medications for prophylaxis of malaria. Washington, DC; 2013 Apr 15. [cited 2014 Sept 13]. Available from: http://www.health.mil/~/media/MHS/Policy%20Files/Import/13-002.ashx.
6. Townell N, Looke D, McDougall D, McCarthy JS. Relapse of imported Plasmodium vivax malaria is related to primaquine dose: a retrospective study. Malaria J. 2012 Jun 22;11(1):214.
7. US Africa Command. Force Health Protection procedures for deployment and travel. 2011 [cited 2014 Sep 13]. Available from: http://www.med.navy.mil/sites/nepmu2/Documents/threat_assessment/AFRICOM-FHP-Guidance-22SEP11.pdf.
8. US Department of Defense. Department of Defense directive: Force Health Protection (FHP), no. 6200.04. Washington, DC: US Department of Defense; 2004 [updated 2007 Apr 23; cited 2014 Sep 13]. Available from: http://www.dtic.mil/whs/directives/corres/pdf/620004p.pdf
9. US Department of Defense. Department of Defense instruction: application of Food and Drug Administration (FDA) rules to Department of Defense Force Health Protection programs, no 6200.02. Washington, DC: US Department of Defense; 2008 [cited 2014 Sep 13]. Available from: http://www.dtic.mil/whs/directives/corres/pdf/620002p.pdf.
10. Whitman TJ, Coyne PE, Magill AJ, Blazes DL, Green MD, Milhous WK, et al. An outbreak of Plasmodium falciparum malaria in US Marines deployed to Liberia. Am J Trop Med Hyg. 2010 Aug;83(2):258–65.

STUDY ABROAD & OTHER INTERNATIONAL STUDENT TRAVEL

Gary Rhodes, Inés DeRomaña, Bettina N. Pedone

US student participation in study abroad has more than tripled in the past 2 decades. In the 2011–2012 academic year, 283,332 US students studied abroad for academic credit—an increase of 3.4% over the previous academic year. Although the top 4 destinations were European countries, 15 of the top 25 were outside Europe. The percentage of students choosing destinations in sub-Saharan Africa, Asia, or the Middle East has approximately doubled over the past decade. Substantial numbers of students are studying in countries where health concerns and endemic diseases differ from those in the United States and Western Europe. Along with students going abroad as a part of their US college or university degree program, a number of US students earn a full undergraduate or graduate degree outside the United States.

Study abroad and international travel can be life-changing and positive experiences. However, students and families must plan for and understand health and safety risks. Part of the plan should include obtaining, before departure, health care and advice from a medical specialist, an assessment of potential local health and safety risks, mitigation strategies, and knowledge of local resources to support a healthy and safe stay abroad. Further resources are included in Table 8-5.

ADMINISTRATION OF STUDY-ABROAD PROGRAMS

The largest number of study-abroad programs for US students are ≤1 year and are integrated as a part of the US degree program. Study-abroad programs vary by administrative structure. Some are administered overseas by a local university, with no US staff support onsite. Others are administered by US colleges and universities that obtain legal status in the country where the program is offered and bring faculty and staff from the United States to run or teach in the program. Others hire local staff or resident directors to administer their centers abroad

Table 8-5. Study-abroad resources

ORGANIZATION	DESCRIPTION
NAFSA: Association of International Educators www.nafsa.org	Useful information for institutions implementing study-abroad programs, as well as information for students to support their health and safety
Responsible Study Abroad: Good Practices for Health & Safety, by the Interorganizational Task Force for Safety and Responsibility in Study Abroad http://www.nafsa.org/Find_Resources/ Supporting_Study_Abroad/Network_Resources/ Education_Abroad/Responsible_Study_Abroad__ Good_Practices_for_Health___Safety/	Advice for developing plans and procedures to implement good practices for program sponsors, students, and parents/guardians/ families, especially those pertaining to health and safety issues
Council on Standards for International Educational Travel (CSIET), http://csiet.org/about/standards.html	Standards for exchange programs for US high- and middle-school students going abroad
Keeping Our Students Safe: Exchange Student Safety Guidelines http://csiet.org/publications-resources/docs/ CSIET_Student_Safety_Guidelines-Final_6-23-09.pdf	Health and safety good practices
Center for Global Education, SAFETI (Safety Abroad First–Educational Travel Information) Clearinghouse http://globaled.us/safeti	Resources to support study-abroad program development and implementation, emphasizing health and safety issues and resources for US colleges and universities supporting study abroad
SAFETI Program Audit Checklist http://globaled. us/SAFETI/program_audit_checklist.asp	List of health and safety and study-abroad issues to guide institutions' policies and procedures
http://studentsabroad.com	Resource website for students that includes a country-specific handbook
GlobalScholar and GlobalStudent: Online Learning for Study Abroad, http://globalscholar.us, http:// globalstudent.us	University- and high school-level online courses that provide students with helpful information, including health and safety information before, during, and after study abroad
Forum on Education Abroad, www.forumea.org/ index.cfm	Standards of good practice, a code of ethics, and resources for institutions and organizations that sponsor and support study-abroad programs

or partner with nonprofit or for-profit companies that provide study-abroad programs (often referred to as third-party providers). Some US universities have developed branch campuses outside the United States where students can obtain a complete US degree. Hybrid versions combine formal connections to international universities with parts of programs administered by the US campus or a third-party provider.

Institutional administrative structures in the United States can vary as well. Some institutions have several study-abroad staff, while others have no full-time staff members. Some universities hire specialized professionals to focus on health and safety issues, while others have no staff dedicated to health and safety support. Some institutions require health insurance that integrates comprehensive medical care, 24-hour assistance, emergency evacuation, and repatriation. Other institutions may recommend obtaining comprehensive health insurance for study abroad but may provide limited or no information about available options.

Some colleges and universities recommend or require that students meet with a travel health specialist before travel to selected countries, in addition to obtaining a predeparture health reviews for all countries. Whether or not a university offers pre-travel health clinic support, students should consult with a medical professional as a part of the planning process before study abroad. This consultation should help students understand how to prepare for a safe and healthy stay in their host country. It should include information on endemic health issues in the host country, availability of medications commonly prescribed in the United States, and information on how to obtain medical care abroad.

PREDEPARTURE PLANNING

Study-abroad program advisors should collaborate with institutional medical professionals to provide students with a comprehensive pre-travel consultation that includes an assessment of the student's health and immunization history, length of program, activities, and other travel that the student will be engaging in during the academic term abroad, in addition to the following:

- Country- and region-specific health and environmental information
- Gender-specific health information
- Required, recommended, and routine vaccinations
- Recommended prophylactic and self-treatment medications and first aid kit (see Chapter 2, Travel Health Kits)
- Advice and resources for students with special needs and disabilities, including a specific plan for students with preexisting conditions that includes provisions for medications, ongoing care, and emergency treatment
- Information about physiologic and psychological consequences they may encounter as a result of culture shock or changes in their routine
- General advice on nutrition and dietary deficiencies
- Cautions about alcohol and drug use and a specific plan for those with preexisting dependency issues
- Rabies education (avoid feeding or petting animals, and postexposure measures)
- Bloodborne pathogens precautions (needles, blood products, tattoos, piercing, surgeries, acupuncture) and safe sex (including emergency contraception)
- General instructions for emergency medical situations, including locating a physician abroad (see Chapter 2, Obtaining Health Care Abroad for the Ill Traveler)
- Full health and accident insurance policies and emergency assistance coverage information, including medical and evacuation insurance
- Pre-travel medical and dental exams

Before departure, study-abroad advisors and health professionals should encourage students to continue learning about the countries they will visit, to understand the health and safety issues as well as the cultural and political climate.

The information in the Humanitarian Aid Workers section earlier in this chapter can be useful for students participating in study abroad, internships, field studies, community service projects, or research in the developing world.

The Department of State's online resource for students (http://studentsabroad. state.gov) includes comprehensive information to help students plan healthy and safe experiences abroad. Their travel website (http://travel.state.gov) provides country-specific information, including issues like crime and transportation safety. Students should check to see whether there is a travel warning or travel alert for the countries they will visit, and take this information into account when making travel decisions. They should have enough background information about the countries they will visit and know how to get help at a US embassy or consulate during an emergency. Before departure, students should be encouraged to register with the Department of State's Smart Traveler Enrollment Program (STEP, available at https://step.state.gov/step/). College and university representatives can also register their students as a group with STEP.

The CDC Travelers' Health website (www.cdc.gov/travel) contains advice for travelers on the most current health recommendations for international destinations.

HEALTH AND SAFETY WHILE ABROAD
Food and Water Safety
Food and water contamination is one of the leading causes of illness for travelers. Basic precautions can minimize the risk of diarrhea and other illnesses. Specific food and water recommendations depend on the destination country. In most developing countries, students should drink only beverages from factory-sealed bottles or water that has been purified (see Chapter 2, Water Disinfection for Travelers). Students should also be advised to avoid ice in drinks, as the ice may have been made with unsafe water.

Cooked foods should be eaten hot; raw fruits and vegetables should be eaten only if they can be washed in clean water or peeled by the traveler. Poor refrigeration, undercooked meat, and food purchased from street vendors could pose problems related to food contamination. See Chapter 2, Food and Water Precautions for more information. Travelers may also wish to download CDC's *Can I Eat This?* app (wwwnc.cdc.gov/travel/page/apps-about) for on-the-go safe food and water guidance.

Adherence to Host Country Laws and Codes of Conduct
Study-abroad professionals and others working with student travelers should advise students that host country and host institution rules and regulations may differ from those on a home campus and in the United States. Students must abide by the legal system of their host country. Additional information on host country laws may be found on the Department of State website (http://travel.state.gov).

Mental and Physical Health
Students must consider their own mental and physical health when applying to a study-abroad program and discuss any existing medical or mental-health issues with their families and health professionals to minimize potential problems.

The NAFSA: Association of International Educators' publication, "Best Practices in Addressing Mental Health Issues Affecting Education Abroad Participants," available at www.nafsa.org/mentalhealth, encourages study-abroad programs "to sensitively offer support that connects the student to professional help before a problem reaches a crisis state or seriously derails the student's academic and career plans." US college and university campuses continue to see an increase in the numbers of students with mental health issues who go abroad. Dealing with stressful situations abroad may be difficult for students away from their familiar support system, which may trigger mental and physical issues. Students should be encouraged to disclose any chronic physical or mental health conditions or accommodation needs before departure. Advisors can encourage students' disclosure by assuring confidentiality and explaining that the information is needed to facilitate a safe experience while abroad—not to prevent them from going.

Mobility International USA (www.miusa.org) provides information and resources to support study abroad by students with special needs and can be contacted directly for assistance.

Prescription Medication
Students must travel with a signed prescription for all medications that indicates the name of the student, the name of the medication (both brand name and generic, as well as the international name if different), the dosage and quantity prescribed, as

well as a letter from the US treating physician explaining the recommended dosage, the student's diagnosis, and the treatment. This is especially important for controlled substances and injectable medications. Translations of these documents to the host country language may be helpful. It is a good idea to leave copies of prescriptions with a family member or friend at home. In most countries, arriving with quantities exceeding those prescribed for personal use is prohibited.

Medications commonly prescribed in the United States may not be legal in the host country. Students should check with the US embassy or consulate before traveling regarding the legality of their prescription medications, discuss with their health care providers whether some medications should be changed, and allow sufficient time to make adjustments before study abroad. Students should avoid switching medications immediately before departure and should not discontinue prescribed medications while abroad unless instructed by a health care professional.

US prescriptions are not accepted by pharmacies overseas, and some prescription medications may not be available in host countries. Students are highly recommended to fill prescriptions in the United States before departure, reducing the need to purchase medication overseas and decreasing potential exposure to counterfeit and poor-quality medications (see Chapter 2, *Perspectives:* Pharmaceutical Quality & Counterfeit Drugs). Shipping or mailing medications may not be a viable option because many countries' laws prohibit the mailing of drugs, including prescription medicines.

Students should pack all medications in the original, labeled containers in their carry-on baggage.

Emergency Contacts

Students should print and fill out an emergency information card (if one is not provided by the program, a sample can be found at http://studentsabroad.com/emergencycard.asp) with contact numbers and personal information, and carry a copy with them at all times. Students should share information on overseas contacts with their emergency contacts in the United States and share information for emergency contacts in the United States with the study-abroad program and the host school.

Students should keep both their program staff and their emergency contacts at home informed of their whereabouts and activities and provide them with copies of their travel documents (passport, visa, plane tickets, and prescriptions) and itinerary.

Transportation and Pedestrian Safety

Traffic crashes are a major cause of injury to students while traveling abroad. Students must understand what safe and legitimate modes of travel are available in their host country. A good source of information is the Association for Safe International Road Travel at www.asirt.org.

Alcohol and Drugs

The misuse and abuse of alcohol and drugs abroad can increase the risk of accidents, injury, unwanted attention, and theft. Being in a foreign environment requires the ability to respond to new and changing circumstances, which is impaired under the influence of drugs or alcohol. Many students are not of legal drinking age in the United States but are in the host country. Many do not receive adequate alcohol- and drug-prevention education explaining the consequences of risky drinking and drug abuse before departure. Violating drug laws abroad may result in serious consequences. In some countries, being found guilty of violating drug laws can lead to life in prison or the death penalty. Study-abroad professionals, in collaboration with institutional experts, should conduct a proper orientation about the risks associated with drinking and abusing drugs abroad.

BIBLIOGRAPHY

1. Forum on Education Abroad. Code of ethics for education abroad. Carlisle, PA: Forum on Education Abroad; 2008 [cited 2012 Sep 24]. Available from: http://www.forumea.org/documents/ForumonEducationAbroadCodeofEthics.pdf.

2. Gore J, Green J. Issues and advising responsibilities. NAFSA's Guide to Education Abroad for Advisors

and Administrators. 3rd ed. Washington, DC: NAFSA Association of International Educators; 2005. p. 261.

3. Institute of International Education. Americans study abroad in increasing numbers. New York: Institute of International Education; 2009 [cited 2014 Sep 24]. Available from: http://www.iie.org/en/Who-We-Are/News-and-Events/Press-Center/Press-Releases/2009/2009-11-16-Americans-Study-Abroad-Increasing.

4. Institute of International Education. Host regions of US study abroad students, 2000/01–2011/12. New York: Institute of International Education; 2013 [cited 2014 Sep 24]. Available from: http://www.iie.org/Research-and-Publications/Open-Doors/Data/US-Study-Abroad/Host-Regions/2001-12.

5. Interorganizational Task Force on Safety and Responsibility in Study Abroad. Responsible study abroad: good practices for health and safety. Washington, DC: NAFSA: Association of International Educators; 2002 [cited 2014 Sep 24]. Available from: http://www.nafsa.org/Find_Resources/Supporting_Study_Abroad/Network_Resources/Education_Abroad/Responsible_Study_Abroad__Good_Practices_for_Health___Safety/.

6. NAFSA: Association of International Educators. Best practices in addressing mental health issues affecting education abroad participants. Washington, DC: NAFSA: Association of International Educators; 2006 [cited 2014 Sep 24]. Available from: http://www.nafsa.org/mentalhealth.

7. Pedersen ER, LaBrie JW, Hummer JF. Perceived behavioral alcohol norms predict drinking for college students while studying abroad. J Stud Alcohol Drugs. 2009;70(6):924–8.

TRAVEL TO MASS GATHERINGS

Joanna Gaines, Gary W. Brunette

OVERVIEW

Mass gatherings are typically defined as a large number of people (ranging from 1,000 to >25,000) at a specific location, for a specific purpose, for a defined time frame. More practically speaking, a mass gathering can be thought of as any gathering of people that is large enough to strain local resources. Travelers to mass gatherings face unique risks because these events are associated with increased infectious disease transmission due to the influx of attendees, crowding at venues, poor hygiene from temporary food and sanitation facilities, and challenging security situations.

CHARACTERISTICS OF MASS GATHERINGS

Medical providers preparing travelers and travelers themselves should understand the characteristics of any mass gathering a patient will attend. These events can be spontaneous, such as the 2013 funeral for Nelson Mandela, which was attended by thousands from around the world; others are planned events. Some mass gatherings regularly occur at different locations, such as the Olympic Games or the FIFA World Cup, while others recur in the same location, such as the Hajj or Wimbledon. Mass gatherings can be effectively described in terms of their location, venue, purpose, size, participants, duration, timing, activities, and capacity.

- **Location:** Factors to consider include identifying the host, what local infrastructure is like, what the environment is like, and whether or not security will be adequate.
- **Venue:** Facilities vary widely, and events may be held indoors or outdoors. The venue's facilities, including food, water, and sanitation, may be of varying quality. Some mass gatherings are also mobile, where attendees move from one place to another, such as during a pilgrimage.
- **Purpose:** Understanding why people will attend an event is important. Mass gatherings can be political, religious, social, or athletic; the purpose of an event can affect the activities and mood of participants.
- **Size:** Organizers must be prepared to manage large crowds, and densely packed crowds may facilitate disease spread

or may promote problems such as riots, stampedes, and resulting injuries.

- **Participants:** Attendees may represent a unique demographic or may vary by features such as sex or age.
- **Duration:** The longer an event lasts, the higher the likelihood that local resources will become strained.
- **Timing:** Mass gatherings and local capacity are affected by the timing of an event. Weather, as well as factors such as high tourist season, can affect the ability of a host to organize a safe mass gathering.
- **Activities:** Understand the activities that participants will be participating in: some activities may be risky or strenuous behaviors or may involve alcohol or drug use.
- **Capacity:** Hosts differ in terms of their ability to detect, respond to, and prevent public health emergencies. Understanding what health outcomes have been previously associated with recurring mass gatherings can help travelers prepare for future events.

HEALTH CONCERNS RELATED TO MASS GATHERINGS

Mass gatherings pose a risk to attendees in the form of exacerbation of existing medical conditions, injuries, and the potential spread of infectious diseases. Emergency medical services are often involved in preparations for mass gatherings and are usually equipped to address acute medical conditions such as myocardial infarction and asthma. Conditions such as heat exhaustion, dehydration, hypothermia, or sunburn can also affect attendees and are usually handled on site.

Because of the possibility of a catastrophic incident, safety is of particular concern with mass gatherings. A number of casualties at mass gatherings have occurred as the result of poor crowd management, structural collapses, fires, and violence. Mass gathering attendees are also at risk for infectious disease. Previously, mass gatherings have been associated with outbreaks of influenza, meningococcal disease, and norovirus. Mass gatherings have implications for global health security. More than 2 million pilgrims attended the Hajj in 2009 during the H1N1 pandemic and in 2013 during the outbreak of Middle East respiratory syndrome

(MERS) in the Arabian Peninsula. Travelers to mass gatherings may import diseases to a host site as well as spread disease upon their return home. In 2010, measles outbreaks in Germany were linked to travelers who had attended a mass gathering event in Taizé, France.

GUIDANCE FOR CLINICIANS

Clinicians can prepare travelers for the unique health risks associated with mass gatherings.

Assessing Risk:

- **Ask travelers about their itineraries and activities.** Verify a traveler's itinerary to identify additional risks beyond those associated with the event. Patients may add side trips or extend travel beyond the mass gathering. For example, if a patient indicates that he will be attending the 2016 Olympic Games in Rio de Janeiro, malaria prophylaxis and yellow fever vaccination would not be a consideration. However, if the traveler chooses to also visit the Amazon rainforest (where malaria and yellow fever are endemic) while in Brazil, he would be at risk. CDC's Travelers' Health website posts travel notices to educate travelers and medical providers about health issues associated with specific destinations (www.cdc.gov/travel).
- **Consider your patient's unique characteristics.** Chronic health conditions may be exacerbated by the activities associated with a mass gathering. Patients should ensure they have adequate supplies of medication for the duration of their trip as well as documentation for any prescriptions.

Mitigating Risk:

- **Identify requirements** for mass gathering attendees beyond those required for entry to a country. For example, all pilgrims to the Hajj are required to have meningococcal vaccinations, whereas other travelers to Saudi Arabia are not required to have these.
- **Identify recommendations** for attendees, as host sites may make additional recommendations on the basis of public

health concerns. In response to the emergence in 2013 of MERS coronavirus, Saudi Arabia recommended that elderly or immunocompromised people delay their pilgrimage.

- **Educate travelers on preventive measures.** These may include the use of insect repellent or advice on how to choose safe food and water from vendors. All travelers to mass gatherings should be educated on the importance of regular handwashing and the use of alcohol-based sanitizer when sanitation facilities are not available.
- **Visit the CDC's Travelers' Health website at www.cdc.gov/travel.** This website is regularly updated with travel health notices; information may also be provided on mass gatherings such as the Hajj or Olympic Games.

GUIDANCE FOR TRAVELERS

- **Consult a travel medicine provider at least 4–6 weeks before the departure date.** This should allow adequate time to receive most vaccinations. Discuss your itinerary and any planned activities with your provider so that he or she can make more accurate recommendations to ensure a traveler's health and safety. If a travel medicine provider is not locally available, a primary care provider should be able to assist you with ensuring you have the adequate vaccinations and health information necessary.
- **Register travel plans with the Department of State's Smart Traveler Enrollment Program (STEP)** (https://step.state.gov/step/). Travelers can subscribe for notifications on Travel Warnings, Travel Alerts, and other information for their specific destination(s), as well as ensure that the Department of State is aware of a traveler's presence should they have serious legal, medical, or financial difficulties while traveling. In the event of an emergency at home, STEP can also help friends and family at home reach travelers abroad.
- **Ensure any existing medical conditions are well controlled before departure.** Travelers should discuss their medical history with their medical provider during the pre-travel consultation.
- **Visit the CDC's Travelers' Health website at www.cdc.gov/travel.** Learn more about specific destinations and view any travel notices for your destination.

BIBLIOGRAPHY

1. Abubakar I, Gautret P, Brunette GW, Blumberg L, Johnson D, Poumerol G, et al. Global perspectives for prevention of infectious diseases associated with mass gatherings. Lancet Infect Dis. 2012 Jan;12(1):66–74.
2. Arbon P. Mass-gathering medicine: a review of the evidence and future directions for research. Prehosp Disaster Med. 2007 Mar–Apr;22(2):131–5.
3. Emergency Management Australia. Safe and healthy mass gatherings: a health, medical and safety planning manual for public events. Fyshwick, Australia: Commonwealth of Australia; 1999 [cited 2014 Sep 24]. Available from: http://www.health.sa.gov.au/pehs/publications/ema-mass-gatherings-manual.pdf.
4. Lombardo JS, Sniegoski CA, Loschen WA, Westercamp M, Wade M, Dearth S, et al. Public health surveillance for mass gatherings. Johns Hopkins APL Technical Digest. 2008;27(4):1–9.
5. McCloskey B, Endericks T. Learning from London 2012: a practical guide to public health and mass gatherings. London: Health Protection Agency; 2013 [cited 2014 Sep 24]. Available from: http://webarchive.nationalarchives.gov.uk/20140714084352/http://www.hpa.org.uk/webc/HPAwebFile/HPAweb_C/1317138422305.
6. Milsten AM, Maguire BJ, Bissell RA, Seaman KG. Mass-gathering medical care: a review of the literature. Prehosp Disaster Med. 2002 Jul–Sep;17(3):151–62.
7. Steffen R, Bouchama A, Johansson A, Dvorak J, Isla N, Smallwood C, et al. Non-communicable health risks during mass gatherings. Lancet Infect Dis. 2012 Feb;12(2):142–9.
8. World Health Organization. Communicable disease alert and response for mass gatherings: key considerations. Geneva: World Health Organization; 2008 [cited 2014 Sep 24]. Available from: http://www.who.int/csr/Mass_gatherings2.pdf.

NEWLY ARRIVED IMMIGRANTS & REFUGEES

Christine K. Olson, William M. Stauffer, Elizabeth D. Barnett

According to the Department of Homeland Security, approximately 58,000 refugees were admitted into the United States during fiscal year (FY) 2012. In addition, >1 million immigrants obtained legal permanent resident status during FY 2012; 547,559 of these were already living in the United States, and 484,072 came directly from overseas. Tables 8-6 and 8-7 list the top 10 countries of origin for refugee and new immigrant arrivals in FY 2012.

The Immigration and Nationality Act (INA), which encompasses the immigration, temporary admission, naturalization, and removal of foreign nationals, mandates that all refugees and applicants for US immigration undergo a medical screening examination, performed by an authorized physician, for inadmissible conditions. Refugees undergo the examination overseas, whereas immigrants are examined in the United States or overseas depending on their place of residence. A panel physician is a medical doctor practicing overseas who has an agreement with a local US embassy or consulate general to perform immigration

Table 8-6. Top 10 countries of birth for newly arriving refugees, fiscal year 2012

COUNTRY OF BIRTH	NUMBER OF ARRIVING REFUGEES
Bhutan	15,070
Burma	14,160
Iraq	12,163
Somalia	4,911
Cuba	1,948
Congo, Democratic Republic	1,863
Iran	1,758
Eritrea	1,346
Sudan	1,077
Ethiopia	620

Table 8-7. Top 10 countries of birth for newly arriving immigrants, fiscal year 2012

COUNTRY OF BIRTH	NUMBER OF ARRIVING IMMIGRANTS
Mexico	75,997
China	38,920
Philippines	37,069
Dominican Republic	33,627
India	24,625
Vietnam	23,446
Haiti	16,995
Bangladesh	13,489
Jamaica	11,640
Pakistan	9,874

medical examinations; more than 760 panel physicians perform these examinations. A civil surgeon is a special designation for a US physician authorized to perform official immigration medical examinations required for adjustment of status (the process of becoming a permanent US resident). CDC's Division of Global Migration and Quarantine (DGMQ) works closely with the Department of State, which has agreements with panel physicians, and US Citizenship and Immigration Services within the Department of Homeland Security, which designates physicians as civil surgeons. DGMQ provides technical instructions for conducting the required medical examinations, including mandated screening for specific diseases (such as tuberculosis). In addition, for special populations such as refugees, the CDC issues health recommendations (such as treatment for parasitic diseases). These health recommendations are implemented when funding and logistical support are available but do not have to be completed prior to migration.

Most immigrants are not required to undergo any health screening following arrival in the United States, although there are systems for certain groups who will routinely undergo a new-arrival medical examination (such as refugees). These new-arrival screenings may be carried out by any qualified health professional.

BEFORE ARRIVAL IN THE UNITED STATES
Overseas Medical Examination and Treatment

CDC provides technical instructions to panel physicians and monitors the quality of the overseas medical examination process. The purpose of the mandated medical examination is to detect inadmissible conditions, including communicable diseases of public health significance, mental disorders associated with harmful behavior, and substance use or substance-induced disorders (www.cdc.gov/immigrantrefugeehealth/exams/ti/panel/technical-instructions-panel-physicians.html). For certain refugee populations, the visit to the panel physician additionally provides an opportunity for preventive medical interventions, such as immunizing against vaccine-preventable diseases and administering presumptive therapy for parasitic diseases, including nematode infections and malaria (www.cdc.gov/immigrantrefugeehealth/guidelines/refugee-guidelines.html).

The medical examination includes a physical examination, mental health evaluation, syphilis serologic testing, review of vaccination records, and chest radiography, followed by acid-fast bacillus smears and sputum cultures if the chest radiograph suggests tuberculosis. Treatment is required before immigration for certain conditions, such as tuberculosis, specified sexually transmitted diseases, and Hansen disease.

For people diagnosed with tuberculosis infection, technical instructions require *Mycobacterium tuberculosis* culture, drug susceptibility testing, and directly observed therapy through the end of treatment before immigration. With the addition of culture to the tuberculosis screening requirements, the yield of screening approximately tripled (in 2012, over 60% of those identified with tuberculosis disease had smear-negative, culture-positive sputum results).

Proof of Vaccination

People seeking immigrant visas for permanent residency must show proof that they received all vaccination series recommended by the Advisory Committee on Immunization Practices (ACIP) (www.cdc.gov/vaccines/hcp/acip-recs/vacc-specific/index.html). In 2009, CDC adopted revised vaccination criteria to determine which vaccines recommended by ACIP should be required for immigrant visa applicants. These criteria allow CDC the flexibility to adapt vaccination requirements according to public health needs (www.cdc.gov/immigrantrefugeehealth/laws-regs/vaccination-immigration/revised-vaccination-criteria-immigration.html). The vaccination criteria state that the vaccine must

- Be age-appropriate
- Protect against a disease that has the potential to cause an outbreak
- Protect against a disease that has been eliminated or is in the process of being eliminated in the United States

These requirements apply to all adult immigrants and most immigrant children. However, internationally adopted children who are aged ≤10 years may be exempted. Clusters of imported measles cases in unvaccinated children were reported in adoptees from China in 2004, 2006, and 2013. Adopting families should be aware that vaccinating children while still overseas reduces the risk of importing disease.

Refugees are not required to meet the INA immunization requirements at the time of entry into the United States. Instead, they must show proof of vaccination at the time they apply for permanent US residence, typically 1 year after arrival. Technical instructions regarding vaccination requirements are available at www.cdc.gov/immigrantrefugeehealth/exams/ti/panel/vaccination-panel-technical-instructions.html.

Classification of Applicants

To determine the inadmissibility of an applicant, the medical conditions of public health significance are categorized as class A or B. Class A conditions preclude an immigrant or refugee from entering the United States. An immigrant or refugee who has an inadmissible condition may still be issued a visa after the illness has been treated or after a waiver of the visa ineligibility has been approved by the United States Citizenship and Immigration Services. Class B conditions are defined as physical or mental abnormalities, diseases, or disabilities serious enough or permanent in nature as to amount to a substantial departure from normal well-being. Follow-up evaluation soon after US arrival is recommended for immigrants or refugees with class B conditions.

Notifications and Follow-Up

The Department of State forms completed by panel physicians are collected at US ports of entry when immigrants and refugees arrive. These forms summarize the results of the overseas medical examination and include classification of health conditions. On the basis of this information, CDC notifies state or local health departments of all arriving refugees, immigrants with class A conditions (with waiver), and immigrants with class B tuberculosis classifications who are resettling in their jurisdictions and need follow-up evaluation and possible treatment. The notification and Department of State form data are transmitted to state and local health departments electronically through CDC's Electronic Disease Notification System (EDN).

State and local health departments are asked to report to CDC through EDN the results of these US follow-up evaluations, as well as any serious public health conditions identified among recently arrived immigrants and refugees. Reporting allows a better understanding of epidemiologic patterns of disease in recently arrived immigrants and refugees and is a way of monitoring the quality of the overseas medical examination.

AFTER ARRIVAL IN THE UNITED STATES: HEALTH STATUS & SCREENING OF IMMIGRANTS

Although an overseas medical examination is mandatory for all immigrants, the primary focus of this examination is to identify applicants with inadmissible health-related conditions. Increasingly, US-bound refugees are receiving enhanced health screening, immunizations, and presumptive treatment for such disorders as hepatitis B, anemia, malaria, and other parasitic diseases. Medical screening after arrival is recommended but not required for all refugees and international adoptees (a category of immigrants). The more comprehensive postarrival screening represents an opportunity to screen for communicable and noncommunicable diseases, to provide preventive services (such as immunizations and treatment for latent tuberculosis) and individual counseling (such as nutritional and mental health), and to establish ongoing primary care and a medical home. Nonrefugee immigrants with class B conditions are also advised to be evaluated after their arrival; however, these evaluations are targeted for particular conditions such as tuberculosis.

Routine postarrival medical screenings are generally conducted at state or local health departments, contracted private clinics, or community health centers. Many clinicians are unfamiliar with screening recommendations and diseases endemic to immigrants' countries of origin and may feel unprepared to deal with medical issues affecting these populations. In addition, clinicians and health systems are frequently unprepared to cope with language, social, and cultural barriers in caring for new arrivals. Further, refugees and immigrants often have other priorities related to their new environment, such as English classes, schooling, housing, and work, which may take precedence over accessing health care services. However, several organizations can facilitate health screening (such as the Association of Refugee Health Coordinators [ARHC], www.refugee healthcoordinators.org/default.html), and the networks of clinicians who serve these populations are growing (a clinical e-mail list is available at www.globalhealth. umn.edu/community-initiatives/index. html). Additional resources are provided in Appendix C, Migrant Health Resources.

Clinicians should be aware that a single dose of a vaccine series fulfills the requirement for proof of vaccination for immigration purposes (a completed series is not required before immigration). Therefore, vaccination records should be reviewed to ensure that any additional doses to complete a vaccine series, as well as any age-appropriate vaccinations not required for immigration purposes, are recommended.

A point for clinicians to bear in mind is that immigrant populations often return to their countries of origin to visit friends and relatives. These people, sometimes referred to as VFR travelers, are at higher risk of travel-related infectious diseases (malaria, tuberculosis, typhoid, hepatitis A) than other groups of international travelers and access pre-travel health care less frequently than other groups. Additional resources for counseling this population can be found in this chapter, Immigrants Returning Home to Visit Friends and Relatives (VFRs).

Medical Screening for Newly Arrived Refugees

Many refugees and immigrants originate from countries with a high prevalence of tropical and other infectious diseases that may present a threat to individual or public health. In addition, untreated chronic health conditions, such as hypertension, diabetes, and obesity, are increasingly common. Identifying infectious diseases with long latency periods, including tuberculosis; hepatitis B; certain intestinal nematodes, such as *Strongyloides stercoralis*; and other parasites, such as *Schistosoma* spp. can be particularly challenging. Recommendations for the postarrival medical evaluation should be tailored to the specific population and based on such factors as country of origin; race; receipt of predeparture interventions, including vaccinations and presumptive therapy for malaria and intestinal parasites; and epidemiologic risks in the country of origin, as well as the country or countries of first asylum.

Medical screening should include a detailed medical and social history as well as a physical examination. Evidence-based screening guidelines for refugees have been developed by CDC in collaboration with the Administration for Children and Families'

Office of Refugee Resettlement (ORR), clinical and subject matter experts outside of CDC, and with representatives of ARHC. The basic components of these guidelines are outlined in Box 8-7. Full guidelines, as well as a summary checklist of the components and recommended testing, are available at www.cdc.gov/immigrantrefugeehealth/guidelines/domestic/domestic-guidelines.html. Population-specific guidelines do not exist, which emphasizes the importance of local epidemiologic data. However, population-specific health profiles are being developed to highlight specific health issues that clinicians should be aware of in each population (www.cdc.gov/immigrantrefugeehealth/profiles/index.html).

An additional function of the postarrival medical screening is to arrange and coordinate ongoing primary care. Many refugees have not had age-appropriate cancer screening, such as a Papanicolaou test, mammography, or colon cancer screening, and these needs should be addressed at early follow-up visits. Clinicians should be

---

BOX 8-7. RECOMMENDED COMPONENTS OF REFUGEE DOMESTIC HEALTH ASSESSMENTS[1,2]

- Review all available records, including chest radiograph (ask for overseas records)
- Complete a history and physical examination, including vision, hearing, and dental evaluation
- Conduct mental health screening and, when clinically indicated, a more detailed social history, including any history of trauma, torture, or rape
- Evaluate for infectious disease, including tuberculosis, HIV and other sexually transmitted infections, and malaria and other parasitic infections (schistosomiasis and intestinal nematodes, including *Strongyloides*), depending on local epidemiology
- Review overseas records for presumptive therapy for strongyloidiasis, schistosomiasis, or malaria, depending on point of departure
- Evaluate for chronic diseases, including obesity, hypertension, diabetes, and nutritional deficiencies, such as vitamin B_{12} deficiency in select populations
- Perform age-appropriate cancer screening, such as mammography, colonoscopy, or Papanicolaou test
- Update immunizations as needed
- Complete laboratory testing as clinically appropriate: hematologic testing, urinalysis, lead, HIV testing, hepatitis B testing for those arriving from countries with prevalence >2%, specific sexually transmitted infection testing, or other screening, such as basic metabolic panel and liver function testing

---

[1] A more detailed discussion of the medical examination of immigrants and refugees is available at www.cdc.gov/immigrantrefugeehealth/guidelines/refugee-guidelines.html.
[2] Full refugee health domestic screening guidelines are available at www.cdc.gov/immigrantrefugeehealth/guidelines/domestic/domestic-guidelines.html.

aware of cancers with a higher prevalence in many immigrant populations, such as cervical, liver, stomach, and nasopharyngeal cancer.

HIV testing was removed from the requirements for US admission in January 2010, but **HIV screening is highly encouraged in all newly arriving immigrants and refugees.** Culturally sensitive counseling regarding HIV testing is critical.

Nutritional deficiencies occur more commonly in refugee populations, such as B_{12} deficiency in Bhutanese Nepali new arrivals. Prevalence ranged from 64% in people tested before migration to 27%–32% in people tested in the United States after arrival. Clinicians should be aware of the possibility of malnutrition and micronutrient deficiencies and screen and treat accordingly.

In areas of the world from which many refugees originate, potential lead exposures include using lead-containing gasoline, burning fossil fuels and waste, and using lead-containing traditional remedies, foods, ceramics, or utensils. Ongoing lead exposure among refugee children in the United States has also been well documented. For these reasons, CDC recommends checking blood lead levels of all refugee children aged 6 months to 16 years of age at the time of arrival, with follow-up blood lead testing to be done 3–6 months after settling into a permanent residence.

In addition to CDC's postarrival domestic medical screening guidelines for refugees, other published resources are available to the clinician. Most recently, the Public Health Authority of Canada has produced consensus documents on evidence-based screening for newly arriving refugees to Canada. A list of resources can be found in Appendix C.

Refugees may qualify for state Medicaid programs to cover this medical screening and any needed ongoing medical care. Refugees determined ineligible for Medicaid are eligible for Refugee Medical Assistance in many states, which provides for their medical care needs for up to 8 months from the date of arrival in the United States. For more information, clinicians and refugees can contact their state health departments and can also access more information through the ORR, which administers this program (www.acf.hhs.gov/programs/orr/programs/cma).

Medical Screening for Immigrants and International Adoptees

For immigrants, no formal mechanism or funding source is available for medical screening; therefore, immigrants, with the exception of international adoptees, do not routinely receive any postarrival medical screening beyond the recommendation that they be evaluated for class B conditions. All newly arrived immigrants, however, would benefit from comprehensive postarrival health screening.

Formal postarrival medical examination is recommended for internationally adopted children. There are many similarities in health conditions on arrival between international adoptees and refugees. A distinction is that refugees generally remain within their own cultural group for some time after arrival and may have limited interactions with the wider community, whereas international adoptees frequently enter households and communities that are clinically naïve to infections common in resource-poor settings. This distinction is particularly pertinent for conditions that may continue to be infectious for weeks to months after arrival (such as hepatitis A or B and *Giardia*). The American Academy of Pediatrics offers guidance in the Red Book: Report of the Committee on Infectious Diseases for clinicians who will serve this population after their arrival in the United States; the Red Book may be accessed at http://aapredbook.aappublications.org. Clinicians should encourage updating immunizations for those who travel internationally to meet their adopted children and travel home with them, as well as close family members and caregivers, to ensure optimal protection from vaccine-preventable diseases. More information is available in Chapter 7, International Adoption and at www.cdc.gov/vaccines/parents/adoptions.html.

BIBLIOGRAPHY

1. Barnett ED. Immunizations and infectious disease screening for internationally adopted children. Pediatr Clin North Am. 2005 Oct;52(5):1287–309, vi.

2. CDC. Technical instructions for panel physicians. Atlanta: CDC; 2014 [cited 2014 Sep 24]. Available from: http://www.cdc.gov/immigrantrefugeehealth/exams/ti/panel/technical-instructions-panel-physicians.html.

3. CDC. Vitamin B12 deficiency in resettled Bhutanese refugees—United States, 2008–2011. MMWR Morb Mortal Wkly Rep. 2011 Mar 25;60(11):343–6.

4. Lowenthal P, Westenhouse J, Moore M, Posey DL, Watt JP, Flood J. Reduced importation of tuberculosis after the implementation of an enhanced pre-immigration screening protocol. Int J Tuberc Lung Dis. 2011 Jun;15(6):761–6.

5. Maloney SA, Fielding KL, Laserson KF, Jones W, Nguyen TN, Dang QA, et al. Assessing the performance of overseas tuberculosis screening programs: a study among US-bound immigrants in Vietnam. Arch Intern Med. 2006 Jan 23;166(2):234–40.

6. Miller LC. International adoption: infectious diseases issues. Clin Infect Dis. 2005 Jan 15;40(2):286–93.

7. Minnesota Department of Health. Lead poisoning in Minnesota refugee children, 2000–2002. Disease Control Newsletter [Internet]. 2004;32(2):13–5. Available from: http://www.health.state.mn.us/divs/idepc/newsletters/dcn/2004/0402dcn.pdf.

8. Nyangoma EN, Olson CK, Benoit SR, Bos J, Debolt C, Kay M, et al. Measles outbreak associated with adopted children from China—Missouri, Minnesota, and Washington, July 2013. MMWR Morb Mortal Wkly Rep. 2014 Apr 11;63(14):301–4.

9. Office of Immigration Statistics. Yearbook of Immigration Statistics: 2012. Washington, DC: US Department of Homeland Security; 2014 [cited 2014 Sep 24]. Available from: http://www.dhs.gov/yearbook-immigration-statistics-2012-legal-permanent-residents.

10. Posey DL, Blackburn BG, Weinberg M, Flagg EW, Ortega L, Wilson M, et al. High prevalence and presumptive treatment of schistosomiasis and strongyloidiasis among African refugees. Clin Infect Dis. 2007 Nov 15;45(10):1310–5.

11. Posey DL, Naughton MP, Willacy EA, Russell M, Olson CK, Godwin CM, et al. Implementation of new TB screening requirements for U.S.-bound immigrants and refugees—2007–2014. MMWR Morb Mortal Wkly Rep. 2014 Mar 21;63(11):234–6.

12. Pottie K, Greenaway C, Feightner J, Welch V, Swinkels H, Rashid M, et al. Evidence-based clinical guidelines for immigrants and refugees. CMAJ. 2011 Sep 6;183(12):e824–925.

13. Walker PF, Barnett ED, editors. Immigrant Medicine. Philadelphia: Saunders Elsevier; 2007.

IMMUNOCOMPROMISED TRAVELERS

Camille Nelson Kotton, David O. Freedman

APPROACH TO THE IMMUNOCOMPROMISED TRAVELER

The pre-travel preparation of travelers with immune suppression due to any medical condition, drug, or treatment must address several categories of concern:

- What is the cause of the immune suppression? Different conditions and medications produce widely varying degrees of compromise, and there are many unknowns in this field. Guidance regarding vaccination of immunocompromised travelers is less evidence based than

guidance for other categories of travelers but is the best available.

- Is the traveler's underlying medical condition stable? The travel health care provider may need to contact the traveler's primary and specialty care providers (with the patient's permission) to discuss the traveler's fitness to travel, give specific medical advice for the proposed itinerary, and verify the drugs and doses composing their usual maintenance regimen.

- Do the conditions, medications, and treatments of the traveler constitute contraindications to, decrease the effectiveness of, or increase the risk for adverse events of any of the disease-prevention measures recommended for the proposed trip? Depending on the destination, these measures include but are not limited to immunizations and drugs used for malaria chemoprophylaxis and management of travelers' diarrhea.

- Could any of the disease-prevention measures recommended for the proposed trip destabilize the underlying medical condition, directly or through drug interactions?
- Are there specific health hazards at the destination that would exacerbate the underlying condition or be more severe in an immunocompromised traveler? If so, can specific interventions be recommended to mitigate these risks?
- If an immunocompromised traveler were to become ill while traveling, what would be the health care options (see Chapter 2, Obtaining Health Care Abroad for the Ill Traveler)? What would the traveler do should medical evacuation be required? An immunocompromised traveler must have a plan for when and how to seek care overseas and how to pay for it.

The traveler's immune status is particularly relevant to immunizations. Overall considerations for vaccine recommendations, such as destination and the likely risk of exposure to disease, are the same for immunocompromised travelers as for other travelers. The risk of severe illness or death from a vaccine-preventable disease must be weighed against potential adverse events from administering a live vaccine to an immunocompromised patient. In some complex cases when travelers cannot tolerate recommended immunizations or prophylaxis, the traveler should consider changing the itinerary, altering the activities planned during travel, or deferring the trip.

For purposes of clinical assessment and approach to immunizations, immunocompromised travelers fall into 1 of 4 groups, based on mechanism and level of immune suppression. Vaccine recommendations for different categories of immunocompromised adults are shown in Table 8-8.

MEDICAL CONDITIONS WITHOUT SIGNIFICANT IMMUNOLOGIC COMPROMISE

With regard to travel immunizations, travelers whose health status places them in one of the following groups are not considered significantly immunocompromised and should be prepared as any other traveler, although the nature of the previous or underlying disease needs to be kept in mind.

1. Travelers receiving corticosteroid therapy under any of the following circumstances:
   > Short- or long-term daily or alternate-day therapy with <20 mg of prednisone or equivalent.[1]
   > Long-term, alternate-day treatment with short-acting preparations.
   > Maintenance physiologic doses (replacement therapy).
   > Steroid inhalers.
   > Topical steroids (skin, ears, or eyes).
   > Intraarticular, bursal, or tendon injection of steroids.
   > If >1 month has passed since high-dose steroids (≥20 mg per day of prednisone or equivalent for >2 weeks) have been used. However, after short-term (<2 weeks) therapy with daily or alternate-day dosing of ≥20 mg of prednisone or equivalent, some experts will still wait 2 weeks before administering live vaccines.
2. HIV patients without severe immunosuppression (for definitions of severe immunosuppression, see the individual vaccine recommendations at http://www.cdc.gov/vaccines/hcp/acip-recs/index.html).
3. Travelers with a history of cancer who received their last chemotherapy treatment ≥3 months previously and whose malignancy is in remission.
4. Hematopoietic stem cell transplant recipients who are >2 years posttransplant, not on immunosuppressive drugs, with no evidence of ongoing malignancy, and without graft-versus-host disease.
5. Travelers with autoimmune disease (such as systemic lupus erythematosus, inflammatory bowel disease, or rheumatoid arthritis) who are not being treated with

---

[1] The Infectious Diseases Society of America suggests a 1-month interval between low immunosuppressive corticosteroids/alternate-day dosing corticosteroids and live vaccines, but this is controversial.

Table 8-8. Immunization of immunocompromised adults

	HIV INFECTION, CD4 CELLS ≥200/mm³	SEVERE IMMUNOSUPPRESSION (HIV/AIDS), CD4 CELLS <200/mm³	SEVERE IMMUNOSUPPRESSION (NOT HIV-RELATED)	ASPLENIA	RENAL FAILURE	CHRONIC LIVER DISEASE, DIABETES
Live Vaccines						
Bacillus Calmette-Guérin (BCG)	X	X	X	U	U	U
Influenza, live attenuated (LAIV)	X	X	X	U	P	P
Measles-mumps-rubella (MMR)	R[1]	X[1]	X[1]	U	U	U
Typhoid, Ty21a	X	X	X	U	U	U
Varicella (adults)[2]	C	X	X	U	U	U
Yellow fever[3]	P[3]	X[3]	X	U	OC[4]	OC[4]
Zoster	C[5]	X[5]	X	U	U	U
Inactivated Vaccines						
Haemophilus influenzae type b (Hib)	U	U	R[6]	R[7]	U	U
Hepatitis A[8]	U	U	U	U	U	U (diabetes), R (liver disease)
Hepatitis B[9]	R[10]	R[10]	U[10]	U[10]	R[10]	R[10, 11]
Influenza (inactivated)	R	R	R	R	R	R
Japanese encephalitis[12]	ND	ND	ND	ND	ND	ND

Meningococcal conjugate	U¹³	U¹³	U	R¹³	U	U
PCV13 followed by PPSV23¹⁴	R	R	R	R	R	C
Polio (IPV)	U	U	U	U	U	U
Rabies	U	U	U	U	U	U
Td or Tdap	R	R	R	R	R	R
Typhoid, Vi	U	U	U	U	U	U

Abbreviations: X, Contraindicated (per the Advisory Committee on Immunization Practices [ACIP]); U, Use as indicated for normal hosts; R, Recommended for all in this patient category; P, Precaution (per ACIP); OC, Other considerations; C, Consider; ND, No data; PCV13, 13-valent pneumococcal conjugate vaccine; PPSV23, 23-valent pneumococcal polysaccharide vaccine.

[1] MMR vaccination is recommended for all HIV-infected patients with CD4 counts ≥200/mm³ for ≥6 months if they are without evidence of measles immunity. Immune globulin may be administered for short-term protection of those facing high risk of measles and for whom MMR vaccine is contraindicated.

[2] Varicella vaccine should not be administered to people who have cellular immunodeficiencies, but people with impaired humoral immunity (including congenital or acquired hypoglobulinemia or dysglobulinemia) may be vaccinated. Immunocompromised hosts should receive 2 doses of vaccine spaced at 3-month intervals.

[3] See details in Chapter 3, Yellow Fever. Yellow fever (YF) vaccination is a precaution for asymptomatic HIV-infected people with CD4 cell counts of 200–499/mm³. YF vaccination is not a precaution for people with asymptomatic HIV infection and CD4 cell counts ≥500/mm³. YF vaccine is also considered contraindicated by ACIP for symptomatic HIV patients without AIDS and with CD4 counts ≥200/mm³.

[4] No data suggest increased risk of serious adverse events after use of YF vaccine in people with these conditions; however, varying degrees of immune deficit might be present, and providers should carefully weigh vaccine risks and benefits before deciding to vaccinate people with these conditions.

[5] Also contraindicated by ACIP for symptomatic HIV patients without AIDS and with CD4 counts ≥200/mm³.

[6] Recipients of a hematopoietic stem cell transplant should be vaccinated with a 3-dose regimen 6–12 months after a successful transplant, regardless of vaccination history; at least 4 weeks should separate doses.

[7] Only recommended for asplenic adults who have not previously received Hib vaccine.

[8] Routinely indicated for all men who have sex with men, people with multiple sexual partners, hemophiliacs, patients with chronic hepatitis, injection drug users, and others.

[9] Hepatitis B vaccination is indicated for people at risk for infection by sexual exposure, including sex partners of hepatitis B surface antigen (HBsAg)–positive people, sexually active people who are not in a long-term, mutually monogamous relationship, people seeking evaluation or treatment for a sexually transmitted disease, men who have sex with men, people at risk for infection by percutaneous or mucosal exposure to blood, current or recent injection-drug users, household contacts of HBsAg-positive people, residents and staff of facilities for developmentally disabled people, health care and public safety workers with reasonably anticipated risk for exposure to blood or blood-contaminated body fluids, people with end-stage renal disease, international travelers to regions with high or intermediate levels (HBsAg prevalence >2%) of endemic HBV infection, people with chronic liver disease, and people with HIV infection.

[10] Adult patients receiving hemodialysis or with other immunocompromising conditions should receive 1 dose of 40 µg/mL Recombivax HB administered on a 3-dose schedule at 0, 1, and 6 months or 2 doses of 20 µg/mL [Engerix-B] administered simultaneously on a 4-dose schedule at 0, 1, 2, and 6 months. Test for antibodies to hepatitis B virus surface antigen serum after vaccination and revaccinate if initial antibody response is absent or suboptimal (<10 mIU/mL). HIV-infected nonresponders may react to a subsequent vaccine course if CD4 cell counts rise to 500/mm³ after institution of highly active antiretroviral therapy. See text for discussion of other immunocompromised groups.

[11] People with diabetes who are younger than 60 years as soon as feasible after diagnosis; people with diabetes who are age 60 years or older at the discretion of the treating clinician based on the likelihood of acquiring HBV infection, including the risk posed by an increased need for assisted blood glucose monitoring in long-term care facilities, the likelihood of experiencing chronic sequelae if infected with HBV, and the likelihood of immune response to vaccination; all people with chronic liver disease not caused by hepatitis B. At present, routine testing of antibody response after vaccination in people with diabetes or chronic liver disease is not recommended.

[12] No safety or efficacy data exist regarding the use of Ixiaro in immunocompromised people. In general, inactivated vaccines can be administered safely to people with altered immunocompetence, using the usual doses and schedules, but the effectiveness might be suboptimal. The inactivated, Vero cell–derived Japanese encephalitis vaccine, Ixiaro, is the only Japanese encephalitis vaccine available in the United States; other types of Japanese encephalitis vaccines, including live vaccines, are available internationally but are not included here.

[13] Two doses ≥2 months apart for asplenic people and people with terminal complement deficiency.

[14] Previously unimmunized asplenic, HIV-infected, or immunocompromised adults aged ≥19 years should receive 1 dose of 13-valent pneumococcal conjugate vaccine (PCV13) followed by 1 dose of pneumococcal polysaccharide vaccine (PPSV23) ≥8 weeks later. People with these conditions previously immunized with PPSV23 should follow catch-up guidelines per ACIP.

immunosuppressive or immunomodulatory drugs, although definitive data are lacking.

6. Travelers with multiple sclerosis (MS) who are not on immunosuppressive or immunomodulatory agents and those who are not experiencing an exacerbation of disease. Although the risks of using live-virus vaccines for those with MS have been debated, the National MS Society and CDC recommend following CDC guidelines for vaccination in those who lack prior immunity, who are not on immunosuppressive or immunomodulatory agents, and who are not experiencing an exacerbation of disease.

MEDICAL CONDITIONS AND TREATMENTS ASSOCIATED WITH LIMITED IMMUNE DEFICITS
Asymptomatic HIV Infection
Asymptomatic HIV-infected adults with CD4 cell counts of 200–500/mm^3 are considered to have limited immune deficits and should be vaccinated according to the guidelines in Table 8-8. (More specific recommendations are available for MMR [measles-mumps-rubella] vaccine. Detailed information is available at http://www.cdc.gov/mmwr/preview/mmwrhtml/rr6204a1.htm and http://www.cdc.gov/mmwr/preview/mmwrhtml/rr6002a1.htm.) CD4 counts while on antiretroviral drugs, rather than nadir counts, should be used to categorize HIV-infected people. The exact time at which reconstituted lymphocytes are fully functional is not well defined. To achieve a maximal vaccine response with minimal risk, many clinicians advise a delay of 3 months after immune reconstitution, if possible, before immunizations are administered. (For MMR vaccine, the recommendation is ≥6 months on antiretroviral therapy with the age- and CD4-based criteria in footnote 2.) Although seroconversion rates and geometric mean titers of antibody in response to vaccines may be less than those measured in healthy controls, most vaccines can elicit seroprotective levels of antibody in many HIV-infected patients in this category.

Transient increases in HIV viral load, which return quickly to baseline, have been observed after administration of several different vaccines to asymptomatic HIV-infected people. The clinical significance of these increases is not known, but they do not preclude the use of any vaccine.

Multiple Sclerosis
Inactivated vaccines are generally considered safe for people with MS, although vaccination should be delayed during clinically significant relapses until patients have stabilized or begun to improve from the relapse, typically 4–6 weeks after it began. Administration of tetanus, hepatitis B, or influenza vaccines does not appear to increase the short-term risk of relapses in people with MS. However, published studies are lacking on the safety and efficacy of other vaccines (such as those against hepatitis A, human papilloma virus, meningitis, pertussis, pneumonia, polio, and typhoid). Inactivated vaccines are theoretically safe for people being treated with an interferon medication, glatiramer acetate, mitoxantrone, fingolimod, or natalizumab, although efficacy data are lacking.

Modern MS therapy often includes aggressive and early immunomodulatory therapy for many MS patients, even those with stable disease. Live-virus vaccines should not be given to people with MS during therapy with immunosuppressants, such as mitoxantrone, azathioprine, methotrexate, or cyclophosphamide; during chronic corticosteroid therapy; or during therapy with immune-suppressing biologic agents. Patients on glatiramer acetate and interferons have more limited immune deficits.

A few published studies suggest that mumps, measles, rubella, varicella, and zoster vaccines may be safe in people with stable MS if administered 1 month before starting or 1 month after discontinuing immunosuppressive therapy. One study suggests yellow fever vaccine can exacerbate symptoms in MS patients; this risk should be considered in consultation with the patient's neurologist before administering the vaccine.

Other Chronic Conditions
Chronic medical conditions that may be associated with varying degrees of immune deficit include asplenia, chronic renal disease, chronic liver disease (including hepatitis C), and diabetes mellitus. These patients should be vaccinated according to the guidelines in Table 8-8. Patients with complement deficiencies can

receive any live or inactivated vaccine. Factors to consider in assessing the general level of immune competence of patients with chronic diseases include disease severity, duration, clinical stability, complications, comorbidities, and any potentially immune-suppressing treatment (see the next section in this chapter, Travelers with Chronic Illnesses).

Adults aged ≥19 years with immunocompromising conditions (including chronic renal failure and nephrotic syndrome), those on the immunocompromising drugs listed below, transplant recipients, and those with functional or anatomic asplenia, malignancy, cerebrospinal fluid leaks, or cochlear implants who have not previously received the 13-valent pneumococcal conjugate vaccine (PCV13) or the 23-valent pnuemococcal polysaccharide vaccine (PPSV23) should receive a single dose of PCV13 followed by a dose of PPSV23 ≥8 weeks later; those who have previously received ≥1 dose of PPSV23 should receive a dose of PCV13 ≥1 year after the last PPSV23 dose was received. For adults who require additional doses of PPSV23, the first such dose should be given no sooner than 8 weeks after PCV13 and ≥5 years after the most recent dose of PPSV23.

A blunted response to hepatitis B vaccine has been reported in patients with chronic renal disease; a decreased response to hepatitis B vaccine has also been observed in patients with diabetes. Additional doses of hepatitis B vaccine beyond the primary series may be necessary. Higher-dose hepatitis B vaccine preparations are used to promote optimal immunization of people undergoing hemodialysis and those with other immunocompromising conditions.

Asplenic patients are susceptible to overwhelming sepsis with encapsulated bacterial pathogens. Although response to vaccines may be less than in people with a functioning spleen, many clinical guidelines recommend immunization against meningococcal, pneumococcal, and *Haemophilus influenzae* disease in these patients, regardless of travel plans.

- Limited data show that vaccine response in people who have had a splenectomy was more impaired if splenectomy was performed because of hematologic malignancy rather than for splenic trauma.

- The Menactra meningococcal A/C/Y/W conjugate vaccine is indicated for both pediatric and adult populations at risk, with 2 doses separated by ≥2 months in asplenic patients; booster vaccinations should be repeated every 5 years if risk is ongoing.
- The Menveo meningococcal A/C/Y/W conjugate vaccine is recommended on a 2-dose schedule for asplenic adults and a 4-dose schedule at ages 2 and 12–15 months.
- The polysaccharide-protein conjugate vaccine against disease due to *H. influenzae* type b (Hib conjugate vaccine) appears to elicit an increased immune response and duration of protection in vaccine recipients, and many experienced clinicians recommend supplemental doses for splenectomized patients with incomplete Hib vaccination histories.
- PCV13 vaccine is recommended for asplenic patients and should be followed by PPSV23 8 weeks and 5 years later (see above and Table 8-8).

People with terminal complement deficiencies and those receiving eculizumab have increased susceptibility to meningococcal infections and should be immunized against meningococcal disease.

MEDICAL CONDITIONS AND TREATMENTS ASSOCIATED WITH SEVERE IMMUNE COMPROMISE
Severe Immune Compromise (Non-HIV)
Severely immunocompromised people include those who have active leukemia or lymphoma, generalized malignancy, aplastic anemia, graft-versus-host disease, or congenital immunodeficiency; others in this category include people who have received recent radiation therapy, those who have had solid-organ transplants and who are on active immunosuppression, and hematopoietic stem cell transplant recipients (within 2 years of transplantation or still taking immunosuppressive drugs). People who are severely immunocompromised may not receive live vaccines, and inactivated vaccines are not likely to be effective; these patients should consider postponing travel until their immune function improves.

People with chronic lymphocytic leukemia have poor humoral immunity, even early in the disease course, and rarely respond to vaccines. Complete revaccination with standard childhood vaccines should begin 12 months after hematopoietic stem cell transplantation. However, MMR and varicella vaccines should be administered 24 months after transplant if the recipient is assumed to be immunocompetent. Inactivated influenza vaccine should be administered beginning ≥6 months after hematopoietic stem cell transplant and annually thereafter; a dose of inactivated influenza vaccine can be given as early as 4 months after transplant, although a booster dose should be considered in this situation.

For solid-organ transplants, the risk of infection is highest in the first year after transplant, so travel to high-risk destinations should be postponed until after that time.

Doses of inactivated vaccines received while concurrently receiving potent immunosuppressive therapy (see below) or during the 2 weeks before starting therapy are not considered valid. At least 3 months after therapy is discontinued, patients should be revaccinated with all inactivated vaccines that are still indicated.

People taking any of the following categories of medications are considered severely immunocompromised:

- **High-dose corticosteroids**—Most clinicians consider a dose of either >2 mg/kg of body weight or ≥20 mg per day of prednisone or equivalent in people who weigh >10 kg, when administered for ≥2 weeks, as sufficiently immunosuppressive to raise concern about the safety of vaccination with live-virus vaccines. Furthermore, the immune response to vaccines may be impaired. Clinicians should wait ≥1 month after discontinuation of high-dose systemic corticosteroid therapy before administering a live-virus vaccine.
- **Alkylating agents** (such as cyclophosphamide).
- **Antimetabolites** (such as azathioprine, 6-mercaptopurine).
- **Transplant-related immunosuppressive drugs** (such as cyclosporine, tacrolimus, sirolimus, azathioprine, and mycophenolate mofetil).

- **Cancer chemotherapeutic agents**, excluding tamoxifen but including low-dose methotrexate weekly regimens, are classified as severely immunosuppressive, as evidenced by increased rates of opportunistic infections and blunting of responses to certain vaccines among patient groups. Limited studies show that methotrexate monotherapy had no effect on the response to influenza vaccine, but it did impair the response to pneumococcal vaccine.
- **Tumor necrosis factor (TNF) blockers** such as etanercept, adalimumab, certolizumabpegol, golimumab, and infliximab blunt the immune response to certain vaccines and certain chronic infections. When used alone or in combination regimens with methotrexate to treat rheumatoid disease, TNF blockers were associated with an impaired response to hepatitis A, influenza, and pneumococcal vaccines.
  > Despite measurable impairment of the immune response, postvaccination antibody titers were often sufficient to provide protection for most people; therefore, treatment with TNF blockers does not preclude immunization against hepatitis A, influenza, and pneumococcal disease. If possible, both doses in the hepatitis A series should be given before travel.
  > The use of live vaccines is contraindicated according to the prescribing information for most of these therapies.
- **Other biologic agents** that are immunosuppressive or immunomodulatory may result in significant immunocompromise. In particular, certain monoclonal antibodies, such as rituximab or alemtuzumab, are more significantly immunosuppressive, and neither inactivated or live vaccines should be administered for at least 6 months—and perhaps longer—after cessation of therapy with these agents.

Severe Immune Compromise due to Symptomatic HIV/AIDS

Knowledge of the HIV-infected traveler's current CD4 T-lymphocyte count is necessary for pre-travel consultation. HIV-infected people with CD4 cell counts <200/mm³, history of an AIDS-defining illness without immune reconstitution, or clinical manifestations of symptomatic HIV are considered to have severe immunosuppression (see Chapter 3, HIV Infection) and should not receive live attenuated viral or bacterial vaccines because of the risk that the vaccine could cause serious systemic disease.[2] The response to inactivated vaccines also will be suboptimal; thus, vaccine doses received by HIV-infected people while CD4 cell counts are <200/mm³ should be ignored, and the person should be revaccinated ≥3 months after immune reconstitution with antiretroviral therapy.

In newly diagnosed, treatment-naïve patients with CD4 cell counts <200/mm³, travel should be delayed pending reconstitution of CD4 cell counts with antiretroviral therapy. Such postponement helps minimize risk of infection and avoid immune reconstitution illness during travel.

Household Contacts

Household contacts of severely immunocompromised patients may be given live-virus vaccines such as yellow fever, MMR, or varicella/zoster vaccines but should not be given the live attenuated influenza vaccine. Immunocompromised patients should be aware of the risk of transmission of oral polio vaccine virus by the fecal-oral route in parts of the world where that vaccine is still given. Smallpox vaccine (mostly for military personnel) is also transmissible to immunocompromised household and intimate contacts.

SPECIAL CONSIDERATIONS FOR IMMUNOCOMPROMISED TRAVELERS
Yellow Fever Vaccine

Travelers with severe immune compromise should be strongly discouraged from travel to destinations that present a true risk for yellow fever (YF). They should not undergo YF vaccination, as there is a risk of developing a serious adverse event, such as life-threatening yellow fever vaccine–associated viscerotropic disease. If travel is unavoidable to an area where YF vaccine is recommended (see Maps 3-16 and 3-17) and the vaccine is not given, these travelers should be informed of the risk of YF, carefully instructed in methods to avoid mosquito bites, and be provided with a vaccination medical waiver (see Chapter 3, Yellow Fever).

Patients with conditions that the Advisory Committee on Immunization Practices considers precautions to administration of YF vaccine, such as asymptomatic HIV (see "Precautions" in Chapter 3, Yellow Fever), may be offered YF vaccine if travel to YF-endemic areas is unavoidable; recipients should be monitored closely for possible adverse effects. As vaccine response may be suboptimal, such vaccinees are candidates for serologic testing 1 month after vaccination. For information about serologic testing, contact your state health department or CDC's Division of Vector-Borne Diseases at 970-221-6400. Data from clinical and epidemiologic studies are insufficient at this time to evaluate the actual risk of severe adverse effects associated with YF vaccine among recipients with limited immune deficits.

If international travel requirements, and not true exposure risk, are the only reasons to vaccinate a traveler with asymptomatic HIV infection or a limited immune deficit, the physician should provide a waiver letter. Travelers should be warned that vaccination waiver documents might not be accepted by some countries; if the waiver is rejected, the option of deportation might be preferable to receipt of YF vaccine at the destination.

Response to Vaccination

Response to vaccination may be muted in immunocompromised hosts, and potential travelers should be informed about this. The decrease in response to vaccination is not particularly predictable based on the immunosuppressive regimen. Encouragingly, recent data in solid organ transplant recipients vaccinated before transplant suggests that a prolonged phase of protective antibody titers can exist after transplant. In general, serologic testing for response to most travel-related vaccines is neither clinically recommended nor readily available to practicing clinicians.

---

[2] For MMR vaccine, severe immunosuppression is defined as CD4 percentages <15% at any age or CD4 count <200/mm³ for people aged >5 years. See http://www.cdc.gov/mmwr/preview/mmwrhtml/rr6204a1.htm.

 IMMUNOCOMPROMISED TRAVELERS

Malaria Chemoprophylaxis

Immunocompromised travelers to malaria-endemic areas should be prescribed drugs for malaria chemoprophylaxis and receive counseling about mosquito bite avoidance—the same as for immunocompetent travelers (see Chapter 3, Malaria). Special concerns for immunocompromised travelers include any of the following possibilities:

- Drugs used for malaria chemoprophylaxis may interact with drugs in the traveler's maintenance regimen, including leading to prolongation of the cardiac QTc interval, arrhythmia, and death.
- The underlying medical condition or immunosuppressive regimen may predispose the immunocompromised traveler to more serious disease from malaria infection.
- A malaria infection and the drugs used to treat the malaria infection may exacerbate the underlying disease.
- The severity of malaria is increased in HIV-infected people: malaria infection increases HIV viral load and thus may exacerbate disease progression.

People with HIV on HAART face particularly large numbers of potential drug interactions with drugs prescribed for malaria chemoprophylaxis. Table 8-9 highlights potential interactions for the most commonly used HAART combinations, but it should be emphasized that these are based on pharmacokinetic or metabolism considerations only and not on any evidence of clinical failure.

- Integrase inhibitor (raltegravir, dolutegravir, elvitegravir)/NRTI combinations have no known interactions with CDC-recommended chemoprophylactic drugs, although the cobicistat booster co-formulated with elvitegravir may theoretically increase mefloquine levels.
- Concurrent use of emtricitabine/tenofovir/efavirenz (Atripla) with chloroquine, mefloquine, or doxycycline has not been associated with drug interactions. Efavirenz lowers serum levels of both atovaquone and proguanil, but there is no evidence for clinical failure of these agents when used concurrently.

- Protease inhibitor (PI)-containing combinations are associated with many drug interactions. Lopinavir/ritonavir (Kaletra) used in combination with tenofovir/emtricatabine (Truvada) or any other PI-containing combination can lower serum levels of both atovaquone/proguanil and mefloquine. Doxycycline is a preferred antimalarial chemoprophylactic agent in patients on such a regimen.
- For less commonly used combinations or drugs not specifically included in Table 8-9, an interactive web-based resource for checking on drug interactions involving HAART drugs is found at the University of Liverpool website (www.hiv-druginteractions.org).

Antimalaria treatment regimens including artemisinin derivatives, quinine/quinidine, lumefantrine (part of the artemether/lumefantrine combination, Coartem), and atovaquone and proguanil may have potential interactions with many NNRTIs, PIs, and with the CCR5 receptor antagonist maraviroc. Expert advice should be sought when treating patients for malaria who are also on HAART.

Organ transplant recipients may have drug interactions between their chronic immunosuppression and agents used for malaria prophylaxis and treatment. Mefloquine, doxycycline, chloroquine, and primaquine may increase calcineurin inhibitor levels (tacrolimus and cyclosporine A), and sulfadoxine-pyrimethamine may decrease their levels. Some travel-related prophylactic medications need to be dose-adjusted according to altered hepatic or renal function.

Some clinical case reports suggest that asplenic people may be at higher risk of acquisition and complications of malaria, so asplenic travelers to malaria areas should be counseled to adhere conscientiously to the malaria chemoprophylaxis regimen prescribed for them.

ENTERIC INFECTIONS

Many foodborne and waterborne infections, such as those caused by *Salmonella*, *Campylobacter*, *Giardia*, *Listeria*, and *Cryptosporidium*, can be severe or become chronic in immunocompromised people.

Table 8-9. Potential interactions between malaria chemoprophylaxis drugs and commonly used HIV or transplant-related drugs[1]

DRUG	PROTEASE INHIBITORS	NRTIs	NNRTIs	INTEGRASE AND ENTRY INHIBITORS	CALCINEURIN INHIBITORS (TACROLIMUS, CYCLOSPORINE A)
Mefloquine	Decreases serum levels of all protease inhibitors, no effect of combination on mefloquine levels	None known or expected	None known or expected with efavirenz or others	Theoretical increase of mefloquine levels by elvitegravir/cobicistat	Could cause prolonged QT interval or elevated calcineurin inhibitor levels
Atovaquone-proguanil	All protease inhibitors including ritonavir, lopinavir, atazanavir lowers serum levels of both atovaquone and proguanil	No known or theortical interactions	Efavirenz lowers serum levels of both atovaquone and proguanil	None known or expected	No available data
Doxycycline	None known or expected	None known or expected	Not studied. Theoretical decrease of doxycycline levels by efavirenz	None known or expected	Could cause elevated calcineurin inhibitor levels
Chloroquine	None known or expected	None known or expected	None known or expected	None known or expected	Could cause prolonged QT interval or elevated calcineurin inhibitor levels
Primaquine	None known or expected	None known or expected	Not studied. Theoretical decrease in primaquine levels by efavirenz	None known or expected	Could cause elevated calcineurin inhibitor levels

Abbreviations: NRTI, nucleoside reverse transcriptase inhibitor; NNRTI, nonnucleoside reverse transcriptase inhibitor.

[1] Potential interactions are based on pharmacokinetic or metabolic considerations only and not evidence of clinical failure. This table highlights interactions associated with the most commonly used antiretroviral combinations, including integrase inhibitor (raltegravir, dolutegravir, elvitegravir)/NRTI combinations, maraviroc/NRTI combinations, emtricitabine/tenofovir/efavirenz (Atripla), and lopinavir/ritonavir/tenofovir/emtricitabine (Kaletra/Truvada). Consult www.hiv-druginteractions.org for comprehensive information.

Safe food and beverage precautions should be followed by all travelers; travelers' diarrhea can nonetheless occur despite strict adherence. Selection of antimicrobials to be used for self-treatment of travelers' diarrhea may require special consideration of potential drug interactions among patients already taking medications for chronic medical conditions. Fluoroquinolones and rifaximin are active against several enteric bacterial pathogens and are not known to have significant interactions with HAART drugs. Macrolide antibiotics may have significant interactions with HAART drugs (Table 8-10) and with organ transplant–related immunosuppression. Waterborne infections might result from swallowing water during recreational activities. To reduce the risk of cryptosporidiosis and giardiasis, patients should avoid swallowing water during swimming and should not swim in water that might be contaminated (with sewage or animal waste, for example). Travelers with liver disease should avoid direct exposure to salt water that may contain *Vibrio* spp.

Attention to hand hygiene, including frequent and thorough handwashing, is the best prevention against gastroenteritis. Hands should be washed after contact with public surfaces and also after any contact with animals or their living areas.

Reducing Risk for Other Diseases

Geographically focal infections that pose an increased risk of severe outcome for immunocompromised people include visceral leishmaniasis and several fungal infections

Table 8-10. Potential interactions between antibiotics for travelers' diarrhea and HIV or transplant-related drugs

DRUG	PROTEASE INHIBITORS	NRTIs	NNRTIs	INTEGRASE AND ENTRY INHIBITORS	CALCINEURIN INHIBITORS (TACROLIMUS, CYCLOSPORINE A)
Fluoroquinolones	No interactions of ciprofloxacin. Potential interactions of other quinolones with atazanavir, saquinavir, and lopinavir	No known or expected interactions	No interactions of ciprofloxacin. Potential interactions of other quinolones with rilpivirine	No known or expected interactions	Could cause prolonged QT interval or elevated fluoroquinolone levels; dose per renal function
Azithromycin	No known or expected interactions	No known or expected interactions	No known or expected interactions	No known or expected interactions	Possible increased levels of calcineurin inhibitors
Rifaximin	No available data but nonabsorbable antibiotic	No available data but nonabsorbable antibiotic	No available data but nonabsorbable antibiotic	No available data but nonabsorbable antibiotic	No available data; could decrease levels of calcineurin inhibitors

Abbreviations: NRTI, nucleoside reverse transcriptase inhibitor; NNRTI, nonnucleoside reverse transcriptase inhibitor.

acquired by inhalation (such as *Penicillium marneffei* infection in Southeast Asia and coccidioidomycosis in the Americas). Many developing areas have high rates of tuberculosis (TB), and establishing the TB status of immunocompromised travelers going to such destinations may be helpful in the evaluation of any subsequent travel-associated illness. Depending on the traveler's degree of immune suppression, the baseline TB status may be assessed by obtaining a tuberculin skin test, *Mycobacterium tuberculosis* antigen-specific interferon-γ assay, or chest radiograph.

Patients with advanced HIV and transplant recipients frequently take either primary or secondary prophylaxis for one or more opportunistic infections (such as *Pneumocystis*, *Mycobacterium*, and *Toxoplasma* spp.). Complete adherence to all indicated regimens should be confirmed before travel (see Chapter 3, HIV Infection).

BIBLIOGRAPHY

1. Agarwal N, Ollington K, Kaneshiro M, Frenck R, Melmed GY. Are immunosuppressive medications associated with decreased responses to routine immunizations? A systematic review. Vaccine. 2012 Feb 14;30(8):1413–24.

2. Askling HH, Rombo L, van Vollenhoven R. Hepatitis A vaccine for immunosuppressed patients with rheumatoid arthritis: a prospective, open-label, multi-centre study. Travel Med Infect Dis. 2014 Mar–Apr;12(2):134–42.

3. Barte HL, Horvath TH, Rutherford GW. Yellow fever vaccine for patients with HIV infection. Cochrane Database Syst Rev. 2014 Jan 23;1:CD010929.

4. Farez MF, Correale J. Yellow fever vaccination and increased relapse rate in travelers with multiple sclerosis. Arch Neurol. 2011 Oct;68(10):1267–71.

5. Geretti AM, Doyle T. Immunization for HIV-positive individuals. CurrOpin Infect Dis. 2010 Feb;23(1):32–8.

6. Kaplan JE, Benson C, Holmes KH, Brooks JT, Pau A, Masur H, et al. Guidelines for prevention and treatment of opportunistic infections in HIV-infected adults and adolescents: recommendations from CDC, the National Institutes of Health, and the HIV Medicine Association of the Infectious Diseases Society of America. MMWR Recomm Rep. 2009 Apr 10;58(RR-4): 1–207.

7. Kotton CN, Hibberd PL, AST Infectious Diseases Community of Practice. Travel medicine and the solid organ transplant recipient. Am J Transplant. 2009 Dec 9;(Suppl 4):S273–81.

8. Loebermann M, Winkelmann A, Hartung HP, Hengel H, Reisinger EC, Zettl UK. Vaccination against infection in patients with multiple sclerosis. Nat Rev Neurol. 2011;8(3):143–51.

9. Rubin LG, Levin MJ, Ljungman P. 2013 IDSA clinical practice guideline for vaccination of the immunocompromised host. Clin Infect Dis. 2014 Feb;58(3):309–18.

10. Visser LG. TNF-α antagonists and immunization. Curr Infect Dis Rep. 2011 Jun;13(3):243–7.

11. Wyplosz B, Burdet C, François H, et al, Persistence of yellow fever vaccine-induced antibodies after solid organ transplantation. Am J Transplant. 2013 Sep;13(9):2458–61.

Appendices

APPENDIX A: PROMOTING QUALITY IN THE PRACTICE OF TRAVEL MEDICINE
Stephen M. Ostroff

Travel medicine remains a young area of medical practice, but even as the field continues to mature based on a growing body of scientific and medical information, there remains no recognized specialty or subspecialty of travel medicine anywhere in the world, including the United States. Clinicians offering travel medicine services are not "board certified" in travel medicine. Instead, travel medicine providers generally have credentials in other disciplines, including infectious diseases, internal medicine, pediatrics, nursing, pharmacy, or family practice. Clinics in the United States that offer travel medicine services are also not specifically credentialed for this purpose.

Given these circumstances, how can travelers maximize the likelihood their provider will deliver quality travel-related medical care and that the advice, preventive measures, and treatment services they are given fall within accepted standards? Similarly, how can providers assure patients they have sufficient knowledge of the subject matter relevant to travel medicine?

Research into the quality of travel health care is limited, but several studies suggest that travelers who visit a clinician with training in travel medicine are more likely to receive pre- and post-travel advice and care than if they see other clinicians for such services. Similarly, 2006 guidelines on travel medicine published by the Infectious Diseases Society of America (Box A-1) recommend that pre- and post-travel care be obtained from a clinician with expertise in travel medicine. This is especially relevant for travelers going to exotic destinations, engaging in adventure travel, or who have special needs or medical problems.

Below is a partial list of resources for clinicians who wish to enhance their knowledge of travel medicine. People seeking travel-related medical services may want to inquire whether their provider or clinic participates in these organizations or activities.

TRAVEL MEDICINE–RELATED PROFESSIONAL ORGANIZATIONS
International Society of Travel Medicine (ISTM)
Founded in 1991, ISTM (www.istm.org) is the preeminent multinational organization dealing exclusively with travel medicine. ISTM has >3,200 members worldwide.

ISTM activities include the following:

- *Journal of Travel Medicine*
- An active listserv (TravelMed) where members share information and can ask questions

- Special-interest groups that include travel medicine nurses and travel medicine pharmacists
- A biennial travel medicine meeting and annual regional submeetings
- A directory of domestic and international travel clinics affiliated with ISTM members in 89 countries
- An online learning curriculum of 60 programs that cover a wide range of topics
- An examination leading to a Certificate of Knowledge in Travel Medicine, available to physicians, nurses, pharmacists, and other professionals offering travel advice
- ISTM Travel Medicine Continuous Professional Development Program

The Certificate of Knowledge in Travel Medicine has been administered by ISTM since 2003. The Body of Knowledge, which covers the scope of the specialty of travel medicine, forms the basis for examination questions. It is updated on a continual basis by the ISTM Exam Committee. Content areas in the Body of Knowledge include the following:

- Epidemiology related to travel medicine
- Immunology and vaccinology (including travel-related vaccines)
  - Pre-travel consultation and management
  - Patient evaluation
  - Travelers with special needs
  - Special itineraries
  - Prevention and self-treatment
  - Precautions
- Diseases contracted during travel
  - Vectorborne diseases
  - Diseases transmitted from person to person
  - Foodborne and waterborne diseases
  - Diseases related to bites and stings
  - Diseases due to environmental hazards
- Other conditions associated with travel
  - Conditions occurring during or after travel
  - Conditions due to environmental factors
  - Threats to personal safety and security
  - Psychocultural issues
- Post-travel management
- General travel medicine issues
  - Medical care abroad
  - Travel clinic management
  - Travel medicine information resources

Since it was introduced, the Certificate of Knowledge in Travel Medicine examination has been taken by >2,600 practitioners. The society hosts a periodic 2-day intensive exam preparation course. Those who are successful in the examination are awarded a Certificate in Travel Health (CTH). Beginning with CTHs awarded in 2011, the certificate is good for 10 years and the awardee must be recertified either through professional development activities or by retaking the examination. Practitioners offering travel medicine services or interested in the subject should strongly consider membership in ISTM. ISTM practitioners are listed on the organization's website, and those who have the CTH are designated as such. ISTM currently recognizes >1,000 members with the CTH designation.

ISTM also offers research programs. These include research grants, travel awards, and support for such efforts as the GeoSentinel Surveillance Network.

American Society of Tropical Medicine and Hygiene (ASTMH)

Formed in 1951 through the merger of predecessor organizations dating back to 1903,

ASTMH (www.astmh.org) has a subsection that deals exclusively with tropical and travel medicine, known as the American Committee on Clinical Tropical Medicine and Travelers' Health.

ASTMH activities include the following:

- *The American Journal of Tropical Medicine and Hygiene*
- An annual meeting
- An electronic distribution list
- A tropical and travel medicine consultant directory
- A biennial examination leading to a Certificate of Knowledge in Clinical Tropical Medicine and Travelers' Health, available to those who have passed an ASTMH-approved tropical medicine diploma course or have sufficient tropical medicine experience

The content areas of the ASTMH Certificate of Knowledge in Clinical Tropic Medicine and Travelers' Health are as follows:

- Basic science and fundamentals
- Infectious and tropical diseases (including parasites, bacteria, fungi, and viruses)
- Other diseases and conditions
- Diagnostic and therapeutic approach to clinical syndromes
- Travelers' health
- Public health in the tropics
- Epidemiology and control of disease
- Laboratory diagnosis

More than 750 people who have passed the ASTMH examination are listed on the ASTMH website. The society offers an annual intensive update course in clinical tropical medicine and travelers' health, which is in part designed to prepare those planning to take the Certificate of Knowledge examination.

Wilderness Medical Society

Organized in 1983, this society (www.wms.org) focuses on adventure travel, including wilderness travel and diving medicine. Its activities include the following:

- The journal *Wilderness and Environmental Medicine*

- Practice guidelines for emergency care in wilderness settings
- Annual meetings, a world congress, and subspecialty meetings
- Courses leading to certification in advanced wilderness life support
- Participation in courses that lead to a diploma in mountain medicine
- A wilderness medical curriculum that, when successfully completed, qualifies members for fellowship in the Academy of Wilderness Medicine

Infectious Diseases Society of America (IDSA)

IDSA (www.idsociety.org) is the largest organization representing infectious disease clinicians in the United States. Although IDSA does not deal exclusively with travel medicine, it has many active members with expertise in tropical and travel medicine or strong interests in these disciplines. In 2006, IDSA published extensive evidence-based guidelines on the practice of travel medicine in the United States (Box A-1). IDSA also publishes travel-related research in its journals: *The Journal of Infectious Diseases, Clinical Infectious Diseases,* and *Open Forum Infectious Diseases.*

International Society for Infectious Diseases (ISID)

ISID (www.isid.org) was formed in 1986 and has approximately 20,000 members in 155 countries around the world. Like IDSA, ISID does not specifically focus on travel medicine. However, its international reach, particularly in low-resource countries, makes travel medicine an important topic in ISID and a valuable source of information for infectious diseases clinicians in many overseas travel destinations. Activities relevant to travel medicine that are supported by ISID include the following:

- *International Journal of Infectious Diseases*
- The biennial meeting International Congress on Infectious Diseases
- The Program for Monitoring Emerging Diseases (Pro-MED), an open-source electronic reporting system for reports of emerging infectious diseases and toxins, including outbreaks (www.promedmail.org)

Aerospace Medical Association

This organization (www.asma.org) represents professionals in the fields of aviation, space, and environmental medicine who deal with air and space travelers. Its activities include the following:

- The journal *Aviation, Space, and Environmental Medicine*
- An annual meeting
- Continuing medical education in topics related to aerospace medicine

FINDING CARE WHILE TRAVELING OUTSIDE THE UNITED STATES

Both the ISTM and ASTMH websites contain the names of non-US-based clinics and health care providers affiliated with members of these organizations. Travelers are advised to review these lists before departure to identify health care resources at their travel destination. A number of countries or national travel medicine societies have websites related to travel medicine that also provide access to clinicians, including the following:

- Canada: Health Canada (www.phac-aspc.gc.ca/tmp-pmv/yf-fj/index-eng.php and travel.gc.ca)
- Great Britain: National Travel Health Network and Centre (www.nathnac.org) and British Global and Travel Health Association (www.bgtha.org)
- South Africa: South African Society of Travel Medicine (www.sastm.org.za)
- Australia: Travel Medicine Alliance (www.travelmedicine.com.au)
- China: International Travel Healthcare Association (http://en.itha.org.cn)

Emergency travel-related medical care may also be accessed through contact with US embassies that may be able to provide a listing of physicians. Travelers are also urged to consider contracting with one of a number of private companies that provide physician services abroad as well as medical evacuations. One example is International SOS, which operates throughout the world. Provider locations and details may be found at www.internationalsos.com.

BIBLIOGRAPHY

1. Boddington NL, Simons H, Launders N, Hill DR. Quality improvement in travel medicine: a programme for yellow fever vaccination centres in England, Wales and Northern Ireland. Qual Prim Care. 2011;19(6):391–8.
2. Chiodini JH, Anderson E, Driver C, Field VK, Flaherty GT, Grieve AM, et al. Recommendations for the practice of travel medicine. Travel Med Infect Dis. 2012 May;10(3):109–28.
3. Hill DR, Ericsson CD, Pearson RD, Keystone JS, Freedman DO, Kozarsky PE, et al. The practice of travel medicine: guidelines by the Infectious Diseases Society of America. Clin Infect Dis. 2006 Dec 15;43(12):1499–539.
4. Kozarsky P. The Body of Knowledge for the practice of travel medicine—2006. J Travel Med. 2006 Sep–Oct;13(5):251–4.
5. LaRocque RC, Jentes ES. Health recommendations for international travel: a review of the evidence base of travel medicine. Curr Opin Infect Dis. 2011 Oct; 24(5):403–9.
6. Ruis JR, van Rijckevorsel GG, van den Hoek A, Koeman SC, Sonder GJ. Does registration of professionals improve the quality of travelers' health advice? J Travel Med. 2009 Jul–Aug;16(4):263–6.
7. Schlagenhauf P, Santos-O'Connor F, Parola P. The practice of travel medicine in Europe. Clin Microbiol Infect. 2010 Mar;16(3):203–8.
8. Sistenich V. International emergency medicine: how to train for it. Emerg Med Australas. 2012 Aug;24(4):435–41.
9. Spira A. Setting the standard. J Travel Med. 2003 Jan–Feb;10(1):1–3.

APPENDIX B: TRAVEL VACCINE SUMMARY TABLE

David R. Shlim

Table B-1 is a quick reference for administering or prescribing travel-related vaccines. Before administering any vaccine, please pay particular attention to the dose and whether it is to be administered intramuscularly or subcutaneously. Also review detailed instructions, contraindications, precautions, and side effects under the specific vaccines discussed in this book or in the manufacturer's prescribing information. For other immunizations, refer to the corresponding disease section in Chapter 3.

Table B-1 Travel Vaccine Summary

VACCINE	TRADE NAME (MANUFACTURER)	AGE	DOSE	ROUTE	SCHEDULE	BOOSTER
Hepatitis A vaccine, inactivated	Havrix (GlaxoSmithKline)	1–18 y	0.5 mL (720 ELU)	IM	0, 6–12 mo	None
		≥19 y	1.0 mL (1,440 ELU)	IM	0, 6–12 mo	None
Hepatitis A vaccine, inactivated	Vaqta (Merck & Co., Inc.)	1–18 y	0.5 mL (25 U)	IM	0, 6–18 mo	None
		≥19 y	1.0 mL (50 U)	IM	0, 6–18 mo	None
Combined hepatitis A and B vaccine	Twinrix (GlaxoSmithKline)	≥18 y (primary)	1.0 mL (720 ELU HAV + 20 μg HBsAg)	IM	0, 1, 6 mo	None
		≥18 y (accelerated)	Same as above	IM	0, 7, 21–30 d	12 mo
Hepatitis B vaccine, recombinant[1]	Engerix-B (GlaxoSmithKline)	0–19 y (primary)	0.5 mL (10 μg HBsAg)	IM	0, 1, 6 mo	None
		0–10 y (accelerated)	0.5 mL (10 μg HBsAg)	IM	0, 1, 2 mo	12 mo
		11–19 y (accelerated)	1.0 mL (20 μg HBsAg)	IM	0, 1, 2 mo	12 mo
		≥20 y (primary)	1.0 mL (20 μg HBsAg)	IM	0, 1, 6 mo	None
		≥20 y (accelerated)	1.0 mL (20 μg HBsAg)	IM	0, 1, 2 mo	12 mo
Hepatitis B vaccine, recombinant[1]	Recombivax HB (Merck & Co., Inc.)	0–19 y (primary)	0.5 mL (5 μg HBsAg)	IM	0, 1, 6 mo	None
		11–15 y (adolescent accelerated)	1.0 mL (10 μg HBsAg)	IM	0, 4–6 mo	None
		≥20 y (primary)	1.0 mL (10 μg HBsAg)	IM	0, 1, 6 mo	None

continued

A

TABLE B-1 TRAVEL VACCINE SUMMARY (continued)

VACCINE	TRADE NAME (MANUFACTURER)	AGE	DOSE	ROUTE	SCHEDULE	BOOSTER
Combined hepatitis A and B vaccine	Twinrix (GlaxoSmithKline)	≥18 y (primary)	1.0 mL (720 ELU HAV + 20 µg HBsAg)	IM	0, 1, 6 mo	None
		≥18 y (accelerated)	Same as above	IM	0, 7, 21–30 d	12 mo
Japanese encephalitis vaccine, inactivated	Ixiaro (Valneval)	≥17 y	0.5 mL	IM	0, 28 d	>1 y after primary series[2]
		3–16 y	0.5 mL	IM	0, 28 d	Data not available
		2 mo–2 y	0.25 mL	IM	0, 28 d	Data not available
Meningococcal polysaccharide diphtheria toxoid conjugate vaccine (MenACWY-D)[3]	Menactra (Sanofi Pasteur)	9–23 mo	0.5 mL	IM	0, 3 mo	If at continued risk[4]
		2–55 y	0.5 mL	IM	1 dose	
Meningococcal oligosaccharide diphtheria CRM$_{197}$ conjugate vaccine (MenACWY-CRM)[3]	Menveo (Novartis)	2–12 mo	0.5 mL	IM	0, 2, 4, 10–13 mo	If at continued risk[4]
		7–23 mo	0.5 mL	IM	0, 3 mo (2nd dose administered in 2nd year of life)	
		2–55 y	0.5 mL	IM	1 dose	
Meningococcal and Haemophilus influenzae type B polysaccharide tetanus toxoid conjugated vaccine[5]	MenHibrix (GSK)	6 wk–18 mo	0.5 mL	IM	0, 2, 4, 10–13 mo	If at continued risk[4]
Meningococcal polysaccharide vaccine (MPSV4)	Menomune (Sanofi Pasteur)	≥2 y	0.5 mL	SC	1 dose	If at continued risk[6]

Vaccine	Product (manufacturer)	Age	Dose	Route	Schedule	Booster
Polio vaccine, inactivated	Ipol (Sanofi Pasteur)	≥18 y	0.5 mL	SC or IM	1 dose if the patient has completed a pediatric series	Repeat boosters may be needed for long-term travelers to polio-affected countries; see Chapter 3, Poliomyelitis
Rabies vaccine (human diploid cell)	Imovax (Sanofi Pasteur)	Any	1.0 mL	IM	Preexposure series: 0, 7, and 21 or 28 d	None; see Chapter 3, Rabies for postexposure immunization
Rabies vaccine (purified chick embryo cell)	RabAvert (Novartis)	Any	1.0 mL	IM	Preexposure series: 0, 7, and 21 or 28 d	None; see Chapter 3, Rabies for postexposure immunization
Typhoid vaccine (oral, live, attenuated)	Vivotif (PaxVax)	≥6 y	1 capsule[7]	Oral	0, 2, 4, 6 d	Repeat primary series after 5 y
Typhoid vaccine (Vi capsular polysaccharide)	Typhim Vi (Sanofi Pasteur)	≥2 y	0.5 mL	IM	1 dose	2 y
Yellow fever	YF-Vax (Sanofi Pasteur)	≥9 mo[8]	0.5 mL	SC	1 dose	10 y[9]

Abbreviations: ELU, ELISA units of inactivated HAV; HAV, hepatitis A virus; HBsAg, hepatitis B surface antigen; IM, intramuscular; U, units HAV antigen; SC, subcutaneous.

[1] Consult the prescribing information for differences in dosing for hemodialysis and other immunocompromised patients.

[2] If potential for Japanese encephalitis virus exposure continues, a booster dose administered ≥2 years after the primary series are not available. Data on the need for and timing of additional booster doses are also not available.

[3] If an infant is receiving the vaccine before travel, 2 doses may be administered as early as 8 weeks apart.

[4] Revaccination with meningococcal conjugate vaccine (MenACWY-D or MenACWY-CRM) is recommended after 3 years for children who were previously vaccinated at ages 9 months through 6 years. Revaccination with meningococcal conjugate vaccine is recommended after 5 years for people who were previously vaccinated at ages 7–55 years and every 5 years thereafter for people who are at continued risk.

[5] Infants and children who received HibMenCY-TT and are traveling to areas with high endemic rates of meningococcal disease such as the African meningitis belt are not protected against serogroups A and W and should receive a quadrivalent meningococcal vaccine before travel.

[6] Revaccination with meningococcal polysaccharide vaccine is recommended for adults aged >55 years who remain at increased risk 5 years after the last dose.

[7] Must be kept refrigerated at 35.6°F–46.4°F [2°C–8°C]; administer with cool liquid no warmer than 98.6°F (37°C).

[8] Special considerations apply in deciding whether to administer yellow fever vaccine to people aged <9 months or ≥60 years. Please review Chapter 3, Yellow Fever before administration.

[9] In 2014, the World Health Assembly (of the World Health Organization) adopted the recommendation to remove the 10 year booster dose requirement from the International Health Regulations as of June 2016. Once this change is instituted, a completed International Certificate of Vaccination or Prophylaxis will be valid for the lifetime of the vaccinee. It is uncertain when and if all countries with yellow fever vaccination entry requirements will adopt this change. In the United States, the Advisory Committee on Immunization Practices (ACIP) is considering the issue of the continued need for yellow fever vaccine boosters. Until the ACIP issues updated recommendations, CDC recommends that US travelers receive booster doses of yellow fever vaccine every 10 years if traveling to an area with risk of exposure to yellow fever virus. For the most up-to-date information about the need for yellow fever vaccine boosters, consult the CDC Travelers' Health website at www.cdc.gov/travel.

APPENDIX C: MIGRANT HEALTH RESOURCES

William M. Stauffer

Historically, the Yellow Book has addressed travel health issues for US residents visiting countries outside the United States. In this increasingly mobile world, the discipline of travel medicine is evolving to recognize non-traditional groups who cross international boundaries into and out of the United States. One such group includes people who originate in other countries and migrate to the United States, either temporarily or permanently. Recognized migrants to the United States include immigrants (documented and undoc-umented), refugees, asylum seekers, and international adoptees. In addition, students and corporate workers are frequent visitors to the United States. Many clinics serving the traditional travel population also function as contact points with the US medical system for these populations, particularly for immi-grants and refugees. This section provides resources to assist clinicians and organiza-tions that serve these populations to access up-to-date patient care guidelines, online education materials, and print resources.

CLINICAL REFERENCES
Organizational Guidelines
- Centers for Disease Control and Preven-tion: predeparture and postarrival pre-sumptive treatment and medical screening guidelines for refugees relocating to the United States, available at www.cdc.gov/immigrantrefugeehealth/guidelines/refu-gee-guidelines.html
- American Academy of Pediatrics: guid-ance on medical screening and vac-cination issues in adoptees, refugees, and immigrants, available in the online Red Book at http://aapredbook.aappublic-ations.org
- Canadian Collaboration for Immigrant and Refugee Health: clinical preventive guidelines for primary care for newly arriving immigrants and refugees, avail-able at www.ccirh.uottawa.ca

Websites
- Centers for Disease Control and Prevention
  - > Immigrant and Refugee Health: information on immigrants and refugees who are resettling in the United States and resources, at www.cdc.gov/immigrantrefugeehealth/index.html
  - > Travelers' Health: health information for international travelers, at www.cdc.gov/travel
  - > Malaria and other parasitic diseases: clinical and public policy information on parasitic diseases, at www.cdc.gov/parasites and www.cdc.gov/malaria
  - > International emergency and refugee health: health information pertaining to complex humanitarian emergencies, at www.cdc.gov/globalhealth/ierh
- Refugee Health Technical Assistance Center: multiple refugee resources and online education, at www.refugeehealthta.org
- Minnesota Department of Health: mul-tiple resources for clinicians in refu-gee health at www.health.state.mn.us/divs/idepc/refugee/hcp/index.html, as well as refugee topics, at www.health.state.mn.us/divs/idepc/refugee/topics/index.html
- Healthy Roads Media: health education materials, including video, in a vari-ety of languages, at http://healthyroadsmedia.org
- EthnoMed: information about cultural beliefs, medical issues, and other related issues pertinent to the health care of recent immigrants, at http://ethnomed.org/ethnomed
- Health Information Translations: com-mon hospital signs with multiple transla-tions, at www.healthinfotranslations.com
- MedicalLeadership.org: database of patient information resources in a

variety of languages and organizations providing services in languages other than English, at www.medicalleadership. org/patient-educations/

- Refugee Health Information Network: multilingual information for clinicians, refugees, and asylum seekers in print, audio, and video formats, at www.rhin.org
- US Committee for Refugees and Immigrants: toolkits on multiple health issues for clinicians, migrants, and communities in multiple languages, at www. refugees.org
- US Citizenship and Immigration Services: information regarding adjustment of status, at www.uscis.gov
- United Nations High Commissioner for Refugees, Health Information System (HIS): information about health issues in specific refugee camps or populations where refugees are originating, at www. unhcr.org/pages/49c3646ce0.html

Reference Books
Textbooks with a Focus on Migrant Health
- Immigrant Medicine. Walker PF, Barnett ED, editors. Philadelphia: Saunders Elsevier; 2007.
- Migration Medicine and Health: Principles and Practice. Gushulak BD, MacPherson D, editors. Hamilton, ON: BC Decker; 2006.
- Travel Medicine and Migrant Health. Lockie C, Walker E, Calvert L, Cossar J, Knill-Jones R, Raeside F, editors. Edinburgh: Churchill Livingstone; 2000.
- Refugee and Immigrant Health. A Handbook for Health Professionals. Kemp C, Rasbridge LA, editors. New York: Cambridge University Press; 2004.

Textbooks with a Focus on Tropical Diseases
- Atlas of Tropical Medicine and Parasitology. 6th ed. Peters W, Pasvol G, editors. Edinburgh: Mosby; 2007.
- Mandell, Douglas, and Bennett's Principles & Practice of Infectious Diseases. 7th ed. Mandell GL, Bennett JE, Dolin R, editors. Philadelphia: Churchill Livingstone; 2010.
- Hunter's Tropical Medicine and Emerging Infectious Diseases. 9th ed. Magill AJ, Ryan ET, Hill D, Solomon T, editors. Philadelphia: Saunders Elsevier; 2012.

- Manson's Tropical Diseases. 22nd ed. Cook GC, Zumla AI, editors. Edinburgh, UK: Saunders Ltd; 2008.
- Tropical Infectious Diseases: Principles, Pathogens and Practice. 3rd ed. Guerrant RL, Walker DH, Weller PF, editors. Philadelphia: Churchill Livingstone; 2011.

GENERAL RESOURCES
Reading Lists
- University of Minnesota reading list on refugee and immigrant health: comprehensive reading list for people interested in refugee and immigrant health, at www. globalhealth.umn.edu/free-intro-course/ immigrant-refugee-health-short-course-resources/index.htm

Educational Opportunities
- University of Minnesota/CDC: American Society of Tropical Medicine and Hygiene (ASTMH)-accredited course in global health—open access to lectures and online content with a focus on immigrant and refugee health, at www.globalhealth. umn.edu
- ASTMH-accredited courses in tropical and travel medicine: list of ASTMH-accredited tropical and travel medicine courses, at www.astmh.org/Approved_Diploma_Courses/2867.htm
- Harvard Program in Refugee Trauma: http://hprt-cambridge.org

Organization Websites with Migrant Information
- US Department of Health and Human Services
  > Office of Refugee Resettlement: www. acf.hhs.gov/programs/orr
  > Office of Global Health Affairs: www. globalhealth.gov
- Centers for Disease Control and Prevention, Immigrant and Refugee Health: www.cdc. gov/immigrantrefugeehealth
- United Nations High Commissioner for Refugees: www.unhcr.org/cgi-bin/texis/ vtx/home
- World Health Organization refugee page: www.who.int/topics/refugees/en
- American Society of Tropical Medicine and Hygiene: www.astmh.org
- International Organization for Migration: www.iom.int

 MIGRANT HEALTH RESOURCES

- International Society of Travel Medicine, Migrants and Refugee Health Interest Group Committee: http://www.istm.org/migrantgroup
- Global Health Council: www.globalhealth.org
- Consortium of Universities for Global Health: www.cugh.org

Other Resources
- The Providers' Guide to Quality and Culture: http://erc.msh.org/mainpage.cfm?file=1.0.htm&module=provider&language=English

Index

Note: Page numbers followed by the letter b refer to boxes; those followed by the letter f refer to figures; those followed by the letter m refer to maps; and those followed by the letter t refer to tables.

Middle East respiratory syndrome (MERS), 16–17m, 268–9
military populations and deployments. *See* US military deployments
mold contamination, 119
Moldova, 399
Monaco, 399
Mongolia, 399
   Lyme disease, 235
   rickettsial infections, 296t
   tickborne encephalitis in, 320
monkeypox, 315, 316, 535
Montenegro, 399
Montserrat (UK)
   no reported cases of rabies, 287t
   yellow fever information for, 399
Moorea. *See* French Polynesia
Morbidity and Mortality Weekly Report (CDC), 13, 42, 43b
Morocco, 399
   rickettsial infections, 295t
morphine, 77t
mosquitoes, avoidance of, 94–8, 115, 243–4, 542–3
motion sickness, 8, 35, 76–8
Mozambique
   dengue distribution in, 173m
   malaria information for, 238m, 399
   yellow fever information for, 399
MPSV4. *See* meningococcal vaccine
multiple sclerosis, 626
mumps, 269–10
   traveler's role in translocation of, 20
   vaccine, 31t. *See also* measles-mumps-rubella (MMR) vaccine; measles-mumps-rubella-varicella (MMRV) vaccine
murine typhus, 296t, 297
Myanmar. *See* Burma (Myanmar)
myiasis, 13, 426, 508t, 509

N

Namibia
   malaria information for, 238m, 400, 400m
   yellow fever information, 399–400
naproxen, 77t
natural disasters, 117–18
Nauru, 401
Neisseria gonorrhoeae, 309
Neisseria meningitidis, 263, 265, 492, 521, 546, 547
nematode eggs, size and susceptibility to filtration, 88t
Neorickettsia, 294, 295t, 298. *See also* rickettsial infections
Nepal
   altitude illness in, 73
   dengue distribution in, 174m
   destination map, 473m
   destination overview, 472–4
   health issues in, 474–5
   Japanese encephalitis risk in, 220m, 225t
   leishmaniasis in, 232
   malaria information for, 401, 474
   yellow fever information for, 401
The Netherlands, 401
neurotoxic shellfish poisoning, 93
New Caledonia (France)
   no reported cases of rabies, 287t
   yellow fever information for, 401

NDM-1, 41, 470, 504
New Zealand. *See also* Cook Islands (New Zealand); Niue (New Zealand); Tokelau (New Zealand)
   no reported cases of rabies, 287t
Nicaragua
   dengue distribution in, 172m
   malaria information for, 237m, 401, 402m
   yellow fever information for, 401
niclosamide, 318
nifedipine, 70, 71t, 105
Niger
   malaria information for, 238m, 401
   yellow fever information for, 347t, 355t, 358m, 401
Nigeria
   dengue distribution in, 173m
   Lassa virus in, 344
   malaria information for, 238m, 256, 402
   meningococcal meningitis in, 264m
   yellow fever information for, 347t, 358m, 401
Nile River cruises. *See* Egypt
nitazoxanide, 167, 184, 186
Niue (New Zealand), 402
N,N-diethyl-3-methyl-benzamide or *N,N*-diethyl-*m*-toluamide (DEET), 96–8, 101, 131
nontyphoidal salmonellosis, 300–302
Norfolk Island (Australia), 402
norovirus, 270–72
North America
   chronic hepatitis B virus prevalence, 194m
   chronic hepatitis C virus prevalence, 200m
   countries reporting no indigenous cases of rabies, 287t
   ehrlichiosis in, 295t
   malaria-endemic countries, 237m
   rickettsial infections, 295–6t
   tuberculosis in, 328m 330m,
Northern Mariana Islands (US), 402
   no reported cases of rabies, 287t
North Korea
   Japanese encephalitis risk in, 220m, 224t
   malaria information for, 402–3
   yellow fever information for, 402
Norway, 403
   no reported cases of rabies, 287t
   tickborne encephalitis in, 320

O

occupational exposure to HIV, 35, 578, 580–82. *See also* human immunodeficiency virus (HIV)
Oceania, 13f, 240
   countries reporting no indigenous cases of rabies, 287t
   dengue in, 174m
Ocean Island. *See* Kiribati
oil of lemon eucalyptus (OLE), 96, 542
Oman, 403
onchocerciasis, 272–3, 509
oral contraceptives, 77t
oral rehydration salts (ORS), 63, 540–41
oseltamivir, 213, 216t
oxyuriasis, 275–6

P

Pakistan
   dengue distribution in, 174m
   Japanese encephalitis risk in, 220m, 225t
   malaria information for, 238m, 403
   yellow fever information for, 403
Palau, 403
   no reported cases of rabies, 287t
Panama
   dengue in, 11t
   malaria information for, 237m, 403, 405m
   reference map, 405m
   yellow fever information for, 347t, 359m, 403, 404m
Papua New Guinea
   dengue distribution in, 174m
   Japanese encephalitis risk in, 220m, 225t
   malaria information for, 246, 404
   no reported cases of rabies, 287t
   yellow fever information for, 404
Paraguay
   dengue distribution in, 172m
   malaria information for, 237m, 404, 406, 406m
   yellow fever information for, 347t, 404
paralytic shellfish poisoning, 93
parasitic diseases, screening asymptomatic travelers, 513–15
paratyphoid fever, 336–9
paromomycin, 186
paroxetine, 77t
Peace Corps, 167, 230, 271, 293, 306, 586
penicillin, 154, 157, 178, 234
permethrin, 95, 96b, 97–8, 244, 303, 325, 425, 542
pernio, 105
persistent travelers' diarrhea, 505–7
pertussis, 273–5. *See also* tetanus-diphtheria-pertussis (Tdap)
   immunization of children, 546, 554, 558
   vaccine, 31t, 42, 48t, 50t, 52t
Peru, 405. *See also* Cusco-Machu Picchu
   dengue distribution in, 172m
   destination map, 453m
   destination overview, 452–3
   health issues in, 454, 455–6
   malaria information for, 237m, 255, 408m
   reference map, 407–8m
   yellow fever information for, 347t, 405, 407m
pharmaceutical quality drugs, 141–3, 145
Philippines
   child sex tourists, 312
   dengue distribution in, 174m
   Ebola-Reston virus, 343
   Japanese encephalitis risk in, 220m, 225t
   malaria information for, 406
   yellow fever information for, 406
phosphodiesterase-5 inhibitors, 70
phytophotodermatitis, 510
picaridin, 96
picornavirus, 189
pinworm, 275–6

Photography Credits

COVER IMAGES
Rio de Janeiro, Brazil
Photos by Julia Raposo

BANNER IMAGES FOR SELECT DESTINATIONS

East Africa: Safaris (p. 423): Michelle Russell/Personal Collection

South Africa (p. 427): Kelly Holton/Personal Collection

Tanzania: Kilimanjaro (p. 430): Kevin Kain/Personal Collection

Brazil (p. 434): Julia Raposo/Personal Collection

Dominican Republic (p. 439): Jeffrey Wages/Personal Collection

Haiti (p. 443): Amethyst Auza/Personal Collection

Mexico (p. 447): Natalia Castells-Esquivel/Personal Collection

Peru: Cusco–Machu Picchu (p. 452): Kelly Holton/Personal Collection

Cambodia (p. 456): Emily Jentes/Personal Collection

China (p. 461): Marco Obando/Personal Collection

India (p. 467): Tiffany Eberhard/Personal Collection

Nepal (p. 472): David R. Shlim/Personal Collection

Thailand (p. 476): Michelle Russell/Personal Collection

Vietnam (p. 481): BK Kapella/Personal Collection

Egypt & Nile River Cruises (p. 486): Geoff Boyer/Personal Collection

Saudi Arabia: Hajj Pilgrimage (p. 490): Ziad A. Memish/Personal Collection